Stem Cells in Health and Disease

Stem Cells in Health and Disease

Editor: Bruce Powell

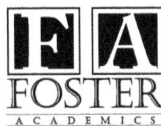

FA
FOSTER
ACADEMICS

www.fosteracademics.com

www.fosteracademics.com

FA
FOSTER
ACADEMICS

Cataloging-in-Publication Data

Stem cells in health and disease / edited by Bruce Powell.
    p. cm.
Includes bibliographical references and index.
ISBN 978-1-63242-915-5
1. Stem cells. 2. Stem cells--Research. 3. Cells. 4. Health. 5. Diseases. I. Powell, Bruce.
QH588.S83 S74 2020
616.027 74-dc23

Foster Academics,
118-35 Queens Blvd., Suite 400,
Forest Hills, NY 11375, USA

ISBN 978-1-63242-915-5 (Hardback)

Contents

Preface

Stem cells are cells with the ability to differentiate into specific cell types. They also self-renew perpetually. Stem cells are of two kinds- embryonic stem cells and adult stem cells. Embryonic stem cells are pluripotent cells that can become any cell in the adult body, while adult stem cells give rise to similar cell types only. Stem cells have immense potential in tissue repair and regeneration. Stem cell therapy, which is also called regenerative medicine, promotes the repair response of dysfunctional, diseased or injured tissues. This is done using stem cells or their derivatives. Stem cells that are manipulated to specialize into specific cell types, like blood cells, nerve cells, heart muscle cells, etc. are then implanted into a person. Stem cell transplants may also be performed to replace cells damaged due to disease or chemotherapy. It can also be done as a strategy to enable the donor's immune system to fight cancers and other blood-related disorders, such as lymphoma, leukemia, neuroblastoma and multiple myeloma. This book covers in detail some existing theories and innovative concepts revolving around stem cell therapy. Some of the diverse topics covered herein address the role of stem cells in health and disease. As this field is emerging at a fast pace, this book will help the readers to better understand the advanced concepts of this field.

This book is a result of research of several months to collate the most relevant data in the field.

When I was approached with the idea of this book and the proposal to edit it, I was overwhelmed. It gave me an opportunity to reach out to all those who share a common interest with me in this field. I had 3 main parameters for editing this text:

1. Accuracy – The data and information provided in this book should be up-to-date and valuable to the readers.

2. Structure – The data must be presented in a structured format for easy understanding and better grasping of the readers.

3. Universal Approach – This book not only targets students but also experts and innovators in the field, thus my aim was to present topics which are of use to all.

Thus, it took me a couple of months to finish the editing of this book.

I would like to make a special mention of my publisher who considered me worthy of this opportunity and also supported me throughout the editing process. I would also like to thank the editing team at the back-end who extended their help whenever required.

Editor

Hydrogen Peroxide-Induced DNA Damage and Repair through the Differentiation of Human Adipose-Derived Mesenchymal Stem Cells

Mahara Valverde ⓘ,[1,2] **Jonathan Lozano-Salgado,**[1] **Paola Fortini,**[2]
Maria Alexandra Rodriguez-Sastre,[1] **Emilio Rojas,**[1] **and Eugenia Dogliotti**[2]

[1]*Instituto de Investigaciones Biomédicas, Universidad Nacional Autónoma de México, C.U. 04510, Mexico*
[2]*Department of Environment and Health, Istituto Superiore di Sanità, Viale Regina Elena 299, 00161 Roma, Italy*

Correspondence should be addressed to Mahara Valverde; mahara@biomedicas.unam.mx

Academic Editor: Heinrich Sauer

Human adipose-derived mesenchymal stem cells (hADMSCs) are recognized as a potential tool in cell tissue therapy because of their capacity to proliferate and differentiate in vitro. Several studies have addressed their use in regenerative medicine; however, little is known regarding their response to DNA damage and in particular to the reactive oxygen species (ROS) that are present in the microenvironment of implantation. In this study, we used the ROS-inducing agent hydrogen peroxide to explore the responses of (1) hADMSCs and (2) derived terminally differentiated adipocytes to oxidatively generated DNA damage. Using single cell gel electrophoresis, a dose-related increase was found for both DNA breaks and oxidative lesions (formamidopyrimidine DNA glycosylase-sensitive sites) upon exposure of hADMSCs to hydrogen peroxide. DNA repair capacity of hADMSCs was affected in cells exposed to 150 and 200 μM of hydrogen peroxide. An increase in the basal levels of DNA breaks and oxidative DNA lesions was observed through adipocyte differentiation. In addition, hydrogen peroxide-induced DNA damage increased through adipocyte differentiation; DNA repair capacity also decreased. This study is the first follow-up report on DNA repair capacity during adipogenic differentiation. Remarkably, in terminally differentiated adipocytes, DNA breakage repair is abolished while the repair of DNA oxidative lesions remains efficient.

1. Introduction

Before the 1980s, adipose tissue was considered only a passive energy storage reservoir. However, when its participation in the metabolism of sex hormones was confirmed, adipose tissue was recognized as an important endocrine organ [1]. A substantial breakthrough occurred when a new source of adult stem cells, called adipose-derived stem cells, was described for the first time by Zuk et al. [2] as self-renewing multipotent cells [3]. Human adipose-derived mesenchymal stem cells (hADMSCs) are isolated from adipose (fat) tissues by lipoaspiration or biopsy. Lipoaspirates represent a heterogeneous mixture of cell types, including adipocytes, endothelial cells, smooth muscle, pericytes, and progenitor cells [2]. Such properties make hADMSCs a

potential tool for therapy in clinics [4] and, in particular, for autologous cell transplantation. However, the low survival rate and increased cell death after implantation into injured tissue suggest that hADMSCs are damaged by the local microenvironment likely due to sustained oxidative stress with the overproduction of reactive oxygen species (ROS) [5, 6]. ROS are well known to play a role in the growth and homeostasis of MSCs even when they are generated as byproducts of normal energy metabolism. Chemically, hydrogen peroxide (H_2O_2) is a poorly reactive ROS in the absence of ions of transition metals; however, because in biological systems it is ubiquitously produced and presents a relatively long half-life, H_2O_2 fulfills the prerequisites for serving as an intracellular messenger and acting as a cell signaling molecule [7]. In chemical terms, H_2O_2 can act as a mild oxidizing agent or as a mild reducing agent, but it does not readily oxidize most biological molecules, including lipids, DNA, and proteins, unless the latter have hyperreactive thiol groups or methionine residues [8]. Because of its mode of action, H_2O_2 can induce distinct responses depending on the cell type. In this study, we explored the capacity of H_2O_2 to induce DNA damage and repair in hADMSCs when proliferating and in different stages of adipocyte differentiation. Although all living cells are provided with a plethora of DNA repair mechanisms to address different DNA lesions and to preserve genomic integrity, mesenchymal stem cells are expected to have a strong response to DNA damage because of their remarkable abilities of self-renewal and differentiation into different functional cell types. In the present study, we specifically investigated whether the response to oxidatively generated DNA damage is modulated during the adipogenic differentiation of hADMSCs. We show that hADMSCs repair DNA breaks and alkali labile sites very efficiently when proliferating but that their repair capacity declines during adipocyte differentiation. Interestingly, adipocytes maintain their ability to repair formamidopyrimidine DNA glycosylase (Fpg) sites, including 7,8-dihydro-8-oxoguanine (8-oxoguanine), 8-oxoadenine, aflatoxin B1-fapy-guanine, 5-hydroxy-cytosine, and 5-hydroxy-uracil [9, 10].

2. Material and Methods

2.1. hADMSC Cell Culture. Normal hADMSCs (ATCC® PCS-500-011™) were cultured at an early passage (passage 4). Cell cultures were made using Gibco MesenPRO RS™ Medium (cat. number 12746-012) prepared according to the supplier's specifications and incubated at 37°C and 5% CO_2. Medium changes were performed every 48 hours and treated at ~85% confluence. For harvesting, the cultures were treated with 0.05% Trypsin-EDTA (Gibco, cat. number 25300-054) at 37°C and 5% CO_2 for 3 minutes (sufficient time to obtain a total suspension of the culture). They were then transferred to PBS and centrifuged at 300 ×g for 5 minutes. They were subsequently handled depending on the test to be performed.

2.2. hADMSC Surface Markers. Anti-CD45, anti-CD146, anti-CD105, and anti-CD90 (Human Mesenchymal Stem Cell Multi-Color Flow Cytometry Kit, R&D Systems; cat. number FMC002) were used for immunophenotype determination of hADMSCs before and after adipocyte differentiation, following the recommendations of the International Society for Cellular Therapy [11]. The protocol indicated by the provider was followed; cell samples were washed with staining buffer and then blocked. The antibody or the corresponding isotype control antibody was then added. Incubation was carried out by 30 minutes at room temperature in the dark, and any excess antibody was removed by washing with staining buffer before analysis. The acquisitions were performed on a Blue/Red Attune (BD Biosystems) flow cytometer.

2.3. Hydrogen Peroxide Treatment. hADMSCs were treated at a density of 4000/cm². H_2O_2 bolus treatment (0, 50, 100,

150, and 200 μM) lasted for 2 hours, and the recovery time in fresh medium was 24 h posttreatment. To be precise, the corresponding incipient toxic doses of H_2O_2 were 0, 152.5, 305, 457.5, and 600 nmol of H_2O_2/mg cell protein.

Cells at different differentiation durations (days 6, 12, and 14) were treated for 2 hours with H_2O_2 100 μM (305 nmol/ mg cell protein), and the recovery time was 24 h posttreatment in fresh medium.

Cells were harvested with trypsin-EDTA; the cell suspension obtained was used to perform the lysosomal activity test, determination of DNA damage (breaks and oxidative lesions), and DNA repair capacity.

2.4. Lysosomal Activity Test. A lysosomal activity test was used to determine cell viability and was performed using the FDA-Et-Br (fluorescein diacetate-ethidium bromide) stain. The cell suspension was mixed 1 : 1 with stain solution, and the analysis was performed by fluorescence microscopy (Olympus BMX-60 with a UM61002 filter). FDA is taken up by cells that through esterase activity transform nonfluorescent FDA into a green fluorescent metabolite. The nuclei of the dead cells are then stained with ethidium bromide and visualized as red fluorescence.

2.5. Reactive Oxygen Species. This technique is based on the ROS-dependent oxidation of dihydrorhodamine 123 (DHR123, Calbiochem, cat. number 309825) to rhodamine 123 (Sigma-Aldrich, cat. number R-8004). hADMSCs or adipocyte cells were grown under the required conditions. The medium was then removed and washed with PBS. Cells were harvested and counted in a Moxi automated cell counter (ORFLO, Montana, US). Aliquots equivalent to 2×10^5 cells were collected and centrifuged at 1200 rpm for 5 minutes. The supernatant was poured, and 180 μl of buffer A (140 mM NaCl, 5 mM KCl, 0.8 mM $MgSO_4 \cdot 7H_2O$, 1.8 mM $CaCl_2$, 5 mM glucose, and 15 mM HEPES) and 20 μl of dihydrorhodamine 123 (1 mM) were added to the pellet. This mixture was placed in a 96-well plate and read using a fluorescence reader (BioTek FLx8000) at a wavelength of 505 nm. The results were interpolated in a curve of rhodamine 123 in buffer A at concentrations of 0–10 μM. Data were expressed as nmol of rhodamine $123/2 \times 10^5$ cells.

2.6. DNA Breaks and DNA Oxidative Damage. DNA damage was determined by alkaline single cell gel electrophoresis assay to evaluate the presence of DNA breaks produced, which includes single and double strand breaks, as well as alkali labile sites in hADMSC cells either proliferating or during differentiation (control, H_2O_2 treatment, and 24 h posttreatment) [12, 13]. For each experimental condition, at least 10,000 cells were mixed with 75 μl of 0.5% low melting point (LMP) agarose. The cells were loaded onto microscope slides prelayered with 200 μl of 0.5% normal melting point agarose and covered with a third layer of LMP agarose 0.5%. Briefly, after lysis of the cells at 4°C for at least 1 h in a buffer consisting of 2.5 M NaCl, 100 mM EDTA, and 10 mM Tris, pH 10, supplemented with 10% DMSO and 1% Triton X-100, the slides were placed in a horizontal electrophoresis chamber with running buffer solution (300 mM

NaOH, 1 mM Na_2EDTA, pH > 13). The slides remained in the electrophoresis buffer for 20 minutes to allow the DNA to unwind and reveal alkali-labile sites (AP sites). Electrophoresis was performed for 20 min at 300 mA and 25 V, ~0.8 V/cm. All steps were performed in the dark to avoid direct light. After electrophoresis, the slides were gently removed and rinsed with neutralization buffer (0.4 M Tris, pH 7.5) at room temperature for 15 min, dehydrated with absolute ethanol for 15 min, and air-dried. Ethidium bromide (20 μl of 20 mg/ml solution) was added to each slide and a coverslip was placed on the gel. Individual cells were visualized at 20x magnification with an Olympus BX-60 microscope with fluorescence attachments (515–560 nm excitation filter, 590 nm barrier filter), and the DNA damage was determined using Komet 5.0 software (Kinetic Imaging Ltd.). To evaluate DNA migration, 50 nucleoids per slide (300 nucleoids total per condition) were scored for each experimental condition. The data were divided into five categories according to the Olive tail moment (OTM) score. The total number of nucleoids in each category was counted and multiplied by an assigned value of 0–4 according to the damage class. The sum of all the categories was calculated and considered the damage index. The overall score was expected to vary between 0 and 400 arbitrary units. Alternatively, the OTM score obtained by the software was employed.

DNA oxidative damage was identified via incubation with formamidopyrimidine DNA glycosylase (Fpg) to reveal 7,8-dihydro-8-oxoguanine (8-oxoguanine), 8-oxoadenine, aflatoxin B1-fapy-guanine, 5-hydroxy-cytosine, and 5-hydroxy-uracil [9, 10]. Briefly, after treatment, the cells immersed in LMP agarose 1% were layered on microscope slides precoated with 1% normal melting point agarose and immersed in lysis buffer for at least 1 h at 4°C. The slides were then rinsed with buffer solution (50 mM Tris-base, 10 mM EDTA, pH 7.6) for 5 minutes. Oxidative lesions were digested by Fpg (Trevigen, CA, USA), under ideal conditions of pH and temperature suggested by the provider. Coverslips were placed on the slides and were incubated for 30 min at 37°C in a humidified atmosphere. A set of slides with cells of every experimental condition in buffer (without enzyme) was included to confirm that the DNA strand breaks were enzyme specific. Following enzyme incubation, the slides were rinsed with solution buffer (50 mM Tris-base, 200 mM EDTA, pH 7.6) and subjected to conventional comet electrophoresis (~0.8 V/cm) for 20 min without unwinding incubation. Dehydration, stain, and analysis were performed as previously described.

To determine the DNA repair capacity, we apply

$$\% \text{ DNA repair capacity} = \frac{[\text{remaining DNA damage (OTM)} \times 100]}{\text{net-induced DNA damage (OTM)}},$$

Remaining damage = DNA damage induced by H_2O_2 (OTM) – posttreatment DNA damage (OTM), (1)

Net induced DNA damage = DNA damage induced by H_2O_2 (OTM) – DNA damage of control.

2.7. Adipocyte Differentiation. Cultures of hADMSCs (pass 4) reached ~80% confluence. They were then passaged into a plate at a density of 18,000 cells/cm^2 in MesenPRO RS™ Medium Gibco (cat. number 12746-012). The cells were incubated at 37°C and 5% CO_2 for 48 h before initiating differentiation. Thereafter, a wash with PBS was performed to remove components from the previous medium and adding the StemPro® Adipogenesis Differentiation Kit, Gibco (cat. number A10070-01). The media changes were established every 72 h and incubated at 37°C and 5% CO_2 until day 14 of adipocyte differentiation. For harvest, the cultures at day 6, 12, and 14 were treated with 0.25% Trypsin-EDTA (Gibco, cat. number 25200-056) at 37°C and 5% CO_2 for 3 minutes. With the help of a plastic scraper, a culture suspension was obtained, which was transferred to PBS to be centrifuged at 300 ×g for 5 minutes. They were subsequently handled depending on the test to be performed.

2.8. hFATP-1. Anti-hFATP-1 (human fat acid transporter protein 1) (R&D Systems; cat. number IC3304P) was used as the surface marker of adipocyte differentiation [14]. Determination of hFATP-1 before and after adipocyte differentiation. The protocol indicated by the provider was followed. A solution of saponin (0.1% w/v saponin and 0.05% NaN_3 in PBS) was used for permeabilization. The antibody or the corresponding isotype control antibody was then added. Incubation was carried out by 30 minutes at room temperature in the dark, and any excess antibody was removed by washing with staining buffer before analysis. The acquisitions were performed on a Blue/Red Attune (BD Biosystems) flow cytometer.

2.9. Cell Cycle Analysis. The cell cycle was evaluated using a DNA intercalating agent (propidium iodide; IP) and RNase A to decrease nonspecificity (Muse Cell Cycle Kit, cat. number MCH100106). After harvesting, the cells were washed with PBS and then fixed with 70% ethanol for at least 48 h. The cells were then centrifuged 300 ×g for 5 minutes and washed with PBS. The IP was added and incubated for 30 minutes at room temperature in the dark. Finally, the acquisition was performed using a FACScan cytometer (BD Biosystems) from the cytofluorometry unit of the Instituto de Investigaciones Biomédicas, UNAM. The cell cycle phase of the cell populations was then determined according to the deoxyribonucleic content.

2.10. Oil Red O Stain. To confirm adipocyte differentiation, the hADMSCs were seeded in 12-well plates. Differentiation

Positive and negative Mesenchymal stem cell (MSC) surface marker and proportion change after adipocyte differentiation

MSC surface markers (positive +, negative −)	hADMSC % positive cells (Mean ± SD)	Adipocytes % positive cells (Mean ± SD)
CD 90 (+)	99	99
CD 105 (+)	82	79
CD 146 (−)	<0,5	3[***]
CD 45 (−)	<0,5	ND
hFATP-1	10	94[****]

ND: nondetermined. Student's t-test hADMSC versus adipocytes. ***$p < 0.01$, ****$p < 0.001$.

(a)

Percentageof cell distribution through cell cycle phases before and after adipocyte differentiation.

Cells	Percentage of cells G1	Percentage of cells S	Percentage of cells G2/M
hADMSC	82	7	11
Adipocytes	95***	2***	3***

Mean ± SE, Student's t-test performed hADMSC versus adipocytes.***$p < 0.01$.

(b)

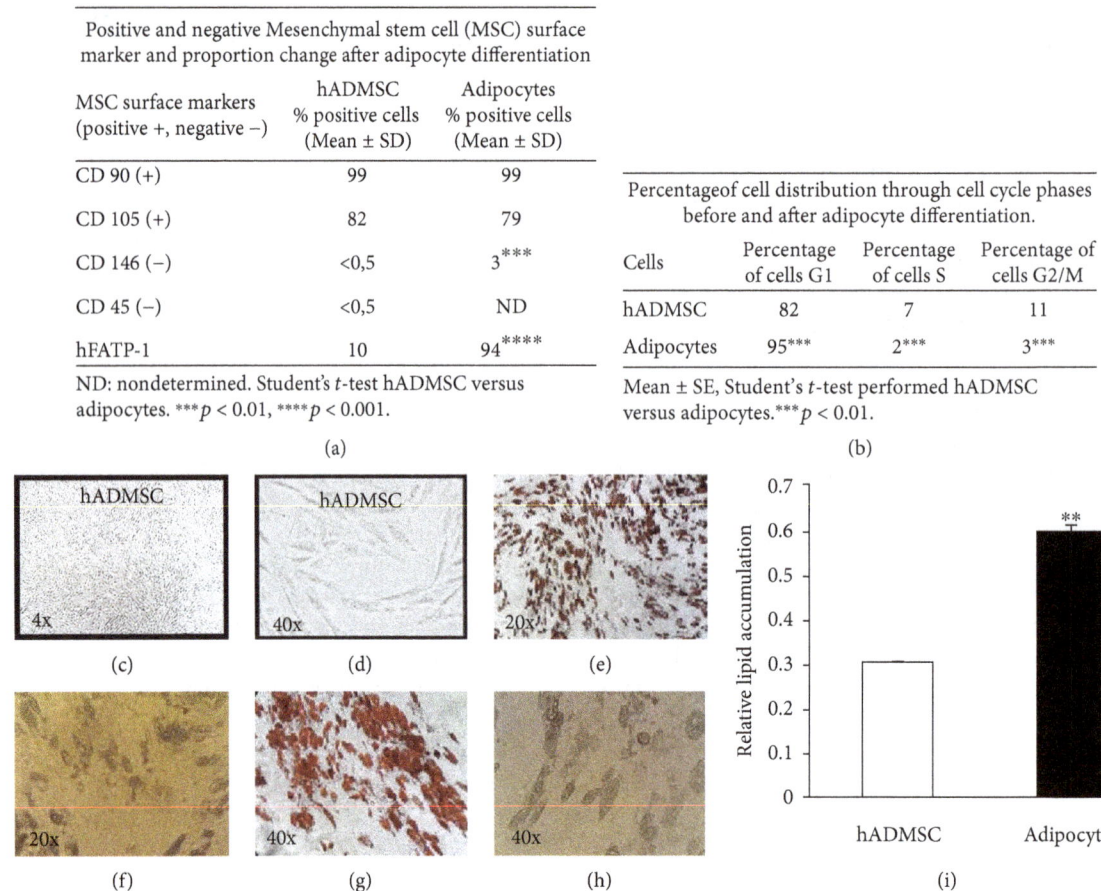

(c)　(d)　(e)

(f)　(g)　(h)

(i)

FIGURE 1: hADMSC immunophenotype and characterization of adipocyte differentiation. Positive and negative surface markers of MSCs and adipocyte differentiation marker hFATP-1 in (a). Cell cycle and G1 arrest of adipocytes in (b). hADMSC representative morphology at 4x magnification in (c) and 40x magnification in (d). Adipocyte differentiation after 14 days evidenced by Oil Red O staining. (e) and (g) are representative images at 20x and 40x magnification, respectively. Light microscopy images at day 14 of differentiation are represented in (f) and (h), corresponding to 20x and 40x magnification, respectively. The increase in the relative lipid accumulation between hADMSCs and adipocytes was determined by Student's t-test, *$p < 0.05$ (i).

was initiated when confluence was 80%. The corresponding stains were carried out at day 14 of differentiation. The cells were washed twice with PBS and then fixed with 10% paraformaldehyde for 30 minutes at room temperature. Finally, two washes were performed with PBS, and Oil Red O (Trevigen cat. number 5010-024-05) prepared according to the supplier was added followed by incubation for 30 minutes with gentle shaking and protection from light. Two additional washes were then carried out, and PBS was added for the inverted microscope display (Olympus IX50-S8F2). For quantification, the PBS was then removed, and the dye was extracted with isopropanol and incubated for 10 minutes with shaking and protection from light. The supernatant was finally placed in a quartz cell (Quartz Spectrophotometer Cell Semi Micro, 9-Q-10 mm, Bio-Rad Laboratories), and the absorbance of the sample was measured on a spectrophotometer (Ultrospec 3000, Pharmacia Biotech) at 500 nm using isopropanol as a blank to obtain the relative lipid accumulation.

2.11. Statistical Analysis. Statistical analysis was performed using the software SigmaStat 3.5 and SigmaPlot

10.0. Nonparametric tests were used for single cell gel electrophoresis analyses, Kruskal-Wallis (one-way ANOVA on ranks) was used for all pairwise multiple comparison procedures (Dunn's test), and for data with normal distribution, Student's t-tests were performed to assess lysosomal activity, ROS levels, surface markers, and the cell cycle.

3. Results

3.1. hADMSC Immunophenotype and Characterization of Adipocyte Differentiation. Mesenchymal stem cells (MSCs) are functionally defined by their capacity to self-renew and their ability to differentiate into multiple cell types (adipocytes, chondrocytes, and osteocytes), which are phenotypically characterized as positive for CD105 and CD90 and negative for CD146 and CD45. The percentage of cells that present these characteristic surface markers are shown in Figure 1(a). The percentage of cells positive for the human fatty acid transporter protein 1 (hFATP1) is also presented to show the tissue source as well as the degree of adipogenic differentiation. The distribution of cells along the cell cycle further confirm that an efficient differentiation is achieved

hADMSCs' viability determined as lysosomal activity and percentage of intracellular ROS levels after H_2O_2 treatment (2 h).		
H_2O_2 nM	% viablity ± SD	% ROS ± SD
0	100 ± 0.7	100 ± 0.5
50	96 ± 2.4	112 ± 0.3
100	88 ± 3.4	114 ± 0.4*
150	71 ± 3.7*	125 ± 0.5**
200	65 ± 7.9*	131 ± 0.5**

Student's t-test versus control = H_2O_2 (0 mM), *$p < 0.05$ and **$p < 0.01$.

(a)

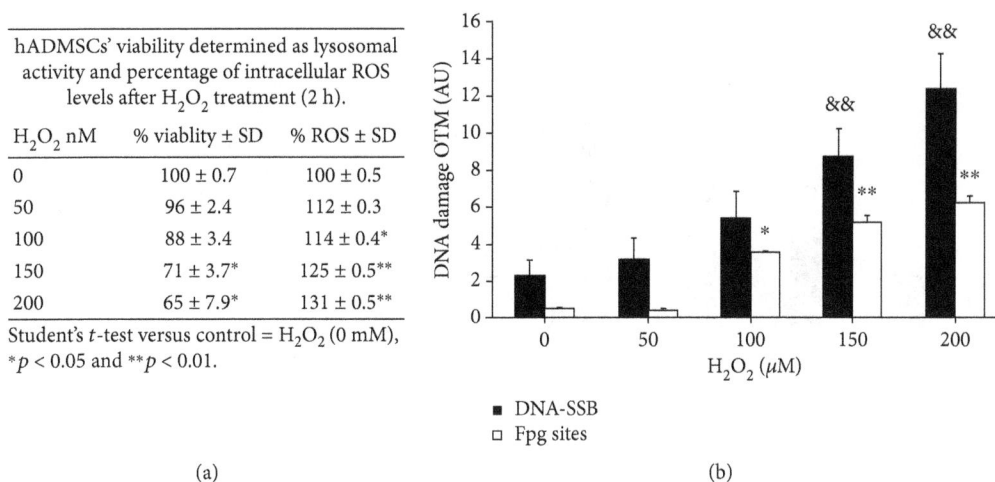

- DNA-SSB
- □ Fpg sites

(b)

FIGURE 2: H_2O_2 dose response in human adipose-derived mesenchymal stem cells. Percentage of cell viability and reactive oxygen species (ROS) in human adipose-derived mesenchymal stem cells (hADMSC) (a). DNA damage induced after 2 h of hydrogen peroxide, expressed as Olive tail moment (OTM) and corresponding to DNA breaks and alkali labile sites (DNA-SSB) and Fpg sites (7,8-dihydro-8-oxoguanine (8-oxoguanine), 8-oxoadenine, aflatoxin B1-fapy-guanine, 5-hydroxy-cytosine, and 5-hydroxy-uracil) in (b) (mean ± SD) (Supplementary Figure 1, comet assay images). To be precise, the corresponding incipient toxic doses of H_2O_2 were 0, 152.5, 305, 457.5, and 600 nmol of H_2O_2/mg cell protein. Data represent 3 independent duplicate experiments ($N = 3$). Nonparametric tests were performed using the Kruskal-Wallis test (one-way ANOVA on ranks), and all pairwise multiple comparison procedures were performed with Dunn's test. DNA-SSB difference versus control (0 μM or 0 nmol/mg cell protein), &&$p < 0.01$. Fpg site difference versus control (0 μM), **$p < 0.01$.

as shown by the increase in the percentage of cells in G1 and a decrease in the percentage of cells in the S and G2/M phases in adipocytes compared with the undifferentiated cells (hADMSCs) (Figure 1(b)). In addition, the relative lipid accumulation as measured by body fat stain with Oil Red O (Figures 1(e)–1(h)) shows lipid accumulation after 14 days (when adipocyte differentiation is complete) compared with that of hADMSCs (Figure 1(i)).

3.2. H_2O_2-Induced DNA Damage and Repair Capacity in hADMSCs.
hADMSCs exposed to H_2O_2 for 2 h showed a dose-dependent response in the metabolic viability test as well as the ROS level assay. In particular, a slight decrease in esterase activity was observed at concentrations higher than 100 μM and was paralleled by an increase in the ROS level (Figure 2(a)). The DNA damage induced by H_2O_2 as both DNA breaks and alkali labile sites as well as oxidative lesions shows a clear dose-dependent response (Figure 2(b)). A relatively higher induction of DNA breaks and alkali labile sites is observed with respect to oxidative DNA lesions. DNA damage may lead to genome instability when it is not repaired. We therefore determined the DNA repair capacity through the level of persistent DNA damage, both via DNA breaks and oxidative DNA lesions, after 24 h posttreatment (Figures 3(a) and 3(b), representative images in Supplementary Material 1). The analysis of the repair rate is shown in Figures 3(c) and 3(d). Notably, in hADMSCs, the DNA breaks induced by H_2O_2 were repaired more efficiently than oxidative lesions (77% versus 45% repair for DNA breaks and oxidative DNA lesions, respectively, upon exposure to 200 μM H_2O_2) (Figures 3(c) and 3(d)). Notably, 24 h after treatment with 100 μM H_2O_2, a concentration that could be reached in engrafted MSCs, repair was complete for both types of lesions.

3.3. DNA Breaks and Oxidative Lesion Accumulation through Adipocyte Differentiation.
DNA damage determined as breaks through adipocyte differentiation shows an increase as a function of the differentiation time with a significant increase already after 6 days (hADMSC 6D) (Figure 4(a), images in Supplementary Figure 2). Similarly, oxidative DNA lesions also increased, although this increase was significant in the final stages of differentiation, since day 12, and to the complete differentiation (14 days) (Figure 4(b), image in Supplementary Figure 2). As observed in the case of hADMSCs, the level of DNA breaks is relatively higher than that of Fpg-sensitive sites. Additionally, we demonstrate the contrast between the basal DNA damage and oxidative lesions according to categories showing undifferentiated (U) and terminally differentiated adipocytes (D) (Figure 4(c)) and increment of ROS levels (Figure 4(d), comet images in Supplementary Figure 2).

3.4. H_2O_2-Induced DNA Damage and Repair Capacity through Adipocyte Differentiation.
The relevance of the DNA damage accumulated through adipocyte differentiation was evaluated by the adipocyte response to H_2O_2 and the measurement of DNA repair capacity 24 h after treatment. The exposure to 100 μM H_2O_2 does not affect hADMSC viability (Table 1); therefore, this experimental condition was selected to monitor DNA damage induction and repair (Figures 5(a) and 5(b), images in Supplementary Figure 3). The capacity of H_2O_2 to induce DNA breaks has shown similar behavior during differentiation even though the values were higher than in undifferentiated hADMSCs (Figure 5(a)); meanwhile, the capacity of H_2O_2 to induce DNA oxidative lesions was higher only in the latest stages of adipocyte differentiation (hADMSC 12D and adipocytes) (Figure 5(b)).

(a)

(b)

(c)

(d)

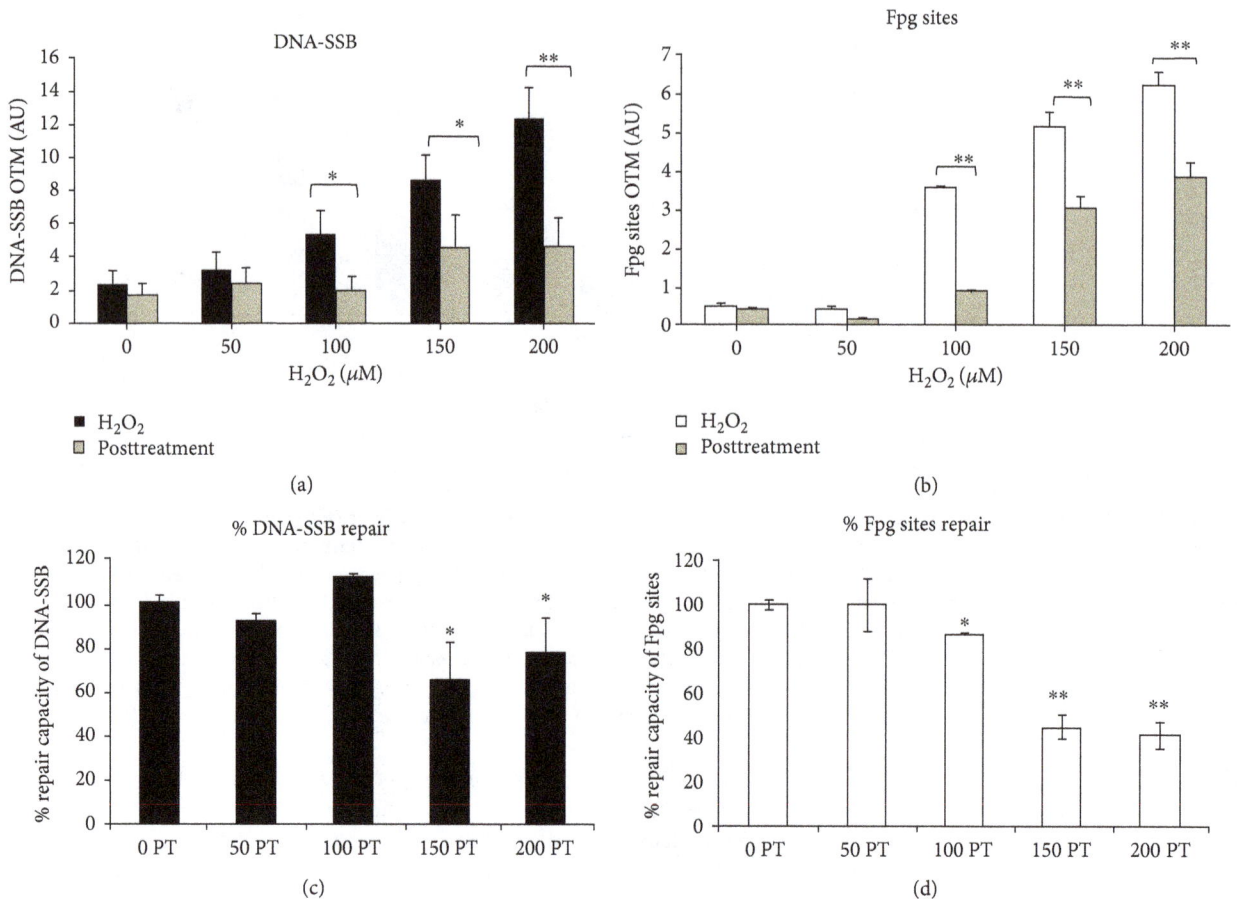

FIGURE 3: DNA repair capacity of H_2O_2 treatment in human adipose-derived mesenchymal stem cells (hADMSCs). DNA damage induced and remnant after 24 h posttreatment (PT), expressed as Olive tail moment (OTM) corresponding to DNA breaks and alkali labile sites in (a) (mean ± SD). DNA-Fpg sites (7,8-dihydro-8-oxoguanine (8-oxoguanine), 8-oxoadenine, aflatoxin B1-fapy-guanine, 5-hydroxy-cytosine, and 5-hydroxy-uracil) in (b) (mean ± SD). Percentage of DNA repair capacity of DNA breaks and alkali labile sites in (c) (percentage ± SD) and percentage of DNA-Fpg sites' repair capacity in (d) (percentage ± SD). 0 PT = control PT; 50 PT = 50 μM H_2O_2 PT; 100 PT = 100 μM H_2O_2 PT; 150 PT = 150 μM H_2O_2 PT; and 200 PT = 200 μM H_2O_2 PT. All data were obtained in 3 independent duplicate experiments ($N = 3$). Kruskal-Wallis was performed with one-way ANOVA on ranks, and all pairwise multiple comparison procedures were performed with Dunn's test. Differences between induced damage and remnant damage were obtained per (a) and (b), $^*p < 0.05$ and $^{**}p < 0.01$. Student's t-test versus control was applied for data in (c) and (d), $^*p < 0.05$ and $^{**}p < 0.01$. Images in Supplementary Figure 3.

The DNA repair capacity indicates that while breaks are fully repaired in undifferentiated hADMSCs, repairs of this type of damage in adipocytes drop drastically to 10% (Figure 5(c)). Less dramatic changes were observed for the repair of oxidative lesions with repair rates of 92% and 50% in undifferentiated hADMSCs and adipocytes, respectively (Figure 5(d)).

4. Discussion

hADMSCs represent a potential source of MSCs for cell therapy [4]. As expected, these cells maintain the ability to be differentiated into chondrocytes, osteoblasts, or adipocytes, as shown by the expression of specific surface markers [11, 14]. Moreover, they express the human fatty acid transport protein-1 (hFATP-1), which is stimulated by insulin and facilitates the transport of fatty acids across the cell membrane to promote the accumulation of long chain fatty acids (LCFAs). This explains the formation of fat vesicles during adipocyte differentiation (Figure 1). Notably, we found an increase in the expression of CD146⁻ in hADMSCs compared with adipocytes, which is also known as melanoma adhesion molecule and could account for the increased adhesion capacity characteristics of the adipocytes. DNA damage is expected to be efficiently removed in stem cells [15, 16], and indeed, hADMSCs efficiently repair DNA breaks and oxidative DNA lesions. Our results were obtained using an early cell passage (4th passage) and are in line with other studies that employed adipose-derived stem cells obtained by bone marrow or femoral/abdominal liposuction [17, 18].

To provide new insights into the use of hADMSC in cell therapy, we investigated its response to oxidative damage generated in DNA induced by a physiological flow of hydrogen peroxide. Experimentally *in vitro*, the reproduction of the flow of hydrogen peroxide is complex; however, it is closer to

(a)

(b)

(c)

(d)

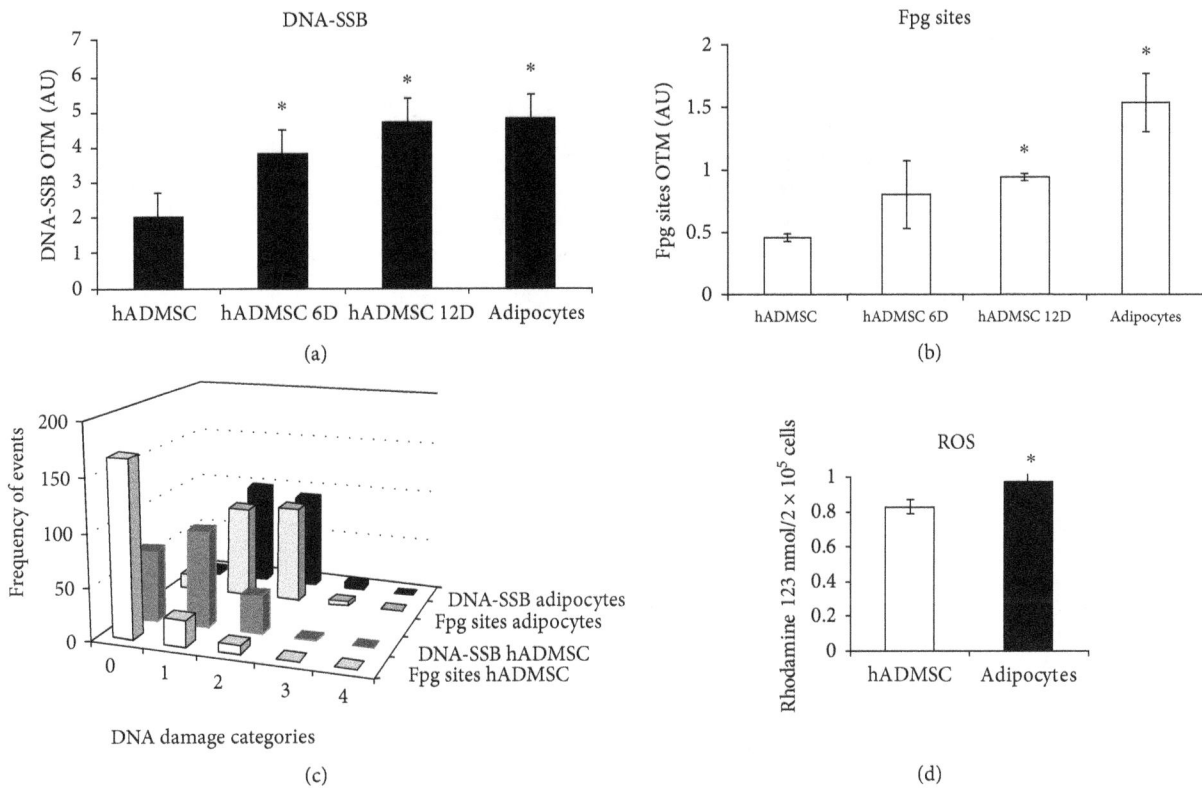

FIGURE 4: DNA damage accumulation through adipocyte differentiation of hADMSCs. DNA damage corresponding to DNA breaks and alkali labile sites accumulated over 14 days of adipocyte differentiation was expressed as Olive tail moment (OTM), (a) (mean ± SD). DNA oxidative damage accumulation, corresponding to DNA-Fpg sites (7,8-dihydro-8-oxoguanine (8-oxoguanine), 8-oxoadenine, aflatoxin B1-fapy-guanine, 5-hydroxy-cytosine, and 5-hydroxy-uracil) expressed as OTM, is represented in (b) (mean ± SD). Basal DNA damage (breaks + alkali labile sites) and basal DNA oxidative damage (Fpg-sensitive sites) of hADMSCs (U = undifferentiated) and adipocytes (D = differentiated) are represented in categories of damage (0, without damage to 4, highest damage) in (c). ROS intracellular levels in hADMSCs and adipocytes are shown in (d) (mean ± SD). Data represent 3 or 4 independent experiments with duplicates. Nonparametric tests were used for single cell gel electrophoresis analyses, Kruskal-Wallis (one-way ANOVA on ranks), and all pairwise multiple comparison procedures (Dunn's test). Differences versus hADMSCs (undifferentiated), $^*p < 0.05$. Images in Supplementary Figure 4.

TABLE 1: Cell viability after H_2O_2 treatment (2 h) in hADMSCs through adipocyte differentiation and 24 h posttreatment.

	Control	H_2O_2 (100 μM)	Posttreatment
hADMSC	96 ± 1	89 ± 4	92 ± 3
hADMSC 6D	98 ± 0	88 ± 1	89 ± 1
hADMSC 12D	99 ± 0.5	85 ± 0.5*	85 ± 0*
Adipocytes	95 ± 1	80 ± 1*	86 ± 0.5*

Mean ± SD, Student's t-test versus control $^*p < 0.05$.

what cells *in vivo* are likely to experience. In this work, we only studied the effect triggered by a single dose of 100 μM. These cells, as well as their differentiated counterpart, appear to be relatively resistant to H_2O_2 because no cytotoxicity was observed up to 100 μM (Table 1 and Figure 2(a)), a dose that is cytotoxic in a wide variety of animals, plants, and bacterial cells in culture [8, 13]. In terms of DNA repair capacity, hADMSCs are fully proficient in the repair of breaks and oxidative lesions induced by hydrogen peroxide levels up to 100 μM. Above this dose (>100 μM), a significant inhibition

of DNA repair is observed (Figure 3), suggesting that the control of the ROS environment is a key factor for stem cell survival. Some studies report that stem cells and MSCs require DSB (double strand break) repair to address DNA damage [13, 15, 18]. Khan et al. recently suggested that only cells with an efficient response to DNA damage are allowed to enter adipogenic differentiation; they proposed that SNEV (senescence evasion factor) regulates adipogenesis, acting as a checkpoint for DNA damage accumulation in human adipocyte-derived stem cells after acute treatment with hydrogen peroxide [17]. A cross talk between DDR and differentiation would therefore provide stem cells with a stringent control of genetic stability before undergoing self-renewal and differentiation [18, 19]. Here, we addressed how hADMSCs respond to an oxidative insult (H_2O_2 100 μM) when proliferating and during adipocyte differentiation. The response to endogenous DNA damage as well as to H_2O_2-induced DNA damage reflects a gradual decrease in repair capacity during the differentiation program. This decrease in repair capacity is more marked than the changes in intracellular ROS levels, which are only slightly modified. Similarly, a decrease in the repair capacity of oxidative

(a)

(b)

(c)

(d)

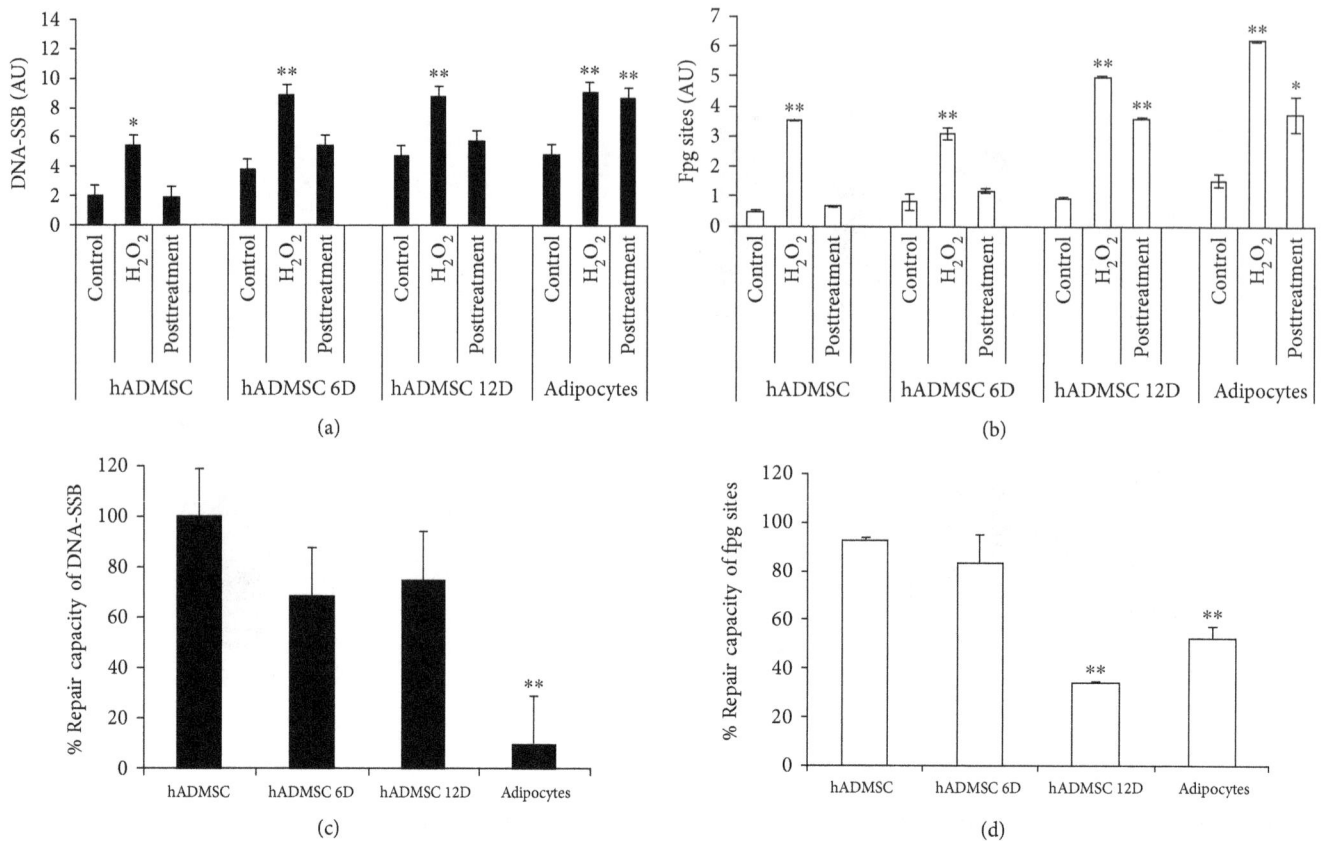

FIGURE 5: H_2O_2-related DNA damage induction and DNA kinetic repair through adipocyte differentiation of hADMSCs. DNA breaks and alkali labile sites are represented in (a) (mean ± SD); DNA-Fpg sites (7,8-dihydro-8-oxoguanine (8-oxoguanine), 8-oxoadenine, aflatoxin B1-fapy-guanine, 5-hydroxy-cytosine, and 5-hydroxy-uracil) are shown in (b) (mean ± SD). Data represent 3 or 4 independent experiments with duplicates. Nonparametric tests were used for single cell gel electrophoresis analyses, the Kruskal-Wallis test employed one-way ANOVA on ranks, and all pairwise multiple comparison procedures used Dunn's test. Differences versus controls correspond to the differentiation stage, $^*p < 0.05$ and $^{**}p < 0.01$. The repair capacity of DNA breaks and alkali labile sites is shown in (c) (mean ± SD). The repair capacity of DNA-Fpg sites (7,8-dihydro-8-oxoguanine (8-oxoguanine), 8-oxoadenine, aflatoxin B1-fapy-guanine, 5-hydroxy-cytosine, and 5-hydroxy-uracil) is shown in (d) (mean ± SD). Student's t-test versus hADMSCs, $^*p < 0.05$ and $^{**}p < 0.01$. Images in Supplementary Figure 5.

damage has been previously reported during myogenesis as well as during neuronal differentiation [13, 20]. Additionally, we want to emphasize that our protocol only reflects the sites sensitive to the Fpg, since we only do the enzymatic digestion immediately after the cell lysis and perform the electrophoretic shift; that is, we do not perform alkaline incubation for unwinding; this avoids the generation of AP sites together with the oxidative lesions digested by the Fpg. When the repair capacity along adipogenesis is analyzed as a function of the DNA lesion type, an interesting scenario emerges: while DNA break repair is fully impaired, the removal of Fpg-sensitive sites is decreased but remains active (50% reduction) in adipocytes. Diverse DNA base lesions are removed by specific repair enzymes to avoid harmful consequences. Abasic sites are repaired by APE1 to avoid mutagenic bypass, replication fork stalling, or conversion to double strand breaks. 7-Methylguanine and 3-methyladenine are repaired by N-methylpurine DNA glycosylase to generate abasic site formation, ring opening to FaPy-G, replication stalling, or chromosomal instability.

SSB are repaired by the single strand break repair (SSBR) machinery to avoid replication fork collapse or conversion to DSB. 8-Oxoguanine is the most common and mutagenic oxidized DNA lesion and is repaired by OGG1 to avoid mutagenic base mispairing. However, oxidatively generated DNA lesions are not only a mutagenic risk factor but also a regulatory marker (for a review, see [21]). Therefore, the accumulation of DNA oxidative lesions may also be of great concern for cells that do not replicate, such as terminally differentiated adipocytes that have to maintain the integrity of the genes essential for their function. This may explain why the repair of oxidatively generated DNA lesions remains active (although reduced) in adipocytes. Whether the transcription-coupled repair of oxidized base lesions [22, 23] is involved warrants further investigation.

5. Conclusions

In regenerative medicine, the use of human adipose-derived mesenchymal stem cells is extensive; however, little is known regarding their response to DNA damage and in particular to the reactive oxygen species (ROS) that are present in the microenvironment of implantation. The role of these ROS in the microenvironment can be partly addressed experimentally by the treatment of a hydrogen peroxide bolus. The present study is the first evidence of DNA breaks and oxidative DNA damage accumulated through adipogenesis, in concordance with the increase of adipogenic biomarkers such as hFATP-1, CD 146, and lipid droplet formation. In addition, we show the increased vulnerability to hydrogen peroxide in the adipogenic differentiation and some interesting particularities in DNA repair capacity which emerge depending on the specific DNA lesions. While DNA break repair is fully impaired, the removal of Fpg-sensitive sites is decreased but remains active (50% reduction) in adipocytes. The removal of oxidative DNA lesions has a primarily protective function; however, our proposal is that all remaining Fpg-sensitive sites realize the regulatory functions in signal transduction and transcriptional regulation required by specialized cells, such as terminally differentiated adipocytes.

Acknowledgments

This work is derived from the sabbatical stay of Mahara Valverde at the Istituto Superiore di Sanità, Rome and was realized with the support of PASPA-DGAPA-UNAM. Jonathan Lozano-Salgado received a CONACyT fellowship. The authors thank Dr. Carlos Castellanos for cytometry acquisition support.

Supplementary Materials

Supplementary Figure 1: H_2O_2-induced DNA damage and repair capacity in hADMSCs. 2 h hydrogen peroxide treatment using 0 to 200 μM and repair capacity presented as DNA damage remnant after 24 h posttreatment. Comet images at 4x magnification acquired by Komet 5.0 (Kinetic Imaging Ltd.). Methodological details are shown in the Material and Methods section. Supplementary Figure 2: DNA damage accumulation through adipocyte differentiation of hADMSCs. Differentiation follow-up at day 0 = hADMSC, day 6 = hADMSC 6D, day 12 = hADMSC 12D, and day 14 = adipocytes. Comet images at 4x magnification acquired by Komet 5.0 (Kinetic Imaging Ltd.). Methodological details are shown in the Material and Methods section. Supplementary Figure 3: H_2O_2-induced DNA damage and repair capacity through adipocyte differentiation. Hydrogen peroxide treatment using 100 μM during 2 h and repair capacity presented as DNA damage remnant after 24 h posttreatment. Differentiation follow-up at day 0 = hADMSC, day 6 = hADMSC 6D, day 12 = hADMSC 12D, and day 14 = adipocytes. Comet images at 4x magnification acquired by Komet 5.0 (Kinetic Imaging Ltd.). Methodological details are shown in the Material and Methods section. *(Supplementary Materials)*

References

[1] A. Bajek, N. Gurtowska, J. Olkowska, L. Kazmierski, M. Maj, and T. Drewa, "Adipose-derived stem cells as a tool in cell-based therapies," *Archivum Immunologiae et Therapiae Experimentalis*, vol. 64, no. 6, pp. 443–454, 2016.

[2] P. A. Zuk, M. Zhu, H. Mizuno et al., "Multilineage cells from human adipose tissue: implications for cell-based therapies," *Tissue Engineering*, vol. 7, no. 2, pp. 211–228, 2001.

[3] P. A. Zuk, M. Zhu, P. Ashjian et al., "Human adipose tissue is a source of multipotent stem cells," *Molecular Biology of the Cell*, vol. 13, no. 12, pp. 4279–4295, 2002.

[4] C.-J. Li, L.-Y. Sun, and C.-Y. Pang, "Synergistic protection of N-acetylcysteine and ascorbic acid 2-phosphate on human mesenchymal stem cells against mitoptosis, necroptosis and apoptosis," *Scientific Reports*, vol. 5, no. 1, article 9819, 2015.

[5] K. Froelich, J. Mickler, G. Steusloff et al., "Chromosomal aberrations and deoxyribonucleic acid single-strand breaks in adipose-derived stem cells during long-term expansion *in vitro*," *Cytotherapy*, vol. 15, no. 7, pp. 767–781, 2013.

[6] K. B. Choo, L. Tai, K. S. Hymavathee et al., "Oxidative stress-induced premature senescence in Wharton's jelly-derived mesenchymal stem cells," *International Journal of Medical Sciences*, vol. 11, no. 11, pp. 1201–1207, 2014.

[7] R. Breton-Romero and S. Lamas, "Hydrogen peroxide signaling in vascular endothelial cells," *Redox Biology*, vol. 2, pp. 529–534, 2014.

[8] B. Halliwell, M. V. Clement, and L. H. Long, "Hydrogen peroxide in the human body," *FEBS Letters*, vol. 486, no. 1, pp. 10–13, 2000.

[9] J. Tchou, V. Bodepudi, S. Shibutani et al., "Substrate specificity of Fpg protein. Recognition and cleavage of oxidatively damaged DNA," *The Journal of Biological Chemistry*, vol. 269, no. 21, pp. 15318–15324, 1994.

[10] Z. Hatahet, Y. W. Kow, A. A. Purmal, R. P. Cunningham, and S. S. Wallace, "New substrates for old enzymes. 5-Hydroxy-2$'$-deoxycytidine and 5-hydroxy-2$'$-deoxyuridine are substrates for Escherichia coli endonuclease III and formamidopyrimidine DNA N-glycosylase, while 5-hydroxy-2$'$-deoxyuridine is a substrate for uracil DNA N-glycosylase," *The Journal of Biological Chemistry*, vol. 269, no. 29, pp. 18814–18820, 1994.

[11] P. Bourin, B. A. Bunnell, L. Casteilla et al., "Stromal cells from the adipose tissue-derived stromal vascular fraction and culture expanded adipose tissue-derived stromal/stem cells: a joint statement of the International Federation for Adipose Therapeutics and Science (IFATS) and the International Society for Cellular Therapy (ISCT)," *Cytotherapy*, vol. 15, no. 6, pp. 641–648, 2013.

[12] E. Rojas, M. C. Lopez, and M. Valverde, "Single cell gel electrophoresis assay methodology and applications," *Journal of Chromatography B: Biomedical Sciences and Applications*, vol. 722, no. 1-2, pp. 225–254, 1999.

[13] P. Ramos-Espinosa, E. Rojas, and M. Valverde, "Differential DNA damage response to UV and hydrogen peroxide depending of differentiation stage in a neuroblastoma model," *Neuro-Toxicology*, vol. 33, no. 5, pp. 1086–1095, 2012.

[14] L. Badimon, B. Oñate, and G. Vilahur, "Adipose-derived mesenchymal stem cells and their reparative potential in ischemic heart disease," *Revista Española de Cardiología*, vol. 68, no. 7, pp. 599–611, 2015.

[15] E. D. Tichy and P. J. Stambrook, "DNA repair in murine embryonic stem cells and differentiated cells," *Experimental Cell Research*, vol. 314, no. 9, pp. 1929–1936, 2008.

[16] P. Fortini, C. Ferretti, and E. Dogliotti, "The response to DNA damage during differentiation: pathways and consequences," *Mutation Research*, vol. 743-744, pp. 160–168, 2013.

[17] A. Khan, H. Dellago, L. Terlecki-Zaniewicz et al., "SNEV[hPrp19/hPso4] regulates adipogenesis of human adipose stromal cells," *Stem Cell Reports*, vol. 8, no. 1, pp. 21–29, 2017.

[18] L. Oliver, E. Hue, Q. Séry et al., "Differentiation-related response to DNA breaks in human mesenchymal stem cells," *Stem Cells*, vol. 31, no. 4, pp. 800–807, 2013.

[19] C. R. R. Rocha, L. K. Lerner, O. K. Okamoto, M. C. Marchetto, and C. F. M. Menck, "The role of DNA repair in the pluripotency and differentiation of human stem cells," *Mutation Research*, vol. 752, no. 1, pp. 25–35, 2013.

[20] L. Narciso, P. Fortini, D. Pajalunga et al., "Terminally differentiated muscle cells are defective in base excision DNA repair and hypersensitive to oxygen injury," *PNAS*, vol. 104, no. 43, pp. 17010–17015, 2007.

[21] M. Seifermann and B. Epe, "Oxidatively generated base modifications in DNA: not only carcinogenic risk factor but also regulatory mark?," *Free Radical Biology & Medicine*, vol. 107, pp. 258–265, 2017.

[22] E. Parlanti, M. D'Errico, P. Degan et al., "The cross talk between pathways in the repair of 8-oxo-7,8-dihydroguanine in mouse and human cells," *Free Radical Biology & Medicine*, vol. 53, no. 11, pp. 2171–2177, 2012.

[23] G. Spivak, "Transcription coupled repair: an update," *Archives of Toxicology*, vol. 90, no. 11, pp. 2583–2594, 2016.

2

Dorsal Root Ganglion Maintains Stemness of Bone Marrow Mesenchymal Stem Cells by Enhancing Autophagy through the AMPK/mTOR Pathway in a Coculture System

Shuaishuai Zhang,[1] Junqin Li,[1] Huijie Jiang,[1] Yi Gao,[1] Pengzhen Cheng,[1] Tianqing Cao,[1] Donglin Li,[2] Jimeng Wang,[3] Yue Song,[1] Bin Liu,[1] Hao Wu,[1] Chunmei Wang,[1] Liu Yang🆔,[1] and Guoxian Pei🆔[1]

[1]*Department of Orthopaedics, Xijing Hospital, Fourth Military Medical University, Xi'an 710032, China*
[2]*Department of Orthopaedics, The 463rd Hospital of PLA, Shenyang 110042, China*
[3]*Department of Orthopaedics, The 251st Hospital of PLA, Zhangjiakou 075000, China*

Correspondence should be addressed to Liu Yang; yangliu@fmmu.edu.cn and Guoxian Pei; nfperry@163.com

Academic Editor: Stefania Bruno

Our previous studies found that sensory nerve tracts implanted in tissue-engineered bone (TEB) could result in better osteogenesis. To explore the mechanism of the sensory nerve promoting osteogenesis in TEB in vitro, a transwell coculture experiment was designed between dorsal root ganglion (DRG) cells and bone marrow mesenchymal stem cells (BMSCs). BMSC proliferation was determined by CCK8 assay, and osteo-, chondro-, and adipogenic differentiation were assessed by alizarin red, alcian blue, and oil red staining. We found that the proliferation and multipotent differentiation of BMSCs were all enhanced in the coculture group compared to the BMSCs group. Crystal violet staining showed that the clone-forming ability of BMSCs in the coculture group was also enhanced and mRNA levels of Sox2, Nanog, and Oct4 were significantly upregulated in the coculture group. Moreover, the autophagy level of BMSCs, regulating their stemness, was promoted in the coculture group, mediated by the AMPK/mTOR pathway. In addition, AMPK inhibitor compound C could significantly downregulate the protein expression of LC3 and the mRNA level of stemness genes in the coculture group. Finally, we found that the NK1 receptor antagonist, aprepitant, could partly block this effect, which indicated that substance P played an important role in the effect. Together, we conclude that DRG could maintain the stemness of BMSCs by enhancing autophagy through the AMPK/mTOR pathway in a transwell coculture system, which may help explain the better osteogenesis after implantation of the sensory nerve into TEB.

1. Introduction

Bone tissue engineering has provided a promising resolution for the treatment of large bone defect, although there are still many problems to be solved [1–3], such as low survival rate and poor osteogenic differentiation of BMSCs. Previously, we found that the sensory nerve tract preimplanted in the tissue-engineered bone (TEB) could significantly improve osteogenesis of the TEB [4, 5], but the underlying mechanism was still largely unknown.

The sensory nerve has been reported to play critical roles in bone metabolism and regeneration in vivo [6–9]. Some studies found that sensory nerve innervation contributed to the maintenance of trabecular bone mass and its mechanical properties by inhibiting bone resorption [8]. Besides, sensory nerves had efferent functions in the tissues they innervated, mediated by transmitters released from the peripheral nerve terminals, which helped to maintain trabecular bone integrity [10]. Recently, sensory neuron-derived Sema3A was found to be responsible for the bone mass loss in Sema3a$^{-/-}$ mice, and Sema3A regulated bone remodelling indirectly by modulating sensory nerve innervation, not directly by acting on osteoblasts [7].

Studies in vitro indicated that neuropeptides, such as substance P and CGRP [11], could influence preosteoblast cells. For example, SP significantly increased proliferation of BMSCs in vitro in a dose-dependent manner [12]. And SP could induce osteoblastic differentiation of BMSCs via the Wnt/β-catenin pathway and promote the angiogenic ability of BMSCs [13]. In addition, CGRP was reported to exert its anabolic action on human osteoblasts by stimulating canonical Wnt signaling and inhibiting human osteoblast apoptosis [14].

Taken together, these findings in vivo and in vitro suggested that the sensory nerve played a vital role in bone metabolism and regeneration. However, the mechanism at the cellular level is rarely studied, and one kind of neuropeptide may not reflect the overall effect of the sensory nerve on bone cells. Therefore, the overall regulation of the sensory nerve on bone cells and its underlying molecular mechanisms need further studies.

In this study, we used a transwell coculture system to investigate the effect of DRG cells on BMSCs. Our results indicated that DRG could help maintain the stemness of BMSCs through improving the basal autophagy level by activating AMPK/mTOR signaling in this coculture system.

2. Materials and Methods

2.1. Isolation and Characterization of GFP Rat BMSCs. BMSCs from 2-week-old GFP Sprague–Dawley (SD) rats were harvested using a well-characterized protocol with slight modification [15]. Briefly, primary cultures of BMSCs were obtained from a 2-week-old GFP rat under sterile conditions. The rats were sacrificed with an overdose of 2% pentobarbital sodium (w/v). After immersing in 75% ethanol (v/v) for 5 min, both the femurs and tibias were isolated and excised with the attached soft tissues, and then epiphyses were cut off with aseptic scissors. Then, the marrow was flushed from the diaphysis with a syringe and collected in a primary culture medium (α-MEM containing 10% FBS and 1% antibiotics (penicillin and streptomycin)). The collected medium containing marrow cells was cultured in 6-well culture plates with 2 ml α-MEM containing 10% FBS each well. After 24 hours, nonadherent cells were carefully removed. The cell growth medium was changed every 2 days, and cells were subcultured until reaching 80% confluence. Passage 3 BMSCs were seeded in a 6-well culture plate at a concentration of 2×10^3 cells/ml for coculture with DRG. BMSCs from passage 3 were characterized with flow cytometry and pluripotent differentiation.

2.2. Flow Cytometry. BMSCs from passage 3 were trypsinized, centrifuged, and suspended in cold PBS, and the cell number was calculated. Then, BMSCs were blocked with 2% BSA for 30 min at room temperature. Meanwhile, the antibodies were diluted to the recommended concentration with PBS. After that, cell density was adjusted to 1×10^6 each tube. Then, cells were incubated for 40 min at 4°C with a

PerCP anti-rat CD90 antibody (202512, BioLegend), PE anti-rat CD11b/c antibody (201807, BioLegend), PE anti-rat CD34 antibody (ab187284, Abcam), and PE-Cy7 anti-rat CD45 antibody (202214, BioLegend). The incubated cells were analyzed by flow cytometry (cytomics FC 500, Beckman Coulter) using isotype-identical antibodies as controls.

2.3. Preparation of DRG and Coculture between BMSCs and DRG Cells. One-day-old postnatal SD rats were sacrificed, and isolation of DRG was based on the previous study [16]. The vertebral column was exposed and opened from the thoracic to the lumbar region. Then, DRG was dissected from the lumbar spinal cord and washed with ice-cold PBS. The connective tissue was carefully removed. DRG was pooled in α-MEM medium on ice until further procedure. The collected DRG was cut mechanically with scissors for 2 minutes and then incubated for 30 minutes at 37°C with 0.1% (v/v) trypsin. Then, cells were filtered through a $100\,\mu m$ cell strainer and centrifuged at $180\,g$ for 5 minutes. The harvested DRG cells were planted in the transwell cell insert (Lot 3450, Corning, USA), which had already been put into the 6-well culture plate, at a concentration of 1×10^4 cells per well. Then, 1 ml of the cell growth medium was added into the transwell insert, which meant that there was 3 ml of the cell growth medium in all 6 wells of the plate. BMSCs cultured without DRG cells were used as the control group. They were cultured at 37°C in 5% CO_2 atmosphere. The use of transwell cell inserts allowed DRG cells and BMSCs to share the same cell growth medium but had no direct contact.

2.4. BMSC Osteogenic Differentiation and Alizarin Red Staining. The osteogenic differentiation medium (RASMX-90021) was purchased from Cyagen Biosciences Inc., and the procedure was performed according to the products' user manual. Briefly, after coculture for 8 days, BMSCs were detached and seeded on a new 12-well culture plate at the density of 2×10^4 cells/well. The osteogenic medium consisted of DMEM with 10% FBS, 50 mg/ml ascorbic acid-2phosphate, 100 nM dexamethasone, and 10 mM β-glycerol phosphate in the presence of 100 U/ml penicillin and 100 mg/ml streptomycin. When cells were approximately 60–70% confluent, the growth mediums were carefully aspirated off from each well and 2 ml of the osteogenic differentiation medium was added. The osteogenic induction mediums were changed every 3 days. After 14 days, cells could be fixed with 4% paraformaldehyde and stained with Alizarin red S (Cyagen Biosciences Inc.) for 3 to 5 min, and then cells were observed under the microscope.

2.5. BMSC Chondrogenic Differentiation and Alcian Blue Staining. For chondrogenic differentiation, 0.5 ml BMSCs containing 2.5×10^5 cells is needed to form one chondrogenic pellet in 15 ml polypropylene culture tubes with the differentiation induction medium (RASMX-90041, Cyagen Biosciences, USA). The caps of the tubes were loosened in order to allow gas exchange, and cells were incubated at 37°C in a humidified atmosphere of 5% CO_2. The pellets were not disturbed for 24 hours. The chondrogenic induction mediums were changed every 2–3 days in each tube (to avoid aspirating the pellets when aspirating the medium, attach a sterile 1–200 μl pipette tip to the end of the aspirating pipette). 0.5 ml of the freshly prepared complete chondrogenic medium was added to each tube. To ensure that the pellet was free floating, the bottom of the tube was flicked several times. Chondrogenic pellets were harvested after 20 days of culture. Pellets were formalin-fixed, and frozen sections of 8 μm thickness were obtained for alcian blue staining analysis.

2.6. Adipogenic Differentiation and Oil Red Staining. For adipogenic differentiation, the differentiation induction medium (RASMD-90031, 1 μM DEX, 1 μg/ml insulin, and 0.5 mM 3-isobutyl-1-methylxanthine) and differentiation basal medium (glutamine, insulin) were prepared according to the user's manual. On the 8th day of experiment, BMSCs were reseeded at 2×10^4 cells/cm^2 in a 6-well tissue culture plate with a medium volume of 2 ml per well. Upon reaching 100% confluent or postconfluent, 2 ml of the induction medium was added per well. Three days later, the medium was changed to a maintenance medium. 24 hours later, the medium was changed back to the induction medium. After repeating the cycle for 4 times, the maintenance medium was continuously used for 4 to 7 days. After the cells had differentiated, cells were rinsed and fixed with 4% paraformaldehyde. 1 ml of oil red O (Cyagen Biosciences Inc.) working solution was added (diluted to 3 : 2 with distilled water and filtered with a filter paper) for 30 minutes to each well. Then, cells were observed under a microscope.

2.7. Cell Proliferation Assay. Cell proliferation assay was performed as previously described [17]. Briefly, cells were seeded on 6-well plates (10^4 cells/well) and cultured with or without DRG for indicated time lengths. At days 1, 2, 4, 6, 8, and 10, the Cell Counting Kit-8 (Dojindo) was applied and incubated for 2 hours, and then absorbance of formazan dye produced by living cells at 450 nm was measured with a microplate reader (Synergy H1, BioTek, USA). All experiments were performed three separate times.

2.8. Colony-Forming Unit (CFU) Assay. CFU assay was conducted to measure the self-renewal ability of BMSCs with or without DRG cells. Briefly, BMSCs, after coculture with DRG for 8 days, were seeded at the number of 50 cells in a 60 mm plate and cultured for 10 days, then stained with crystal violet staining solution. Colonies containing more than 50 cells were counted under a microscope. Monocultured BMSCs were recognized as the control in all the experiments. All experiments were performed three separate times.

2.9. Real-Time Quantitative PCR. All procedures were performed according to products' instruction and referring to a well-documented method in a previous study [15]. Briefly, total RNA from BMSCs was extracted using OMEGA Total RNA Kit I (lot R6834-01, OMEGA bio-tek, USA) according to the manufacturer's protocol. Concentration and purity of the RNA were determined by measuring the absorbance in TE buffer (10 mM Tris-HCl, pH 8.0, and 1 mM EDTA) at 260 and 280 nm. Then, cDNA was

synthesized from the total RNA using a Takara PrimeScript™ RT Master Mix (Perfect Real Time) kit (Lot RR036, Takara, Japan) following the supplier's instructions. The levels of mRNA of Sox2, Nanog, and Oct4 in BMSCs were determined by quantitative real-time RT-PCR using the Takara SYBR Green I kit according to the user manual (Bio-Rad, CFX96, Real-Time System, USA). The sequences of the primers are as follows: for Sox2, forward primer 5′-GTCAGCGCCCT GCAGTACAA-3′ and reverse primer 5′-GCGAGTAGGAC ATGCTGTAGGTG-3′; for Oct4, forward primer 5′-GAC AACCATCTGCCGCTTC-3′ and reverse primer 5′-TCC TCCACCCACTTCTCCA-3′; for Nanog, forward primer 5′-TGGACACTGGCTGAATCCTTC-3′ and reverse primer 5′-CGCTGATTAGGCTCCAACCAT-3′; and for GADPH (as the internal control), forward primer 5′-ACAGGGCTA TCAGGGAGCA-3′ and reverse primer 5′-GGAGCGAGA TCCCTCCAAAAT-3′.

2.10. Western Blotting Analysis. Western blotting analysis was conducted as previously described [18]. Briefly, BMSCs in the 6-well plate were washed in cold-buffered PBS and lysed in RIPA buffer with 1 mm PMSF on ice. Cell lysates were centrifuged (12000 rpm, 10 min) at 4°C, and the protein supernatant was transferred into new tubes. The concentration of the protein samples was determined with the BCA Protein Assay Kit (PC0020, Solarbio, Beijing, China). A 20 μg sample of the total protein was resolved using 12% SDS-PAGE and transferred onto PVDF membranes. The membranes were blocked in Tris-buffered saline containing Tween 20 with 5% BSA at room temperature for 2 h. Primary antibodies (LC3A/B, 50 μg/50 μl, AF5402, anti-LC3A/B antibody, 1 : 1000, Affinity, USA; AMPK, ab32047, 1 : 2500, Abcam, USA; p-AMPK, ab133448, 1 : 5000, Abcam, USA; P-AKT, ab81283, 1 : 7000, Abcam, USA; AKT, ab8805, 1 : 500, Abcam, USA; mTOR, ab2732, 1 : 2000, Abcam, USA; P-mTOR, ab137133, 1 : 5000, Abcam, USA; and β-actin, 66009-1-lg, 1 : 20000, Proteintech Group, USA) were incubated overnight with the membranes at 4°C. Membranes were incubated with horseradish peroxidase-conjugated anti-rabbit secondary antibodies (Goat Anti-Rabbit IgG (HRP), Abcam, ab6721, USA), and proteins were detected by enhanced chemiluminescence (Beyotime, Shanghai, China) using Amersham Imager 600 (General Electric Company, USA). β-Actin was used as the internal control to normalize the loading materials.

2.11. Immunofluorescence. Cells were immobilized with 4% paraformaldehyde and permeabilized with 1% triton X-100 for 10 min, followed by blocking with 2% bovine serum albumin for 30 minutes. Then, the primary antibody, rabbit polyclonal antibody (LC3A/B, 50 μg/50 μl, AF5402, anti-LC3A/B antibody, 1 : 100, Affinity, USA), was used for incubation overnight at 4°C. Then, cells were incubated with a secondary antibody Alexa Fluor 647 donkey anti-rabbit (ab150075, 1 : 200, Abcam, USA) away from light for 1 hour. After that, cells were mounted with DAPI (1 : 1000, 32670-5MG-F, Sigma, USA) for 5 minutes. Immunofluorescent

(a)　(b)　(c)　(d)

(e)

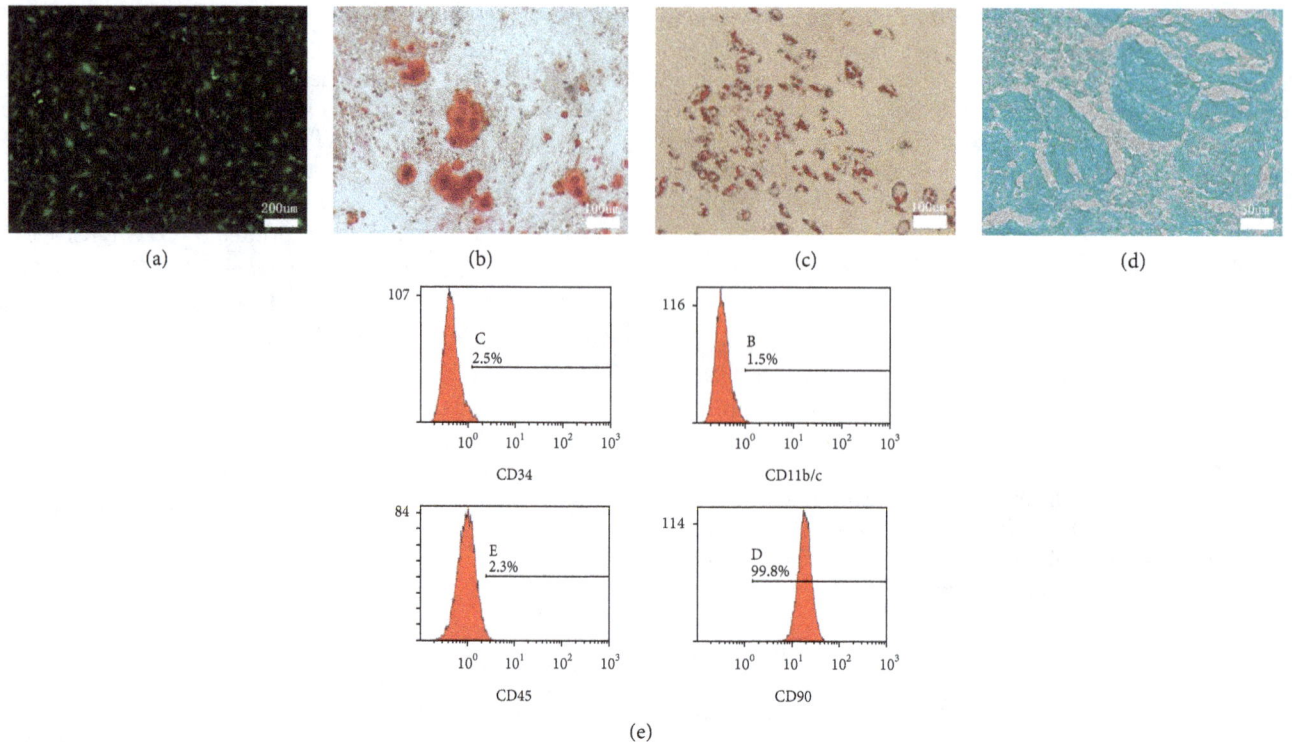

FIGURE 1: Characterization of GFP BMSCs. (a) Morphology of P3 GFP BMSCs. (b) Alizarin red staining of BMSCs after osteogenic induction for 14 days. (c) Oil red staining of BMSCs after adipogenic induction for 10 days. (d) Alcian blue staining of BMSCs after chondrogenic induction for 20 days. (e) Representative results of flow cytometry analysis of P3 BMSCs indicating abundant expression of CD90 and the absence of CD 34, CD11b/c, and CD45.

images were captured and analyzed with a confocal microscope (Olympus, FV10-ASW3.1, JPN).

2.12. Drug Treatment. The AMPK inhibitor, compound C, was purchased from Millipore (Merck, Billerica, MA, USA), and the dose of compound C was $20\,\mu$M [19, 20]. Compound C was added into the system for 24 hours after coculture for 8 days. The NK1 receptor antagonist, aprepitant, was purchased from Sigma-Aldrich (SML2215-5MG, Shanghai, China). The dose of aprepitant was $50\,\mu$M [21, 22]. After coculture for 8 days, DRG and BMSCs were treated with aprepitant for 48 hours. Then, BMSCs were collected for the following analysis.

2.13. Statistical Analysis. All data were expressed as means ± standard deviation and analyzed by SPSS software (version 13.0). The difference between groups was compared by Student's *t*-test, and *P* value less than 0.05 was considered to be statistically significant.

3. Results

3.1. Characterization of GFP Rat BMSCs. BMSCs appeared to have fusiform morphology with green fluorescence, the classical form of them (Figure 1(a)). The multipotential differentiation of BMSCs was verified by alizarin red staining (Figure 1(b)), oil red O staining (Figure 1(c)), and alcian blue staining (Figure 1(d)), which showed that BMSCs used in this study could differentiate into osteoblasts,

adipocytes, and chondrocytes under induction condition. The flow cytometry analysis suggested that P3 cells used in this experiment had abundant expression of CD90 (99.8%) and the absence of CD34 (2.5%), CD11b/c (1.5%), and CD45 (2.3%) (Figure 1(e)). Together, BMSCs in this study had multiple potential for differentiation, and the purity of BMSCs was very high, so P3 BMSCs could be used for the following experiments.

3.2. Coculturing with DRG Promoted Proliferation and Enhanced Multipotential Differentiation of BMSCs. Here, we analyzed the effect of coculturing with DRG on BMSC proliferation and multipotential differentiation. We found that coculturing with DRG significantly promoted BMSC proliferation and elevated their osteogenic, adipogenic, and chondrogenic differentiations. Rat GFP-BMSCs in the coculture group showed similar fibroblastic morphology to those from the control group (Figure 2(a)). However, the density of BMSCs in the coculture group was larger than that in the control group at distinct time points (day 3, day 5, and day 8) (Figure 2(a)). To assess the proliferation of the two groups, CCK8 analysis was conducted until day 10, and the BMSC proliferation curve showed that BMSC coculturing with DRG proliferated more significantly at each time point, especially at day 6 and day 8, compared with the control BMSC group (Figure 2(b)). So we chose BMSCs at coculture day 8 to analyze the effect of DRG on multiple differentiation of BMSCs. The results of alizarin red, oil red O, and alcian blue stainings showed that osteogenic, adipogenic, and

(a)

(b)

(c)

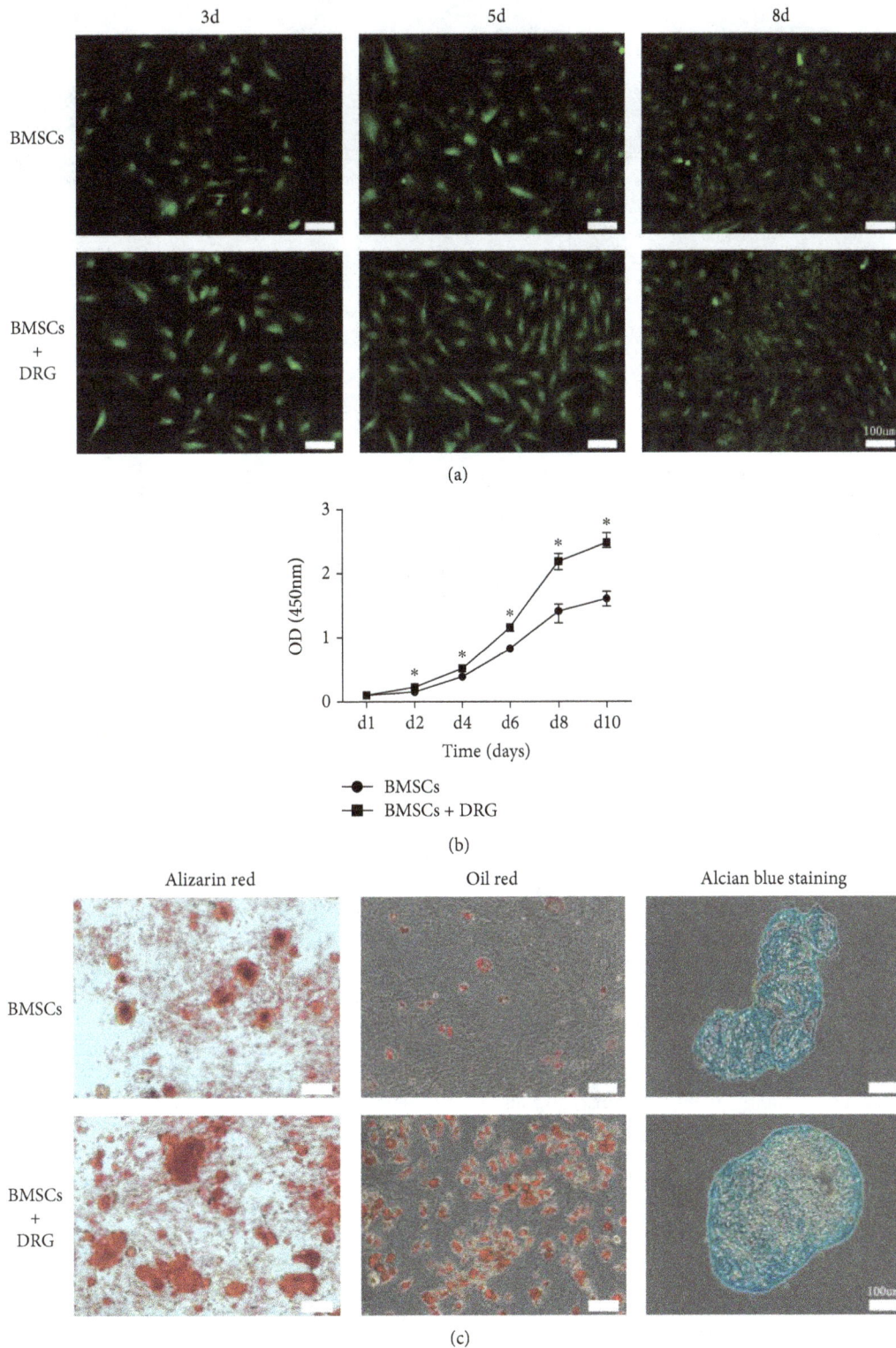

FIGURE 2: Coculturing with DRG promoted proliferation and enhanced multipotential differentiation of BMSCs. (a) Morphology and density of GFP BMSCs at days 3, 5, and 8. (b) Proliferation curves of BMSCs after coculture with DRG by the CCK8 assay. (c) Osteogenic, adipogenic, and chondrogenic differentiation of BMSCs were significantly promoted after coculture with DRG for 8 days.

chondrogenic differentiations of BMSCs were all enhanced in the DRG + BMSC group, compared with the BMSC group (Figure 2(c)). These findings suggested that coculture with DRG could not only enhance proliferation but also promote multiple differentiation of BMSCs, which hinted that coculture with DRG may have an effect on stemness of BMSCs.

(a)

(b)

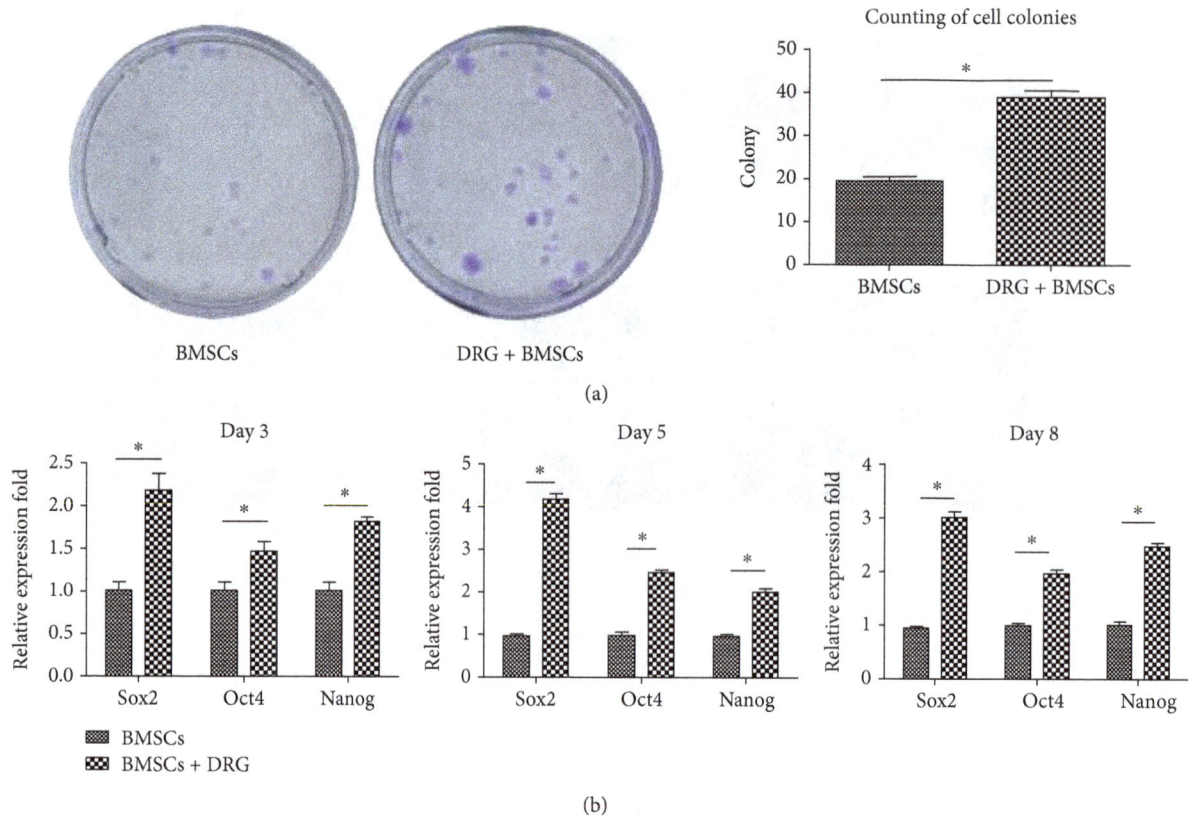

FIGURE 3: Coculturing with DRG promoted the self-renewal ability and stem cell-related gene expression of BMSCs. (a) CFU assay of the BMSCs and BMSCs + DRG groups. Purple dots refer to cell colonies. (b) Stem cell-related gene expression after coculture for 3, 5, and 8 days. ∗ denotes that differences are statistically significant between BMSCs + DRG and BMSCs groups.

3.3. Coculturing with DRG Promoted the Self-Renewal Ability and Stem Cell-Related Gene Expression of BMSCs. To investigate the effect of coculturing with DRG on stemness of BMSCs, CFU assay, which detected the self-renewal ability of BMSCs, was conducted. BMSCs at day 8 were used and cultured for 10 days. Compared with the BMSC group, more colonies were formed and the colony area was much larger in the DRG + BMSC group ($P < 0.05$, Figure 3(a)). To verify the effect of DRG on BMSC stemness, we detected the expression of stem cell-related genes, Nanog, Oct4, and Sox2, and all of them were significantly upregulated after coculture for 3, 5, and 8 days, especially at days 5 and 8 ($P < 0.05$, Figure 3(b)), which was in line with the result of BMSC proliferation. These findings indicated that coculture with DRG could maintain the stemness of BMSCs.

3.4. Coculturing with DRG Enhanced BMSC Autophagy. As was indicated by mounting evidence, autophagy plays a critical role in the stemness maintenance of stem cells. To verify whether autophagy was involved in the process of stemness maintenance of BMSCs in the coculture group, we detected the protein expression of autophagic markers LC3II and LC3I by Western blot and immunofluorescence at day 8. BMSCs in the coculture group displayed stronger LC3 fluorescence intensity than BMSCs in the control group (Figure 4(a)). The conversion of soluble LC3I to lipid-bound LC3II is an indicator of autophagosome formation,

so the LC3II/LC3I ratio means the level of autophagy activation. Western blot results showed that there was much more LC3II protein expression in the coculture group and the LC3II/LC3I ratio was predominantly larger in the coculture group than in the control group (Figure 4(b)). These results suggested that autophagy was activated in BMSCs during the process of coculture with DRG.

3.5. AMPK/mTOR Signaling Was Activated in the Coculture Group. In order to identify the mechanism of autophagy activation of BMSCs in the coculture group, we next investigated two classical signaling pathways involved in autophagy activation, including AMPK/mTOR and AKT/mTOR signaling pathways, by Western blot after coculture for 8 days. The activation of mTOR could inhibit the autophagy, and phosphorylation of AMPK inhibited the activation of mTOR, so the activation of AMPK would promote the level of autophagy. The results showed that the protein expression of p-AMPK in the coculture group was significantly upregulated compared to that in the control group, while the expression of P-AKT remained unchanged between two groups (Figure 5). These results provided evidence that autophagy activation of BMSCs in the coculture group may be mediated through AMPK/mTOR signaling but not through AKT/mTOR signaling.

3.6. Compound C Treatment Downregulated Autophagy and Stem Cell-Related Genes in the Coculture Group. To further

(a)

(b)

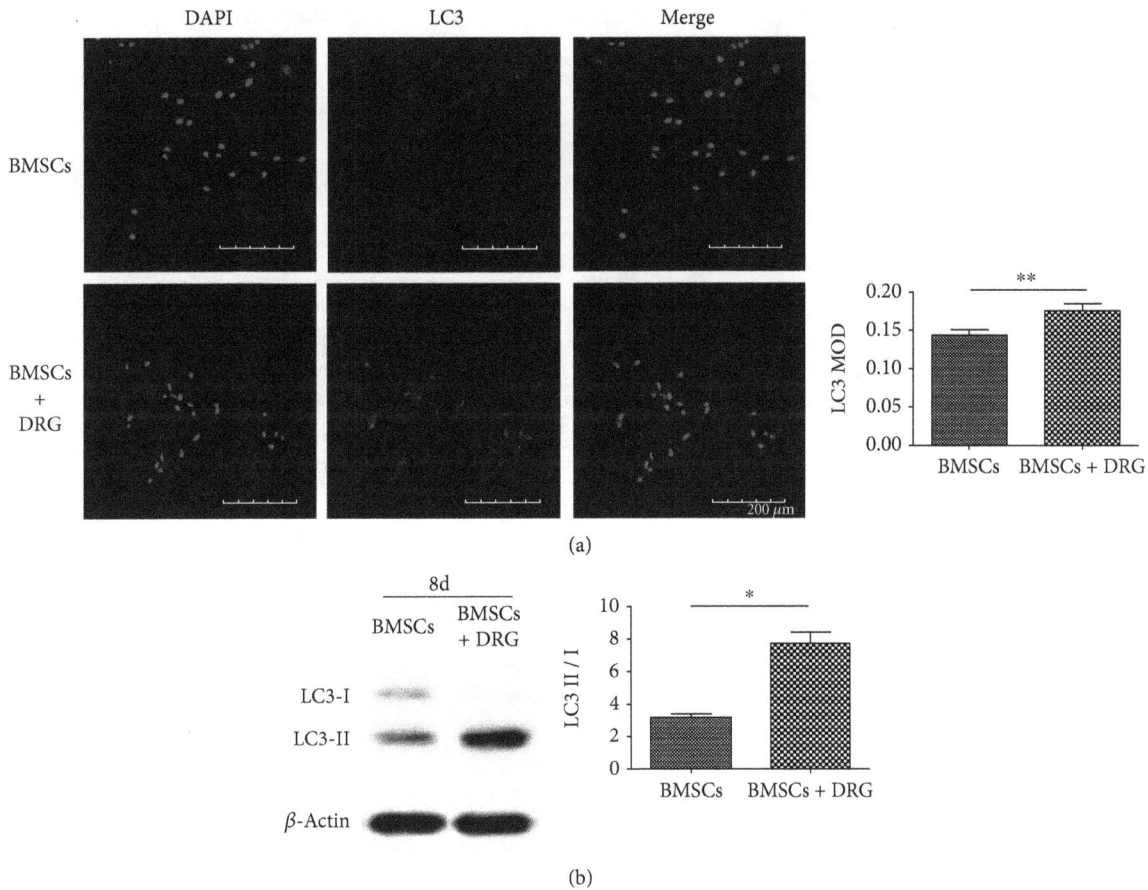

FIGURE 4: Coculturing with DRG enhanced BMSCs autophagy. (a) LC3 immunofluorescence images after coculture for 8 days. (b) Western blot analysis of LC3II and LC3I and the LC3II/LC3I ratio analysis after coculture for 8 days. MOD: mean optical density. ∗ denotes that differences are statistically significant between BMSCs + DRG and BMSCs groups.

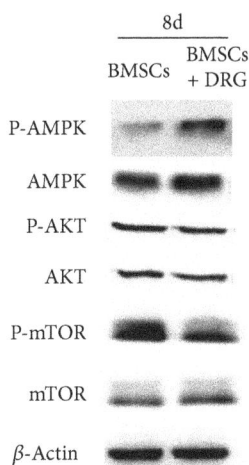

FIGURE 5: AMPK signaling pathway, not the AKT signaling pathway, was activated in BMSCs after coculture for 8 days.

confirm whether AMPK/mTOR signaling mediated the autophagy and maintenance of BMSC stemness, we treated BMSCs with compound C, an AMPK-specific inhibitor, in the coculture group. After treatment with compound C for 8 days, the protein expression of LC3II and LC3I was significantly decreased compared with the coculture group without compound C ($P < 0.05$, Figures 6(a) and 6(b)). This indicated that AMPK/mTOR signaling mediated the autophagy of BMSCs in the coculture system. Moreover, the mRNA levels of stemness genes, Sox2, Oct4, and Nanog, were predominantly downregulated, yet still higher than those of the control group ($P < 0.05$, Figure 6(c)). These data demonstrated that autophagy mediated by AMPK/mTOR signaling took an active part in BMSC stemness maintenance in the coculture group, although not the whole part, as the expression of stem cell-related genes in the coculture + compound C group was still higher than that in the control group.

To identify the factors involved in the effects of DRG-derived cells on BMSCs, DRG and BMSCs were cocultured for 8 days and then were treated with aprepitant, an NK1 receptor antagonist, for 48 h at the concentration of $50 \mu M$. Then, BMSCs were collected, and autophagy-related proteins LC3I and LC3II and stemness gene expressions in the three groups, BMSCs + DRG, BMSCs + DRG + aprepitant, and BMSCs, were detected. We found that the expression of autophagy-related proteins and the ratio of LC3II/I decreased after adding aprepitant into the coculture system (Figures 7(a) and 7(b)), but the autophagy protein expression

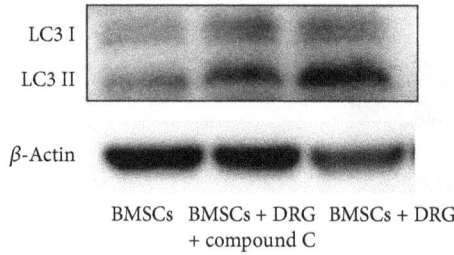

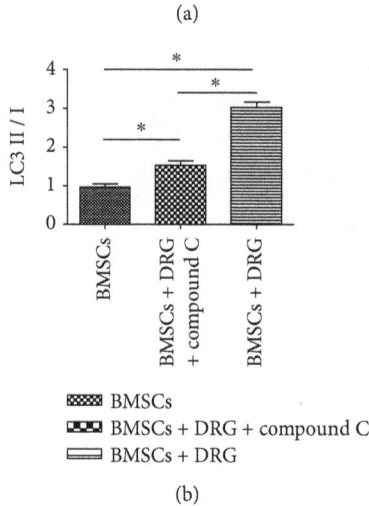

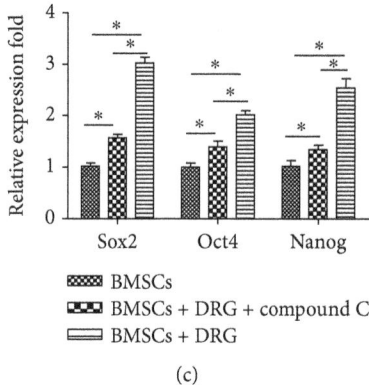

FIGURE 6: Compound C treatment downregulated autophagy and stem cell-related genes in the coculture group. (a) Western blot analysis of LC3II and LC3I after treatment with compound C. (b) Analysis of LC3II/LC3I among the three groups. (c) Stem cell-related gene expression after treatment with compound C. * denotes that differences are statistically significant between two groups. Compound C alone did not change the autophagy level or stemness genes of BMSCs (Fig S1).

FIGURE 7: Effect of aprepitant on autophagy and stemness genes in the coculture system. (a) Western blot analysis of LC3I and LC3II after treatment with aprepitant. (b) Analysis of LC3II/LC3I among the three groups. (c) Stemness gene expression after treatment with aprepitant. * denotes that differences are statistically significant between two groups.

and the ratio of LC3II/I were still higher than those of the control group (Figures 7(a) and 7(b)). Similar to the autophagy level, the stemness genes were also downregulated after treatment with aprepitant compared with the coculture group but were still higher than those of the control group (Figure 7(c)). These results showed that aprepitant could partly block the effect of DRG-derived cells on BMSCs, which indicated that substance P might play an important role in the effect of DRG-derived cells on BMSCs in the coculture system.

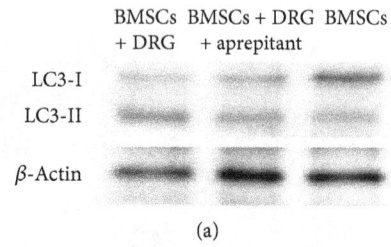

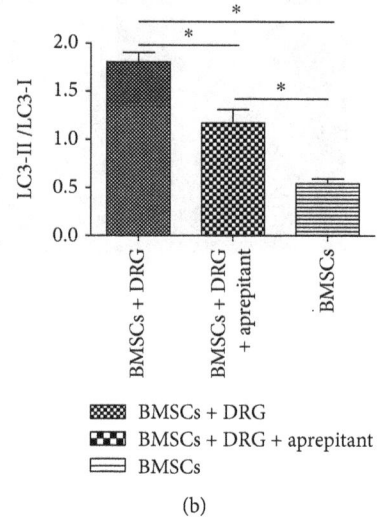

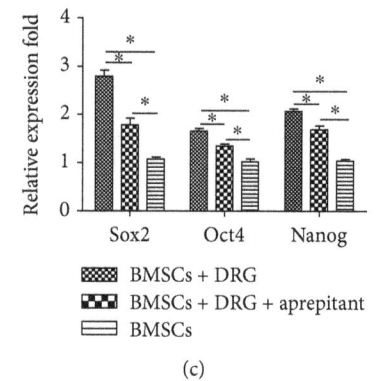

4. Discussion

A number of studies, both in vivo and in vitro, have explored the diverse roles of the sensory nerve in bone physiology [6–10]. However, the direct effect of the sensory nerve on bone cells at the cellular level and its underlying molecular mechanisms were still unclear. In order to investigate the overall effect of the sensory nerve on cell biological behavior of BMSCs, we designed a transwell coculture system between DRG and BMSCs, considering that there was no direct contact between DRG and BMSCs in the bone in vivo. We found that DRG could promote the proliferation and self-renewal ability of BMSCs. What is more, multipotential differentiation of BMSCs was more significant in the coculture group. Since the ability of self-renewal and multiple differentiation potential were two major characteristics of stem cells [23], we assumed that coculture with DRG might help keep the stemness of BMSCs. Next, we found that stem cell-related genes, Sox2, Nanog, and Oct4, were upregulated in the coculture group, which further confirmed the role of DRG in stemness maintenance of BMSCs in this coculture system.

As was reported, the stemness maintenance of stem cells had a close relationship with autophagy [24–27]. Autophagy is a process of self-degradation of cellular components in which double-membrane autophagosomes sequester organelles or portions of cytosol and fuse with lysosomes or vacuoles for breakdown by resident hydrolases [28]. The mechanism of autophagy maintaining stemness was studied in many researches. They concluded that autophagy helped maintain stemness through suppressing stem cell metabolism by clearing active, healthy mitochondria [25], clearing away toxic cellular waste [26], and preventing reactive oxygen species (ROS) accumulation [27]. In the process of autophagy, LC3 was reported to be a well-known marker of autophagosomes, and the ratio of LC3II/LC3I reflected the level of autophagy [26]. In our study, to confirm whether autophagy played a role in the maintenance of stemness of BMSCs in the coculture system, the expression of LC3 was detected and the ratio of LC3II/LC3I was analyzed. Our results proved that the basal autophagy level in the coculture group was higher than that in the control group, but we still could not conclude that the higher autophagy level resulted in the maintenance of BMSCs in this study.

Mounts of evidences have revealed the signaling regulation of autophagy [29, 30], among which AMPK/mTOR and AKT/mTOR were two most studied pathways [31–34]. So we examined the protein expression of AMPK, AKT, and mTOR at day 8 during coculture, and we found that, compared to the control group, p-AMPK was upregulated and mTOR was downregulated, while AKT was unchanged in the coculture group. Therefore, AMPK/mTOR signaling mediated the enhancing autophagy. What is more, compound C, an AMPK inhibitor [35, 36], downregulated the autophagy and stem cell-related genes in the coculture group, which demonstrated that autophagy maintained the stemness of BMSCs in the coculture group mediated by the AMPK/mTOR pathway. In addition, the stemness genes in the compound C group, although lower than those in the DRG coculture group, were still higher than those in the BMSC monoculture group, which might suggest that there existed other mechanisms of stemness maintenance in the coculture group except the enhanced autophagy.

In order to further determine the factors by which DRG acts on BMSCs, two major sensory neuropeptides, SP and CGRP, were taken into consideration. However, according to some researches, CGRP receptors exist not only in BMSCs but also in DRG and Schwann cells, and CGRP can play an important role in the function of Schwann cells and DRG [37–39]. Therefore, in the coculture system, if the CGRP receptor inhibitor is added, it would not only block the CGRP receptors of BMSCs but also block the CGRP receptors of

Schwann cells and DRG neurons, which would totally change the original system and make the results hard to analyze. Since we did not find that SP had any effect on DRG and Schwann cells, we used the NK1 receptor antagonist, aprepitant [21, 22], to explore the role of SP in this coculture system.

In several studies, the coculture system had been used to investigate the communication between neurons and other cells [16, 40–43]. It was reported that DRG could promote the proliferation of osteoblasts differentiated from BMSCs and the osteogenic gene expression under direct contact condition [40]. And the sensory neuron could regulate MC3T3-E1 cells through exocytosis of glutamate and substance P, and it was confirmed that the peptidergic neurons were involved in this process [43]. More recently, Silva et al. [41] designed a microfluidic device where only the neurites from DRG neurons reached the MSCs to study the direct effect of sensory neurons on BMSCs. They found that DRG neurons enhanced osteogenic differentiation of MSCs through the activation of the Wnt/β-catenin signaling pathway, which was proved by the upregulation of osteogenic genes and cytoplasmic accumulation and translocation into the nucleus of β-catenin in BMSCs, but DRG was found to have the ability to maintain stemness of BMSCs in the coculture system in our study. It seemed different from our results. However, the BMSCs in their studies were cultured in the presence of dexamethasone, ascorbic acid, and β-glycerol phosphate, which could induce the osteogenic differentiation themselves without other factors [44, 45], while we did not add an osteogenic inducer in our study. Also, there was no difference in osteoblast marker genes between mono- and coculture groups without the osteogenic induction medium, which meant that the effect of the DRG neuron per se was not sufficient to induce the osteoblastogenesis in vitro. They concluded that DRG could only enhance the osteogenic differentiation in the presence of the osteogenic induction medium but could not start it. This finding was in accord with our results. In our study, the mechanism of promoting osteogenesis was that transwell coculture with DRG helped maintain the stemness of BMSCs; then, the osteogenic induction medium would show a more significant effect on osteogenic differentiation.

As was reported, in vitro culture impaired the stemness of BMSCs [46, 47] and resulted in impaired self-renewal and multilineage differentiation ability, which was not good for their use as seed cells in bone tissue engineering. Besides, the mechanism of BMSC stemness maintenance was the enhancement of their basal autophagy level in our study. This suggested that the moderate enhancement of autophagy might be beneficial to the culture of stem cells in vitro, which cleared away the impaired cellular components and kept cell homeostasis [48, 49]. Moreover, the intensity of autophagy could be regulated by certain drugs, such as rapamycin [50, 51] and bafilomycin A1 [52, 53]. Since BMSCs are widely applied as seed cells in bone tissue engineering [54], our study may provide a new strategy to expand BMSCs abundantly in vitro by regulating their autophagy intensity without impairing their self-renewal and pluripotent differentiation abilities.

It should be noted that DRG cells contained both sensory neurons and Schwann cells in our experiment, although DRG explants had been shredded and digested. These two components are similar to the sensory nerve in vivo, where sensory neurites are wrapped around by the Schwann cells [55]. Therefore, the phenomenon of stemness enhancement observed in this experiment should be considered the synthetic effects of sensory neurons and Schwann cells. In another study, it was found that Schwann cells secreted extracellular vesicles to promote and maintain the proliferation and multipotency of human dental pulp cells (hDPCs), and through proteome and Western blot analysis, they detected abundant enrichment of Oct4 and TGFβs in Schwann cell-derived extracellular vesicles, which explained the upregulation of stem cell-related genes and the acceleration of proliferation in hDPCs [17]. As hDPCs showed common features with BMSCs in many aspects, this result might partly explicate the stemness enhancement of BMSCs in a coculture system containing Schwann cells in our study. At the same time, it might also explain why stemness enhancement of BMSCs still existed even after blocking autophagy with compound C in the coculture group.

In our study, we used a transwell coculture system to explore the effect of DRG on BMSCs, which mimicked the implanted sensory nerve and BMSCs in TEB. And we found that DRG could help maintain the stemness of BMSCs in vitro, in which the process of secreting substance P from DRG neurons played an important role. Based on this finding, it could be hypothesized that the sensory nerves implanted into the tissue-engineered bone enhanced the autophagy of BMSCs and helped maintain their stemness, which would keep the self-renewal and multilineage differentiation abilities of BMSCs. Therefore, BMSCs would be more ready to proliferate and differentiate into other kinds of cells, such as osteoblasts, chondrocytes, vascular endothelial cells, and even Schwann cells, under the induction condition [56–58]. These cells were all critical for bone repair and regeneration. In addition, BMSCs have powerful paracrine function, including growth factors and neurotrophic factors [59–61]. And the maintenance of stemness is important for keeping this ability. Moreover, this study presented a new perspective for understanding neuronal regulation of the bone, but it still needs further study regarding which factors, except substance P, in DRG acted on BMSCs and how they worked on BMSCs.

5. Conclusion

DRG was helpful in maintaining the stemness of BMSCs in a transwell coculture system, and this function was achieved by enhancing the autophagy level of BSMCs through AMPK/mTOR signaling, which may explain the mechanism of the sensory nerve promoting osteogenesis, and substance P plays an important role in the process.

Authors' Contributions

Liu Yang, Guoxian Pei, Chunmei Wang, and Shuaishuai Zhang designed the experiments. Shuaishuai Zhang, Junqin Li, Yi Gao, and Huijie Jiang performed the CCK8 and differentiation induction experiments. Shuaishuai Zhang, Pengzhen Cheng, Tianqing Cao, and Jimeng Wang performed the RT-PCR and Western blot experiments. Yue Song, Bin Liu, and Hao Wu performed the primary BMSC culture experiment. Shuaishuai Zhang collected the data. Liu Yang, Shuaishuai Zhang, and Junqin Li analyzed the data and generated figures. Shuaishuai Zhang, Liu Yang, and Guoxian Pei wrote and revised the manuscript.

Acknowledgments

This study was financially supported by the key project of National Natural Science Foundation of China (81430049 and 81772377).

References

[1] I. Dumic-Cule, M. Pecina, M. Jelic et al., "Biological aspects of segmental bone defects management," *International Orthopaedics*, vol. 39, no. 5, pp. 1005–1011, 2015.

[2] M. B. Nair, J. D. Kretlow, A. G. Mikos, and F. K. Kasper, "Infection and tissue engineering in segmental bone defects—a mini review," *Current Opinion in Biotechnology*, vol. 22, no. 5, pp. 721–725, 2011.

[3] S. G. Pneumaticos, G. K. Triantafyllopoulos, E. K. Basdra, and A. G. Papavassiliou, "Segmental bone defects: from cellular and molecular pathways to the development of novel biological treatments," *Journal of Cellular and Molecular Medicine*, vol. 14, no. 11, pp. 2561–2569, 2010.

[4] S. Y. Chen, J. J. Qin, L. Wang et al., "Different effects of implanting vascular bundles and sensory nerve tracts on the expression of neuropeptide receptors in tissue-engineered bone *in vivo*," *Biomedical Materials*, vol. 5, no. 5, article 055002, 2010.

[5] J. J. Fan, T. W. Mu, J. J. Qin, L. Bi, and G. X. Pei, "Different effects of implanting sensory nerve or blood vessel on the vascularization, neurotization, and osteogenesis of tissue-engineered bone in vivo," *BioMed Research International*, vol. 2014, Article ID 412570, 10 pages, 2014.

[6] S. Grässel, "The role of peripheral nerve fibers and their neurotransmitters in cartilage and bone physiology and pathophysiology," *Arthritis Research & Therapy*, vol. 16, no. 6, p. 485, 2014.

[7] T. Fukuda, S. Takeda, R. Xu et al., "Sema3A regulates bone-mass accrual through sensory innervations," *Nature*, vol. 497, no. 7450, pp. 490–493, 2013.

[8] Y. Ding, M. Arai, H. Kondo, and A. Togari, "Effects of capsaicin-induced sensory denervation on bone metabolism in adult rats," *Bone*, vol. 46, no. 6, pp. 1591–1596, 2010.

[9] E. Salisbury, E. Rodenberg, C. Sonnet et al., "Sensory nerve induced inflammation contributes to heterotopic ossification," *Journal of Cellular Biochemistry*, vol. 112, no. 10, pp. 2748–2758, 2011.

[10] S. C. Offley, T. Z. Guo, T. Wei et al., "Capsaicin-sensitive sensory neurons contribute to the maintenance of trabecular bone integrity," *Journal of Bone and Mineral Research*, vol. 20, no. 2, pp. 257–267, 2005.

[11] W. Deng, T. J. Bivalacqua, N. N. Chattergoon, J. R. Jeter Jr., and P. J. Kadowitz, "Engineering ex vivo-expanded marrow stromal cells to secrete calcitonin gene-related peptide using adenoviral vector," *Stem Cells*, vol. 22, no. 7, pp. 1279–1291, 2004.

[12] L. Wang, R. Zhao, X. Shi et al., "Substance P stimulates bone marrow stromal cell osteogenic activity, osteoclast differentiation, and resorption activity in vitro," *Bone*, vol. 45, no. 2, pp. 309–320, 2009.

[13] S. Fu, G. Mei, Z. Wang et al., "Neuropeptide substance P improves osteoblastic and angiogenic differentiation capacity of bone marrow stem cells *in vitro*," *BioMed Research International*, vol. 2014, Article ID 596023, 10 pages, 2014.

[14] E. Mrak, F. Guidobono, G. Moro, G. Fraschini, A. Rubinacci, and I. Villa, "Calcitonin gene-related peptide (CGRP) inhibits apoptosis in human osteoblasts by β-catenin stabilization," *Journal of Cellular Physiology*, vol. 225, no. 3, pp. 701–708, 2010.

[15] J. J. Cao, P. A. Singleton, S. Majumdar et al., "Hyaluronan increases RANKL expression in bone marrow stromal cells through CD44," *Journal of Bone and Mineral Research*, vol. 20, no. 1, pp. 30–40, 2005.

[16] J. M. Mehnert, T. Kisch, and M. Brandenburger, "Co-culture systems of human sweat gland derived stem cells and peripheral nerve cells: an *in vitro* approach for peripheral nerve regeneration," *Cellular Physiology and Biochemistry*, vol. 34, no. 4, pp. 1027–1037, 2014.

[17] Z. Li, Y. Liang, K. Pan et al., "Schwann cells secrete extracellular vesicles to promote and maintain the proliferation and multipotency of hDPCs," *Cell Proliferation*, vol. 50, no. 4, 2017.

[18] J. Hou, Z. P. Han, Y. Y. Jing et al., "Autophagy prevents irradiation injury and maintains stemness through decreasing ROS generation in mesenchymal stem cells," *Cell Death & Disease*, vol. 4, no. 10, article e844, 2013.

[19] A. Pedram, M. Razandi, B. Blumberg, and E. R. Levin, "Membrane and nuclear estrogen receptor α collaborate to suppress adipogenesis but not triglyceride content," *The FASEB Journal*, vol. 30, no. 1, pp. 230–240, 2016.

[20] B. Lv, F. Li, J. Han et al., "Hif-1α overexpression improves transplanted bone mesenchymal stem cells survival in rat MCAO stroke model," *Frontiers in Molecular Neuroscience*, vol. 10, p. 80, 2017.

[21] M. Muñoz, M. Rosso, M. J. Robles-Frias et al., "The NK-1 receptor is expressed in human melanoma and is involved in the antitumor action of the NK-1 receptor antagonist aprepitant on melanoma cell lines," *Laboratory Investigation*, vol. 90, no. 8, pp. 1259–1269, 2010.

[22] M. Berger, O. Neth, M. Ilmer et al., "Hepatoblastoma cells express truncated neurokinin-1 receptor and can be growth inhibited by aprepitant *in vitro* and *in vivo*," *Journal of Hepatology*, vol. 60, no. 5, pp. 985–994, 2014.

[23] A. E. Almada and A. J. Wagers, "Molecular circuitry of stem cell fate in skeletal muscle regeneration, ageing and disease," *Nature Reviews. Molecular Cell Biology*, vol. 17, no. 5, pp. 267–279, 2016.

[24] H. Pan, N. Cai, M. Li, G. H. Liu, and J. C. Izpisua Belmonte, "Autophagic control of cell 'stemness'," *EMBO Molecular Medicine*, vol. 5, no. 3, pp. 327–331, 2013.

[25] T. T. Ho, M. R. Warr, E. R. Adelman et al., "Autophagy maintains the metabolism and function of young and old stem cells," *Nature*, vol. 543, no. 7644, pp. 205–210, 2017.

[26] L. García-Prat, M. Martínez-Vicente, E. Perdiguero et al., "Autophagy maintains stemness by preventing senescence," *Nature*, vol. 529, no. 7584, pp. 37–42, 2016.

[27] H. Chen, H. A. Ge, G. B. Wu, B. Cheng, Y. Lu, and C. Jiang, "Autophagy prevents oxidative stress-induced loss of self-renewal capacity and stemness in human tendon stem cells by reducing ROS accumulation," *Cellular Physiology and Biochemistry*, vol. 39, no. 6, pp. 2227–2238, 2016.

[28] C. He and D. J. Klionsky, "Regulation mechanisms and signaling pathways of autophagy," *Annual Review of Genetics*, vol. 43, no. 1, pp. 67–93, 2009.

[29] I. Dikic, "Proteasomal and autophagic degradation systems," *Annual Review of Biochemistry*, vol. 86, no. 1, pp. 193–224, 2017.

[30] K. Cadwell, "Crosstalk between autophagy and inflammatory signalling pathways: balancing defence and homeostasis," *Nature Reviews. Immunology*, vol. 16, no. 11, pp. 661–675, 2016.

[31] R. A. Saxton and D. M. Sabatini, "mTOR signaling in growth, metabolism, and disease," *Cell*, vol. 168, no. 6, pp. 960–976, 2017.

[32] D. Garcia and R. J. Shaw, "AMPK: mechanisms of cellular energy sensing and restoration of metabolic balance," *Molecular Cell*, vol. 66, no. 6, pp. 789–800, 2017.

[33] V. B. Pillai, N. R. Sundaresan, and M. P. Gupta, "Regulation of Akt signaling by sirtuins: its implication in cardiac hypertrophy and aging," *Circulation Research*, vol. 114, no. 2, pp. 368–378, 2014.

[34] G. J. Yoshida, "Therapeutic strategies of drug repositioning targeting autophagy to induce cancer cell death: from pathophysiology to treatment," *Journal of Hematology & Oncology*, vol. 10, no. 1, p. 67, 2017.

[35] J. E. Jang, J. I. Eom, H. K. Jeung et al., "AMPK-ULK1-mediated autophagy confers resistance to BET inhibitor JQ1 in acute myeloid leukemia stem cells," *Clinical Cancer Research*, vol. 23, no. 11, pp. 2781–2794, 2017.

[36] S. Gallolu Kankanamalage, A. Y. Lee, C. Wichaidit et al., "WNK1 is an unexpected autophagy inhibitor," *Autophagy*, vol. 13, no. 5, pp. 969–970, 2017.

[37] C. C. Toth, D. Willis, J. L. Twiss et al., "Locally synthesized calcitonin gene-related peptide has a critical role in peripheral nerve regeneration," *Journal of Neuropathology and Experimental Neurology*, vol. 68, no. 3, pp. 326–337, 2009.

[38] K. R. Jessen and R. Mirsky, "The repair Schwann cell and its function in regenerating nerves," *The Journal of Physiology*, vol. 594, no. 13, pp. 3521–3531, 2016.

[39] A. M. Chung, "Calcitonin gene-related peptide (CGRP): role in peripheral nerve regeneration," *Reviews in the Neurosciences*, vol. 29, no. 4, pp. 369–376, 2018.

[40] P. X. Zhang, X. R. Jiang, L. Wang, F. M. Chen, L. Xu, and F. Huang, "Dorsal root ganglion neurons promote proliferation and osteogenic differentiation of bone marrow mesenchymal stem cells," *Neural Regeneration Research*, vol. 10, no. 1, pp. 119–123, 2015.

[41] D. I. Silva, B. P. . Santos, J. Leng, H. Oliveira, and J. Amédée, "Dorsal root ganglion neurons regulate the transcriptional

and translational programs of osteoblast differentiation in a microfluidic platform," *Cell Death & Disease*, vol. 8, no. 12, p. 3209, 2017.

[42] K. Obata, T. Furuno, M. Nakanishi, and A. Togari, "Direct neurite-osteoblastic cell communication, as demonstrated by use of an in vitro co-culture system," *FEBS Letters*, vol. 581, no. 30, pp. 5917–5922, 2007.

[43] D. Kodama, T. Hirai, H. Kondo, K. Hamamura, and A. Togari, "Bidirectional communication between sensory neurons and osteoblasts in an in vitro coculture system," *FEBS Letters*, vol. 591, no. 3, pp. 527–539, 2017.

[44] J. M. Anderson, J. B. Vines, J. L. Patterson, H. Chen, A. Javed, and H. W. Jun, "Osteogenic differentiation of human mesenchymal stem cells synergistically enhanced by biomimetic peptide amphiphiles combined with conditioned medium," *Acta Biomaterialia*, vol. 7, no. 2, pp. 675–682, 2011.

[45] E. Luzi, F. Marini, S. C. Sala, I. Tognarini, G. Galli, and M. L. Brandi, "Osteogenic differentiation of human adipose tissue-derived stem cells is modulated by the miR-26a targeting of the SMAD1 transcription factor," *Journal of Bone and Mineral Research*, vol. 23, no. 2, pp. 287–295, 2008.

[46] T. Jiang, G. Xu, Q. Wang et al., "*In vitro* expansion impaired the stemness of early passage mesenchymal stem cells for treatment of cartilage defects," *Cell Death & Disease*, vol. 8, no. 6, article e2851, 2017.

[47] Y. Shuai, L. Liao, X. Su et al., "Melatonin treatment improves mesenchymal stem cells therapy by preserving stemness during long-term *in vitro* expansion," *Theranostics*, vol. 6, no. 11, pp. 1899–1917, 2016.

[48] S. Wang, P. Xia, M. Rehm, and Z. Fan, "Autophagy and cell reprogramming," *Cellular and Molecular Life Sciences*, vol. 72, no. 9, pp. 1699–1713, 2015.

[49] L. Oliver, E. Hue, M. Priault, and F. M. Vallette, "Basal autophagy decreased during the differentiation of human adult mesenchymal stem cells," *Stem Cells and Development*, vol. 21, no. 15, pp. 2779–2788, 2012.

[50] A. Sotthibundhu, K. McDonagh, A. von Kriegsheim et al., "Rapamycin regulates autophagy and cell adhesion in induced pluripotent stem cells," *Stem Cell Research & Therapy*, vol. 7, no. 1, p. 166, 2016.

[51] H. Y. Chiu, Y. G. Tsay, and S. C. Hung, "Involvement of mTOR-autophagy in the selection of primitive mesenchymal stem cells in chitosan film 3-dimensional culture," *Scientific Reports*, vol. 7, no. 1, article 10113, 2017.

[52] A. I. Masyuk, T. V. Masyuk, M. J. Lorenzo Pisarello et al., "Cholangiocyte autophagy contributes to hepatic cystogenesis in polycystic liver disease and represents a potential therapeutic target," *Hepatology*, vol. 67, no. 3, pp. 1088–1108, 2018.

[53] S. I. Choi, K. S. Kim, J. Y. Oh, J. Y. Jin, G. H. Lee, and E. K. Kim, "Melatonin induces autophagy via an mTOR-dependent pathway and enhances clearance of mutant-TGFBIp," *Journal of Pineal Research*, vol. 54, no. 4, pp. 361–372, 2013.

[54] Z. Man, L. Yin, Z. Shao et al., "The effects of co-delivery of BMSC-affinity peptide and rhTGF-β1 from coaxial electrospun scaffolds on chondrogenic differentiation," *Biomaterials*, vol. 35, no. 19, pp. 5250–5260, 2014.

[55] M. Blais, M. Grenier, and F. Berthod, "Improvement of nerve regeneration in tissue-engineered skin enriched with schwann cells," *The Journal of Investigative Dermatology*, vol. 129, no. 12, pp. 2895–2900, 2009.

[56] S. Cai, Y. P. Tsui, K. W. Tam et al., "Directed differentiation of human bone marrow stromal cells to fate-committed Schwann cells," *Stem Cell Reports*, vol. 9, no. 4, pp. 1097–1108, 2017.

[57] J. Xue, J. Yang, D. M. O'Connor et al., "Differentiation of bone marrow stem cells into Schwann cells for the promotion of neurite outgrowth on electrospun fibers," *ACS Applied Materials & Interfaces*, vol. 9, no. 14, pp. 12299–12310, 2017.

[58] B. Movaghar, T. Tiraihi, M. Javan, T. Taheri, and H. Kazemi, "Progesterone-induced transdifferentiation of bone marrow stromal cells into Schwann cells improves sciatic nerve transection outcome in a rat model," *Journal of Neurosurgical Sciences*, vol. 61, no. 5, pp. 504–513, 2017.

[59] R. Uemura, M. Xu, N. Ahmad, and M. Ashraf, "Bone marrow stem cells prevent left ventricular remodeling of ischemic heart through paracrine signaling," *Circulation Research*, vol. 98, no. 11, pp. 1414–1421, 2006.

[60] E. Blondiaux, L. Pidial, G. Autret et al., "Bone marrow-derived mesenchymal stem cell-loaded fibrin patches act as a reservoir of paracrine factors in chronic myocardial infarction," *Journal of Tissue Engineering and Regenerative Medicine*, vol. 11, no. 12, pp. 3417–3427, 2017.

[61] G. Chen, C. K. Park, R. G. Xie, and R. R. Ji, "Intrathecal bone marrow stromal cells inhibit neuropathic pain via TGF-β secretion," *The Journal of Clinical Investigation*, vol. 125, no. 8, pp. 3226–3240, 2015.

3

Cobalt Chloride Enhances the Anti-Inflammatory Potency of Human Umbilical Cord Blood-Derived Mesenchymal Stem Cells through the ERK-HIF-1α-MicroRNA-146a-Mediated Signaling Pathway

Jihye Kwak, Soo Jin Choi, Wonil Oh, Yoon Sun Yang, Hong Bae Jeon ⓘ, and Eun Su Jeon ⓘ

Biomedical Research Institute, R&D Center, and MEDIPOST Co., Ltd., 21 Daewangpangyo-ro 644 Beon-gil, Bundang-gu, Seongnam-si, 13494 Gyeonggi-do, Republic of Korea

Correspondence should be addressed to Hong Bae Jeon; jhb@medi-post.co.kr and Eun Su Jeon; esjeon@medi-post.co.kr

Academic Editor: Andrzej Lange

Human mesenchymal stem cells (hMSCs), including human umbilical cord blood-derived mesenchymal stem cells (hUCB-MSCs), which have high proliferation capacity and immunomodulatory properties, are considered to be a good candidate for cell-based therapies. hMSCs show enhanced therapeutic effects via paracrine secretion or cell-to-cell contact that modulates inflammatory or immune reactions. Here, treatment with cobalt chloride ($CoCl_2$) was more effective than naïve hUCB-MSCs in suppressing inflammatory responses in a coculture system with phytohemagglutinin- (PHA-) activated human peripheral blood mononuclear cells (hPBMCs). Furthermore, the effect of $CoCl_2$ is exerted by promoting the expression of anti-inflammatory mediators (e.g., PGE_2) and inhibiting that of inflammatory cytokines (e.g., TNF-α and IFN-γ). Treatment of hUCB-MSCs with $CoCl_2$ leads to increased expression of microRNA- (miR-) 146a, which was reported to modulate anti-inflammatory responses. Hypoxia-inducible factor- (HIF-) 1α silencing and ERK inhibition abolished $CoCl_2$-induced miR-146a expression, suggesting that ERK and HIF-1α signals are required for $CoCl_2$-induced miR-146a expression in hUCB-MSCs. These data suggest that treatment with $CoCl_2$ enhances the immunosuppressive capacity of hUCB-MSCs through the ERK-HIF-1α-miR-146a-mediated signaling pathway. Furthermore, pretreatment of transplanted MSCs with $CoCl_2$ can suppress lung inflammation more than naïve MSCs can in a mouse model of asthma. These findings suggest that $CoCl_2$ may improve the therapeutic effects of hUCB-MSCs for the treatment of inflammatory diseases.

1. Introduction

Human mesenchymal stem cells (hMSCs), also termed as stromal cells, are isolated from a variety of tissues, including bone marrow, adipose tissue, and umbilical cord blood and are recognized as a promising therapeutic agent for clinical application because of their high proliferative capacity, multilineage differentiation potential, and immunomodulatory properties [1–3]. The release of paracrine/autocrine factors is a key mechanism of action of hMSCs [4–6]. Many studies have demonstrated that transplanted MSCs help prepare the inflammatory microenvironment by producing immunomodulatory factors that modulate the progression of inflammation [1, 2, 7]. Improvement of immunomodulating properties is expected to enhance the therapeutic effects of hMSCs. Hence, the aim of the present study was to develop a method to enhance the immunosuppression of hMSCs and clarify the therapeutic effects of modified hMSCs.

Hypoxia plays pivotal roles in the maintenance of hMSCs and is regulated by several transcriptional factors, including various hypoxia-inducible factors (HIFs) [8]. Of these, HIF-1α plays a key role in the cellular response against hypoxia by activating the transcription of various genes involved in the differentiation, colony formation, proliferation, and paracrine action of hMSCs [9]. Cobalt chloride ($CoCl_2$) is a hypoxia-mimetic compound that induces biochemical and molecular responses similar to those observed under hypoxic conditions [10]. Treatment with the hypoxia-mimetic $CoCl_2$ is used to evaluate the effect of immune responses and delineate the underlying signaling mechanisms [11]. Also, $CoCl_2$ has been shown to confer a protective effect on TNF-α/IFN-γ-induced inflammation *in vitro* [12].

In the present study, the role of $CoCl_2$ in the immunomodulation of human umbilical cord blood-derived mesenchymal stem cells (hUCB-MSCs) was examined. Treatment with $CoCl_2$ was found to increase the anti-inflammatory effects of hUCB-MSCs in a HIF-1α- and ERK-dependent manner. Furthermore, $CoCl_2$-induced microRNA- (miR-) 146a expression regulated the secretion of inflammatory cytokines, whereas anti-miR-146a abolished $CoCl_2$-induced anti-inflammatory properties of hUCB-MSCs. These results demonstrate for the first time that miR-146a is critical for the $CoCl_2$-induced anti-inflammatory properties of hUCB-MSCs.

Studies of rodent asthma models demonstrated that intravenous administration of MSCs attenuated the major pathologic features of asthma, including airway inflammation [13, 14] and remodeling, and the enhanced anti-inflammatory capacity of MSCs increased the therapeutic effect in an *in vivo* asthma model [15, 16]. Moreover, $CoCl_2$ preconditioning was shown to improve the therapeutic effects of hUCB-MSC in asthma. These results suggest that $CoCl_2$ signaling may improve the therapeutic effects of hUCB-MSCs.

2. Materials and Methods

2.1. Materials. Alpha-minimum essential medium (MEM) and fetal bovine serum (FBS) were purchased from Gibco (Carlsbad, CA, USA). Trypsin, phosphate-buffered saline (PBS), and distilled water were purchased from Biowest (Carlsbad, CA, USA). Lipofectamine™ 3000 reagent was purchased from Invitrogen Corporation (Carlsbad, CA, USA). Antibodies against phospho-ERK and ERK were obtained from Cell Signaling Technology (Beverly, MA, USA), those against HIF-1α were purchased from BD Biosciences (Oxford, UK), and those against glyceraldehyde 3-phosphate dehydrogenase (GAPDH) were obtained from Gwangju Institute of Science and Technology (Gwangju, Korea). $CoCl_2$ was purchased from Sigma-Aldrich Corporation (St. Louis, MO, USA). U0126 and peroxidase-labeled secondary antibodies were purchased from Cell Signaling Technology (Beverly, MA, USA).

2.2. Cell Culture and Treatment. hUCB-MSCs were collected from the umbilical cord vein of a newborn baby, with the consent of the mother. To isolate and expand MSCs from cord blood, mononuclear cells were removed using Ficoll–Hypaque solution ($d = 1.077 \text{ g/cm}^3$; Sigma-Aldrich Corporation) and MSCs were then seeded at 5×10^5 cells/cm^2 in culture flasks. After the formation of colonies, spindle-shaped cells were reseeded for expansion.

hUCB-MSCs were cultured in alpha-MEM supplemented with 10% FBS and gentamicin in a humidified 5% CO_2 atmosphere at 37°C. Cells were passaged to 80%–90% confluency and either used for experiments or redistributed to new culture plates. All experiments were performed with cells that were passaged 5–8 times.

To prepare $CoCl_2$ stock solution, the chemical was dissolved directly in distilled water (100 mM). The stock solutions were filter-sterilized (0.22 mm) and stored at −20°C. Cells were cultured in alpha-MEM supplemented with 10% FBS and gentamicin at 37°C under humidified 5% CO_2 atmosphere. $CoCl_2$, a chemical hypoxia-mimetic agent, was added into the medium at 100 μM, and cells were incubated in the presence of $CoCl_2$ for the indicated times and then used for further assays. In order to clarify the role of ERK1/2 in $CoCl_2$-enhanced immunosuppressive capacity of hUCB-MSCs, cells were pretreated with U0126 (ERK1/2 inhibitor) for 60 min prior to treatment with 100 μM $CoCl_2$. The effects of HIF-1α knockdown were observed by treatment with 100 μM $CoCl_2$ at 48 hr posttransfection with HIF-1α-specific siRNA.

2.3. Mixed Lymphocyte Reaction (MLR) and Enzyme-Linked Immunosorbent Assay (ELISA). Prior to the MLR process, stimulator hPBMCs and hUCB-MSCs were inactivated by treatment with 10 μg/mL mitomycin C (Sigma, St. Louis, MO) for 1 hr at 37°C. hUCB-MSCs (1×10^3 cells/well) were seeded and maintained at 37°C in a humidified incubator for 2–4 hr and then cocultured with responder peripheral blood mononuclear cells (PBMCs; 1×10^5 cells/well; All-Cells, Boston, MA, USA) and stimulator PBMCs (1×10^5 cells/well; AllCells) from different donors. Phytohemagglutinin- (PHA-) (5 μg/ml, Roche) treated PBMCs were used as the positive control. After coculturing with MSCs, PBMCs were maintained for 6 days in Roswell Park Memorial Institute 1640 medium (Gibco) supplemented with 10% FBS and gentamicin. Proliferation of PBMCs was measured using a cell proliferation BrdU (colorimetric) ELISA kit (Roche). Supernatant was collected after the MLR assay to measure levels of the immunoregulatory cytokines TNF-α, IFN-γ, and PGE$_2$ using ELISA kits (R&D Systems Inc., Minneapolis, MN, USA).

2.4. Cell Proliferation Assay. The MTS ([3-(4,5-dimethylthiazol-2-yl)-5-(3-carboxymethoxyphenyl)-2-(4-sulfophenyl)-2H-tetrazolium, inner salt]) cell proliferation assay was used to detect the effect of drug sensitivity. Briefly, hUCB-MSCs were seeded in 96-well plates and incubated at 37°C in a 5% CO_2 incubator for 24 hr. The cells were treated with various concentrations of $CoCl_2$ for 72 hr. Then, the MTS assay was performed using CellTiter 96 AQueous One Solution (Promega Corporation, Madison, WI, USA) following the manufacturer's instructions.

2.5. Western Blot Analysis. After treatment as described above, hUCB-MSCs were washed with ice-cold 1x PBS and lysed with radioimmunoprecipitation assay buffer containing protease inhibitors and phosphatase inhibitors (Roche, Basel, Switzerland). Protein concentrations were determined with the Bradford assay. Lysates were separated using Novex®, NuPAGE®, and Bolt® precast gels (Invitrogen Corporation) under denaturing conditions and transferred to nitrocellulose membranes. After blocking with 1% bovine serum albumin solution, membranes were immunoblotted with various antibodies and then probed with horseradish peroxidase-conjugated secondary antibodies. Bands were visualized with an enhanced chemiluminescence immunoblotting system (GE Healthcare Life Sciences, Chicago, IL, USA).

2.6. Transfection with Small Interference RNA (siRNA) or miR and Quantitative Real-Time PCR (RT-qPCR) Analysis. The following oligoribonucleotides for RNA interference were synthesized, desalted, and purified by ST Pharm. Co. Ltd. (Siheung, Gyeonggi, Korea): HIF-1α siRNA S5$'$-GUC CCA UGA AAA GAC UUA AdTdT-3$'$ and A5$'$-UUA AGU CUU UUC AUG GGA CdTdT-3$'$ and nonspecific control siRNA S5$'$-GGA GAA AUG GUG CGA GAA GdTdT-3$'$ and A5$'$-CUU CUC GCA CCA UUU CUC CdTdT-3$'$. For siRNA experiments, hUCB-MSCs were transfected with 100 nM HIF-1α or control siRNAs with Lipofectamine 3000 reagent (Invitrogen Corporation) according to the manufacturer's instructions. Cells were cultured in growth medium for 48 h, and the knockdown efficiency of target genes was confirmed by determining the decrease in the expression level of total HIF-1α.

Precursor miR-146a (pre-miR-146a) and antisense miR-146a (anti-miR-146a) were purchased from Ambion Inc. (Austin, TX, USA) and used for activation or inhibition of miR function, respectively. To determine the expression levels, miR was isolated using TRIzol reagent (Invitrogen Corporation) according to the manufacturer's protocol. The level of miR-146a was determined using stem loop-specific RT primer and TaqMan PCR Master Mix (Applied Biosystems, Carlsbad, CA, USA) and normalized against the level of U6 snRNA.

2.7. Flow Cytometry. For flow cytometry, single-cell suspensions were generated from 1×10^6 cells that were incubated with the indicated monoclonal antibody (mAb) at room temperature for 15 min. The following conjugated antibodies were used for the analyses: fluorescein isothiocyanate-conjugated mAbs against CD14, CD45, CD34, and HLA-DR and phycoerythrin-conjugated mAbs against CD90, CD105, CD73, and CD166 (BD Biosciences). After incubation for 15 min, cells were washed twice with Dulbecco's PBS and fixed with 1% paraformaldehyde. At least 10,000 events were measured using a fluorescence-activated cell sorting (FACS) instrument (FACSCalibur; Becton Dickinson, San Jose, CA, USA), and cell flow cytometry data were analyzed using CellQuest software (Becton Dickinson). A fluorescence histogram for each MSC marker was marked with the control antibody. The percentages of positive cells were subtracted from the isotype control antibody of each conjugate.

2.8. Generation of Asthma Model and Evaluation of Lung Inflammation. BALB/c female mice (6 weeks old) were purchased from Orient Bio Inc. (Seongnam, Korea) and acclimated for 1 week prior to beginning the experiment. To induce asthma, mice were anesthetized and then sensitized with 75 μg of ovalbumin (OVA; Sigma-Aldrich Corporation) and 10 μg of polyinosinic-polycytidylic acid [poly(I:C); Calbiochem-Merck KGaA, Darmstadt, Germany] via intranasal administration on days 0, 1, 2, 3, and 7; they were then intranasally challenged with 50 μg of OVA with 10 μg of poly(I:C) on days 14, 21, 22, and 23. To verify the treatment effect of hUCB-MSCs or CoCl$_2$-MSCs, mice were intravenously injected into the tail vein on day 15 with hUCB-MSCs or CoCl$_2$-MSCs (1×10^5 cells/100 μL/mouse). As the positive control group, several mice were administered equal volumes of PBS. All mice were sacrificed on day 24, and bronchoalveolar lavage fluid (BALF) was obtained from the left lung by lavaging three times with 1 mL of saline via trachea cannula, while the right lung was resected. Then, BALF was centrifuged, precipitated cells were resuspended in 1 mL of PBS, and the number of cells was counted under a biological microscope (Olympus Corporation, Tokyo, Japan). Isolated lungs were fixed with 4% paraformaldehyde, embedded in paraffin, and then cut into sections at a thickness of 3–4 μm, which were stained with hematoxylin and eosin.

2.9. Statistical Analysis. All statistical analyses were performed using SPSS software version 18 (SPSS Inc., Chicago, IL, USA), and data are reported as the mean ± standard deviation (SD). Differences and significance were verified by one-way analysis of variance followed by Fisher's least significant difference post hoc test. A probability (p) value of <0.05 was considered statistically significant.

3. Results

3.1. Effects of CoCl$_2$ on the Anti-Inflammatory Effects of hUCB-MSCs. To investigate the effects of CoCl$_2$ on the immunomodulatory properties of hUCB-MSCs, MLR was performed. CoCl$_2$-treated hUCB-MSCs were prepared as described in Materials and Methods. When CoCl$_2$-treated hUCB-MSCs were cocultured with allogeneic hPBMCs or PHA, the proliferation and cluster formation of T cells decreased compared with that of naïve hUCB-MSCs (Figures 1(a) and 1(b), and Supplementary Figure 1). To confirm the immunomodulatory effect, the supernatant from the MLR assay was obtained, and the production of PGE$_2$, TNF-α, and IFN-γ was confirmed with ELISA. The results showed that CoCl$_2$-treated hUCB-MSCs highly expressed the anti-inflammatory mediator PGE$_2$ (Figure 1(c)), whereas expression levels of the proinflammatory cytokines TNF-α and IFN-γ (Figures 1(d) and 1(e)) were relatively lower than those in the control group.

3.2. The Effects of CoCl$_2$ Treatment on Characterization of hUCB-MSCs. To explore whether CoCl$_2$ can induce morphological and cell viability changes, hUCB-MSCs were treated with CoCl$_2$. As shown in Figures 2(a) and 2(b), treatment with CoCl$_2$ had no effect on the morphology or viability of hUCB-MSCs. FACS analysis showed that CoCl$_2$-treated hUCB-MSCs expressed the MSC-specific markers CD90,

(a)

(b)

(c)

(d)

(e)

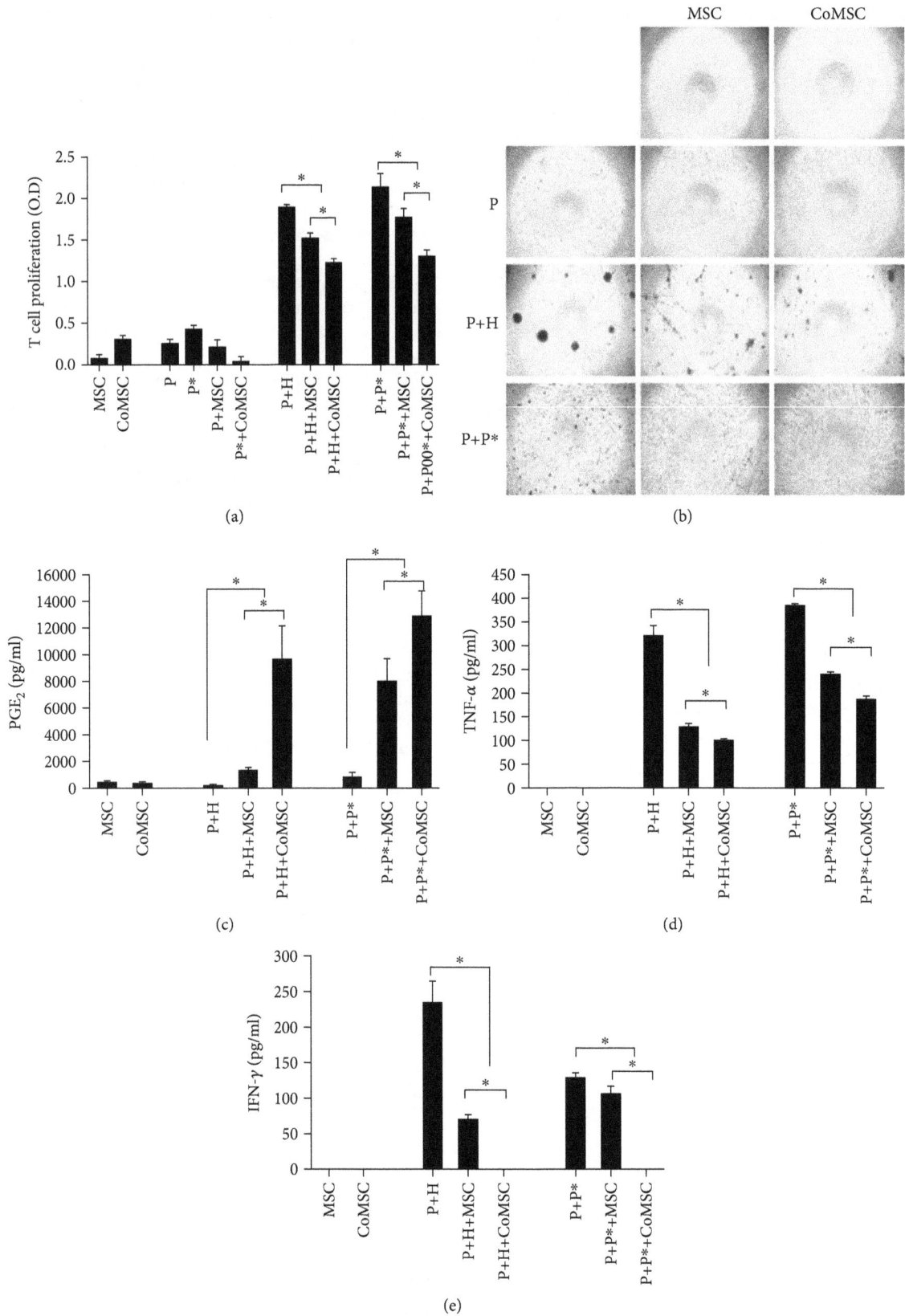

FIGURE 1: Cobalt chloride (CoCl$_2$) stimulates the immunomodulation of human umbilical cord blood-derived mesenchymal stem cells (hUCB-MSCs). (a and b) The immunogenicity of hUCB-MSCs was assessed using the MLR assay. Allogeneic hPBMCs were cocultured with hUCB-MSCs. The proliferation of responding cells was assessed using the MLR assay. PGE$_2$ (c), TNF-α (d), and IFN-γ (e) levels in the MLR culture supernatants were measured by ELISA. Data represent the mean $\pm$ SD, $n = 3$; $^*p < 0.05$. P: hPBMCs; P*: allogeneic hPBMCs as stimulator; H: phytohemagglutinin; MSC: naïve hUCB-MSCs; CoMSC: CoCl$_2$-pretreated hUCB-MSCs.

(a)

(b)

	CD14	CD45	CD34	HLR-DR	CD90	CD105	CD166	CD73
MSC	0.3 ± 0.1	0.1 ± 0.0	0.1 ± 0.0	0.1 ± 0.1	88.5 ± 2.9	98.6 ± 1.2	94.2 ± 1.4	98.0 ± 0.8
CoMSC	0.3 ± 0.1	0.0 ± 0.0	0.1 ± 0.0	0.1 ± 0.0	88.7 ± 2.9	99.9 ± 0.0	95.6 ± 1.5	98.8 ± 0.5

(c)

(d)

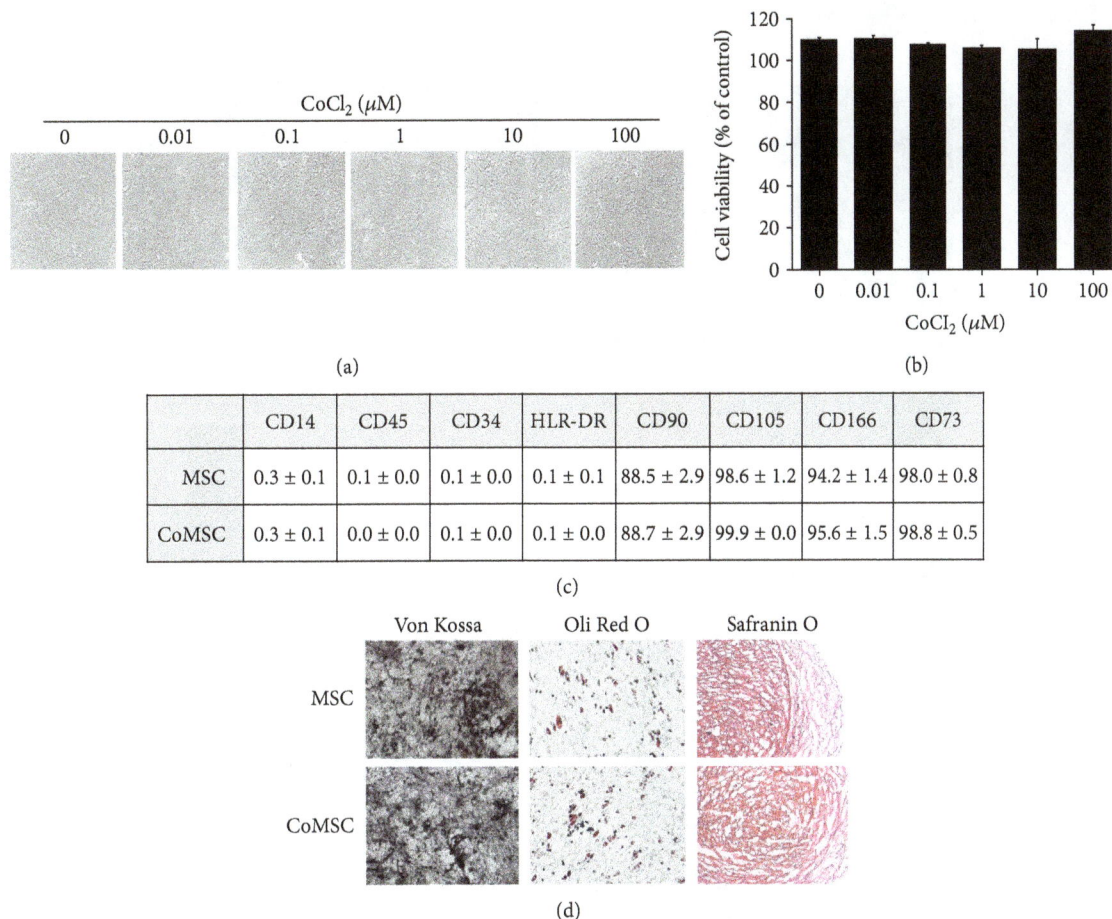

FIGURE 2: Effects of cobalt chloride ($CoCl_2$) on the characterization of hUCB-MSCs. (a and b) The morphology and growth curve of cultured hUCB-MSCs were analyzed. hUCB-MSCs were treated with the indicated concentrations of $CoCl_2$ for 72 hr. Phase-contrast image of hUCB-MSCs were obtained with an inverted microscope equipped with a digital camera. Cell viability was determined with the MTS assay. (c) The immunophenotypic characteristics of naïve hUCB-MSCs and $CoCl_2$-treated hUCB-MSCs were examined by flow cytometry. (d) During incubation in specialized induction media, multilineage differentiation was measured by staining for typical lineage markers. Osteogenic, adipogenic, and chondrogenic lineages were measured by staining for von Kossa, Oil Red O, or safranin O, respectively. Data represent the mean ± SD, $n = 3$. MSC: naïve hUCB-MSCs; CoMSC: $CoCl_2$-pretreated hUCB-MSCs.

CD105, CD166, and CD73, but not CD14, CD45, CD34, and HLA-DR (Figure 2(c) and Supplementary Figure 2). Next, the effects of $CoCl_2$ treatment on the multilineage differentiation of hUCB-MSCs were investigated. MSCs can differentiate into osteoblast, adipocytes, and chondrocytes when cultured in defined media specific for induction of the respective cell types. Osteogenesis was associated with the presence of calcium deposits as shown by von Kossa staining. Adipogenesis was observed by staining of cytoplasmic lipid vacuoles with Oil Red O. Chondrogenesis was observed by an increase in proteoglycans and was demonstrated by safranin O staining (Figure 2(d)). Pretreatment with $CoCl_2$ can successfully differentiate hUCB-MSCs into multiple cell types, including osteoblasts and adipocytes, and chondrocytes. These results suggest that $CoCl_2$ treatment had no influence on the characterization of hUCB-MSCs.

3.3. miR-146a Controls the CoCl_2-Induced Anti-Inflammatory Effects of hUCB-MSCs. Regulation of inflammatory responses

in a disease state is mediated by coordinated control of gene expression via modulation by miRs. To identify potential miR targets, an miR expression profiling experiment was conducted using two cell populations: hMSCs and coculture of hPBMCs with hMSCs (hPBMC + hMSC). miR microarray analysis of these two cell populations was performed using Affymetrix GeneChip miR microarrays (Affymetrix, Santa Clara, CA, USA). The results showed that 21 miRs were significantly upregulated and 28 were significantly downregulated in hPBMC + hMSC compared with those in hMSCs. In particular, miR-146a was upregulated by approximately 53-fold in hPBMC + hMSC (Figure 3(a), Tables 1 and 2). To determine if miRs are involved in $CoCl_2$-induced anti-inflammation, hUCB-MSCs were treated with $CoCl_2$ and the expression of miR-146a was determined by RT-qPCR. As shown in Figure 3(b), miR-146a was significantly upregulated in $CoCl_2$-treated hUCB-MSCs. To determine whether miR-146a expression is critical for $CoCl_2$-induced anti-inflammation, hUCB-MSCs were transfected with control siRNA, pre-miR-146a, or anti-miR-146a (Figure 3(c)), followed by

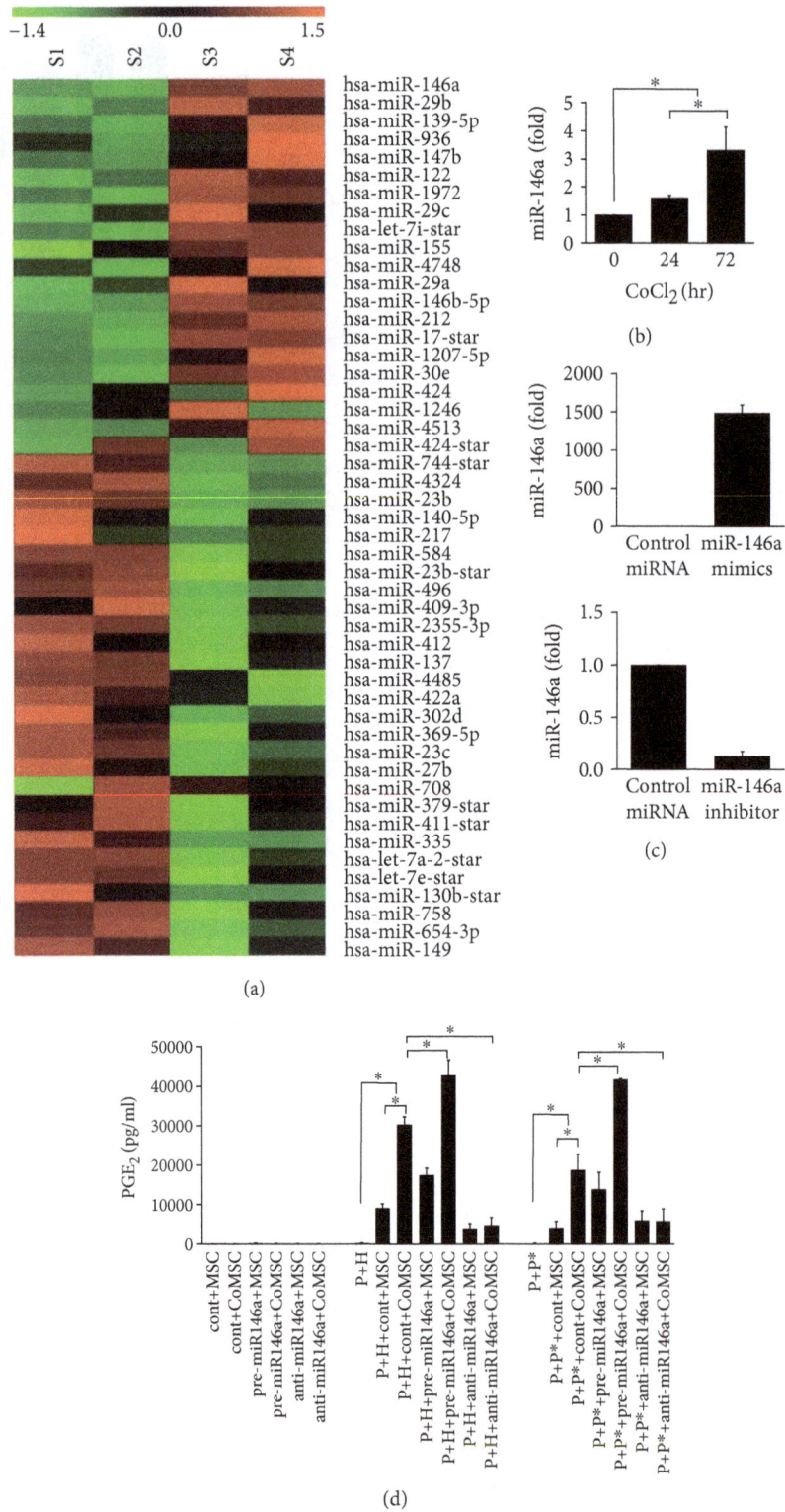

(a)

(b)

(c)

(d)

FIGURE 3: Continued.

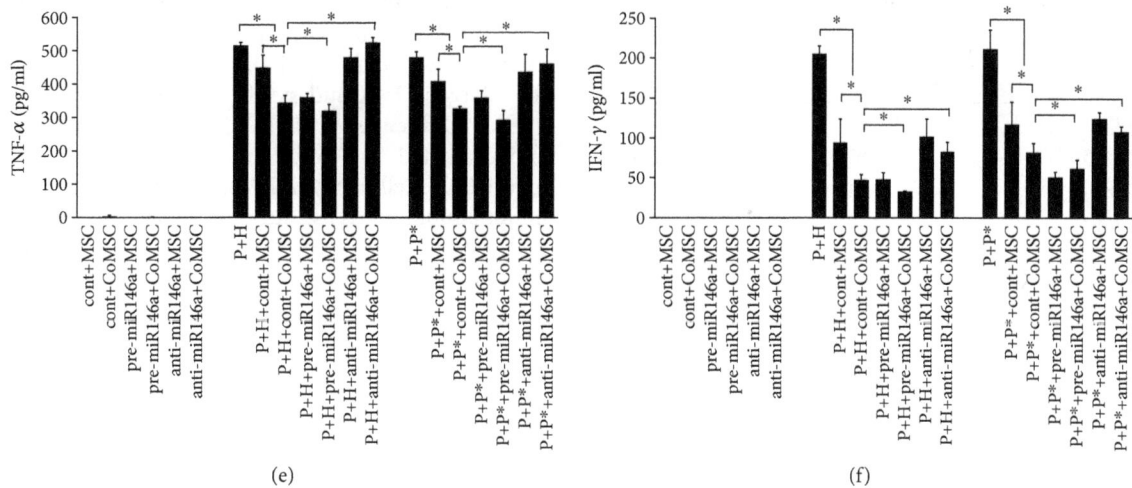

(e)　　　　　　　　　　　　　　　　　　　(f)

FIGURE 3: Cobalt chloride- ($CoCl_2$-) induced expression of miR-146a in immunomodulation of hUCB-MSCs. (a) hUCB-MSCs (S1–2) and coculture of hPBMCs with hUCB-MSCs (hPBMC + hMSC, S3–4) were collected for microRNA (miR) microarray analysis. Normalized log2 miRNA expression for miRNAs that showed significant differences ($p < 0.05$) between groups is listed according to the color scale. (b) hUCB-MSCs were treated with $100\,\mu M$ $CoCl_2$ and then harvested at the indicated times. The expression level of miR-146a was determined by RT-qPCR. (c) hUCB-MSCs were transfected with scrambled miR-control, miR-146a mimics, or inhibitors. The expression level of miR-146a was determined by RT-qPCR. (d–f) hUCB-MSCs were transfected with scrambled miR-control, miR-146a mimics, or inhibitors and exposed to $100\,\mu M$ $CoCl_2$ for 72 h, and then allogeneic hPBMCs were cocultured with hUCB-MSCs. PGE_2, TNF-α, and IFN-γ levels in the culture supernatants were measured by ELISA. Data represent the mean ± SD, $n = 3$; $^*p < 0.05$. P: hPBMCs; P*: allogeneic hPBMCs as stimulator; H: phytohemagglutinin; MSC: naïve hUCB-MSCs; CoMSC: $CoCl_2$-pretreated hUCB-MSCs.

TABLE 1: List of upregulated miRNAs (>2-fold).

miRNA	Upregulated Fold change	p value
hsa-miR-146a	53.58	0.0003
hsa-miR-29b	9.76	0.007
hsa-miR-139-5p	6.79	0.011
hsa-miR-936	4.61	0.065
hsa-miR-147b	4.54	0.143
hsa-miR-122	4.13	0.012
hsa-miR-1972	3.68	0.053
hsa-miR-29c	3.37	0.036
hsa-let-7i*	3.16	0.005
hsa-miR-155	3.10	0.053
hsa-miR-4748	2.79	0.030
hsa-miR-29a	2.74	0.039
hsa-miR-146b-5p	2.73	0.003
hsa-miR-212	2.72	0.103
hsa-miR-17*	2.46	0.002
hsa-miR-1207-5p	2.42	0.015
hsa-miR-30e	2.41	0.038
hsa-miR-424	2.31	0.139
hsa-miR-1246	2.28	0.361
hsa-miR-4513	2.08	0.015
hsa-miR-424*	2.05	0.279

treatment with $CoCl_2$ for 72 hr. As previously shown, expression of an anti-inflammatory mediator, such as PGE_2, increased, whereas that of proinflammatory factors TNF-α and IFN-α decreased in $CoCl_2$-treated hUCB-MSCs. However, as shown in Figures 3(d)–3(f), $CoCl_2$-regulated expression levels of these factors significantly changed in anti-miR-146a-transfected hUCB-MSCs. Furthermore, hUCB-MSCs transfected with pre-miR-146a showed increased expression of PGE_2 and decreased expression of TNF-α and IFN-γ.

3.4. $CoCl_2$ Increased the Expression of miR-146a through ERK-HIF-1α-Dependent Signals.
It is well known that $CoCl_2$ is able towards transcriptional factor HIF-1 (HIF-1) activation by hypoxia [17]. Moreover, it has been reported that hypoxia condition induces the activation of the ERK pathway, which is involved in HIF-1α expression [18]. To explore whether $CoCl_2$ induced ERK phosphorylation and HIF-1α expression, hUCB-MSCs were treated with $100\,\mu M$ $CoCl_2$ for the indicated time periods. As shown in Figure 4(a), hUCB-MSC increased the expression of HIF-1α in a time-dependent manner upon treatment of $100\,\mu M$ $CoCl_2$ and reached the maximum level at 3 hr, and ERK phosphorylation was time-dependent and occurred rather early. Therefore, we next examined the effects of HIF-1α knockdown by treatment of hUCB-MSCs with siRNA, followed by culture under $CoCl_2$-treated conditions. The silencing of HIF-1α significantly inhibited $CoCl_2$-induced HIF-1α expression (Figure 4(b)), as well as regulation of PGE_2, TNF-α, and IFN-γ secretion (Supplementary Figure 3). As shown in Figure 4(c), pretreatment with U0126 prevented $CoCl_2$-induced ERK phosphorylation. In addition, to determine

TABLE 2: List of downregulated miRNAs (>2-fold).

miRNA	Downregulated Fold change	p value
hsa-miR-149	6.06	0.011
hsa-miR-654-3p	3.52	0.003
hsa-miR-758	3.41	0.018
hsa-miR-130b*	3.40	0.022
hsa-let-7e*	3.37	0.028
hsa-let-7a-2*	3.30	0.004
hsa-miR-355	3.21	0.027
hsa-miR-411*	3.14	0.016
hsa-miR-379*	3.00	0.047
hsa-miR-708	3.00	0.721
hsa-miR-27b	2.77	0.015
hsa-miR-23c	2.70	0.004
hsa-miR-369-5p	2.60	0.030
hsa-miR-302d	2.52	0.468
hsa-miR-422a	2.45	0.074
hsa-miR-4485	2.45	0.065
hsa-miR-137	2.41	0.019
hsa-miR-412	2.38	0.049
hsa-miR-2355-3p	2.26	0.004
hsa-miR-409-3p	2.22	0.033
hsa-miR-496	2.20	0.049
hsa-miR-23b*	2.19	0.022
hsa-miR-584	2.15	0.003
hsa-miR-217	2.12	0.089
hsa-miR-140-5p	2.09	0.058
hsa-miR-23b	2.07	0.000
hsa-miR-4324	2.05	0.026
hsa-miR-744*	2.01	0.004

whether the ERK pathway also affects HIF-1α, pretreatment with U0126 significantly inhibited CoCl$_2$-induced HIF-1α expression. By contrast, the CoCl$_2$-induced ERK phosphorylation was not changed by silencing of HIF-1α (Figure 4(b)). Also, CoCl$_2$-induced immunomodulation of hUCB-MSCs, such as the regulation of PGE$_2$, TNF-α, and IFN-γ secretion, was blocked by U0126 (Supplementary Figure 4). To elucidate the underlying mechanism, the role of ERK and HIF-1α signaling in CoCl$_2$-induced miR-146a expression was investigated. The treatment of hUCB-MSCs with CoCl$_2$ increased miR-146a expression, which was significantly inhibited by silencing of HIF-1α (Figure 4(d)) and U0126 (Figure 4(e)). As summarized in Figure 4(f), these results suggested that miR-146a plays a critical role in CoCl$_2$-induced anti-inflammatory effects through the ERK- and HIF-1α-dependent signaling pathway.

3.5. CoCl$_2$ Enhanced the Therapeutic Effects of hUCB-MSCs for the Treatment of Inflammatory Disease. As intravenously injected MSCs are retained for a short period in the lungs, where they exert anti-inflammatory effects, a well-established mouse model of asthma was used to compare the effects of naïve MSCs and CoCl$_2$-treated MSCs. Six-week-old wild-type BalB/C mice were sensitized with the allergen OVA and synthetic dsRNA [poly(I:C)], subsequently challenged with OVA and poly(I:C) for 10 days, and evaluated 24 h after the final challenge, as shown in Figure 5(a). Cellularity in BALF showed that lung infiltration of inflammatory cells, such as macrophages, neutrophils, and lymphocytes, strongly decreased in the CoCl$_2$-MSC-injected mice compared with the naïve MSC-injected mice (Figure 5(b) and Supplementary Figure 5). The inhibitory effects of hMSC administration were also evident histologically, as lung tissue sections from CoCl$_2$-hMSC-treated mice showed greater reduction in inflammatory cells in the airway tissues compared with naïve MSCs (Figure 5(c)).

4. Discussion

Various source-derived MSCs have the ability to modulate the regenerative environment via anti-inflammatory and immunomodulatory mechanisms and are therefore considered to be a good candidate for cell-based therapies. Although adult bone marrow (BM) and adipose tissue (AT) are main source of MSCs for clinical use, they are limited because of the stringent requirements for autologous donors. hUCB-MSCs have a higher rate of cell proliferation, lower senescence, and more extensive anti-inflammatory effects than BM-MSCs and AT-MSCs, along with accessibility, making hUCB-MSCs more suitable than other MSCs for clinical applications [19].

Prostaglandin E$_2$ (PGE$_2$) plays a key role in association of anti-inflammation and immune suppression via EP$_4$ receptor activation [20]. PGE$_2$ produced by MSCs exerts anti-inflammatory effects through the regulation of immune cell activation and maturation [21]. The results of the present study demonstrated that pretreatment with CoCl$_2$ significantly increased the anti-inflammatory potency of hUCB-MSCs, as evidenced by the increased expression of the anti-inflammatory mediator PGE$_2$ and decreased expression of the proinflammatory factors TNF-α and INF-γ. CoCl$_2$ is a hypoxia-mimetic compound that activates HIF-1α and other signaling pathways [10, 17]. Furthermore, siRNA-mediated knockdown of HIF-1α attenuated the CoCl$_2$-induced anti-inflammatory effects.

Mitogen-activated protein kinases (MAPKs) play an important role in numerous cellular processes, which are regulated by various extracellular stimuli, such as cytokines, stress, and growth factors [22]. The results of the present study also showed that CoCl$_2$-induced HIF-1α expression required activation of ERK. Also, CoCl$_2$-induced secretion of anti-inflammatory cytokines was prevented by pretreatment of hUCB-MSCs with the ERK inhibitor U0126, indicating the involvement of ERK in CoCl$_2$-induced anti-inflammatory effects.

miRs are small, single-stranded RNA molecules of 21–23 nucleotides in length that fully or partially bind to their target mRNA and posttranscriptionally regulate the expression of target genes by inducing decay of target mRNA or suppressing translation. Recently, miRs have been found to be an

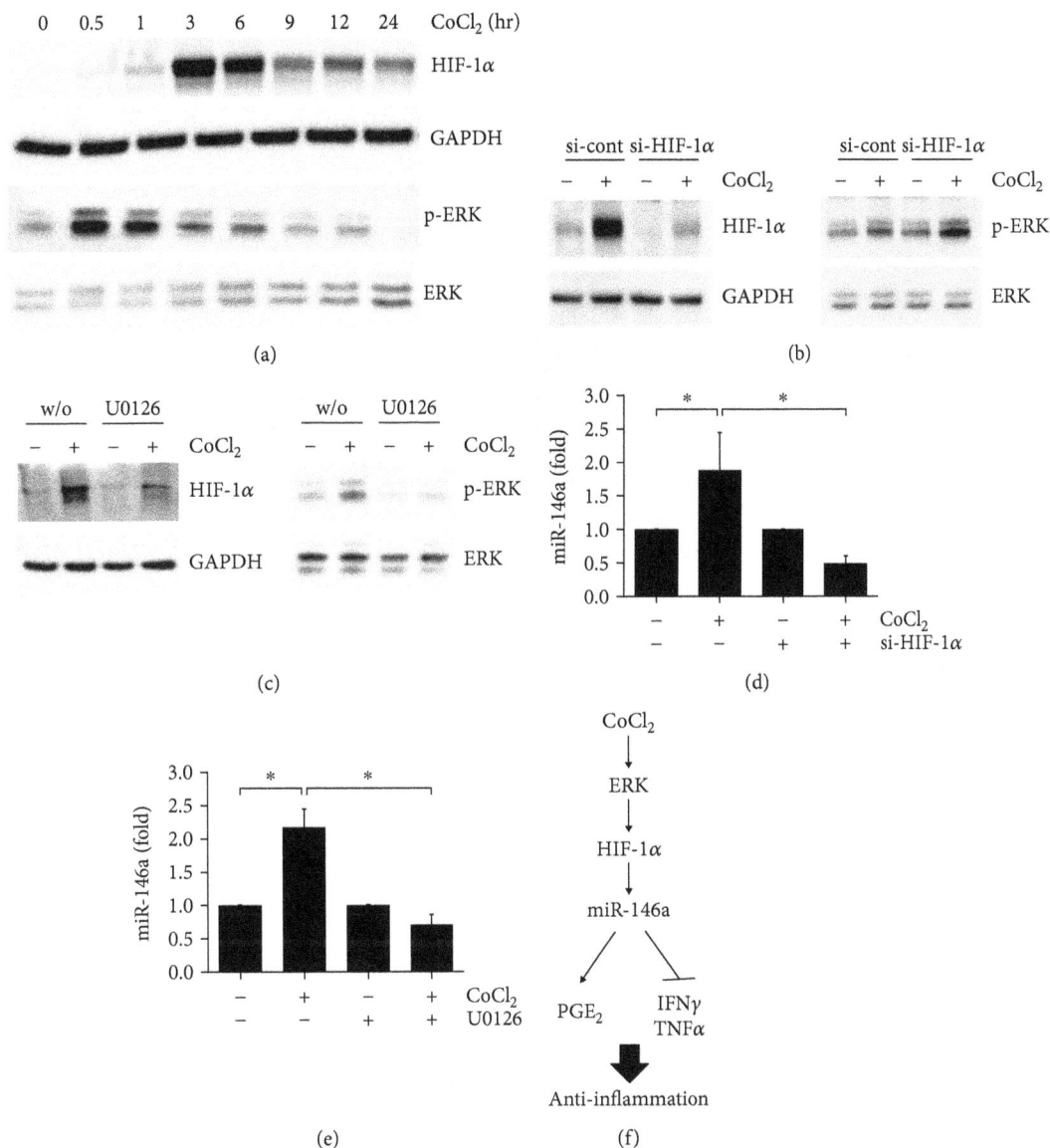

FIGURE 4: Cobalt chloride ($CoCl_2$) stimulates the immunomodulation of hUCB-MSCs through an ERK- and HIF-1α-dependent pathway. (a) hMSCs were treated with 100 μM $CoCl_2$ and then harvested at the indicated times. The protein level of HIF-1α and p-ERK was determined by Western blot analysis. (b) At 48 hr posttransfection with control siRNA (CTRL) or HIF-1α-specific siRNA (si-HIF-1α), hUCB-MSCs were treated with 100 μM $CoCl_2$ for 30 min or 3 hr. (c) hUCB-MSCs were treated with 100 μM $CoCl_2$ for 30 min or 3 hr in the absence or presence of 10 μM U0126. ERK phosphorylation and HIF-1α expression were determined by Western blot analysis. (d) hUCB-MSCs were transfected with control siRNA (si-control) or HIF-1α siRNA (si-HIF-1α) and then treated with 100 μM $CoCl_2$ for 72 h. (e) hUCB-MSCs were pretreated with the vehicle control (DMSO) or the ERK-specific inhibitor 10 μM U0126 for 60 min and then treated with 100 μM $CoCl_2$ for 72 h. The expression level of miR-146a was determined by RT-qPCR. (f) Schematic illustration of the molecular mechanisms involved in the $CoCl_2$-enhanced anti-inflammatory effects. Data represent the mean $\pm$ SD, $n = 3$; $^*p < 0.05$. P: hPBMCs; P*: allogeneic hPBMCs as stimulator; H: phytohemagglutinin; MSC: naïve hUCB-MSCs; CoMSC: $CoCl_2$-pretreated hUCB-MSCs.

important beneficial mechanism in the immune microenvironment. For example, the macrophage inflammatory response to infection involves the upregulation of several miRs, such as miR-155, miR-146, miR-147, miR-21, and miR-9. It has been reported that the induction of miR-29 suppresses host immune response by targeting IFN-γ. Furthermore, miRs have a strong impact on the immunomodulatory activity of MSCs [23–25].

Additional studies are warranted to dissect the effect of specific miRs on the regulatory function of MSC. We

hypothesized that miRs could control the inflammation processes of hUCB-MSCs. To examine this possibility, the potential of miR to regulate hUCB-MSCs in an inflammatory environment was analyzed using the miR array, which revealed altered expression of more than 49 miRs between populations of hUCB-MSCs and hPBMCs + hUCB-MSCs.

The miR-146 family is composed of two members: miR-146a and miR-146b. The roles of miR-146 in the suppression of inflammatory cytokine secretion and negative regulation of inflammation induced via the innate immune response

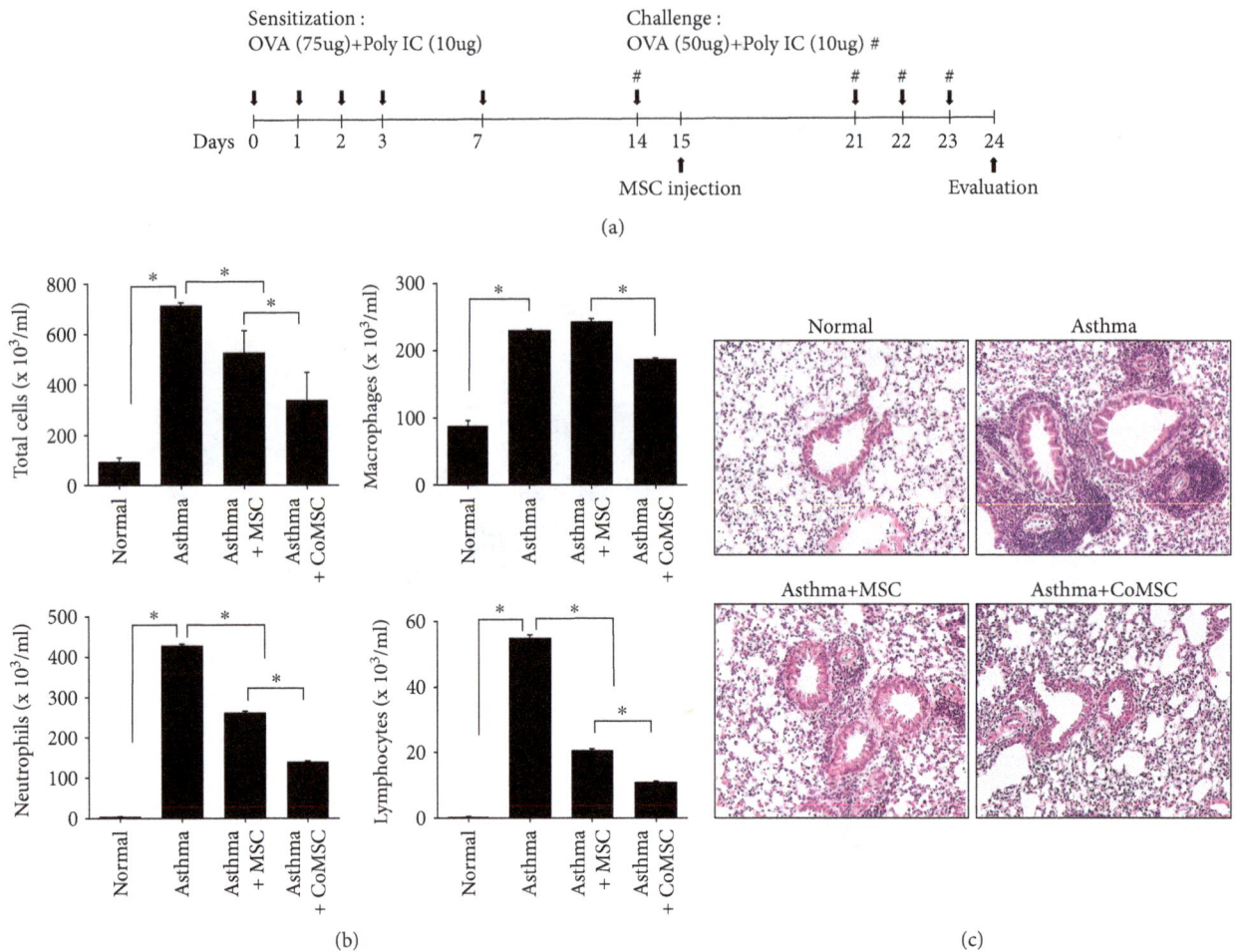

FIGURE 5: Administration of cobalt chloride- ($CoCl_2$-) treated hUCB-MSCs inhibited airway inflammation in a mouse model of asthma. (a) Schematic of the experimental studies. (b) BALF cell differentials in naïve hUCB-MSCs, $CoCl_2$-treated hUCB-MSCs, and PBS-treated asthma mouse models. (c) Representative photomicrographs stained with hematoxylin and eosin depicting histologic inflammation on day 24 for asthma models are depicted for each experimental condition. $^*p < 0.05$. MSC: naïve hUCB-MSCs; CoMSC: $CoCl_2$-pretreated hUCB-MSCs.

have been demonstrated [25–28]. Interestingly, treatment with $CoCl_2$ induced miR-146a expression in hUCB-MSCs, which suppressed the expression of inflammatory factors. Furthermore, overexpression of pre-miR-146a induced the anti-inflammatory potency of hUCB-MSCs. These findings demonstrated that miR-146a creates an anti-inflammatory environment and is required for the effect of $CoCl_2$. Furthermore, MAPKs were shown to positively regulate miR-146a expression, and $CoCl_2$-induced activation of ERK had a significant effect on miR-146a induction in hUCB-MSCs. These results indicate that $CoCl_2$ treatment induces anti-inflammation through ERK-HIF-1α-miR-146a expression in hUCB-MSCs. Although further studies are necessary to elucidate the mechanisms underlying this process, these findings indicate that miR-146a is a novel target of $CoCl_2$ and a key regulator of the $CoCl_2$-enhanced anti-inflammatory potency of hUCB-MSCs. These findings present clues to further understand the immunomodulation role of miR-146a in hUCB-MSCs, and activators of miR-146a expression may be used to develop anti-inflammatory therapeutics. In addition, pretreatment with $CoCl_2$ had no significant effect on the stem

cell properties of hUCB-MSCs, such as morphology, growth, stem cell marker expression, and differentiation abilities. $CoCl_2$ preconditioning enhanced the anti-inflammatory capacity and improved the therapeutic effects of hUCB-MSCs compared with naïve MSCs in an *in vivo* asthma model. These results suggest that $CoCl_2$ signaling may improve the therapeutic effects of hUCB-MSCs, which may be a very useful model for the clinical application of allogeneic cell therapies.

5. Conclusions

In conclusion, we demonstrated that the treatment with $CoCl_2$ enhanced the anti-inflammatory property of hUCB-MSCs through ERK-HIF-1α-dependent miR-146a expression. $CoCl_2$-induced high potency MSCs showed therapeutic effects more than naïve MSCs in the asthma models. These findings suggest that pretreatment of hUCB-MSCs with $CoCl_2$ improves the therapeutic effects of MSCs for the clinical application of allogeneic cell therapies.

Acknowledgments

This research was cosupported by the Global High-tech Biomedicine Technology Development Program of the National Research Foundation (NRF) and Korea Health Industry Development Institute (KHIDI) funded by the Korean Government (Ministry of Science, ICT and Future Planning and Ministry of Health and Welfare) (2015M3D6A1065098) and by the Korean Health Technology R&D Project of Korea Health Industry Development Institute funded by the Ministry of Health and Welfare (HI12C1821).

Supplementary Materials

Figure 1: dose and time dependency of $CoCl_2$ treatment in the immunogenicity of hUCB-MSCs using the MLR assay. Supplementary Figure 2: flow cytometry analysis of naïve human umbilical cord blood-derived hUCB-MSCs and $CoCl_2$-treated hUCB-MSCs. Supplementary Figure 3: the role of HIF-1α in $CoCl_2$-induced immunomodulation of hUCB-MSCs such as PGE_2, TNF-α, and IFN-γ regulation. Supplementary Figure 4: the role of ERK in $CoCl_2$-induced immunomodulation of hUCB-MSCs such as PGE_2, TNF-α, and IFN-γ regulation. Supplementary Figure 5: BALF cell differentials in naïve hUCB-MSCs, $CoCl_2$-treated hUCB-MSCs, and PBS-treated asthma mouse models. Data are presented as the percent of the total cell count. *(Supplementary Materials)*

References

[1] S. Aggarwal and M. F. Pittenger, "Human mesenchymal stem cells modulate allogeneic immune cell responses," *Blood*, vol. 105, no. 4, pp. 1815–1822, 2005.

[2] S. Ma, N. Xie, W. Li, B. Yuan, Y. Shi, and Y. Wang, "Immunobiology of mesenchymal stem cells," *Cell Death and Differentiation*, vol. 21, no. 2, pp. 216–225, 2014.

[3] M. Lee, S. Y. Jeong, J. Ha et al., "Low immunogenicity of allogeneic human umbilical cord blood-derived mesenchymal stem cells in vitro and in vivo," *Biochemical and Biophysical Research Communications*, vol. 446, no. 4, pp. 983–989, 2014.

[4] S. Y. Jeong, J. Ha, M. Lee et al., "Autocrine action of thrombospondin-2 determines the chondrogenic differentiation potential and suppresses hypertrophic maturation of human umbilical cord blood-derived mesenchymal stem cells," *Stem Cells*, vol. 33, no. 11, pp. 3291–3303, 2015.

[5] D. H. Kim, D. Lee, E. H. Chang et al., "GDF-15 secreted from human umbilical cord blood mesenchymal stem cells delivered through the cerebrospinal fluid promotes hippocampal neurogenesis and synaptic activity in an Alzheimer's disease model," *Stem Cells and Development*, vol. 24, no. 20, pp. 2378–2390, 2015.

[6] E. S. Kim, H. B. Jeon, H. Lim et al., "Conditioned media from human umbilical cord blood-derived mesenchymal stem cells inhibits melanogenesis by promoting proteasomal degradation of MITF," *PLoS One*, vol. 10, no. 5, article e0128078, 2015.

[7] Y. Wang, X. Chen, W. Cao, and Y. Shi, "Plasticity of mesenchymal stem cells in immunomodulation: pathological and therapeutic implications," *Nature Immunology*, vol. 15, no. 11, pp. 1009–1016, 2014.

[8] R. Das, H. Jahr, G. J. V. M. van Osch, and E. Farrell, "The role of hypoxia in bone marrow–derived mesenchymal stem cells: considerations for regenerative medicine approaches," *Tissue Engineering Part B: Reviews*, vol. 16, no. 2, pp. 159–168, 2010.

[9] K. Tamama, H. Kawasaki, S. S. Kerpedjieva, J. Guan, R. K. Ganju, and C. K. Sen, "Differential roles of hypoxia inducible factor subunits in multipotential stromal cells under hypoxic condition," *Journal of Cellular Biochemistry*, vol. 112, no. 3, pp. 804–817, 2011.

[10] H. Lee, C. M. Bien, A. L. Hughes, P. J. Espenshade, K. J. Kwon-Chung, and Y. C. Chang, "Cobalt chloride, a hypoxia-mimicking agent, targets sterol synthesis in the pathogenic fungus Cryptococcus neoformans," *Molecular Microbiology*, vol. 65, no. 4, pp. 1018–1033, 2007.

[11] Shweta, K. P. Mishra, S. Chanda, S. B. Singh, and L. Ganju, "A comparative immunological analysis of CoCl2 treated cells with in vitro hypoxic exposure," *Biometals*, vol. 28, no. 1, pp. 175–185, 2015.

[12] S. W. Oh, Y. M. Lee, S. Kim, H. J. Chin, D. W. Chae, and K. Y. Na, "Cobalt chloride attenuates oxidative stress and inflammation through NF-κB inhibition in human renal proximal tubular epithelial cells," *Journal of Korean Medical Science*, vol. 29, Supplement 2, pp. S139–S145, 2014.

[13] T. L. Bonfield, M. Koloze, D. P. Lennon, B. Zuchowski, S. E. Yang, and A. I. Caplan, "Human mesenchymal stem cells suppress chronic airway inflammation in the murine ovalbumin asthma model," *American Journal of Physiology-Lung Cellular and Molecular Physiology*, vol. 299, no. 6, pp. L760–L770, 2010.

[14] H. Kavanagh and B. P. Mahon, "Allogeneic mesenchymal stem cells prevent allergic airway inflammation by inducing murine regulatory T cells," *Allergy*, vol. 66, no. 4, pp. 523–531, 2011.

[15] H. K. Park, K. S. Cho, H. Y. Park et al., "Adipose-derived stromal cells inhibit allergic airway inflammation in mice," *Stem Cells and Development*, vol. 19, no. 11, pp. 1811–1818, 2010.

[16] K. Nemeth, A. Keane-Myers, J. M. Brown et al., "Bone marrow stromal cells use TGF-β to suppress allergic responses in a mouse model of ragweed-induced asthma," *Proceedings of the National Academy of Sciences of the United States of America*, vol. 107, no. 12, pp. 5652–5657, 2010.

[17] A. Lan, X. Liao, L. Mo et al., "Hydrogen sulfide protects against chemical hypoxia-induced injury by inhibiting ROS-activated ERK1/2 and p38MAPK signaling pathways in PC12 cells," *PLoS One*, vol. 6, no. 10, article e25921, 2011.

[18] L. Liu, H. Zhang, L. Sun et al., "ERK/MAPK activation involves hypoxia-induced MGr1-Ag/37LRP expression and contributes to apoptosis resistance in gastric cancer," *International Journal of Cancer*, vol. 127, no. 4, pp. 820–829, 2010.

[19] H. Jin, Y. Bae, M. Kim et al., "Comparative analysis of human mesenchymal stem cells from bone marrow, adipose tissue, and umbilical cord blood as sources of cell therapy," *International Journal of Molecular Sciences*, vol. 14, no. 9, pp. 17986–18001, 2013.

[20] E. H. C. Tang, P. Libby, P. M. Vanhoutte, and A. Xu, "Anti-inflammation therapy by activation of prostaglandin EP4 receptor in cardiovascular and other inflammatory diseases," *Journal of Cardiovascular Pharmacology*, vol. 59, no. 2, pp. 116–123, 2012.

[21] R. Yanez, A. Oviedo, M. Aldea, J. A. Bueren, and M. L. Lamana, "Prostaglandin E2 plays a key role in the immuno-

suppressive properties of adipose and bone marrow tissue-derived mesenchymal stromal cells," *Experimental Cell Research*, vol. 316, no. 19, pp. 3109–3123, 2010.

[22] L. Chang and M. Karin, "Mammalian MAP kinase signalling cascades," *Nature*, vol. 410, no. 6824, pp. 37–40, 2001.

[23] L. T. Jeker and R. Marone, "Targeting microRNAs for immunomodulation," *Current Opinion in Pharmacology*, vol. 23, pp. 25–31, 2015.

[24] C. Xu, G. Ren, G. Cao et al., "miR-155 regulates immune modulatory properties of mesenchymal stem cells by targeting TAK1-binding protein 2," *Journal of Biological Chemistry*, vol. 288, no. 16, pp. 11074–11079, 2013.

[25] Y. F. Xie, R. Shu, S. Y. Jiang et al., "miRNA-146 negatively regulates the production of pro-inflammatory cytokines via NF-κB signalling in human gingival fibroblasts," *Journal of Inflammation*, vol. 11, no. 1, p. 38, 2014.

[26] A. Iyer, E. Zurolo, A. Prabowo et al., "MicroRNA-146a: a key regulator of astrocyte-mediated inflammatory response," *PLoS One*, vol. 7, no. 9, article e44789, 2012.

[27] K. D. Taganov, M. P. Boldin, K. J. Chang, and D. Baltimore, "NF-kappaB-dependent induction of microRNA miR-146, an inhibitor targeted to signaling proteins of innate immune responses," *Proceedings of the National Academy of Sciences*, vol. 103, no. 33, pp. 12481–12486, 2006.

[28] Z. Zeng, H. Gong, Y. Li et al., "Upregulation of miR-146a contributes to the suppression of inflammatory responses in LPS-induced acute lung injury," *Experimental Lung Research*, vol. 39, no. 7, pp. 275–282, 2013.

4

Current Strategies to Generate Human Mesenchymal Stem Cells In Vitro

Jennifer Steens and Diana Klein ⓘD

Institute for Cell Biology (Cancer Research), University Hospital Essen, University of Duisburg-Essen, Essen, Germany

Correspondence should be addressed to Diana Klein; diana.klein@uk-essen.de

Academic Editor: Stan Gronthos

Mesenchymal stem cells (MSCs) are heterogeneous multipotent stem cells that are involved in the development of mesenchyme-derived evolving structures and organs during ontogeny. In the adult organism, reservoirs of MSCs can be found in almost all tissues where MSCs contribute to the maintenance of organ integrity. The use of these different MSCs for cell-based therapies has been extensively studied over the past years, which highlights the use of MSCs as a promising option for the treatment of various diseases including autoimmune and cardiovascular disorders. However, the proportion of MSCs contained in primary isolates of adult tissue biopsies is rather low and, thus, vigorous ex vivo expansion is needed especially for therapies that may require extensive and repetitive cell substitution. Therefore, more easily and accessible sources of MSCs are needed. This review summarizes the current knowledge of the different strategies to generate human MSCs *in vitro* as an alternative method for their applications in regenerative therapy.

1. Introduction

Among the adult stem cells, MSCs are supposed to be the most promising stem cell type for cell-based therapies [1–4]. Compared with less differentiated pluripotent stem cells, in particular embryonic stem cells or induced pluripotent stem cells (iPSCs), MSCs are well tolerated and lack ethical concerns as well as teratoma-formation and histocompatibility issues [5–7] [8, 9]. Adult MSCs are multipotent cells, which are commonly characterized by their ability to adhere on plastic, by the expression of a typical panel of MSC surface markers (CD105(+), CD73(+), CD90(+), CD11b(−), CD79a(−), CD19(−), and human leukocyte antigen (HLA-DR) (−)), and the ability to differentiate into mesenchymal and nonmesenchymal tissues in vitro and in vivo [10, 11].

Once therapeutically applied, MSC can either act directly by homing to particular anatomical sites after transplantation and differentiating into specific cell types to locally restore the damaged tissue. Even more important, MSCs can support tissue regeneration by a paracrine ("hit and run") mechanism of action, such as secretion of multiple bioactive molecules capable of stimulating recovery of injured cells and inhibiting inflammation [12–14]. In addition, MSCs lack immunogenicity and possess the ability to perform immunomodulatory functions [15, 16]. These unique properties have promoted numerous applications of MSCs which currently undergo hundreds of clinical trials (http://www.clinicaltrials.gov) for disease treatments including graft versus host disease, chronic obstructive pulmonary disease, Crohn's disease, or even multiple sclerosis [17–20]. Genetically modified MSCs were further used to enable targeted delivery of a variety of therapeutic agents in malignant diseases [21–23].

The classical known reservoir of MSCs is the bone marrow, but nowadays, MSCs are effectively isolated from almost every organ such as adipose tissue, cartilage, muscle, liver, blood, and blood vessels [4, 24–29]. However, there are several limitations for the vigorous *in vitro* expansion of ex vivo isolated adult MSCs: a decline of their plasticity and *in vivo* potency over time was reported, as well as accumulated DNA abnormalities and replicative senescence [30–35]. In addition, variations of the quality of obtained donor cells and tissue sources have caused numerous inconsistencies in

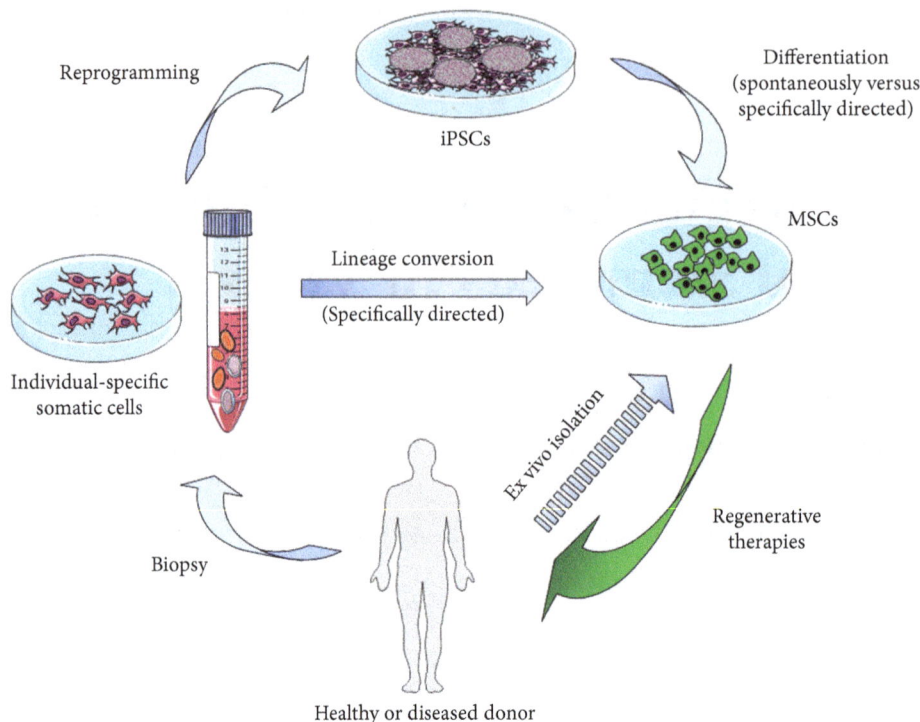

FIGURE 1: Patient-specific adult MSCs. Somatic cells (e.g., fibroblasts and peripheral blood cells) can be isolated from individual healthy or diseased donors (biopsy) and (i) directly converted into MSCs or (ii) reprogrammed into iPSCs by the introduction of the common transcription (Yamanaka) factors *OCT4*, *SOX2*, *KLF4*, and *c-MYC*. iPSCs were characterized by indefinite self-renewal and pluripotent differentiation capacities and, thus, represent an attractive source to generate unlimited cell numbers for targeted differentiation into MSCs. For regenerative therapy, only donor cells that have reached a particular differentiation stage could be used, which means that the iPSCs must first be brought to an ordered differentiation path. MSC differentiation of iPSC is initiated either spontaneously (by deprivation of pluripotent signals) or specifically directed by the induction of mesodermal differentiation, followed by treatment with MSC-specific growth factors that allows then the isolation and expansion of the selected MSCs under chemically defined cell culture conditions. As an alternative pathway, patient-specific somatic cells can directly programmed/transdifferentiated to MSCs which would avoid the need for prior reprogramming those cells back the pluripotent stage. Hypothetically, human MSCs could also be obtained by a direct programming approach, by ectopic expression of MSC-specific transcription factors in iPSCs and somatic cells, or by the introduction of cell type-specific microRNA molecules that functions in RNA silencing and posttranscriptional regulation of MSC gene expression. Morphology-based manual selection and/or sorting for cell type-specific cell surface markers using flow cytometry or immunomagnetic separation might further be used to increase purity of generated MSCs. The generation of patient- and disease-specific iPSCs is a valuable tool for regenerative therapies, for example, restoration of function through transplantation of ex vivo manufactured cells.

the reported *in vivo* effectiveness of MSCs [36–39]. Therefore, more reliable sources of MSCs remain an important problem.

To circumvent many of these issues, alternative methods to generate therapeutically sufficient numbers of MSCs *in vitro* were established. MSCs for autologous cell replacement therapy can be derived from immune-compatible somatic cells, which possesses huge clinical potential. However, the large-scale production of human MSCs for regenerative cell therapies depends on well-defined, highly reproducible culture and differentiation conditions. This review will focus on the different methods to generate therapeutically active MSCs *in vitro*.

2. Patient-Specific MSCs

MSCs can be derived from different donor cells via 2 primary strategies: (1) direct conversion or induced

transdifferentiation of patient-specific somatic cells or (2) differentiation from reprogrammed (pluripotent) somatic cells (iPSCs) (Figure 1). No matter which way of in vitro generation is chosen, MSCs emerge then from the proliferating donor cells in the presence of mesodermal growth factors, growth factor inhibitors, and small molecules. When iPSCs were used, MSCs can even be derived spontaneously by depriving the pluripotent signals from the culture conditions. In an additional, but up to now theoretical approach, derivation of MSCs could also be obtained by direct programming that would mean the ectopic expression of MSC-specific (transcription) factors that regulate MSC gene expressions [40–42]. To enrich the generated MSCs further, some forms of cell sorting and isolation using morphological features and/or antibodies specific for MSC-typical cell surface molecules or genetic tagging of the iPSCs with lineage-specific fluorescent reporter systems are required.

3. Human Embryonic Stem Cell-Derived MSCs

The first reports on MSCs generated from pluripotent stem cells were performed with pluripotent embryonic stem cells before iPSCs came into focus. Xu et al. isolated human embryonic fibroblast-like cells (HEF1 cells) from pluripotent human embryonic H1 stem cells after induction of differentiation by small aggregate formation (embryonic bodies) and subsequent cultivation in HEF1 medium (knockout- (KO-) DMEM supplemented with 10% heat-inactivated fetal bovine serum (FBS) and nonessential amino acids) [43]. The remaining fibroblast-like cells were further infected with a retrovirus expressing human telomerase reverse transcriptase (hTERT) which extended their replicative capacity, resulting in immortal human HEF1-hTERT cells. These cells exhibited a similar marker profile like MSCs and had the capacity to differentiate into cells of the osteogenic lineage, as telomerase expression in human MSCs had already been shown to enhance an osteogenic differentiation potential [44].

Only one year later, a more directed approach for the in vitro generation of MSCs was reported. Barberi et al. used the same embryonic H1 stem cell line (together with H9 embryonic stem cells) and cocultured these cells with the mesoderm embryonic cell line OP9 (mouse bone marrow stromal cells) to induce mesodermal differentiation in the presence of 20% heat-inactivated FBS (in alpha-MEM) for approximately 40 days prior flow-activated cell sorting (FACS) for the MSC marker CD73 [45]. This simple and quite unspecific differentiation protocol yielded multipotent mesenchymal precursors from human embryonic stem cells with typical average of 5% CD73-positive cells (in the mixed culture of OP9 and differentiated embryonic stem cells), which expressed several classical MSC markers and differentiation capabilities [45]. Gene expression profiling in addition confirmed a MSC-typical expression profile of differentiated MSC as compared to primary human bone marrow-derived MSCs including the MSC protein DSC54, neuropilin, hepatocyte growth factor, forkhead box D1, and notch homolog [45]. Thus, the basis for the *in vitro* generation of MSC differentiated from pluripotent stem cells which followed the classical MSC characteristics was made.

A number of reports followed to derive MSCs from human embryonic stem cells. A more specific approach was provided by Lian et al. who established a protocol for the derivation of clinically compliant MSCs, which were derived from Hues9 and H1 human embryonic stem cells without the use of animal products [46]. Mesodermal differentiation was induced by plating trypsinized embryonic stem cells in MSC growth medium supplemented with serum replacement medium, basic fibroblast growth factor (bFGF/FGF2), and platelet-derived growth factor AB (PDGF-AB) on gelatinized tissue culture plates. After one week of culture, CD105(+)- and CD24(−)-differentiated cells that comprised approximately 5% of the culture were sorted via FACS. Classical MSC characteristics were proven including gene expression analysis as compared to bone marrow MSCs [46]. In addition, the CD24-negative isolation allowed for the selection of the desired cells deprived from remaining non- or partially differentiated embryonic stem cells, as CD24 was identified as a human embryonic stem cell marker. Although the authors successfully reduced the unacceptable risks of tumorigenicity or potential xenozootic infection by circumventing the coculture with murine cells, the authors did not completely circumvent the use of animal products, namely, gelantin for coating and antibodies for flow cytometry purification.

This issue was addressed in the following study. Karlsson et al. established an optimized protocol resulting in the simple and reproducible derivation of mesenchymal progenitors from xeno-free, undifferentiated human embryonic stem cell lines [47, 48]. Therefore, undifferentiated embryonic stem cells were removed from the supporting feeder layer, enzymatically dissociated, and plated as high-density cultures on plastic dishes coated with human recombinant gelatin in medium supplemented with human serum (10%) and human recombinant bFGF. After 7 days, the resulting outgrowth of heterogeneous cell types was further passaged and cultured until a homogeneous culture with mesenchymal progenitor morphology (at passage 2-3) was achieved [48, 49]. Resulting MSC characteristics as well as microarray analysis confirmed the MSC nature of generated MSCs as compared to MSCs isolated from human bone marrow aspirates from the iliac crest [49]. Preclinical evaluation of implanted human embryonic stem cell-derived mesenchymal progenitor cells further revealed that generated cells gave rise to homogeneous, well-differentiated tissues that were exclusively of mesenchymal origin while no teratoma formation was observed [48]. The authors successfully established here a robust protocol that does not require cell transfection, coculture, cell sorting, or subjective manual selection for the xeno-free derivation of mesenchymal progenitors from diverse human embryonic stem cell lines that were safe for the use in tissue engineering and cell therapies.

Conclusively, MSCs can either be derived from human embryonic stem cells spontaneously, upon less stringent culture conditions, and in particular upon culturing in medium which is deprived of pluripotent signals, or by a specific stimulus (e.g., growth factors or inhibitors) which directs MSC differentiation. Most of these protocols were consistent and cost-effective, but inefficient, as the MSC population yielded by the unspecific differentiation methods yielded only approximately 5% MSCs. Pure cultures could then be established upon prolonged culturing, by fluorescence-activated cell sorting or by manual selection of cell populations.

4. iPSC-Derived MSCs

Human iPSCs constitute a well-characterized, generally unlimited cell source for the mass generation of lineage- and patient-specific MSCs without any ethical concerns because of their theoretical unlimited growth and differentiation potential. Human iPSC-derived MSCs were already shown to display similar features with mature MSCs at the genetic and functional levels [37, 50–52]. As already stated, the major challenge is here to establish reliable, efficient, and scalable protocols to differentiate functionally mature adult MSCs.

The classical method for differentiating iPSCs towards MSCs is the use of media that contains a high serum concentration or MSC-typical growth factors such as bFGF after mesoderm induction [32, 50, 53–55]. Induction of mesodermal differentiation is usually achieved by embryoid body formation or mesodermal-inductive factor treatments (*bone morphogenetic protein 4*, activin A/nodal, bFGF, and *glycogen synthase kinase 3* inhibitors or WNT ligands) in chemically defined monolayer systems. Successive treatment with MSC-specific growth factors and/or sorting for MSC-specific cell surface markers using flow cytometry or immunomagnetic separation allows then the isolation and expansion of the selected MSCs under chemically defined cell culture conditions.

A clinically compliant protocol for the MSC differentiation of human iPSCs was established by Lian et al. [56]. According to their previously established protocol for the derivation of MSCs from human embryonic stem cells, the authors used three iPSC lines (iPSC(iMR90)-5 and iPSC(iMR90)-4 cells derived from IMR90 fibroblasts as well as iPSC(foreskin)Clone1 cells derived from foreskin fibroblasts), which were cultured on gelatin-coated plastic dishes in KO-DMEM supplemented with 10% serum replacement medium in the presence of bFGF, PDGF-AB, and epidermal growth factor to foster the MSC outgrowth [46, 56]. After 1 week of culturing, CD24(−) and CD105(+) cells were isolated via FACS and clonally expanded. By this, the authors successfully generated therapeutically active MSCs which exhibited the classical MSC characteristics and furthermore the ability for self-renewal in culture for >120 population doublings without obvious loss of plasticity or onset of replicative senescence [56]. The transplanted iPSC-derived MSCs were shown to be superior in attenuation of severe hindlimb ischemia (significantly improved vascular and muscle regeneration) than adult bone marrow MSCs which may result from a better in vivo survival and to their trophic factors that protect endangered cells after ischemic injury [56]. Giuliani et al. confirmed the beneficial role of iPSC-derived MSCs as compared to bone marrow MSCs concerning survival and longevity [57]. The authors used MSC differentiated from 5 iPSC lines (H9-iPS, SA-01-iPS, PB03, PB10, and PB11) using DMEM/F12 medium supplemented with 10% heat-inactivated FBS, bFGF, and nonessential amino acids as differentiation medium. Respective iPSC-derived MSCs displayed remarkable inhibition of natural killer (NK) cell proliferation and cytolytic function, while being more resistant than adult bone marrow MSCs to preactivated NK cells, which highlights their potential to prevent allograft rejection [57]. In line with these findings, a differential expression of ion channels in iPSC-derived MSCs was shown to contribute to their higher proliferation capacity compared with classically bone marrow MSCs [58]. Among the different ion channels, increased expression of the functional *KCNH1*-encoded human ethera`-go-go 1 (hEAG1) potassium channel was identified being responsible for higher cell proliferative rate in iPSC-derived MSCs using the Lian protocol [56, 58].

A new method to rapidly derive MSC-like cells from human iPSCs in one step using thin, fibrillar, type I collagen as matrix that mimics the structure of physiological collagen was reported for the effective differentiation of MSC from the human dermal fibroblast-derived HDFa-YK26 iPSCs [32]. Resilient colonies of homogenous spindle-shaped cells were obtained after 10 days of culturing iPSCs in alpha-MEM supplemented with 10% FBS, magnesium L-ascorbic acid phosphate, and dexamethasone that displayed the classical MSC characteristics [32]. After 2 passages, 82.9% of the cells were CD90-positive, indicating an efficient MSC generation. Prolonged passaging on collagen type I further increased this number to 96.9% of generated MSCs. The advantage for using collagen type I or in general appropriate biomaterial matrices here offers additional means to influence cell fate through physicochemical stimulation, as collagen type I was already known to activate an epithelial-to-mesenchymal transition (EMT) of epithelial cells [32, 59]. Another single-step method to direct mesengenic differentiation of human iPSCs was reported by Chen et al., who used a small molecule inhibitor, the transforming growth factor-β pathway inhibitor SB431542 [60]. iPSCs (MR90CL2 and ES4CL1) were cultured in the presence of this inhibitor for 10 days resulting in MSCs which exhibit typical MSC characteristics that conform to the criteria of the International Society for Cell Therapy (ISCT) for classification of MSCs. Mechanistically, this study revealed that SB431542 treatment triggered both intrinsic and autocrine mechanisms in iPSCs that collectively prime a subset of cells for a mesenchymal stromal cell fate by inducing EMT [60]. This modification in terms of fostering EMT in iPSC cultures resulted in higher MSC numbers of approximately 75–96% [60]. A simplified and reproducible method for inducing iPSC into MSC-like cells that further resulted in increased percentages of generated MSCs was then presented by Hynes et al. [61]. Herein, MSC-like cells were developed from iPSC lines arising from three different somatic tissues (gingiva, periodontal ligament, and lung) by a continuous culturing of respective cells in MSC culture media (alpha-MEM supplemented with 10% FCS, sodium pyruvate, l-ascorbate-2-phosphate, nonessential amino acids, and HEPES). After 2 weeks, the resulting heterogeneous cell types were passaged as a single-cell suspension and clones of arising cells were selected based on their typical morphology. Selected clones expressed key MSC-associated markers (CD73, CD90, CD105, CD146, and CD166) and lacked expression of pluripotent markers (TRA160, TRA181, and alkaline phosphatase) and hematopoietic markers (CD14, CD34, and CD45). *In vitro*, iPSC-MSC-like cells displayed the capacity to differentiate into osteoblasts, adipocytes, and chondrocytes [61]. By this method, the authors reported the generation of 95% pure MSC cultures.

Most of the protocols used fetal bovine serum as supplement which provides multiple growth factors with nonspecific signals to the cultures. In contrast, providing a chemically defined medium with known morphogens that fosters the MSC differentiation is supposed to increase the yield and homogeneity of the derived MSCs. In addition to the more specific and defined medium supplements, the use of xeno-free supplements (e.g., no animal products and no coculturing with mouse cells) would allow the generation of highly identical and clinically compliant MSC cultures from human iPSCs. Luzzani et al. used H9 human embryonic stem cells and iPSCs reprogrammed from human foreskin fibroblasts in combination with platelet lysate as a media supplement to produce pluripotent-derived MSCs (PD-MSC) within 3 to 4 weeks in a robust and consistent way [62]. The authors designed a two-stage protocol for the MSC differentiation from pluripotent stem cells. In the first step, mesodermal differentiation was induced by dissociating the pluripotent stem cell clusters and plating single-cell isolates on a reduced growth factor basement membrane matrix (Matrigel or Geltrex, a soluble and LDEV-free form of basement membrane extracted from murine Engelbreth-Holm-Swarm tumors) for 14 days in the presence of platelet lysate and supplement B27 [63]. After these 14 days, when the cells were transitioned to a mesenchymal state, the prolonged culturing was performed with plastic dishes in alpha MEM supplemented with platelet lysate (10%) for additional 7–14 days [62]. The resulting PD-MSCs were generated more efficiently as compared to cells differentiated in the presence of FBS as supplement (25 cells per pluripotent stem cells when platelet lysate was used versus 10 cells per pluripotent stem cells when FBS was used) and displayed all the MSC characteristics. Conclusively, the presented protocol used simple steps using therapy-grade platelet lysate as supplement and thus yielded significant amounts of MSCs in approximately 1 month [62]. Human serum in general as well as the derived platelet lysate (and thrombin-activated platelet releasate in plasma) turned out to be promising alternatives to FBS as a medium supplement for growing MSCs [64–66]. Although the concentrations of cytokines and growth factors in the respective supplements released by the platelets after lysing vary enormously, PDGF-AB/BB, TGF-β1, and bFGF turned out to be the essential factors (beside HGF and IGF-1) for the strong positive effect on the proliferation of MSCs [67, 68]. A potential but due to the strict protocols for blood testing minimal risk remains that the human material may contain virus or parasites [69].

In summary, robust protocols have been established to obtain patient-specific, therapeutically active MSCs from iPSCs in large amounts which will potentially open avenues towards novel, MSC-based therapies. Another straight forward strategy would be the ectopic overexpression of MSC-related genes or transcription factors in human iPSCs to generate MSCs. The *in vitro* generation of vascular wall-typical MSCs from iPSCs, based on a vascular wall MSC-specific gene code, was reported by our group [55, 70]. Herein, a lentiviral vector expressing a small set of recently identified human vascular wall MSC-specific HOX genes was used to directly program iPSCs into MSCs which displayed classical MSC characteristics, both *in vitro* and *in vivo* [55]. However, this forward programming approach remains limited to murine iPSCs, but it is very likely that our results will also hold true for human iPSCs as the activity of homeotic selector proteins is highly conserved throughout evolution.

5. Direct Conversion of MSCs from Somatic Cells

The main limitation for a possible therapeutic use of pluripotent stem cells and/or their derived MSCs is the medical risk to generate teratomas. Although already robust selection markers and refined experimental protocols have been established to guide human iPSCs reproducibly to MSCs, an additional negative selection against remaining pluripotent cells could be an additional option, to limit the risk of teratoma formation and foster clinical safety. As an alternative, somatic donor cells that have reached a particular differentiation stage could be used.

Meng et al. used CD34-positive cord blood and adult peripheral blood cells in combination with a single factor, namely, OCT4 to demonstrate a direct programming of patient-specific somatic cells into MSCs [71]. An episomal or lentiviral vector-mediated OCT4 expression followed by a subsequent culture of treated cells on fibronectin in commercially available MSC Medium Kit allowed the rapid and efficient programming of human CD34(+) cells directly into MSCs. The generated MSCs were multipotent, being able to differentiate into different types of MSC progenies both *in vitro* and *in vivo*, and were not tumorigenic [71, 72]. Conformingly, Lai et al. established an effective protocol to directly convert primary human dermal fibroblasts into multipotent, induced MSC-like cells (iMSCs) [73]. A cocktail containing six chemical inhibitors (SP600125 (JNK inhibitor), SB202190 (p38 inhibitor), Go6983 (protein kinase C inhibitor), Y-27632 (ROCK inhibitor), PD0325901 (ERK1/2 inhibitor), and CHIR99021 (GSK3β inhibitor)) with or without the addition of three growth factors (TGF-β1, bFGF, and leukemia inhibitory factor (LIF)) efficiently generated functional iMSCs from human primary dermal fibroblasts (primary neonatal foreskin fibroblasts (CRL2097) within 6 days (average rate of 38%)). The generated MSCs shared similar molecular signatures with bone marrow MSCs and fulfilled all of the MSC criteria defined by ISCT, including plastic adherence, marker expressions, and multipotency differentiation. *In vivo*, a markedly attenuation of endotoxin-induced acute lung injury, which was paralleled by a decrease of the amounts of proinflammatory cytokines, was reported [73]. Thus, an efficient conversion method that does not involve any processes that may lead to insertional mutagenesis, resulting in MSCs with lower safety concerns for disease treatments was reported [73].

Conclusively, chemical-induced conversion or direct programming of somatic cells into MSCs is possible and augurs strong clinical potential for respective MSCs but the protocols up to now are limited.

6. The Pros and Cons

Global gene and miRNA profiling of human iPSC- and embryonic stem cell-derived MSCs demonstrated a high degree of similarity between the derived MSCs, in particular as compared to bone marrow MSCs [45, 46, 49]. Bone marrow MSCs generally serve as the gold standard against which other MSC sources are compared [74]. However, there is a convincing evidence that MSCs from diverse tissue are different and display distinct differentiation tendencies, paracrine potential, and immune properties, but the benefit and mechanisms of these MSCs from various sources remain unexplored [75]. The significant heterogeneity in the differentiating potential of MSCs from different sources however may influence their clinical application [74, 76]. Adipose tissue-derived MSCs, for example were, shown to have a stronger inhibitory effect in the suppression of peripheral blood B, T, and NK cells than bone marrow and umbilical cord matrix-derived MSCs [77]. As another example, MSCs isolated from the placenta and adipose tissue were morphologically and immune phenotypically similar to MSCs obtained from the bone marrow, but MSCs derived from the placenta were proven to be a more optimal cellular source for the treatment of ischemic diseases [75]. A proteomic profiling of the three MSC types revealed that the highly upregulated proteins in placenta-derived MSCs, which were related to oxidative stress, peroxiredoxin activity, and apoptosis function, corresponded to the in vivo functional performance [75]. Previous reports have already demonstrated that bone marrow-derived MSCs were less effective after a therapeutically application as compared to other stem cell sources [77–82].

According to the general guidelines, MSCs from distinct tissue origins have a large number of similarities concerning their characteristics, but the isolated MSCs remain a heterogeneous cell population until a clonal expansion. Up to now, it is not clear, whether tissue-resident MSCs are the progenies of one ancestor cell lineage or the results of parallel cell developmental events [83, 84]. The tissue-specific properties of MSCs were related to the expression profiles of HOX genes that are master regulators of regional specification and organ development [46]. These HOX expression profiles can be used to distinguish functionally distinct populations of MSCs, as shown for bone marrow, umbilical cord blood, and blood vessel-derived MSCs [55, 70, 85]. However, the precise mechanisms that regulate lineage specification of the isolated heterogeneous MSCs have been largely unexplored [86, 87]. The transcriptome analyses of human MSCs revealed that expressed transcripts encode for a diverse repertoire of proteins that regulate angiogenesis, hematopoiesis, cell motility, neural activities, and immunity which finally lead to the conclusion that single cells were unlikely to possess all properties. [87–89]. The different functional attributes were relegated then to distinct subpopulations. Therefore, more effort is needed to develop clinical manufacturing protocols that reproducibly generate functionally equivalent MSC populations.

The tissue-specific homing and the activities of isolated and cultured MSCs prior to transfusion are supposed to be based on an underlying transcriptional code caused by epigenetic memory allowing them to home back to the tissue they originally were derived from [53]. In line with these findings, it was shown that vascular wall-derived MSCs were more potent than bone marrow-derived MSCs to protect lung blood vessels from the adverse late effects of radiotherapy, which supports the assumption that tissue-specific stem cells support mainly the tissue type from which they originate

because of their tissue-specific action [90, 91]. Therefore, a central advantage would be the use of tissue-specific MSCs for the protection and curative treatment of the same and/or similar affected tissue that in turn would require protocols for the derivation of tissue-specific MSCs. The generation of tissue-specific MSCs from somatic cells and/or iPSCs reprogrammed from somatic cells could be achieved by transient, ectopic expression of cell type-specific transcription factors, miRNAs, or by using of epigenetic modifiers, as shown for other cell types, such as neurons or hepatocyte-like cells [92–95].

The age of MSCs may also have a major impact on their therapeutic outcome, as the differentiation potential of MSCs decreases with age [96]. Aged MSCs showed decreased proliferation rates, higher oxidative damage, and cell senescence [97]. This would argue against the derivation of MSCs from adult somatic cell types, but MSC derived from pluripotent stem cells may overcome the fact that adult MSCs have limited proliferation and differentiation capabilities. It was already suggested that every pluripotent cell may become a MSC "by default," an event that occurs spontaneously when pluripotent stem cells are cultured under less stringent pluripotent conditions [62, 69]. However, the respective percentages of MSCs generated by these culture conditions were lower (approximately 5%) as compared to more specific culture conditions with mesoderm-specific growth factors. Epigenetic instabilities or phenotypic switches after prolonged culture might also occur because the identity of derived MSCs may not be well inherited in human iPSCs and embryonic stem cell-derived MSCs, and further studies are needed to specify the nature of derived MSCs and if all of the derived MSCs correspond to the similar (tissue-specific) MSC type.

Finally, the use of pluripotent stem cell-derived MSCs could be limited due to allogenic rejection or teratoma formation. In particular, the clinical use of the successful generated MSCs from human iPSCs and embryonic stem cells has been hampered by the tumorigenic potential elicited by undifferentiated iPSCs potentially remaining in the differentiated cell population, the lengthy and inefficient differentiation process, and genomic instability due to suboptimal culture conditions. Observed differences and efficiencies in MSC generation might be based on a somatic memory of the different cell types used for iPSC generation [98–100]. In line with this hypothesis, it was also shown that the cellular origin influences the lineage differentiation propensity of human iPSCs [41, 101]. A possible solution to these drawbacks could be to directly program an easily accessible patient-specific somatic cell types towards MSCs. Although a direct programming of somatic cells into MSCs is possible, robust protocols for this derivation are limited.

7. Conclusion

Beside the abundant origins but low frequencies of tissue-specific MSCs, the potentials to generate patient-individualized MSCs with comparable properties that bypass the immunogenicity and ethical issues in therapeutically relevant numbers are central advantages of using somatic cells and iPSCs as MSC source. Concerning the proliferative and regenerative potency of generated MSC, iPSC-derived MSC may be superior to somatic cell-derived MSC because MSCs differentiated from iPSCs might be closer to fetal MSCs, since pluripotent stem cells represent the early time point in development. In contrast, the tumorigenic potential of undifferentiated iPSCs in a population of iPSC-derived MSCs is a significant safety concern for iPSC-related clinical applications. This risk might be further reduced by the use of MSCs derived from integration-free iPSCs. An alternative quite promising method to gain MSCs *in vitro* is the direct conversion of somatic cells, for example, easily accessible fibroblasts or blood cells. However, respective studies and standardized protocols used to prepare large-scale MSC as well as useful tests to compare their potency are limited up to now. The significant molecular and functional differences in the properties of the generated MSCs according to their different origins influence the respective therapeutic potential. Therefore, the identification of the (tissue-specific) nature of *in vitro* generated MSCs from pluripotent stem cells needs further investigations as well as the establishment of protocols which would allow the generation of tissue-specific MSCs. Finally, the somatic memory of iPSCs should be carefully considered before clinical translation. Up to now, there are no reports on the direct comparison of MSCs generated by different approaches, which must be investigated in future studies together with the clinical safety of different MSC sources. Concerning the patient-derived autologous MSCs generated *in vitro*, the respective genetic background should be a benefit for (disease) modeling studies, but the same genetic or acquired abnormalities that predisposed a patient to a particular disease will be persisted in the respective MSCs which might result in dysfunctional MSCs with reduced therapeutically activities.

Acknowledgments

The Jürgen Manchot Stiftung (Düsseldorf, Germany) supported this work.

References

[1] A. P. Chidgey, D. Layton, A. Trounson, and R. L. Boyd, "Tolerance strategies for stem-cell-based therapies," *Nature*, vol. 453, no. 7193, pp. 330–337, 2008.

[2] B. Kristjansson and S. Honsawek, "Current perspectives in mesenchymal stem cell therapies for osteoarthritis," *Stem Cells International*, vol. 2014, Article ID 194318, 13 pages, 2014.

[3] S. Rafii and D. Lyden, "Therapeutic stem and progenitor cell transplantation for organ vascularization and regeneration," *Nature Medicine*, vol. 9, no. 6, pp. 702–712, 2003.

[4] A. Uccelli, L. Moretta, and V. Pistoia, "Mesenchymal stem cells in health and disease," *Nature Reviews Immunology*, vol. 8, no. 9, pp. 726–736, 2008.

[5] I. B. Copland, "Mesenchymal stromal cells for cardiovascular disease," *Journal of Cardiovascular Disease Research*, vol. 2, no. 1, pp. 3–13, 2011.

[6] K. Komatsu, O. Honmou, J. Suzuki, K. Houkin, H. Hamada, and J. D. Kocsis, "Therapeutic time window of mesenchymal stem cells derived from bone marrow after cerebral ischemia," *Brain Research*, vol. 1334, pp. 84–92, 2010.

[7] Z. Wen, S. Zheng, C. Zhou, J. Wang, and T. Wang, "Repair mechanisms of bone marrow mesenchymal stem cells in myocardial infarction," *Journal of Cellular and Molecular Medicine*, vol. 15, no. 5, pp. 1032–1043, 2011.

[8] W. R. Otto and N. A. Wright, "Mesenchymal stem cells: from experiment to clinic," *Fibrogenesis & Tissue Repair*, vol. 4, no. 1, p. 20, 2011.

[9] R. R. Sharma, K. Pollock, A. Hubel, and D. McKenna, "Mesenchymal stem or stromal cells: a review of clinical applications and manufacturing practices," *Transfusion*, vol. 54, no. 5, pp. 1418–1437, 2014.

[10] M. Dominici, K. le Blanc, I. Mueller et al., "Minimal criteria for defining multipotent mesenchymal stromal cells. The International Society for Cellular Therapy position statement," *Cytotherapy*, vol. 8, no. 4, pp. 315–317, 2006.

[11] V. B. Fernandez Vallone, M. A. Romaniuk, H. Choi, V. Labovsky, J. Otaegui, and N. A. Chasseing, "Mesenchymal stem cells and their use in therapy: what has been achieved?," *Differentiation*, vol. 85, no. 1-2, pp. 1–10, 2013.

[12] M. Conese, A. Carbone, S. Castellani, and S. Di Gioia, "Paracrine effects and heterogeneity of marrow-derived stem/progenitor cells: relevance for the treatment of respiratory diseases," *Cells, Tissues, Organs*, vol. 197, no. 6, pp. 445–473, 2013.

[13] A. De Becker and I. V. Riet, "Homing and migration of mesenchymal stromal cells: how to improve the efficacy of cell therapy?," *World Journal of Stem Cells*, vol. 8, no. 3, pp. 73–87, 2016.

[14] J. Leibacher and R. Henschler, "Biodistribution, migration and homing of systemically applied mesenchymal stem/stromal cells," *Stem Cell Research & Therapy*, vol. 7, no. 1, p. 7, 2016.

[15] E. Mariani and A. Facchini, "Clinical applications and biosafety of human adult mesenchymal stem cells," *Current Pharmaceutical Design*, vol. 18, no. 13, pp. 1821–1845, 2012.

[16] S. Wang, X. Qu, and R. C. Zhao, "Clinical applications of mesenchymal stem cells," *Journal of Hematology & Oncology*, vol. 5, no. 1, p. 19, 2012.

[17] P. Bader, Z. Kuçi, S. Bakhtiar et al., "Effective treatment of steroid and therapy-refractory acute graft-versus-host disease with a novel mesenchymal stromal cell product (MSC-FFM)," *Bone Marrow Transplantation*, vol. 53, no. 7, pp. 852–862, 2018.

[18] P. Connick and S. Chandran, "Mesenchymal stromal cell transplantation modulates neuroinflammatory milieu in amyotrophic lateral sclerosis," *Cytotherapy*, vol. 16, no. 8, pp. 1031-1032, 2014.

[19] P. Connick, M. Kolappan, C. Crawley et al., "Autologous mesenchymal stem cells for the treatment of secondary progressive multiple sclerosis: an open-label phase 2a

proof-of-concept study," *The Lancet Neurology*, vol. 11, no. 2, pp. 150–156, 2012.

[20] S. Fujii, Y. Miura, A. Fujishiro et al., "Graft-versus-host disease amelioration by human bone marrow mesenchymal stromal/stem cell-derived extracellular vesicles is associated with peripheral preservation of naive T cell populations," *Stem Cells*, vol. 36, no. 3, pp. 434–445, 2018.

[21] F. Marofi, G. Vahedi, A. Biglari, A. Esmaeilzadeh, and S. S. Athari, "Mesenchymal stromal/stem cells: a new era in the cell-based targeted gene therapy of cancer," *Frontiers in Immunology*, vol. 8, article 1770, 2017.

[22] E. K. Sage, R. M. Thakrar, and S. M. Janes, "Genetically modified mesenchymal stromal cells in cancer therapy," *Cytotherapy*, vol. 18, no. 11, pp. 1435–1445, 2016.

[23] Y. Yu, Y. Liu, C. Zong et al., "Mesenchymal stem cells with Sirt1 overexpression suppress breast tumor growth via chemokine-dependent natural killer cells recruitment," *Scientific Reports*, vol. 6, no. 1, article 35998, 2016.

[24] M. Crisan, S. Yap, L. Casteilla et al., "A perivascular origin for mesenchymal stem cells in multiple human organs," *Cell Stem Cell*, vol. 3, no. 3, pp. 301–313, 2008.

[25] D. Klein, P. Weisshardt, V. Kleff, H. Jastrow, H. G. Jakob, and S. Ergun, "Vascular wall-resident CD44+ multipotent stem cells give rise to pericytes and smooth muscle cells and contribute to new vessel maturation," *PLoS One*, vol. 6, no. 5, article e20540, 2011.

[26] M. F. Pittenger, A. M. Mackay, S. C. Beck et al., "Multilineage potential of adult human mesenchymal stem cells," *Science*, vol. 284, no. 5411, pp. 143–147, 1999.

[27] V. Tirino, F. Paino, R. d'Aquino, V. Desiderio, A. de Rosa, and G. Papaccio, "Methods for the identification, characterization and banking of human DPSCs: current strategies and perspectives," *Stem Cell Reviews*, vol. 7, no. 3, pp. 608–615, 2011.

[28] S. A. Wexler, C. Donaldson, P. Denning-Kendall, C. Rice, B. Bradley, and J. M. Hows, "Adult bone marrow is a rich source of human mesenchymal 'stem' cells but umbilical cord and mobilized adult blood are not," *British Journal of Haematology*, vol. 121, no. 2, pp. 368–374, 2003.

[29] W. Zhao, D. G. Phinney, D. Bonnet, M. Dominici, and M. Krampera, "Mesenchymal stem cell biodistribution, migration, and homing *in vivo*," *Stem Cells International*, vol. 2014, Article ID 292109, 2 pages, 2014.

[30] P. J. Ho, M. L. Yen, B. C. Tang, C. T. Chen, and B. L. Yen, "H$_2$O$_2$ accumulation mediates differentiation capacity alteration, but not proliferative decline, in senescent human fetal mesenchymal stem cells," *Antioxidants & Redox Signaling*, vol. 18, no. 15, pp. 1895–1905, 2013.

[31] C. Kyriakou, N. Rabin, A. Pizzey, A. Nathwani, and K. Yong, "Factors that influence short-term homing of human bone marrow-derived mesenchymal stem cells in a xenogeneic animal model," *Haematologica*, vol. 93, no. 10, pp. 1457–1465, 2008.

[32] Y. Liu, A. J. Goldberg, J. E. Dennis, G. A. Gronowicz, and L. T. Kuhn, "One-step derivation of mesenchymal stem cell (MSC)-like cells from human pluripotent stem cells on a fibrillar collagen coating," *PLoS One*, vol. 7, no. 3, article e33225, 2012.

[33] M. Mimeault and S. K. Batra, "Recent insights into the molecular mechanisms involved in aging and the malignant transformation of adult stem/progenitor cells and their therapeutic implications," *Ageing Research Reviews*, vol. 8, no. 2, pp. 94–112, 2009.

[34] M. Miura, Y. Miura, H. M. Padilla-Nash et al., "Accumulated chromosomal instability in murine bone marrow mesenchymal stem cells leads to malignant transformation," *Stem Cells*, vol. 24, no. 4, pp. 1095–1103, 2006.

[35] W. J. C. Rombouts and R. E. Ploemacher, "Primary murine MSC show highly efficient homing to the bone marrow but lose homing ability following culture," *Leukemia*, vol. 17, no. 1, pp. 160–170, 2003.

[36] J. Galipeau, "The mesenchymal stromal cells dilemma—does a negative phase III trial of random donor mesenchymal stromal cells in steroid-resistant graft-versus-host disease represent a death knell or a bump in the road?," *Cytotherapy*, vol. 15, no. 1, pp. 2–8, 2013.

[37] E. A. Kimbrel, N. A. Kouris, G. J. Yavanian et al., "Mesenchymal stem cell population derived from human pluripotent stem cells displays potent immunomodulatory and therapeutic properties," *Stem Cells and Development*, vol. 23, no. 14, pp. 1611–1624, 2014.

[38] A. Tyndall, "Mesenchymal stem cell treatments in rheumatology: a glass half full?," *Nature Reviews Rheumatology*, vol. 10, no. 2, pp. 117–124, 2014.

[39] W. Wagner and A. D. Ho, "Mesenchymal stem cell preparations—comparing apples and oranges," *Stem Cell Reviews*, vol. 3, no. 4, pp. 239–248, 2007.

[40] I. Budniatzky and L. Gepstein, "Concise review: reprogramming strategies for cardiovascular regenerative medicine: from induced pluripotent stem cells to direct reprogramming," *Stem Cells Translational Medicine*, vol. 3, no. 4, pp. 448–457, 2014.

[41] D. Klein, "iPSCs-based generation of vascular cells: reprogramming approaches and applications," *Cellular and Molecular Life Sciences: CMLS*, vol. 75, no. 8, pp. 1411–1433, 2018.

[42] L. Kurian, I. Sancho-Martinez, E. Nivet et al., "Conversion of human fibroblasts to angioblast-like progenitor cells," *Nature Methods*, vol. 10, no. 1, pp. 77–83, 2013.

[43] C. Xu, J. Jiang, V. Sottile, J. McWhir, J. Lebkowski, and M. K. Carpenter, "Immortalized fibroblast-like cells derived from human embryonic stem cells support undifferentiated cell growth," *Stem Cells*, vol. 22, no. 6, pp. 972–980, 2004.

[44] S. Shi, S. Gronthos, S. Chen et al., "Bone formation by human postnatal bone marrow stromal stem cells is enhanced by telomerase expression," *Nature Biotechnology*, vol. 20, no. 6, pp. 587–591, 2002.

[45] T. Barberi, L. M. Willis, N. D. Socci, and L. Studer, "Derivation of multipotent mesenchymal precursors from human embryonic stem cells," *PLoS Medicine*, vol. 2, no. 6, article e161, 2005.

[46] Q. Lian, E. Lye, K. Suan Yeo et al., "Derivation of clinically compliant MSCs from CD105+, CD24− differentiated human ESCs," *Stem Cells*, vol. 25, no. 2, pp. 425–436, 2007.

[47] C. Ellerstrom, R. Strehl, K. Moya et al., "Derivation of a xeno-free human embryonic stem cell line," *Stem Cells*, vol. 24, no. 10, pp. 2170–2176, 2006.

[48] C. Karlsson, K. Emanuelsson, F. Wessberg et al., "Human embryonic stem cell-derived mesenchymal progenitors—potential in regenerative medicine," *Stem Cell Research*, vol. 3, no. 1, pp. 39–50, 2009.

[49] G. M. de Peppo, S. Svensson, M. Lenneras et al., "Human embryonic mesodermal progenitors highly resemble human mesenchymal stem cells and display high potential for tissue engineering applications," *Tissue Engineering Part A*, vol. 16, no. 7, pp. 2161–2182, 2010.

[50] Y. Jung, G. Bauer, and J. A. Nolta, "Concise review: induced pluripotent stem cell-derived mesenchymal stem cells: progress toward safe clinical products," *Stem Cells*, vol. 30, no. 1, pp. 42–47, 2012.

[51] T. Ma, M. Xie, T. Laurent, and S. Ding, "Progress in the reprogramming of somatic cells," *Circulation Research*, vol. 112, no. 3, pp. 562–574, 2013.

[52] H. Okano, M. Nakamura, K. Yoshida et al., "Steps toward safe cell therapy using induced pluripotent stem cells," *Circulation Research*, vol. 112, no. 3, pp. 523–533, 2013.

[53] J. Frobel, H. Hemeda, M. Lenz et al., "Epigenetic rejuvenation of mesenchymal stromal cells derived from induced pluripotent stem cells," *Stem Cell Reports*, vol. 3, no. 3, pp. 414–422, 2014.

[54] C. Roux, G. Saviane, J. Pini et al., "Immunosuppressive mesenchymal stromal cells derived from human-induced pluripotent stem cells induce human regulatory T cells *in vitro* and *in vivo*," *Frontiers in Immunology*, vol. 8, 2018.

[55] J. Steens, M. Zuk, M. Benchellal et al., "In vitro generation of vascular wall-resident multipotent stem cells of mesenchymal nature from murine induced pluripotent stem cells," *Stem Cell Reports*, vol. 8, no. 4, pp. 919–932, 2017.

[56] Q. Lian, Y. Zhang, J. Zhang et al., "Functional mesenchymal stem cells derived from human induced pluripotent stem cells attenuate limb ischemia in mice," *Circulation*, vol. 121, no. 9, pp. 1113–1123, 2010.

[57] M. Giuliani, N. Oudrhiri, Z. M. Noman et al., "Human mesenchymal stem cells derived from induced pluripotent stem cells down-regulate NK-cell cytolytic machinery," *Blood*, vol. 118, no. 12, pp. 3254–3262, 2011.

[58] J. Zhang, Y. C. Chan, J. C. Y. Ho, C. W. Siu, Q. Lian, and H. F. Tse, "Regulation of cell proliferation of human induced pluripotent stem cell-derived mesenchymal stem cells via ether-à-go-go 1 (hEAG1) potassium channel," *American Journal of Physiology-Cell Physiology*, vol. 303, no. 2, pp. C115–C125, 2012.

[59] D. Medici and A. Nawshad, "Type I collagen promotes epithelial-mesenchymal transition through ILK-dependent activation of NF-κB and LEF-1," *Matrix Biology*, vol. 29, no. 3, pp. 161–165, 2010.

[60] Y. S. Chen, R. A. Pelekanos, R. L. Ellis, R. Horne, E. J. Wolvetang, and N. M. Fisk, "Small molecule mesengenic induction of human induced pluripotent stem cells to generate mesenchymal stem/stromal cells," *Stem Cells Translational Medicine*, vol. 1, no. 2, pp. 83–95, 2012.

[61] K. Hynes, D. Menicanin, K. Mrozik, S. Gronthos, and P. M. Bartold, "Generation of functional mesenchymal stem cells from different induced pluripotent stem cell lines," *Stem Cells and Development*, vol. 23, no. 10, pp. 1084–1096, 2014.

[62] C. Luzzani, G. Neiman, X. Garate et al., "A therapy-grade protocol for differentiation of pluripotent stem cells into mesenchymal stem cells using platelet lysate as supplement," *Stem Cell Research & Therapy*, vol. 6, no. 1, p. 6, 2015.

[63] Y. Chen, B. Stevens, J. Chang, J. Milbrandt, B. A. Barres, and J. W. Hell, "NS21: re-defined and modified supplement B27 for neuronal cultures," *Journal of Neuroscience Methods*, vol. 171, no. 2, pp. 239–247, 2008.

[64] A. Flemming, K. Schallmoser, D. Strunk, M. Stolk, H. D. Volk, and M. Seifert, "Immunomodulative efficacy of bone marrow-derived mesenchymal stem cells cultured in human platelet lysate," *Journal of Clinical Immunology*, vol. 31, no. 6, pp. 1143–1156, 2011.

[65] P. Iudicone, D. Fioravanti, G. Bonanno et al., "Pathogen-free, plasma-poor platelet lysate and expansion of human mesenchymal stem cells," *Journal of Translational Medicine*, vol. 12, no. 1, p. 28, 2014.

[66] S. Kinzebach, L. Dietz, H. Kluter, H. J. Thierse, and K. Bieback, "Functional and differential proteomic analyses to identify platelet derived factors affecting ex vivo expansion of mesenchymal stromal cells," *BMC Cell Biology*, vol. 14, no. 1, p. 48, 2013.

[67] J. J. Auletta, E. A. Zale, J. F. Welter, and L. A. Solchaga, "Fibroblast growth factor-2 enhances expansion of human bone marrow-derived mesenchymal stromal cells without diminishing their immunosuppressive potential," *Stem Cells International*, vol. 2011, Article ID 235176, 10 pages, 2011.

[68] N. Fekete, M. Gadelorge, D. Fürst et al., "Platelet lysate from whole blood-derived pooled platelet concentrates and apheresis-derived platelet concentrates for the isolation and expansion of human bone marrow mesenchymal stromal cells: production process, content and identification of active components," *Cytotherapy*, vol. 14, no. 5, pp. 540–554, 2012.

[69] C. D. Luzzani and S. G. Miriuka, "Pluripotent stem cells as a robust source of mesenchymal stem cells," *Stem Cell Reviews*, vol. 13, no. 1, pp. 68–78, 2017.

[70] D. Klein, M. Benchellal, V. Kleff, H. G. Jakob, and S. Ergun, "Hox genes are involved in vascular wall-resident multipotent stem cell differentiation into smooth muscle cells," *Scientific Reports*, vol. 3, no. 1, article 2178, 2013.

[71] X. Meng, R. J. Su, D. J. Baylink et al., "Rapid and efficient reprogramming of human fetal and adult blood CD34$^+$ cells into mesenchymal stem cells with a single factor," *Cell Research*, vol. 23, no. 5, pp. 658–672, 2013.

[72] W. Chen, D. J. Baylink, K. H. William Lau, and X. B. Zhang, "Generation of mesenchymal stem cells by blood cell reprogramming," *Current Stem Cell Research & Therapy*, vol. 11, no. 2, pp. 114–121, 2016.

[73] P. L. Lai, H. Lin, S. F. Chen et al., "Efficient generation of chemically induced mesenchymal stem cells from human dermal fibroblasts," *Scientific Reports*, vol. 7, no. 1, article 44534, 2017.

[74] F. Gao, S. M. Chiu, D. A. L. Motan et al., "Mesenchymal stem cells and immunomodulation: current status and future prospects," *Cell Death & Disease*, vol. 7, no. 1, article e2062, 2016.

[75] Y. J. Jeon, J. Kim, J. H. Cho, H. M. Chung, and J. I. Chae, "Comparative analysis of human mesenchymal stem cells derived from bone marrow, placenta, and adipose tissue as sources of cell therapy," *Journal of Cellular Biochemistry*, vol. 117, no. 5, pp. 1112–1125, 2016.

[76] P. S. in 't Anker, W. A. Noort, S. A. Scherjon et al., "Mesenchymal stem cells in human second-trimester bone marrow, liver, lung, and spleen exhibit a similar immunophenotype but a heterogeneous multilineage differentiation potential," *Haematologica*, vol. 88, no. 8, pp. 845–852, 2003.

[77] A. Ribeiro, P. Laranjeira, S. Mendes et al., "Mesenchymal stem cells from umbilical cord matrix, adipose tissue and

bone marrow exhibit different capability to suppress peripheral blood B, natural killer and T cells," *Stem Cell Research & Therapy*, vol. 4, no. 5, p. 125, 2013.

[78] J. J. Montesinos, E. Flores-Figueroa, S. Castillo-Medina et al., "Human mesenchymal stromal cells from adult and neonatal sources: comparative analysis of their morphology, immunophenotype, differentiation patterns and neural protein expression," *Cytotherapy*, vol. 11, no. 2, pp. 163–176, 2009.

[79] S. J. Prasanna, D. Gopalakrishnan, S. R. Shankar, and A. B. Vasandan, "Pro-inflammatory cytokines, IFNγ and TNFα, influence immune properties of human bone marrow and Wharton jelly mesenchymal stem cells differentially," *PLoS One*, vol. 5, no. 2, article e9016, 2010.

[80] X. Wang, E. A. Kimbrel, K. Ijichi et al., "Human ESC-derived MSCs outperform bone marrow MSCs in the treatment of an EAE model of multiple sclerosis," *Stem Cell Reports*, vol. 3, no. 1, pp. 115–130, 2014.

[81] H. Wegmeyer, A. M. Bröske, M. Leddin et al., "Mesenchymal stromal cell characteristics vary depending on their origin," *Stem Cells and Development*, vol. 22, no. 19, pp. 2606–2618, 2013.

[82] Z.-Y. Zhang, S. H. Teoh, M. S. K. Chong et al., "Superior osteogenic capacity for bone tissue engineering of fetal compared with perinatal and adult mesenchymal stem cells," *Stem Cells*, vol. 27, no. 1, pp. 126–137, 2009.

[83] K. B. Ackema and J. Charite, "Mesenchymal stem cells from different organs are characterized by distinct topographic *Hox* codes," *Stem Cells and Development*, vol. 17, no. 5, pp. 979–992, 2008.

[84] B. Sági, P. Maraghechi, V. S. Urbán et al., "Positional identity of murine mesenchymal stem cells resident in different organs is determined in the postsegmentation mesoderm," *Stem Cells and Development*, vol. 21, no. 5, pp. 814–828, 2012.

[85] S. Liedtke, A. Buchheiser, J. Bosch et al., "The *HOX* code as a "biological fingerprint" to distinguish functionally distinct stem cell populations derived from cord blood," *Stem Cell Research*, vol. 5, no. 1, pp. 40–50, 2010.

[86] Z. Hamidouche, K. Rother, J. Przybilla et al., "Bistable epigenetic states explain age-dependent decline in mesenchymal stem cell heterogeneity," *Stem Cells*, vol. 35, no. 3, pp. 694–704, 2017.

[87] D. G. Phinney, "Functional heterogeneity of mesenchymal stem cells: implications for cell therapy," *Journal of Cellular Biochemistry*, vol. 113, no. 9, pp. 2806–2812, 2012.

[88] M. Baddoo, K. Hill, R. Wilkinson et al., "Characterization of mesenchymal stem cells isolated from murine bone marrow by negative selection," *Journal of Cellular Biochemistry*, vol. 89, no. 6, pp. 1235–1249, 2003.

[89] N. Tremain, J. Korkko, D. Ibberson, G. C. Kopen, C. DiGirolamo, and D. G. Phinney, "MicroSAGE analysis of 2,353 expressed genes in a single cell-derived colony of undifferentiated human mesenchymal stem cells reveals mRNAs of multiple cell lineages," *Stem Cells*, vol. 19, no. 5, pp. 408–418, 2001.

[90] D. Klein, A. Schmetter, R. Imsak et al., "Therapy with multipotent mesenchymal stromal cells protects lungs from radiation-induced injury and reduces the risk of lung metastasis," *Antioxidants & Redox Signaling*, vol. 24, no. 2, pp. 53–69, 2016.

[91] D. Klein, J. Steens, A. Wiesemann et al., "Mesenchymal stem cell therapy protects lungs from radiation-induced endothelial cell loss by restoring superoxide dismutase 1 expression," *Antioxidants & Redox Signaling*, vol. 26, no. 11, pp. 563–582, 2017.

[92] S. A. Doppler, M.-A. Deutsch, R. Lange, and M. Krane, "Direct reprogramming—the future of cardiac regeneration?," *International Journal of Molecular Sciences*, vol. 16, no. 8, pp. 17368–17393, 2015.

[93] P. S. Hou, C. Y. Chuang, C. H. Yeh et al., "Direct conversion of human fibroblasts into neural progenitors using transcription factors enriched in human ESC-derived neural progenitors," *Stem Cell Reports*, vol. 8, no. 1, pp. 54–68, 2017.

[94] D. Nakamori, H. Akamine, K. Takayama, F. Sakurai, and H. Mizuguchi, "Direct conversion of human fibroblasts into hepatocyte-like cells by ATF5, PROX1, FOXA2, FOXA3, and HNF4A transduction," *Scientific Reports*, vol. 7, no. 1, article 16675, 2017.

[95] M. B. Victor, M. Richner, H. E. Olsen et al., "Striatal neurons directly converted from Huntington's disease patient fibroblasts recapitulate age-associated disease phenotypes," *Nature Neuroscience*, vol. 21, no. 3, pp. 341–352, 2018.

[96] W. Wagner, S. Bork, P. Horn et al., "Aging and replicative senescence have related effects on human stem and progenitor cells," *PLoS One*, vol. 4, no. 6, article e5846, 2009.

[97] A. Stolzing, E. Jones, D. McGonagle, and A. Scutt, "Age-related changes in human bone marrow-derived mesenchymal stem cells: consequences for cell therapies," *Mechanisms of Ageing and Development*, vol. 129, no. 3, pp. 163–173, 2008.

[98] Z. Ghosh, K. D. Wilson, Y. Wu, S. Hu, T. Quertermous, and J. C. Wu, "Persistent donor cell gene expression among human induced pluripotent stem cells contributes to differences with human embryonic stem cells," *PLoS One*, vol. 5, no. 2, article e8975, 2010.

[99] M. Stadtfeld, E. Apostolou, H. Akutsu et al., "Aberrant silencing of imprinted genes on chromosome 12qF1 in mouse induced pluripotent stem cells," *Nature*, vol. 465, no. 7295, pp. 175–181, 2010.

[100] A. Urbach, O. Bar-Nur, G. Q. Daley, and N. Benvenisty, "Differential modeling of fragile X syndrome by human embryonic stem cells and induced pluripotent stem cells," *Cell Stem Cell*, vol. 6, no. 5, pp. 407–411, 2010.

[101] S. Hu, M. T. Zhao, F. Jahanbani et al., "Effects of cellular origin on differentiation of human induced pluripotent stem cell-derived endothelial cells," *JCI Insight*, vol. 1, no. 8, 2016.

5

Azithromycin Promotes the Osteogenic Differentiation of Human Periodontal Ligament Stem Cells after Stimulation with TNF-α

Tingting Meng,[1] Ying Zhou,[1] Jingkun Li,[1] Meilin Hu,[1] Xiaomeng Li,[2] Pingting Wang,[1] Zhi Jia,[1] Liyu Li ⓘ,[3] and Dayong Liu ⓘ[1]

[1]*Department of Endodontics & Laboratory of Stem Cells and Endocrine Immunology, Tianjin Medical University School of Stomatology, Tianjin 300070, China*
[2]*Department of Prosthodontics, Tianjin Medical University School of Stomatology, Tianjin 300070, China*
[3]*Department of Intensive Care Unit, The Second Hospital of Tianjin Medical University, Tianjin 300211, China*

Correspondence should be addressed to Liyu Li; tjydlly@126.com and Dayong Liu; dyliuperio@tmu.edu.cn

Academic Editor: Peter Zanvit

Background and Objective. This study investigated the effects and underlying mechanisms of azithromycin (AZM) treatment on the osteogenic differentiation of human periodontal ligament stem cells (PDLSCs) after their stimulation with TNF-α *in vitro.* *Methods.* PDLSCs were isolated from periodontal ligaments from extracted teeth, and MTS assay was used to evaluate whether AZM and TNF-α had toxic effects on PDLSCs viability and proliferation. After stimulating PDLSCs with TNF-α and AZM, we analyzed alkaline phosphatase staining, alkaline phosphatase activity, and alizarin red staining to detect osteogenic differentiation. Real-time quantitative polymerase chain reaction (RT-qPCR) analysis was performed to detect the mRNA expression of osteogenic-related genes, including *RUNX2, OCN,* and *BSP.* Western blotting was used to measure the NF-κB signaling pathway proteins p65, phosphorylated p65, IκB-α, phosphorylated IκB-α, and β-catenin as well as the apoptosis-related proteins caspase-8 and caspase-3. Annexin V assay was used to detect PDLSCs apoptosis. *Results.* TNF-α stimulation of PDLSCs decreased alkaline phosphatase and alizarin red staining, alkaline phosphatase activity, and mRNA expression of *RUNX2, OCN,* and *BSP* in osteogenic-conditioned medium. AZM enhanced the osteogenic differentiation of PDLSCs that were stimulated with TNF-α. Western blot analysis showed that β-catenin, phosphorated p65, and phosphorylated IκB-α protein expression decreased in PDLSCs treated with AZM. In addition, pretreatment of PDLSCs with AZM (10 μg/ml, 20 μg/ml) prevented TNF-α-induced apoptosis by decreasing caspase-8 and caspase-3 expression. *Conclusions.* Our results showed that AZM promotes PDLSCs osteogenic differentiation in an inflammatory microenvironment by inhibiting the WNT and NF-κB signaling pathways and by suppressing TNF-α-induced apoptosis. This suggests that AZM has potential as a clinical therapeutic for periodontitis.

1. Introduction

Periodontitis is a chronic infectious disease of the periodontal supportive tissues, and it is the main cause of tooth loss in adults. Its pathological manifestations include gingival and periodontal ligament inflammatory infiltration, periodontal pocket formation, progressive attachment loss, and alveolar bone destruction [1]. Growing evidence demonstrates the correlation between periodontitis and systemic disorders such as diabetes, cardiovascular diseases, preterm birth, and low birth weight [2, 3]. A recent report identified periodontal disease as a risk factor for non-Hodgkin lymphoma and colorectal cancer [4]. Etiological evidence shows that periodontal pathogens in the dental biofilm under the gingival epithelium are necessary but insufficient for periodontitis development. Accumulating evidence shows that host susceptibility rather than bacterial plaque leads to periodontal destruction. Indeed, the host inflammatory response plays an essential role in the pathogenesis of periodontitis [5, 6].

Mesenchymal stem cells (MSCs) were first isolated from bone marrow and possess self-renewal, colony-forming unit, and immunomodulation properties. Notably, MSCs can differentiate into osteoblasts, adipocytes, chondrocytes, and neural cells [7]. MSCs play important roles in tissue hemostasis and in maintaining the balance between effective and regulative immune cells [8], and impaired MSCs in bone marrow or in local tissue may cause disease. We demonstrated previously that MSCs derived from the periodontal ligament tissues of patients with periodontitis showed impaired differentiation and immunomodulation that contributed to the development of periodontal tissue destruction [9–11]. Recent reports indicate the close relationship between impaired MSCs and autoimmune or inflammatory diseases [12]. Indeed, MSC transplantation is a successful therapeutic strategy for treating autoimmune diseases such as SLE [13]; Sjögren syndrome, autoimmune diabetes, and airway inflammation [14]; systemic sclerosis [15]; and periodontitis [16–18]. However, the mechanisms underlying MSC deficiency in periodontitis remain poorly defined and it is unclear how to restore MSC function and achieve periodontal tissue regeneration in an inflammatory microenvironment.

Azithromycin (AZM) is a clinically available macrolide antibiotic like erythromycin A and clarithromycin [19]. In addition to their antimicrobial activity, macrolides can modulate the immune response and inflammation with no effects on homeostatic immunity [20]. In epithelial and immune cells, low-dose macrolides inhibit the secretion of proinflammatory cytokines and chemokines, including IL-6, IL-8, and TNF-α [21, 22]. They also suppress interferon gamma production by memory T cells [23]. CSY0073, an AZM derivative that lacks antibiotic activity, improves the clinical scores of dextran sulfate sodium- (DSS-) induced experimental colitis and collagen-induced arthritis [24]. AZM is reported to be transported into inflamed tissues in the periodontium. After 3 days of daily administration of a single dose of AZM (500 mg), AZM can be detected for up to 6.5 days in the plasma, saliva, and inflamed periodontal tissues of human subjects [25]. Although there are no definitive, controlled clinical studies on the effects of AZM on periodontitis, AZM elicits clinical and microbiological improvement when used in conjunction with nonsurgical periodontal therapy [26–30]. Moreover, one study reported that AZM suppresses human osteoclast differentiation and bone resorption [31]. However, it remains unclear whether AZM affects osteoblasts or the osteogenesis of MSCs in an inflammatory microenvironment.

This study isolated human periodontal ligament stem cells (PDLSCs) and stimulated them with the proinflammatory cytokine TNF-α in vitro. Osteogenic differentiation and cell viability were determined in order to investigate the effects and underlying mechanisms of AZM on the osteogenic differentiation of PDLSCs in an inflammatory microenvironment. Our results showed that AZM promoted PDLSCs osteogenic differentiation after TNF-α stimulation by inhibiting the WNT and NF-κB signaling pathways and by attenuating TNF-α-induced apoptosis.

2. Materials and Methods

2.1. Cell Culture. All researches involving human stem cells complied with the ISSCR "Guidelines for the Conduct of Human Embryonic Stem Cell Research." PDLSCs were isolated from healthy volunteers who had no history of periodontal diseases and who had relatively healthy periodontiums. All of the experiments followed the guidelines of the Tianjin Medical University School of Stomatology. We obtained written informed consent from all volunteers prior to collecting their cells. PDLSCs were isolated, cultured, and identified as described previously [32]. Generally, the middle one-third of the periodontal ligament was extracted from the surface of the tooth root and then subjected to a gradient wash. Next, the chopped tissues were digested in a solution of 3 mg/ml collagenase type I plus 4 mg/ml dispase (Sigma-Aldrich, St. Louis, MO, USA) for 1 h at 37°C.

The PDLSCs from all of the volunteers were pooled. A single-cell suspension was prepared by passing the cells through a 70 μm strainer (Falcon, BD Labware, Franklin Lakes, NJ, USA), and PDLCSs were plated in complete α-MEM (HyClone, Logan, UT, USA) plus 20% FBS (Gibco, Carlsbad, CA, USA), 100 U/ml penicillin, and 100 μg/ml streptomycin (Invitrogen, Carlsbad, CA, USA). The cells were cultured at 37°C in 5% carbon dioxide, and the culture medium was changed every 3 days. Passages 3–6 were used for the experiments. A total of 15 volunteers, aged 18 to 23 years old, provided informed written consent. PDLSCs were identified by flow cytometry using antibodies against STRO-1, CD90, CD45, and CD146. The details are described in the Supplementary Materials and Methods (available here).

2.2. MTS Assay. Cell viability was measured using an MTS assay (Promega, Madison, WI, USA). PDLSCs were seeded in 96-well plates at a density of 3×10^3 cells/well and cultured to approximately 80% confluence. TNF-α (20 ng/ml, 100 ng/ml) and AZM (1 μg/ml, 10 μg/ml, and 20 μg/ml) were added. The cells were cultured in osteogenic medium for 48 h at 37°C and then incubated for 3 h with MTS. The OD_{490} was measured using a microplate reader. The experiments, which had 7 replicates, were repeated at least 3 times.

2.3. Alizarin Red Staining and Quantitative Calcium Analysis. PDLSCs were fixed in 70% ethanol for 1 h and washed with deionized water. We added 40 mM alizarin red staining solution (pH 4.2) into the 6-well plates, incubated the cells at room temperature for 10 min, washed the cells with deionized water 5 times, viewed them under a microscope, and captured the images. For quantitative calcium analysis, the cells were treated with 10% cetylpyridinium chloride solution (Sigma-Aldrich) for 30 min at room temperature. The OD_{562} was used to quantify the degree of mineralization and calcium quantitative analysis for alizarin red staining was normalized to the total protein content before calculation. The experiments were repeated at least 3 times.

2.4. Alkaline Phosphatase Staining. PDLSCs were seeded in 6-well plates. In addition to the control conditions, there were 3 experimental conditions: 100 ng/ml TNF-α, 100 ng/ml TNF-α plus 10 μg/ml AZM, and 100 ng/ml TNF-α plus 20 μg/ml AZM. We examined osteogenesis at 7 days and acquired images. The alkaline phosphatase (ALP) activity assay is described in the Supplementary Materials and Methods.

2.5. Quantitative Real-Time PCR. Total RNA was isolated from PDLSCs using TRIzol reagent (Life Technologies, Carlsbad, CA, USA). We used oligo (dT) primers and reverse transcriptase to amplify cDNA according to the manufacturer's protocol (Invitrogen). RT-qPCR was performed using the SYBR Green PCR kit (Qiagen, Düsseldorf, Germany). Each reaction was repeated at least three times. Supplementary Table 1 shows the primers for specific genes.

2.6. Western Blot Analysis. Total proteins were extracted from PDLSCs by lysing the cells in RIPA buffer (10 mM Tris-HCl, 1 mM EDTA, 1% sodium dodecyl sulfate (SDS), 1% NP-40, 1 : 100 proteinase inhibitor cocktail, 50 mM β-glycerophosphate, and 50 mM sodium fluoride) and 1% PMSF. The proteins were separated on 10% and 12% SDS polyacrylamide gels and then electrotransferred to polyvinylidene fluoride (PVDF) membranes for 2 h at 300 mA. The membranes were incubated overnight with primary antibodies at 4°C. Primary monoclonal antibodies directed against the following were used in this study: phosphorylated p65, p65, phosphorylated IκB-α, IκB-α, the housekeeping protein glyceraldehyde phosphate dehydrogenase (GAPDH, Abcam, Cambridge, MA, USA), caspase-3, and caspase-8 (Cell Signaling Technology Inc.) Blots were then incubated with the secondary antibody (peroxidase-conjugated goat anti-rabbit; 1 : 1000, Abcam) for 2 h at room temperature. GAPDH was used as the internal control. Each experiment had three replicates and was repeated at least three times.

2.7. Cell Apoptosis Assay. Cells were seeded at a density of $2 \times 10^3/cm^2$. After treatment with 100 ng/ml TNF-α or 10 μg/ml AZM plus 20 μg/ml AZM for 24 h, PDLSCs were stained with annexin V-fluorescein isothiocyanate (FITC) and counterstained with propidium iodide (PI). The eBioscience™ annexin V-FITC Apoptosis Detection Kit (Life Technologies) was used. Briefly, cells were washed twice with phosphate-buffered saline (PBS) and then stained with 200 μl binding buffer (1x) and 5 μl annexin V-FITC for 10 min at room temperature in the dark. Finally, 10 μl of PI in 1x binding buffer was added to the cells for 5 minutes. The cells were analyzed using a fluorescence microscope.

2.8. Annexin V Apoptosis Assay. We washed 1×10^5 cells twice with PBS followed by centrifugation at 4°C at 2000 rpm for 5 minutes to collect cell pellets. The cell pellets were resuspended in 200 μl binding buffer (1x) and stained with 5 μl of annexin V-FITC for 10 min at room temperature in the dark, and then 10 μl PI in 1x binding buffer was added to the cell suspension. The cells were analyzed by fluorescence-activated cell sorting (FACs). Each experiment was performed in triplicate.

2.9. Statistical Analysis. The data are reported as means ± SD. We used one-way ANOVA for statistical analysis, and a P value < 0.05 was considered significant.

3. Results

3.1. TNF-α and AZM at Experimental Levels Had No Toxic Effects on PDLSC Viability or Proliferation. PDLSCs have an elongated spindle morphology (Figure S1). Flow cytometry results for biomarkers are shown in Figure S2. To investigate whether different concentrations of TNF-α and AZM affected cell proliferation and viability, we used MTS assay to compare the viability of PDLSCs cultured in osteogenic conditions versus PDLSCs treated with TNF-α and AZM (Figure S3). TNF-α was used at two concentrations (20 ng/ml, 100 ng/ml) and AZM at three concentrations (1 μg/ml, 10 μg/ml, and 20 μg/ml). TNF-α treatment alone tended to reduce the number of viable cells, although this reduction was not significant. Based on these results, we chose to use 20 ng/ml and 100 ng/ml TNF-α and 10 μg/ml and 20 μg/ml AZM as working concentrations for the subsequent experiments.

3.2. Effects of AZM on the Osteogenic Differentiation of PDLSCs. To investigate the effects of AZM on the osteogenic differentiation of PDLSCs, cells were cultured in osteogenic medium for 7 days. Experimental PDLSCs were treated with TNF-α (100 ng/ml) and AZM (10 μg/ml, 20 μg/ml). The ALP staining results (Figure 1) and alizarin red staining results (Figure 2) showed that AZM can restore the ability of PDLSCs to undergo osteogenic differentiation after the cells are impaired by TNF-α (100 ng/ml). Compared to control cells that underwent osteogenic induction, TNF-α treatment decreased staining and calcium nodule formation (Figure 2). Notably, TNF-α is a proinflammatory cytokine that contributes to bone loss in many different diseases. Until now, the mechanisms by which TNF-α inhibits osteogenic differentiation have been unclear and have been thought to be complex. In accordance with previous results, TNF-α reduced osteogenic differentiation and our data suggested that it decreased the number of calcium nodules that were formed as well (Figure 2(e)). Cotreatment of PDLSCs with TNF-α (100 ng/ml) and AZM (20 μg/ml) rescued the cells' ability to undergo osteogenesis compared with the TNF-α group, even though osteogenesis was lower than that for control cells. The higher the AZM concentration, the deeper the blue or red staining is. This suggests that AZM has a positive role in human PDLSC osteogenic differentiation, since cells underwent osteogenesis when they were cultured in the absence or presence of TNF-α and AZM for 0, 3, or 7 days.

Similar to the ALP staining and alizarin red staining results, analysis of ALP activity demonstrated that AZM caused PDLSCs to regain their osteogenic ability (Figure 1(g)). Remarkably, the cells that were treated with TNF-α alone clearly had fewer cells (Figures 1(b) and 2(b)). As the AZM concentration increased, the number of cells increased as well.

We speculated that AZM could promote osteogenesis and could partially restore PDLSC osteogenic capacity in an inflammatory microenvironment. To verify this, we assessed the mRNA expression of the osteogenic differentiation markers *OCN*, *BSP*, and *RUNX2* by real-time PCR (Figure 3). We found that AZM treatment promoted PDLSCs osteogenic differentiation and the mRNA expression of these genes in a dose-dependent manner (Figure 3(a)–3(f)). When cells were exposed to an inflammatory microenvironment (i.e., treated with TNF-α), the mRNA levels of *OCN*, *BSP*, and *RUNX2* were lower than those in control

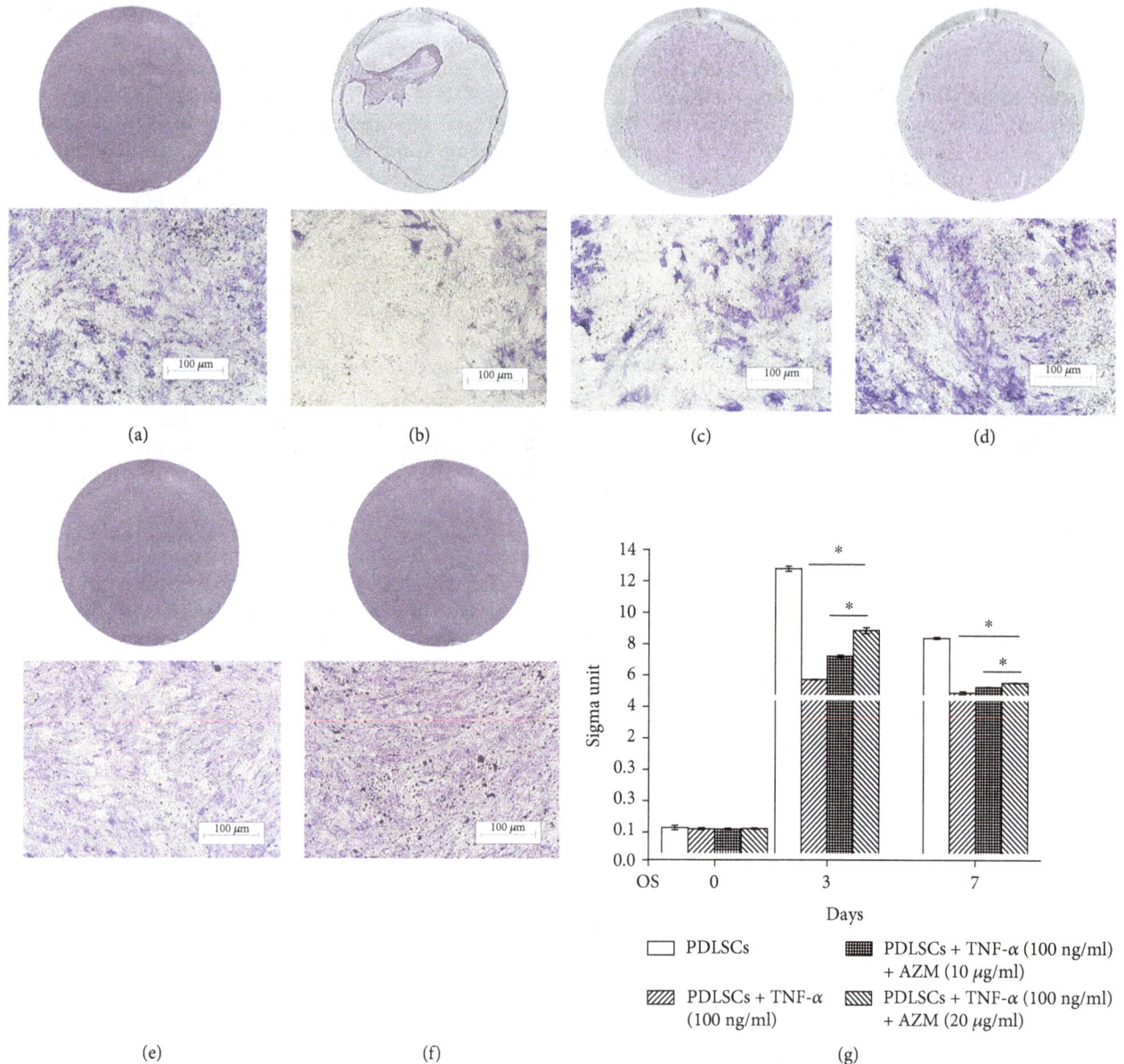

FIGURE 1: Analysis of alkaline phosphatase staining and alkaline phosphatase activity in human PDLSCs after treatment with AZM. (a–f) PDLSCs were cultured in osteogenic medium for 7 days. (a) Control PDLSCs cultured without any additions. (b) PDLSCs treated with TNF-α (100 ng/ml). (c) PDLSCs treated with TNF-α (100 ng/ml) and AZM (10 μg/ml). (d) PDLSCs treated with TNF-α (100 ng/ml) and AZM (20 μg/ml). (e) PDLSCs treated with AZM (10 μg/ml). (f) PDLSCs treated with AZM (20 μg/ml). (g) Alkaline phosphatase activity analysis. PDLSCs were induced to form osteoblasts for 0, 3, or 7 days. The results showed that AZM promoted the ability of PDLSCs to undergo osteogenesis differentiation. *$P < 0.05$ indicates significant differences. Data are presented as means $\pm$ SD.

($P < 0.05$). However, cotreatment with AZM restored the mRNA expression levels (Figure 3(a)–3(f)). The mRNA expression levels of *KDM2A*, *KDM2B*, and *EZH2* were higher in TNF-α-treated cells compared to control cells, and AZM mitigated this effect (Figure 3(g)–3(i)).

3.3. AZM Rescued the Osteogenic Potential of PDLSCs through the WNT and NF-κB Signaling Pathways.
In an inflammatory environment, NF-κB plays a vital role in the osteogenic differentiation of PDLSCs [33]. We next asked whether TNF-α-induced osteogenic inhibition could be partially reversed in the presence of AZM through the suppression of NF-κB signaling. Accordingly, we used Western blotting to analyze the expression of p65, phosphorylated p65, IκB-α, and phosphorylated IκB-α (Figure 4). After 7 days of osteogenic differentiation, TNF-α promoted the expression of phosphorylated p65 and phosphorylated IκB-α in PDLSCs compared with control. However, when PDLSCs were treated with both 100 ng/ml TNF-α and 20 μg/ml AZM, the levels of phosphorylated p65 and phosphorylated IκB-α were lower than those in cells treated with TNF-α alone. We also detected the levels of p65 and IκBα. The protein level is shown in Figure 4.

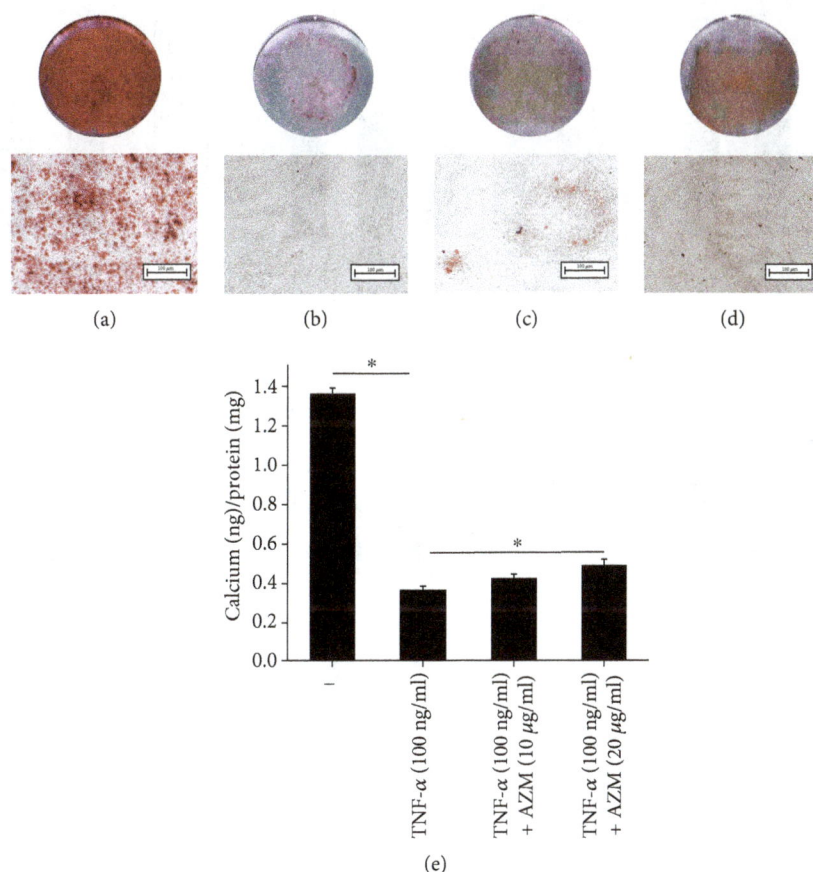

FIGURE 2: Alizarin red staining of human PDLSCs cultured in osteogenic media for 7 days. (a–d) PDLSCs cultured in osteogenic medium for 7 days. (a) Control PDLSCs cultured without any additions. (b) PDLSCs treated with TNF-α (100 ng/ml). (c) PDLSCs treated with TNF-α (100 ng/ml) and AZM (10 μg/ml). (d) PDLSCs treated with TNF-α (100 ng/ml) and AZM (20 μg/ml). (e) Detection of the calcium ion concentration and the calcium quantitative analysis for alizarin red staining were normalized to the total protein content before calculation. Increasing the AZM concentration significantly changed the number of calcium nodules. The results showed that AZM promoted the osteogenic differentiation of PDLSCs. $^*P < 0.05$ indicates significant differences. Data are presented as means $\pm$ SD.

Consistent with the ALP and alizarin staining results, TNF-α inhibited PDLSC osteogenic differentiation, while AZM partially reversed this effect and promoted PDLSC osteogenic differentiation. Phosphorylated p65 reflects the activation of the NF-κB signaling pathway. Thus, the results showed that AZM promoted osteogenic differentiation by suppressing the NF-κB signaling pathway. We then investigated whether WNT signaling plays a role in this process. We found that β-catenin expression increased after cells were treated with TNF-α. These results suggested that AZM promoted the osteogenic differentiation of PDLSCs in an inflammatory microenvironment by inhibiting the activation of the WNT and NF-κB signaling pathways.

3.4. AZM Promotes PDLSC Osteogenic Differentiation by Suppressing TNF-α-Induced Apoptosis.

TNF-α is a strong apoptosis-promoting factor. There were some indications that AZM might repress the TNF-α-induced apoptosis of PDLSCs, since ALP staining showed that TNF-α treatment alone reduced the number of viable cells and that cotreatment with TNF-α plus AZM mitigated this effect (Figures 1 and 2). To investigate the mechanism underlying this phenomenon, we tested whether AZM rescued PDLSC osteogenesis by

suppressing TNF-α-induced apoptosis. PDLSCs were seeded at a density of $2 \times 10^3/\text{cm}^2$ in 6-well plates with or without TNF-α (100 ng/ml) and AZM (10 μg/ml, 20 μg/ml) for 24 hours. Notably, 100 ng/ml TNF-α promoted PDLSCs apoptosis and AZM mitigated this process. In addition, AZM did not promote PDLSCs apoptosis. PI staining and FITC staining were used to follow apoptosis in PDLSCs undergoing osteogenic differentiation and showed that 10 μg/ml or 20 μg/ml AZM had no effect on apoptosis (Figure 5(a)).

In the caspase activation process, the caspase prodomain is cleaved and caspase proteins form a heterotetrameric enzyme in response to proteolytic activation. Next, protein downstream of caspase is activated, resulting in apoptosis [34, 35]. Caspase-8 is an initiator caspase, and caspase-3 is an effector caspase. To further investigate the mechanisms underlying the effects of AZM, we determined the protein levels of caspase-3, caspase-8, cleaved caspase-3, and cleaved caspase-8. The results demonstrated that after PDLSCs underwent osteogenic differentiation for 7 days, the protein levels of caspase-8 and cleaved caspase 3 were high in cells treated with TNF-α alone and lower when AZM was added (Figures 5(b) and 5(c)). PDLSCs treated with 10 μg/ml or

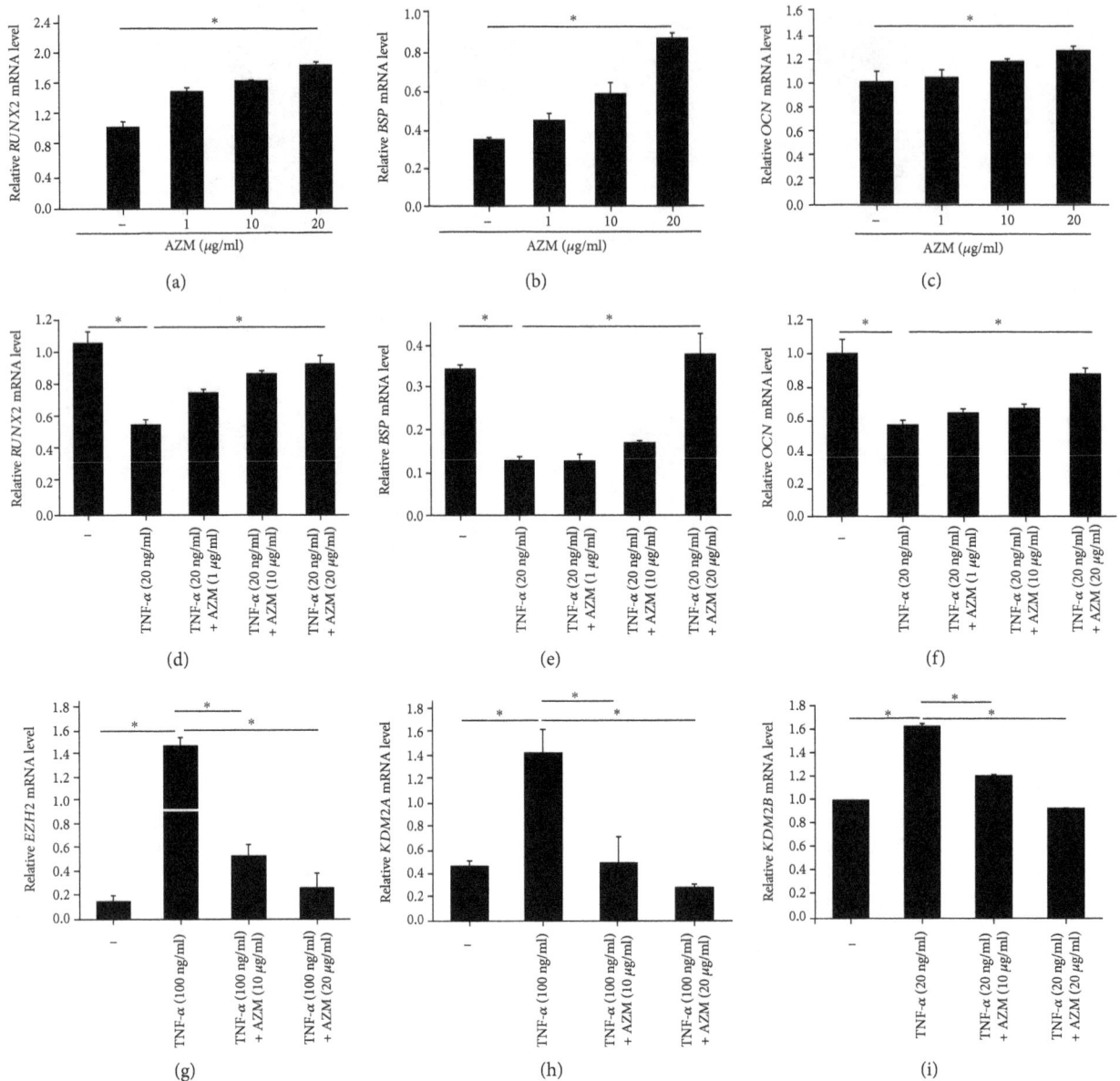

FIGURE 3: RT-qPCR analysis showed that AZM promotes the osteogenic differentiation of human PDLSCs and impacts the mRNA levels of epigenetic-related genes. Quantitative real-time PCR analysis of *RUNX2*, *BSP*, *OCN*, *KDM2A*, *KDM2B*, and *EZH2*. PDLSCs were treated with TNF-α and AZM as indicated. The top three images show the mRNA levels of (a) *RUNX2*, (b) *BSP*, and (c) *OCN* in cells treated with 1 μg/ml, 10 μg/ml, and 20 μg/ml AZM, respectively. The middle three images show the mRNA levels of (d) *RUNX2*, (e) *BSP*, and (f) *OCN* treated with 20 ng/ml TNF-α and 1 μg/ml, 10 μg/ml, or 20 μg/ml AZM. The mRNA levels of (g) *EZH2*, (h) *KDM2A*, and (i) *KDM2B* are shown in the bottom three images. PDLSCs were treated with 20 ng/ml TNF-α and 10 μg/ml AZM or with 20 ng/ml TNF-α and 20 μg/ml AZM. *$P < 0.05$ indicates significant differences. The data are presented as means $\pm$ SD.

20 μg/ml AZM (Figure 5(d)) showed no differences in the protein levels of caspase-3 and caspase-8.

Compared with levels in cells treated with 10 μg/ml AZM, the levels of cleaved caspase-3 and cleaved caspase-8 were higher in cells treated with 20 μg/ml AZM. It is possible that AZM promotes PDLSC differentiation. A more favorable cellular state can increase cell proliferation, although the MTS results showed no statistically significant differences in the proliferation of cells treated with AZM (Figure S3). Compared with cells treated with 10 μg/ml AZM, cells treated with 20 μg/ml AZM showed a slightly increased cell number. The level of apoptosis in cells treated with AZM was lower than in that cells treated with TNF-α and control cells (Figures 5(b) and 5(d)). AZM inhibited apoptosis in a dose-dependent manner (Figures 5(b) and 5(d)). To confirm if AZM promotes human PDLSC osteogenesis differentiation associated with the suppression of TNF-α-induced apoptosis, PDLSCs were cultured in basal medium and then cultured with or without TNF-α (100 ng/ml) and AZM (10 μg/ml, 20 μg/ml) for 24 hours. Annexin V-positive cells were detected by flow cytometry analysis. Moderate levels of TNF-α can promote apoptosis in PDLSCs, but AZM mitigated this effect. Compared with PDLSCs treated with TNF-α alone (Figure 6), the

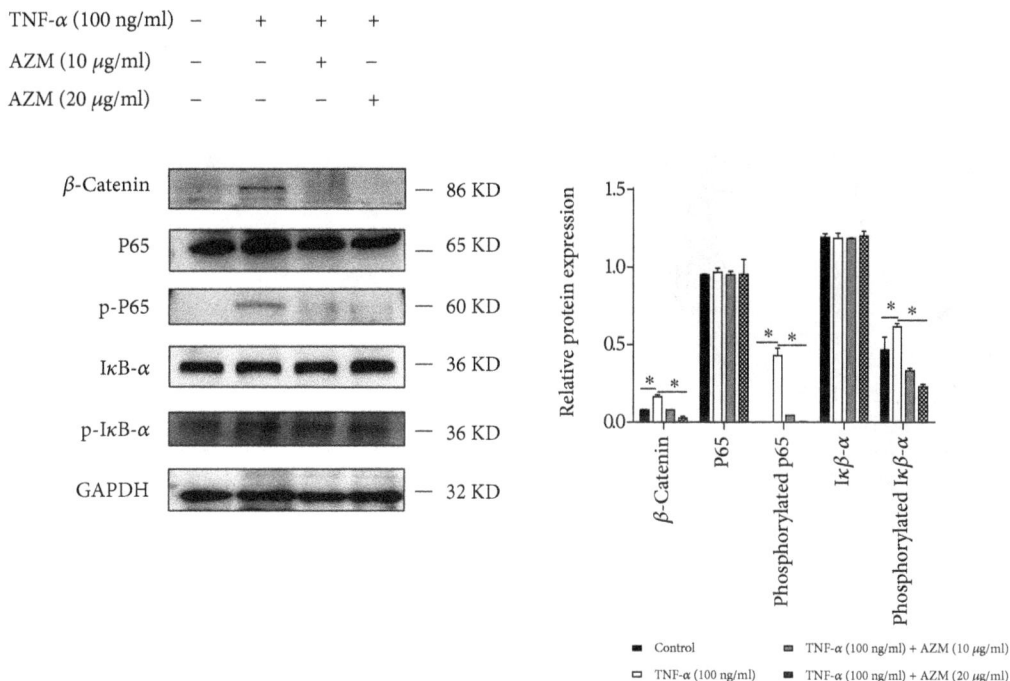

FIGURE 4: AZM restored the osteogenic potential of human PDLSCs through the WNT and NF-κB signaling pathways. PDLSCs were cultured in osteogenic medium and treated with 100 ng/ml TNF-α and AZM (10 μg/ml, 20 μg/ml) for 7 days. The protein levels of p65, phosphorylated p65, β-catenin, IκB-α, and phosphorylated IκB-α were detected by Western blot analysis. *$P < 0.05$ indicates significant differences. Data are presented as means ± SD.

apoptosis level decreased in the presence of AZM. Our data thus showed that AZM can block TNF-α-induced apoptosis.

Taken together, these data demonstrate that AZM promotes the osteogenic differentiation of PDLSCs by suppressing TNF-α-induced apoptosis.

4. Discussion

Periodontitis is a complex progressive inflammatory disease that is more prevalent in adults but also occurs in children and adolescents. Notably, periodontitis can lead to alveolar bone loss and systemic inflammation. Dysbiosis of the dental plaque, which interacts with the host immune defense, initiates periodontitis. Because the underlying mechanism is complex, it is challenging to repair bone loss and improve the deep periodontal pocket to achieve a satisfactory end result [9]. Bartold et al. demonstrated that dental plaque is essential but insufficient for periodontitis [4, 5, 36, 37]. AZM has anti-inflammatory properties and it is reported by several groups [38, 39]. Here, we found that AZM can reverse bone loss and suppress PDLSC apoptosis. PDLSCs that can differentiate into osteoblasts show great potential for treating patients with periodontitis.

TNF-α is a strong apoptosis inducer and a proinflammatory cytokine that contributes to bone loss in local and systemic inflammatory bone diseases [40]. TNF-α inhibits the expression of the osteogenic-related gene *Runx2* in two ways. First, it suppresses *Runx2* gene expression. Second, it promotes *Runx2* degradation [41]. Our data provide

evidence that AZM promotes PDLSCs osteogenic differentiation in an inflammatory microenvironment.

This study had four major findings. First, PDLSCs osteogenesis was strikingly inhibited by TNF-α and clearly enhanced by AZM. Second, Western blot analysis showed that TNF-α increased the expression of phosphorylated p65, phosphorylated IκB-α, and β-catenin. In contrast, the levels of these proteins were inhibited by AZM in a concentration-dependent manner. Third, stimulation with TNF-α activated the cleaved caspase-3 protein and AZM reversed the TNF-α-induced apoptosis of PDLSCs. Fourth, flow cytometry analysis showed that moderate concentrations of TNF-α promoted PDLSC apoptosis and that AZM mitigated this process. Our finding that AZM can inhibit the apoptosis of PDLSCs is consistent with the work of Mizunoe et al. [42] and Stamatiou et al. [43].

Our data shed light on the mechanisms by which AZM promotes osteogenesis. When trimeric TNF-α binds to TNFR1, the TNFR1-associated death domain protein (TRADD) is recruited to TNFR1. TRADD then acts as a bridge to recruit other apoptosis-related proteins, such as receptor-interacting protein (RIP), TNF receptor-associated factor 2 (TRAF2), and the Fas-associated death domain protein (FADD). Next, the integration of TRAF2 and RIP leads to the recruitment of the IKK complex. Intriguingly, phosphorylated-IκBα is then degraded and this activates the NF-κB signaling pathway and mediates cell apoptosis. TNF-α can trigger cell apoptosis in another way, that is, via the caspase pathway. This pathway involves FADD, caspase-8, and caspase-3. Caspase-3 activation allows it to cleave related proteins and results in

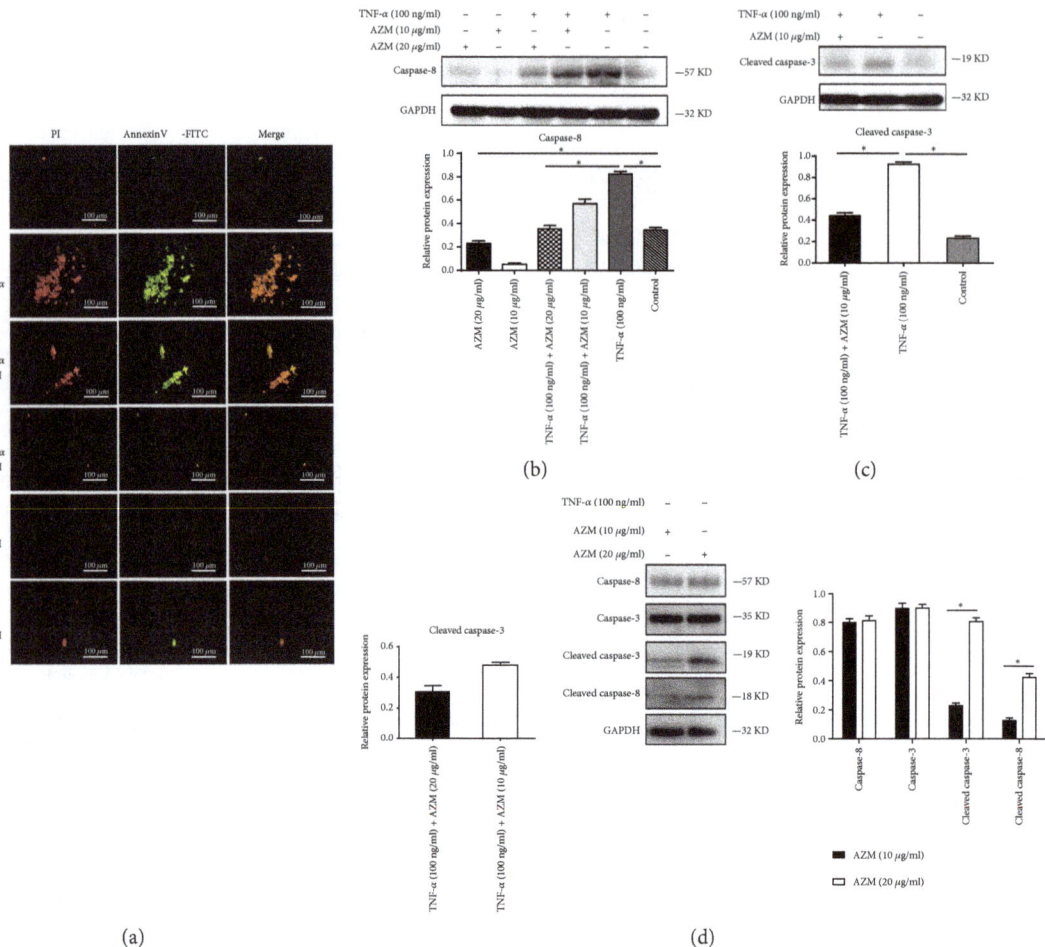

FIGURE 5: Immunocytochemical staining and the expression levels of the apoptosis proteins caspase-3 and caspase-8 in human PDLSCs. (a) Immunofluorescence staining. PDLSCs were incubated in osteogenic medium with or without TNF-α and AZM as indicated for 24 h. (b–d) The expression levels of caspase-3, caspase-8, cleaved caspase-3, and cleaved caspase-8 were detected by Western blot analysis. The results showed that TNF-α induced cell apoptosis and that AZM treatment prevented PDLSCs from undergoing TNF-α-induced apoptosis. AZM alone at 10 or 20 μg/ml had no effect on apoptosis. $^*P < 0.05$ indicates significant differences. Data are presented as means ± SD.

cell death [34]. AZM blocks bone loss induced by TNF-α in two ways. First, it suppresses the activation of NF-κB signaling, and second, it inhibits the cleavage of caspase family proteins.

Increasing evidence shows that the WNT pathway plays an important role in bone metabolism. There are two WNT signaling pathways: the canonical pathway, termed the WNT/β-catenin pathway, and the noncanonical WNT/Ca^{2+} pathway. The activation state of β-catenin is central in the WNT/β-catenin pathway. When WNT proteins bind to Frizzled receptors, β-catenin is activated and accumulates in the cytoplasm. Stable β-catenin is transported into the nucleus and mediates the transcription of downstream genes ([44], Huang, and [45–47]). Notably, high expression of β-catenin decreased the mRNA expression of *Runx2*, *COL1*, and *OCN* in PDLSCs extracted from an inflammatory microenvironment. Some researchers asserted that high β-catenin expression decreases osteogenesis via the noncanonical pathway, while others considered this to occur via the canonical pathway [47, 48]. Because we examined the protein expression of β-catenin, we do not know which

pathway AZM inhibits and additional experiments are needed to determine the precise mechanism.

Epigenetic regulation of gene expression is heritable and reversible. The DNA sequence is not altered in epigenetics; rather, there is methylation of lysine or arginine residues in the histone tails. The methylated lysine residues are considered epigenetic signals that may be related to gene activation, as for methylation at H3K4 and H3K36, or to gene repression, as for methylation at H3K9 and H3K27 [49, 50]. The histone lysine demethylases (KDMs) KDM2A and KDM2B demethylate H3K4me3 and H3K36me1/2 [50]. KDM2B plays an important role in BCOR mutation-associated diseases [51]. Moreover, the interactions between KDM2A and BCOR can inhibit osteogenesis by suppressing epiregulin (EREG) gene transcription, which is required for the expression of osterix (OSX) and distal-less homeobox 5 (DLX5) [52]. Our results are consistent with these reports.

KDM2B is a component of the noncanonical PRC1 (polycomb repressive complex 1), and it recruits Ring1B and Nspc1 to promote H2AK119 monoubiquitylation [53].

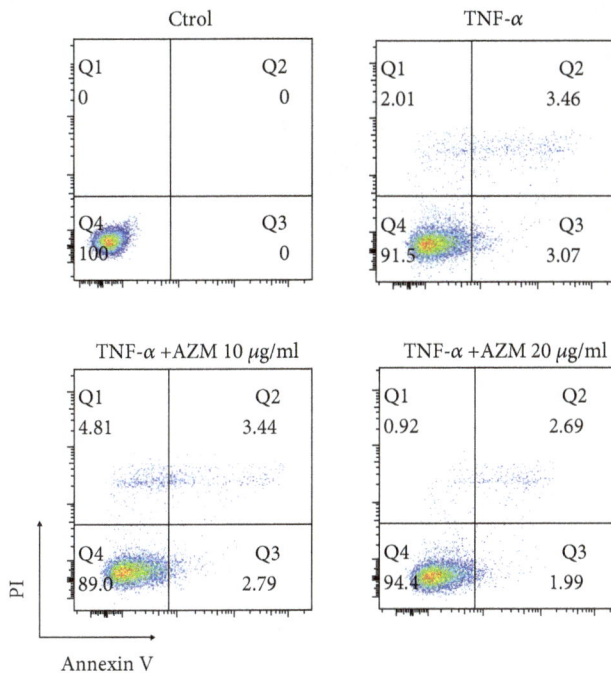

FIGURE 6: Detection of apoptosis in human PDLSCs by flow cytometry. PDLSCs were cultured in standard medium and treated with 100 ng/ml TNF-α and 10 μg/ml or 20 μg/ml AZM as indicated for 24 h. Apoptosis was detected using annexin V apoptosis assay.

The recruited Ring1B may interact with RNA polymerase II (RNAPII), leading to a bivalent state [54]. KDM2B localizes to regions where H3K36me2 levels are low. TNF-α stimulation promotes the removal of the dimethyl markers at H3K36 and inhibits osteogenic-related gene transcription. EZH2, a member of PRC2 (polycomb repressive complex 2), is a type of histone lysine methyltransferase (KMT). EZH2 mainly catalyzes H3K27 trimethyl markers. The canonical PRC1 complex is recruited to the appropriate locations by PRC2, which can recognize H3K27me3 [55]. EZH2 has been known for decades to be a negative mediator of MSC osteogenesis, which is in accordance with our findings. AZM may promote osteogenesis through three ways. First, it can block PRC1 binding to the H2AK119ub promoter and then decrease the level of H2AK119ub. Second, it can increase the level of H3K36me2 and then promote gene transcription. Third, it can decrease the level of H3K27me3 downstream genes.
and reduce the recruitment of PRC2, which can inhibit transcription inhibition and promote the expression of

Periodontal diseases contribute to the formation of a complex inflammatory microenvironment. This study showed that AZM has potential as a new drug for treating periodontal diseases. Although AZM cannot completely reverse bone loss, it is likely to be helpful to have some insights into the putative effects of AZM on periodontal diseases. There may be additional mechanisms involved that we did not explore here. In a TNF-α-induced inflam-

matory microenvironment, we detected the expression of osteoblast-specific genes and cell apoptosis in vitro, and we concluded that AZM promotes the osteogenic differentiation of PDLSCs in an inflammatory microenvironment by inhibiting the WNT and NF-κB signaling pathways and the process associated with suppression of TNF-α-induced apoptosis. This study has some limitations. In particular, this was an in vitro study; animal studies were not conducted. Further experiments focusing on tissue regeneration are needed to better model the environment in humans.

In summary, our study suggested that AZM has potential as a new drug to treat periodontitis diseases and offered some insights into AZM and epigenetics. Further experiments are needed to investigate AZM as a therapeutic drug for periodontitis and bone tissue regeneration.

5. Conclusion

Our results showed that AZM promotes PDLSCs osteogenic differentiation in response to TNF-α stimulation by inhibiting the WNT and NF-κB signaling pathways and by attenuating TNF-α-induced apoptosis.

Abbreviations

BSP:	Bone sialoprotein
EZH2:	Enhancer of zeste homolog 2
FBS:	Fetal bovine serum
FITC:	Fluorescein isothiocyanate
KDM2A:	Lysine-specific demethylase 2A
KDM2B:	Lysine-specific demethylase 2B
OCN:	Osteocalcin
PI:	Propidium iodide
Runx2:	Runt-related transcription factor 2.

Authors' Contributions

Tingting Meng, Ying Zhou, Jingkun Li, Xiaomeng Li, and Pingting Wang performed the collection and/or assembly of data; Tingting Meng and Meilin Hu wrote the manuscript; Zhi Jia, Liyu Li, Dayong Liu performed the data analysis and interpretation; Zhi Jia, Liyu Li and Dayong Liu provided financial support; Dayong Liu performed the conception and design and final approval of the manuscript. Tingting Meng and Ying Zhou contributed equally to this work as first authors. Dayong Liu contributed as lead contact.

Acknowledgments

The authors thank Professor Xudong Wu of Tianjin Medical University for his expert help with data interpretation and the discussion section of the manuscript. This work was supported by grants from the National Natural Science

Foundation of China (81371109 and 81670953 to Dayong Liu), by a grant from Beijing Key Laboratory of Tooth Regeneration and Function Reconstruction Open Project (2014QYZS02 to Dayong Liu), by a grant from the Natural Science Foundation of Tianjin City (15JCYBJC50200 to Zhi Jia), and by the Science Foundation of Tianjin Medical University (2015KYZM11 to Pingting Wang).

Supplementary Materials

The experimental section of alkaline phosphatase (ALP) activity assay and flow cytometric analysis were in the supplementary materials, and primers for specific genes sequences and the supplementary figures were also included. Supplementary Table 1: primers for gene sequences. Fig. S1: the image of PDLSCs under a 10x microscope. PDLSCs have the elongated spindle morphology. Fig. S2: PDLSCs cultured in normal medium. Flow cytometric analysis of PDLSCs showed positive expression of cell markers STRO-1, CD90, and CD146 and negative results for CD45. Fig. S3: appropriate TNF-α and azithromycin have no overt toxic effect on cell viability and proliferation of PDLSCs. Cell viability was measured using MTS assay; there are no significant difference between the 12 groups. (Supplementary Materials)

References

[1] G. C. Armitage, "Learned and unlearned concepts in periodontal diagnostics: a 50-year perspective," *Periodontology 2000*, vol. 62, no. 1, pp. 20–36, 2013.

[2] A. Khocht and J. M. Albandar, "Aggressive forms of periodontitis secondary to systemic disorders," *Periodontology 2000*, vol. 65, no. 1, pp. 134–148, 2014.

[3] D. F. Kinane and P. Mark Bartold, "Clinical relevance of the host responses of periodontitis," *Periodontology 2000*, vol. 43, no. 1, pp. 278–293, 2007.

[4] M. K. Barton, "Evidence accumulates indicating periodontal disease as a risk factor for colorectal cancer or lymphoma," *CA: A Cancer Journal for Clinicians*, vol. 67, no. 3, pp. 173–174, 2017.

[5] P. M. Bartold and T. E. Van Dyke, "Periodontitis: a host-mediated disruption of microbial homeostasis. Unlearning learned concepts," *Periodontology*, vol. 62, no. 1, pp. 203–217, 2013.

[6] R. C. Page and H. E. Schroeder, "Pathogenesis of inflammatory periodontal disease. A summary of current work," *Laboratory Investigation*, vol. 34, no. 3, pp. 235–249, 1976.

[7] A. J. Friedenstein, R. K. Chailakhjan, and K. S. Lalykina, "The development of fibroblast colonies in monolayer cultures of guinea-pig bone marrow and spleen cells," *Cell and Tissue Kinetics*, vol. 3, no. 4, pp. 393–403, 1970.

[8] Y. Wang, X. Chen, W. Cao, and Y. Shi, "Plasticity of mesenchymal stem cells in immunomodulation: pathological and therapeutic implications," *Nature Immunology*, vol. 15, no. 11, pp. 1009–1016, 2014.

[9] Z. Jia, Y. Wang, Y. Xu et al., "Aberrant gene expression profiles and related pathways in chronic periodontitis," *International Journal of Clinical & Experimental Medicine*, vol. 9, no. 11, 2016.

[10] D. Liu, Y. Wang, Z. Jia et al., "Demethylation of *IGFBP5* by histone demethylase KDM6B promotes mesenchymal stem cell-mediated periodontal tissue regeneration by enhancing osteogenic differentiation and anti-inflammation potentials," *Stem Cells*, vol. 33, no. 8, pp. 2523–2536, 2015.

[11] D. Liu, J. Xu, O. Liu et al., "Mesenchymal stem cells derived from inflamed periodontal ligaments exhibit impaired immunomodulation," *Journal of Clinical Periodontology*, vol. 39, no. 12, pp. 1174–1182, 2012.

[12] J. Xu, D. Wang, D. Liu et al., "Allogeneic mesenchymal stem cell treatment alleviates experimental and clinical Sjogren syndrome," *Blood*, vol. 120, no. 15, pp. 3142–3151, 2012.

[13] L. Sun, K. Akiyama, H. Zhang et al., "Mesenchymal stem cell transplantation reverses multiorgan dysfunction in systemic lupus erythematosus mice and humans," *Stem Cells*, vol. 27, no. 6, pp. 1421–1432, 2009.

[14] D. Zhang, C. Chia, X. Jiao et al., "D-mannose induces regulatory T cells and suppresses immunopathology," *Nature Medicine*, vol. 23, no. 9, pp. 1036–1045, 2017.

[15] K. Akiyama, C. Chen, D. Wang et al., "Mesenchymal-stem-cell-induced immunoregulation involves FAS-ligand-/FAS-mediated T cell apoptosis," *Cell Stem Cell*, vol. 10, no. 5, pp. 544–555, 2012.

[16] G. Ding, Y. Liu, W. Wang et al., "Allogeneic periodontal ligament stem cell therapy for periodontitis in swine," *Stem Cells*, vol. 28, no. 10, pp. 1829–1838, 2010.

[17] O. Liu, J. Xu, G. Ding et al., "Periodontal ligament stem cells regulate B lymphocyte function via programmed cell death protein 1," *Stem Cells*, vol. 31, no. 7, pp. 1371–1382, 2013.

[18] Y. Liu, Y. Zheng, G. Ding et al., "Periodontal ligament stem cell-mediated treatment for periodontitis in miniature swine," *Stem Cells*, vol. 26, no. 4, pp. 1065–1073, 2008.

[19] D. J. Payne, M. N. Gwynn, D. J. Holmes, and D. L. Pompliano, "Drugs for bad bugs: confronting the challenges of antibacterial discovery," *Nature Reviews Drug Discovery*, vol. 6, no. 1, pp. 29–40, 2007.

[20] M. Shinkai, M. O. Henke, and B. K. Rubin, "Macrolide antibiotics as immunomodulatory medications: proposed mechanisms of action," *Pharmacology & Therapeutics*, vol. 117, no. 3, pp. 393–405, 2008.

[21] M. Bosnar, B. Bosnjak, S. Cuzic et al., "Azithromycin and clarithromycin inhibit lipopolysaccharide-induced murine pulmonary neutrophilia mainly through effects on macrophage-derived granulocyte-macrophage colony-stimulating factor and interleukin-1β," *The Journal of Pharmacology and Experimental Therapeutics*, vol. 331, no. 1, pp. 104–113, 2009.

[22] M. Yasutomi, Y. Ohshima, N. Omata et al., "Erythromycin differentially inhibits lipopolysaccharide- or poly(I:C)-induced but not peptidoglycan-induced activation of human monocyte-derived dendritic cells," *Journal of Immunology*, vol. 175, no. 12, pp. 8069–8076, 2005.

[23] C. Pragnell and R. Wilson, "Fabricated or induced illness in children. Open mind is needed regarding origins of childhood symptoms and illnesses," *BMJ*, vol. 324, no. 7329, p. 114, 2002.

[24] A. Mencarelli, E. Distrutti, B. Renga et al., "Development of non-antibiotic macrolide that corrects inflammation-driven immune dysfunction in models of inflammatory bowel diseases and arthritis," *European Journal of Pharmacology*, vol. 665, no. 1–3, pp. 29–39, 2011.

[25] C. Blandizzi, T. Malizia, A. Lupetti et al., "Periodontal tissue disposition of azithromycin in patients affected by chronic inflammatory periodontal diseases," *Journal of Periodontology*, vol. 70, no. 9, pp. 960–966, 1999.

[26] S. L. Buset, N. U. Zitzmann, R. Weiger, and C. Walter, "Non-surgical periodontal therapy supplemented with systemically administered azithromycin: a systematic review of RCTs," *Clinical Oral Investigations*, vol. 19, no. 8, pp. 1763–1775, 2015.

[27] X. Feng and J. Liu, "A combination of irsogladine maleate and azithromycin exhibits addictive protective effects in LPS-induced human gingival epithelial cells," *Pharmazie*, vol. 72, no. 2, pp. 91–94, 2017.

[28] L. Gershenfeld, A. Kalos, T. Whittle, and S. Yeung, "Randomized clinical trial of the effects of azithromycin use in the treatment of Peri-implantitis," *Australian Dental Journal*, vol. 63, no. 3, pp. 374–381, 2018.

[29] T. Miyagawa, T. Fujita, H. Yumoto et al., "Azithromycin recovers reductions in barrier function in human gingival epithelial cells stimulated with tumor necrosis factor-α," *Archives of Oral Biology*, vol. 62, pp. 64–69, 2016.

[30] M. Nafar, R. Ataie, B. Einollahi, F. Nematizadeh, A. Firoozan, and F. Poorrezagholi, "A comparison between the efficacy of systemic and local azithromycin therapy in treatment of cyclosporine induced gingival overgrowth in kidney transplant patients," *Transplantation Proceedings*, vol. 35, no. 7, pp. 2727-2728, 2003.

[31] S. C. Gannon, M. D. Cantley, D. R. Haynes, R. Hirsch, and P. M. Bartold, "Azithromycin suppresses human osteoclast formation and activity in vitro," *Journal of Cellular Physiology*, vol. 228, no. 5, pp. 1098–1107, 2013.

[32] B.-M. Seo, M. Miura, S. Gronthos et al., "Investigation of multipotent postnatal stem cells from human periodontal ligament," *The Lancet*, vol. 364, no. 9429, pp. 149–155, 2004.

[33] J. Chang, F. Liu, M. Lee et al., "NF-κB inhibits osteogenic differentiation of mesenchymal stem cells by promoting β-catenin degradation," *Proceedings of the National Academy of Sciences of the United States of America*, vol. 110, no. 23, pp. 9469–9474, 2013.

[34] V. Baud and M. Karin, "Signal transduction by tumor necrosis factor and its relatives," *Trends in Cell Biology*, vol. 11, no. 9, pp. 372–377, 2001.

[35] W. C. Earnshaw, L. M. Martins, and S. H. Kaufmann, "Mammalian caspases: structure, activation, substrates, and functions during apoptosis," *Annual Review of Biochemistry*, vol. 68, no. 1, pp. 383–424, 1999.

[36] K. A. Bertrand, J. Shingala, A. Evens, B. M. Birmann, E. Giovannucci, and D. S. Michaud, "Periodontal disease and risk of non-Hodgkin lymphoma in the health professionals follow-up study," *International Journal of Cancer*, vol. 140, no. 5, pp. 1020–1026, 2017.

[37] P. Mark Bartold and T. E. Van Dyke, "Host modulation: controlling the inflammation to control the infection," *Periodontology 2000*, vol. 75, no. 1, pp. 317–329, 2017.

[38] F. Tang, R. Li, J. Xue et al., "Azithromycin attenuates acute radiation-induced lung injury in mice," *Oncology Letters*, vol. 14, no. 5, pp. 5211–5220, 2017.

[39] Y. F. Wan, Z. H. Huang, K. Jing et al., "Azithromycin attenuates pulmonary inflammation and emphysema in smoking-induced COPD model in rats," *Respiratory Care*, vol. 60, no. 1, pp. 128–134, 2015.

[40] A. Annibaldi and P. Meier, "Checkpoints in TNF-induced cell death: implications in inflammation and cancer," *Trends in Molecular Medicine*, vol. 24, no. 1, pp. 49–65, 2018.

[41] H. Kaneki, R. Guo, D. Chen et al., "Tumor necrosis factor promotes Runx2 degradation through up-regulation of Smurf1 and Smurf2 in osteoblasts," *Journal of Biological Chemistry*, vol. 281, no. 7, pp. 4326–4333, 2006.

[42] S. Mizunoe, J. Kadota, I. Tokimatsu, K. Kishi, H. Nagai, and M. Nasu, "Clarithromycin and azithromycin induce apoptosis of activated lymphocytes via down-regulation of Bcl-xL," *International Immunopharmacology*, vol. 4, no. 9, pp. 1201–1207, 2004.

[43] R. Stamatiou, K. Boukas, E. Paraskeva, P. A. Molyvdas, and A. Hatziefthimiou, "Azithromycin reduces the viability of human bronchial smooth muscle cells," *The Journal of Antibiotics*, vol. 63, no. 2, pp. 71–75, 2010.

[44] R. Nusse, "Wnt signaling," *Cold Spring Harbor Perspectives in Biology*, vol. 4, no. 5, 2012.

[45] M. D. Gordon and R. Nusse, "Wnt signaling: multiple pathways, multiple receptors, and multiple transcription factors," *Journal of Biological Chemistry*, vol. 281, no. 32, pp. 22429–22433, 2006.

[46] H. Huang and X. He, "Wnt/β-catenin signaling: new (and old) players and new insights," *Current Opinion in Cell Biology*, vol. 20, no. 2, pp. 119–125, 2008.

[47] N. Liu, S. Shi, M. Deng et al., "High levels of β-catenin signaling reduce osteogenic differentiation of stem cells in inflammatory microenvironments through inhibition of the noncanonical Wnt pathway," *Journal of Bone and Mineral Research*, vol. 26, no. 9, pp. 2082–2095, 2011.

[48] W. Liu, A. Konermann, T. Guo, A. Jager, L. Zhang, and Y. Jin, "Canonical Wnt signaling differently modulates osteogenic differentiation of mesenchymal stem cells derived from bone marrow and from periodontal ligament under inflammatory conditions," *Biochimica et Biophysica Acta (BBA) - General Subjects*, vol. 1840, no. 3, pp. 1125–1134, 2014.

[49] A. J. Bannister and T. Kouzarides, "Regulation of chromatin by histone modifications," *Cell Research*, vol. 21, no. 3, pp. 381–395, 2011.

[50] P. Deng, Q. M. Chen, C. Hong, and C. Y. Wang, "Histone methyltransferases and demethylases: regulators in balancing osteogenic and adipogenic differentiation of mesenchymal stem cells," *International Journal of Oral Science*, vol. 7, no. 4, pp. 197–204, 2015.

[51] Z. Fan, T. Yamaza, J. S. Lee et al., "BCOR regulates mesenchymal stem cell function by epigenetic mechanisms," *Nature Cell Biology*, vol. 11, no. 8, pp. 1002–1009, 2009.

[52] J. Du, Y. Ma, P. Ma, S. Wang, and Z. Fan, "Demethylation of epiregulin gene by histone demethylase FBXL11 and BCL6 corepressor inhibits osteo/dentinogenic differentiation," *Stem Cells*, vol. 31, no. 1, pp. 126–136, 2013.

[53] X. Wu, J. V. Johansen, and K. Helin, "Fbxl10/Kdm2b recruits polycomb repressive complex 1 to CpG islands and regulates H2A ubiquitylation," *Molecular Cell*, vol. 49, no. 6, pp. 1134–1146, 2013.

[54] E. Brookes, I. de Santiago, D. Hebenstreit et al., "Polycomb associates genome-wide with a specific RNA polymerase II variant, and regulates metabolic genes in ESCs," *Cell Stem Cell*, vol. 10, no. 2, pp. 157–170, 2012.

[55] A. Sparmann and M. van Lohuizen, "Polycomb silencers control cell fate, development and cancer," *Nature Reviews Cancer*, vol. 6, no. 11, pp. 846–856, 2006.

6

Type III Transforming Growth Factor-β Receptor RNA Interference Enhances Transforming Growth Factor β3-Induced Chondrogenesis Signaling in Human Mesenchymal Stem Cells

Shuhui Zheng,[1] Hang Zhou (ID),[2] Zhuohui Chen,[3] Yongyong Li (ID),[1] Taifeng Zhou (ID),[2] Chengjie Lian (ID),[4] Bo Gao (ID),[4] Peiqiang Su (ID),[2] and Caixia Xu (ID)[1]

[1]Research Center for Translational Medicine, The First Affiliated Hospital of Sun Yat-sen University, Guangzhou, China
[2]Department of Orthopedic Surgery, The First Affiliated Hospital of Sun Yat-sen University, Guangzhou, China
[3]Oral and Maxillofacial Surgery, Guanghua School of Stomatology, Hospital of Stomatology, Sun Yat-sen University, Guangzhou, China
[4]Department of Spine Surgery, Sun Yat-Sen Memorial Hospital, Sun Yat-sen University, Guangzhou, China

Correspondence should be addressed to Peiqiang Su; supq@mail.sysu.edu.cn and Caixia Xu; xucx3@mail.sysu.edu.cn

Academic Editor: Kar Wey Yong

The type III transforming growth factor-β (TGF-β) receptor (TβRIII), a coreceptor of the TGF-β superfamily, is known to bind TGF-βs and regulate TGF-β signaling. However, the regulatory roles of TβRIII in TGF-β-induced mesenchymal stem cell (MSC) chondrogenesis have not been explored. The present study examined the effect of TβRIII RNA interference (RNAi) on TGF-β3-induced human MSC (hMSC) chondrogenesis and possible signal mechanisms. A lentiviral expression vector containing TβRIII small interfering RNA (siRNA) (SiTβRIII) or a control siRNA (SiNC) gene was constructed and infected into hMSCs. The cells were cultured in chondrogenic medium containing TGF-β3 or control medium. TβRIII RNAi significantly enhanced TGF-β3-induced chondrogenic differentiation of hMSCs, the ratio of type II (TβRII) to type I (TβRI) TGF-β receptors, and phosphorylation levels of Smad2/3 as compared with cells infected with SiNC. An inhibitor of the TGF-β signal, SB431542, not only inhibited TβRIII RNAi-stimulated TGF-β3-mediated Smad2/3 phosphorylation but also inhibited the effects of TβRIII RNAi on TGF-β3-induced chondrogenic differentiation. These results demonstrate that TβRIII RNAi enhances TGF-β3-induced chondrogenic differentiation in hMSCs by activating TGF-β/Smad2/3 signaling. The finding points to the possibility of modifying MSCs by TβRIII knockdown as a potent future strategy for cell-based cartilage tissue engineering.

1. Introduction

Cell-based cartilage tissue engineering provides a feasible way of regenerating damaged cartilage tissue caused by trauma or joint diseases. Mesenchymal stem cells (MSCs), common precursor cells of chondrocytes, are the basis for the development of cartilage and represent promising cells for use in stem cell therapy [1, 2]. However, cartilage tissue formed by MSC-derived chondrocytes is not the same as that of native articular cartilage and has poor functional properties [3, 4]. Understanding the molecular mechanisms that control chondrogenic differentiation of MSCs and enhancing chondrogenic activities of cells are crucial to improve cartilage regeneration by MSCs.

Chondrogenic differentiation is potently induced by growth factors [2, 5]. Transforming growth factor-β3 (TGF-β3), a member of the transforming growth factor-β (TGF-β) superfamily, induces chondrogenic differentiation of MSCs [6]. TGF-β signaling is initiated by the binding of TGF-β to type II TGF-β receptors (TβRII) and then forms heteromeric complexes with type I receptors (TβRI) [7]. These complexes further phosphorylate cytoplasmic effector molecules Smad2 and Smad3, which are translocated to the nucleus, where they modulate the expression of target genes, such as SOX9 and collagen type II (COL II) [8].

In addition to kinase receptors, the type III TGF-β receptor (TβRIII), also known as betaglycan, participates in ligand binding of the TGF-β superfamily and signaling [9, 10]. TβRIII is a membrane-anchored proteoglycan found in many cell types. The main function of this receptor was thought to be binding members of the TGF-β family, including TGF-β isoforms TGF-β1–TGF-β3, and presenting them to type II receptors [11, 12]. However, according to the recent literature, TβRIII seems to play complex roles in cellular processes. For example, studies reported that in some cell lines, TβRIII significantly enhanced the response to TGF-β by increasing the affinity of TβRII for TGF-β [12, 13]. Studies also showed that TβRIII functioned as a potent inhibitor of TGF-β signaling in other types of cells, such as renal epithelial cells [14, 15]. Our previous study demonstrated that human MSCs (hMSCs) expressed abundant TβRIII and that TGF-β3 stimulation clearly repressed TβRIII expression in MSCs and induced MSC chondrogenic differentiation [16]. These results suggested that the effect of TGF-β3 on MSC chondrogenesis might be associated with low expression of TβRIII. However, the role of TβRIII in TGF-β-induced chondrogenic differentiation of MSCs is unknown.

In the present study, we studied the biological effects of TβRIII on TGF-β3-induced MSC chondrogenesis. We demonstrated that TβRIII RNA interference (RNAi) enhanced TGF-β-induced chondrogenic differentiation of hMSCs by activating TGF-β and Smad2/3 signaling.

2. Materials and Methods

2.1. Isolation and Culture of hMSCs. The study was approved by the ethics committee of the First Affiliated Hospital of Sun Yat-sen University in accordance with the Declaration of Helsinki, and all the subjects provided written informed consent. hMSCs were isolated and purified from bone marrow samples of 3 healthy volunteer donors by density gradient centrifugation, as described previously [17]. Briefly, bone marrow samples (8–10 ml) were diluted with 10 ml phosphate-buffered saline (PBS). Cells were then fractionated using a Lymphoprep (MP Biomedicals LLC., Santa Ana, CA, USA) density gradient by centrifugation at 500 ×g for 20 minutes. Interfacial mononuclears were collected and cultured in low-glucose Dulbecco's modified Eagle medium (L-DMEM) (Gibco; Invitrogen Corporation, NY, USA), supplemented with 10% fetal bovine serum (FBS) (Gibco; Invitrogen Corporation, NY, USA) under 37°C and 5% CO_2. Cells were passaged when they reached approximately 80% confluence. Passages 3 to 5 cells were used for the experimental protocols.

2.2. TβRIII Small Interfering RNA (siRNA) Design and Lentiviral Vector Construction. The human TβRIII cDNA sequence (GenBank accession number: NM_003243) was searched for siRNA target sequences. Four target sequences were selected, AAGCATGAAGGAACCAAAT, TGCTTT ATCTCTCCATATT, ACCTGAAATCGTGGTGTTT, and

AGTTGGTAAAGGGTTAATA. A scrambled sequence, TTCTCCGAACGTGTCACGT, was used as a negative control (NC). DNA oligos containing the target sequence were synthesized, annealed, and inserted into a green fluorescent protein (GFP) lentiviral expression vector GV248 (GeneChem, Shanghai, China). The ligated production was transformed into *Escherichia coli* DH5α cells. Briefly, 100 μl of DH5α cells was mixed with 2 μl ligated product at 42°C for 90 s. The mixtures were added on Luria-Bertani (LB) media (ATCC, USA) containing ampilillin (50 μg/ml) and incubated at 37°C for 16 h. The transformant was identified by polymerase chain reaction (PCR) and DNA sequencing.

2.3. Lentiviral Production and Infection. A lentivirus TβRIII (LV-TβRIII) siRNA-mix and lentivirus normal control (LV-NC) virus were produced by plasmid cotransfection of 293T cells. Briefly, 293T cells were transfected with DNA mix (pGC-LV vector, 20 μg; pHelper 1.0 vector, 15 μg; and pHelper 2.0 vector, 10 μg) (GeneChem, Shanghai, China) and 100 μl of Lipofectamine 2000 reagent (Invitrogen, NY, USA), according to the manufacturer's instructions. The viral supernatant was harvested 48 hours (h) after transfection, and the concentrated viral titer was determined. The viral supernatant was added into target MSCs at multiplicity of infection (MOI 10). Before infection, 5×10^4/ml of MSCs were seeded onto a $60 \, cm^2$ cell culture dish overnight. The cells were then infected with 100 μl of 1×10^8 TU/ml virus and 5 μg/ml of polybrene, following the manufacturer's instructions. Then, 10 h after infection, the cells were incubated with L-DMEM containing 10% FBS. Three days after infection, GFP expression in cells was observed by a fluorescence microscope (Olympus, Japan). TβRIII expression was detected by the real-time polymerase chain reaction (PCR) and Western blot analysis.

2.4. Chondrogenic Differentiation of hMSCs in Micromass Culture. Chondrogenic differentiation of hMSCs was performed using a modified micromass culture system according to a previously described method [18]. Briefly, MSCs being infected with TβRIII siRNA (SiTβRIII) or control siRNA (SiNC), or without infection, were harvested and resuspended at 2×10^7 cells/ml. Cell droplets (4×10^5/20 μl) were placed carefully in each well of 24-well plates for 2 h, followed by the addition of control medium or chondrogenic medium at 37°C/5% CO_2. The control medium consisted of high-glucose DMEM (H-DMEM), supplemented with 50 μg/ml of vitamin C, 100 nM dexamethasone, 1 mM sodium pyruvate, 40 μg/ml of proline, and ITS+Universal Culture Supplement Premix (BD Biosciences, NY, USA). The chondrogenic medium consisted of the control medium, added by 10 ng/ml of TGF-β3 (PeproTech, Rocky Hill, USA). After 24 h, the cell droplets became spherical. The medium was changed every 3 days.

Cell pellets from uninfected MSCs were divided into a control group and TGF-β3 group according to the control medium and chondrogenic medium and used for TβRIII analysis. The cells were harvested on day 7 after chondrogenic induction. The pellets from infected MSCs were divided into the following four groups for identification of

TABLE 1: Primers used for real-time PCR.

Gene	Forward primer (5′ to 3′)	Reverse primer (5′ to 3′)
GAPDH	5′-AGAAAAACCTGCCAAATATGATGAC-3′	5′-TGGGTGTCGCTGTTGAAGTC-3′
β-Actin	5′-GACTTAGTTGCGTTACACCCTTTC-3′	5′-GCTGTCACCTTCACCGTTCC-3′
Col2A1	5′-GGCAATAGCAGGTTCACGTACA-3′	5′-CGATAACAGTCTTGCCCCACTT-3′
SOX 9	5′-AGCGAACGCACATCAAGAC-3′	5′-GCTGTAGTGTGGGAGGTTGAA-3′
TβRI	5′-ATTACCAACTGCCTTATTATGA-3′	5′-CATTACTCTCAAGGCTTCAC-3′
TβRII	5′-ATGGAGGCCCAGAAAGATG-3′	5′-GACTGCACCGTTGTTGTCAG-3′
TβRIII	5′GTGTTCCCTCCAAAGTGCAAC-3′	5′-AGCTCGATGATGTGTACTTCCT-3′

GAPDH: glyceraldehyde-3-phosphate dehydrogenase; COL2A1: collagen type II; SOX9: SRY- (sex determining region Y-) box 9; TβRI/II/III: recombinant human transforming growth factor-β receptor type I/II/III.

chondrogenic differentiation and TGF-β/Smad signaling: C-SiNC group (SiNC-infected cells cultured in control medium), C-SiTβRIII group (SiTβRIII-infected cells cultured in control medium), T-SiNC group (SiNC-infected cells cultured in chondrogenic medium), and T-SiTβRIII group (SiTβRIII-infected cells cultured in chondrogenic medium). The cells were harvested on day 14 for identification of chondrogenic differentiation, and on day 7 for TβRI and TβRII analysis. All experiments were performed by using 3 biological replicate samples each group.

2.5. RNA Extraction and Real-Time PCR Analysis. Total RNA was isolated from transfected MSCs or pellets using an RNAsimple Total RNA Kit (Tiangen, Beijing, China). Total RNA was then converted into cDNA using a PrimeScript® RT Reagent Kit (Takara, Osaka, Japan) according to the manufacturer's instructions. Real-Time PCR assay was performed in triplicate in a Real-Time PCR system (Bio-Rad Laboratories, Hercules, CA, USA) by using SYBR Green I Master Mix (Takara, Osaka, Japan). The following genes were examined: COL II, alpha 1 (COL2A1), SRY- (sex determining region Y-) box 9 [SOX9], TβRI, TβRII, and TβRIII. The primer sequences are listed in Table 1. The relative expression levels for each target gene were calculated by referencing to the internal controls glyceraldehyde-3-phosphate dehydrogenase (GAPDH) and β-actin using the $2^{-\Delta\Delta CT}$ method.

2.6. Histology and Immunohistochemistry. The pellets were fixed in 4% paraformaldehyde and embedded in paraffin. 4 μm sections were deparaffinized, rehydrated through decreasing concentrations of ethanol, and stained with 0.1% Alcian blue (Sigma-Aldrich, St. Louis, USA) for glycosaminoglycan (GAG) analysis. For immunohistochemistry analysis, the sections were blocked with 1/100 diluted goat serum for 15 min and then reacted overnight at 4°C with the appropriate primary antibody against human COL II polyclonal antibodies (Abzoom Biolabs, Dallas, TX, USA) and human TβRIII antibody (Santa Cruz, Dallas, USA) followed by biotinylated goat anti-rabbit immunoglobulin G (IgG) (EarthOx, SFO, USA) for 30 min. The sections were incubated with peroxide-conjugated streptavidin and

stained with 3,3′-diaminobenzidine tetrahydrochloride (DAB) (Jinshan Jinqiao, Beijing, China).

For fluorescent immunohistochemistry, the pellets from transfected MSCs were frozen and then sectioned using a Leica CM1950 microtome (Leica, Germany) on day 7 after chondrogenic induction. Tissue sections that were 4 μm thick were permeabilized with 0.1% Triton X for 5 min and blocked with 5% BSA for 1 h. The sections were then incubated with primary antibodies against TβRI (Santa Cruz, Dallas, USA) and human TβRII antibody (RD Systems, USA), diluted at 1 : 50 at 4°C overnight. FITC-conjugated secondary antibody (K00018968; Dako North America Inc., Dako, Denmark) diluted at 1 : 100 was applied for 1 h. The sections were then stained with 4′-6-diamidino-2-phenylindole (1 mg/ml) and visualized using a Zeiss LSM 710 confocal microscope (Carl Zeiss, Heidelberg, Germany).

2.7. Glycosaminoglycan (GAG) Quantitation. The pellets were harvested on day 14 and papain-digested for 16 h at 65°C. An aliquot of 40 μl lysate was reacted with 1,9-dimethyl-methylene blue (DMMB) (Sigma-Aldrich, St. Louis, USA) for GAG analysis. The absorbance at 525 nm was measured using an Automatic Microplate Reader (Bio-Tek, Winooski, Vermont, USA). Total GAG was calculated by a standard curve obtained with shark chondroitin sulfate (Sigma-Aldrich, MO, USA). The total amount of DNA was quantified by reacting with 0.7 μg/ml Hoechst 33258 solution (Sigma-Aldrich, St. Louis, USA). The reaction product was measured using a Synergy Microplate Reader (BioTek, Winooski, Vermont, USA). The results of GAG quantification were normalized to the DNA content.

2.8. Western Blot. For TβRIII RNAi identification, proteins were extracted from MSCs 72 h after transfection. For detection of Smad2/3 phosphorylation, proteins were extracted from pellets after 24 h of chondrogenic induction. The protein concentration was quantified by a BCA Protein Assay Kit (CWBio, Beijing, China). 100 μg proteins was subjected to 6% SDS-PAGE and electrotransferred onto PVDF membrane (Millipore, Boston, USA) at 250 mV for 100 min. After blocking with 5% skim milk and Tris-buffered saline containing 0.1% Tween-20, the PVDF membranes were incubated with antibodies against human TβRIII antibody (Santa Cruz,

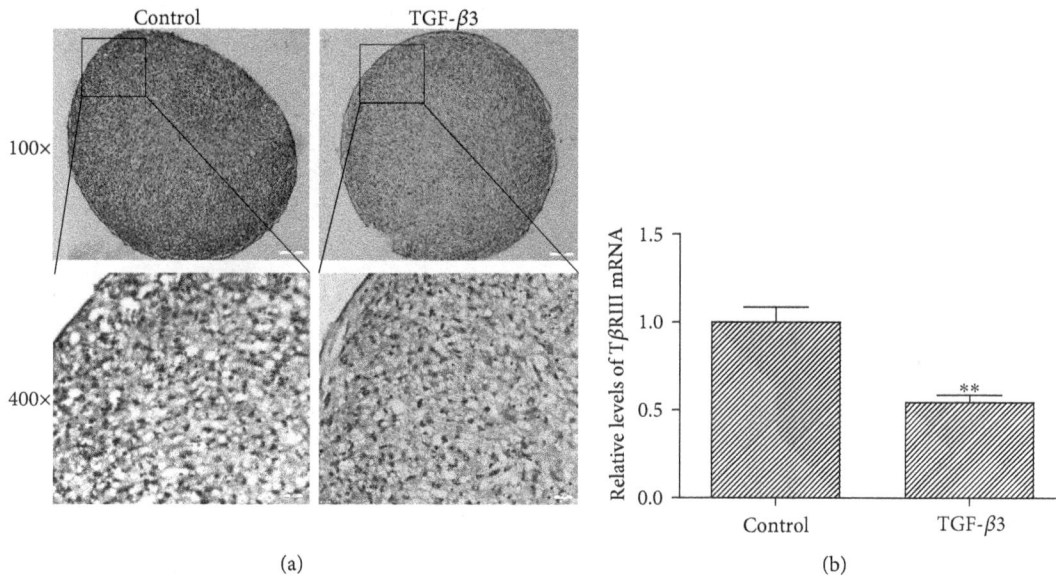

FIGURE 1: TGF-β3 inhibited the expression of TβRIII during chondrogenic differentiation of hMSCs. (a) hMSCs were cultured in chondrogenic medium including TGF-β3 or control medium without TGF-β3 for 7 days and subjected to immunohistochemistry analysis for TβRIII (upper panel, scale bar = 100 μm; lower panel, scale bar = 20 μm; the TβRIII is stained in brown, cell nucleus is stained in blue). (b) qPCR analysis of TβRIII mRNA level in hMSCs cultured in chondrogenic medium or control medium for 7 days. The TβRIII mRNA level was lower in hMSCs cultured in chondrogenic medium containing TGF-β3 as compared with that of cells cultured in control medium. Error bars represent the means ± SD, $n = 3$. $^{**}P < 0.01$ versus control.

Dallas, USA), rabbit anti-phospho-Smad2 (Ser465/467)/Smad3 (Ser423/425) (Cell Signaling, Danvers, USA), rabbit anti-Smad2/3 (Cell Signaling, Danvers, USA), and anti-GAPDH monoclonal antibody (EarthOx, SFO, USA) followed by incubation with HRP-conjugated corresponding secondary antibodies. The signals were detected using SuperSignal West Pico Chemiluminescent Substrate (Pierce, NY, USA). Protein levels in phosphorylated-Smad2/3 (P-Smad2/3) were normalized to those of total Smad2/3 quantities or GAPDH.

2.9. Inhibition of TGF-β/Smad Signaling. The infected cells were treated with or without SB431542 (Sigma-Aldrich, St. Louis, USA), a selective inhibitor of activin receptor-like kinase 5 (ALK5) (TβRI) [19], for 2 h before being cultured in chondrogenic medium or control medium. After 24 h of chondrogenic induction, the cells were collected, and the expression of P-Smad2/3 and that of Smad2/3 was detected by a Western blot. After 14 days of chondrogenic induction, the chondrogenic differentiation ability of hMSCs was assayed by detecting protein and gene expression.

2.10. Statistical Analysis. All quantitative data were presented as mean values ± standard errors (S.E.). All the statistical analysis was performed using SPSS 16.0 statistical software (SPSS, Chicago, IL, USA). For comparisons of two groups, independent student's t-test was performed; for comparisons of multiple groups, one-way ANOVA followed by an LSD t-test was performed. $P < 0.05$ was chosen as the threshold of significance.

3. Results

3.1. TGF-β3 Inhibited the Expression of TβRIII in hMSCs. To ascertain whether hMSCs express TβRIII and TGF-β3 could regulate TβRIII expression level, we detected the expression of TβRIII during TGF-β3-induced hMSC chondrogenesis by immunohistochemistry staining and quantitative PCR. The results showed that hMSCs expressed abundant TβRIII protein (Figure 1(a), left panels) and high TβRIII mRNA ($P < 0.01$, Figure 1(b)). Exogenous TGF-β3 clearly reduced TβRIII expression in hMSCs at protein and mRNA levels (Figures 1(a) and 1(b)).

3.2. Viral Infection and Suppression of TβRIII Expression at mRNA and Protein Levels. In order to investigate the role of TβRIII in hMSC chondrogenesis, we infected hMSCs with LV-TβRIII siRNA-mix and identified the silencing effect on TβRIII. Following viral infection for 72 h, most of the cells exhibited high GFP expression under fluorescence microscopy (Figure 2(a)). As compared with the control group, the expression profile of TβRIII mRNA and that of the TβRIII protein decreased significantly in the SiTβRIII groups, with mRNA expression decreased by 77.65% (Figures 2(b) and 2(c)).

3.3. TβRIII RNAi Enhanced TGF-β3-Induced Chondrogenic Differentiation of hMSCs. We then investigated the effects of TβRIII RNAi on the TGF-β3-induced chondrogenic differentiation of hMSCs. As shown in Figure 3, TβRIII RNAi had no obvious effects on GAG and COL II secretion (Figures 3(a) and 3(b); $P > 0.05$) or any noticeable effects on the expression of cartilage-specific genes (SOX9 and

White GFP

SiNC

SiTβRIII

(a)

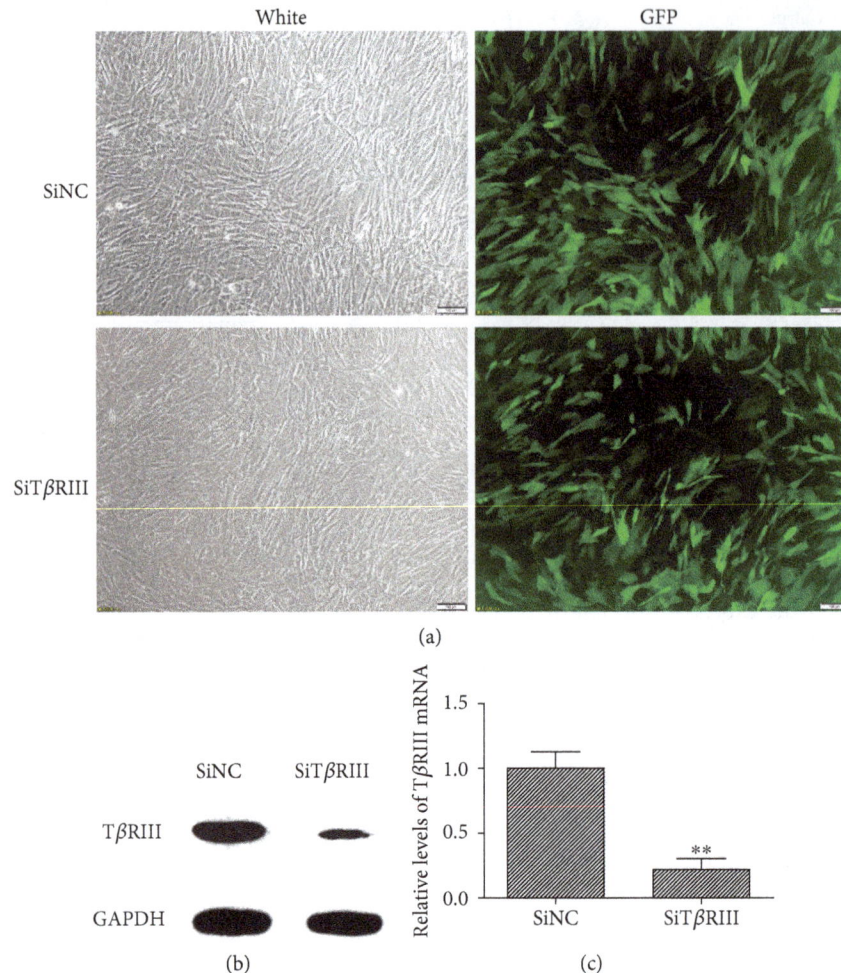

SiNC SiTβRIII

TβRIII

GAPDH

(b)

(c)

FIGURE 2: Identification and efficiency of lentiviral infection. (a) GFP fluorescence imaging confirmed that the majority of hMSCs were GFP positive 72 h after they were infected by TβRIII siRNA (SiTβRIII) or SiNC virus. Scale bar = 100 μm. (b) Western blot showed that TβRIII siRNA clearly inhibited the expression of the TβRIII protein. (c) qPCR confirmed that the expression profiles of TβRIII mRNA decreased significantly in the SiTβRIII groups as compared with those in the SiNC group. Error bars represent the means ± SD, $n = 3$. $^{**}P < 0.01$ versus SiNC group.

COL2A1) when hMSCs were cultured in control medium (Figure 3(c); $P > 0.05$). However, TβRIII RNAi significantly enhanced TGF-β3-induced chondrogenic differentiation of hMSCs as compared with that of cells infected with SiNC (Figures 3(a)–3(c); $P < 0.05$).

3.4. TβRIII RNAi Increased the Ratio of TβRII to TβRI. To explore the mechanism on TβRIII RNAi regulating TGF-β3-induced chondrogenic differentiation of hMSCs, we further analyzed the effect of TβRIII RNAi on TβRI and TβRII expression and downstream Smad2/3 signaling during TGF-β3-induced chondrogenesis. Analysis of TβRI and TβRII expression revealed that both TβRI mRNA levels and protein expression had no difference between the cells in the C-SiNC, C-SiTβRIII, and T-SiNC groups (Figures 4(a) and 4(b); $P > 0.05$). However, TβRI mRNA and protein expression levels were decreased in the T-SiTβRIII group as compared with those in the other groups (Figures 4(a) and 4(b); $P < 0.05$). Neither the expression of the TβRII gene (Figure 4(a)) nor that of the protein (Figure 4(b)) was

increased in the C-SiTβRIII group as compared with that in the C-SiNC group ($P > 0.05$). However, as compared with the C-SiNC group, both the T-SiNC and T-SiTβRIII groups had enhanced mRNA levels of TβRII (Figure 4(a); $P < 0.05$) and TβRII expression (Figure 4(b)). The expression of the TβRII gene, as well as that of the TβRII protein, was higher in the T-SiTβRIII group as compared with that in the T-SiNC group. The ratio of TβRII to TβRI in the T-SiNC and T-SiTβRIII groups was higher than that in the C-SiNC and C-SiTβRIII groups (Figure 4(a); $P < 0.05$ and $P < 0.01$, resp.). TβRII/TβRI levels increased dramatically in the T-SiTβRIII groups as compared with those in other groups (Figure 4(a); $P < 0.05$).

3.5. TβRIII RNAi Strengthened TGF-β3-Mediated Phosphorylation of Smad2/3. Analysis of phosphorylation of Smad2/3 revealed that TβRIII-RNAi did not affect the expression of P-Smad2/3 in control medium. However, phosphorylation of Smad2/3 was obviously activated in T-SiNC and T-SiTβRIII groups. Interestingly, when cells

(a)

(b)

(c)

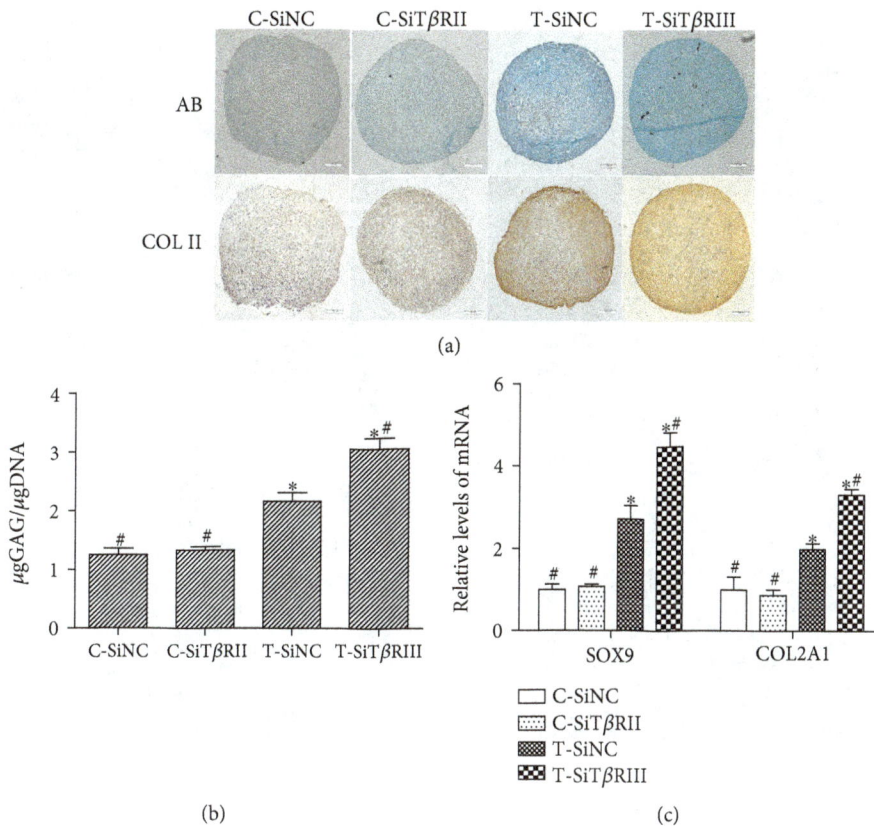

FIGURE 3: TβRIII RNAi enhanced TGF-β3-induced chondrogenic differentiation of hMSCs. SiNC- or SiTβRIII-infected cells were cultured in control medium (C-SiNC group; C-SiTβRIII group) or chondrogenic medium containing TGF-β3 (T-SiNC group; T-SiTβRIII group) for 14 days. (a) Upper panels show glycosaminoglycan (GAG) expression by Alcian blue staining; lower panels show COL II expression by immunohistochemistry. Scale bar = 100 μm. (b) GAG content was quantitatively analyzed and normalized by DNA content. (c) Real-time PCR analysis of COL2A1 and SOX9 mRNA levels in hMSCs from different groups. Error bars represent the means ± SD, $n = 3$. $^{*}P < 0.05$ versus C-SiNC group; $^{\#}P < 0.05$ versus T-SiNC group.

were infected with SiTβRIII, the activation of P-Smad2/3 was further enhanced (Figures 5(a) and 5(b)).

3.6. SB431542 Blocked TβRIII RNAi-Activated TGF-β3-Mediated Phosphorylation of Smad2/3. SB431542 was identified as a specific inhibitor of TβRI and TGF-β signaling [19]. Therefore, we tested whether SB431542 blocked TβRIII RNAi-activated TGF-β signaling. The results showed that SB431542 inhibited both TGF-β3-activated Smad2/3 phosphorylation and TβRIII RNAi-activated TGF-β3-mediated Smad2/3 phosphorylation (Figure 6(a)). The results of the statistical analysis revealed decreased ratios of P-Smad2/3 to Smad2/3 and P-Smad2/3 to GAPDH in the T-SiNC + SB and T-SiTβRIII + SB groups as compared with those in the T-SiNC and T-SiTβRIII groups ($P < 0.05$), as shown in Figure 6(b). There was no statistical difference in P-Smad2/3 levels in the T-SiNC + SB group versus those in the T-SiTβRIII + SB group ($P > 0.05$) (Figure 6(b)). These data showed that SB431542 completely inhibited TGF-β3-mediated Smad2/3 phosphorylation, activated by TβRIII RNAi.

3.7. SB431542 Inhibited TβRIII RNAi-Enhanced TGF-β3-Induced Chondrogenic Differentiation of hMSCs. We have shown that SB431542 blocked TβRIII RNAi-activated TGF-

β signaling. We next investigated whether it was sufficient to inhibit the ability of TβRIII RNAi-enhanced TGF-β3-induced chondrogenic differentiation of hMSCs. As shown in Figure 7, GAG and COL II secretion increased significantly in the T-SiTβRIII group (Figures 7(a) and 7(b)), as well as mRNA levels of cartilage-specific genes (SOX9 and COL2A1), as compared with that in the T-SiNC group (Figure 7(c); $P < 0.05$). Cartilage-specific protein and gene expression decreased in the T-SiNC + SB and T-SiTβRIII + SB groups as compared with cartilage-specific protein and gene expression in the T-SiNC and T-SiTβRIII groups (Figures 7(a)–7(c); $P < 0.05$).

4. Discussion

TβRIII is an abundant TGF-β receptor, which is present in many cell types [9, 13]. We previously demonstrated that hMSCs expressed high levels of TβRIII and that TGF-β3 reduced the expression of TβRIII at mRNA and protein levels [15]. Other studies demonstrated the specific role of TGF-β1 in decreasing TβRIII mRNA and protein levels in cancer cells [20, 21]. These findings were similar to those of our own study. Hempel et al. [21] showed the TGF-β1-mediated downregulation of TβRIII mRNA expression by

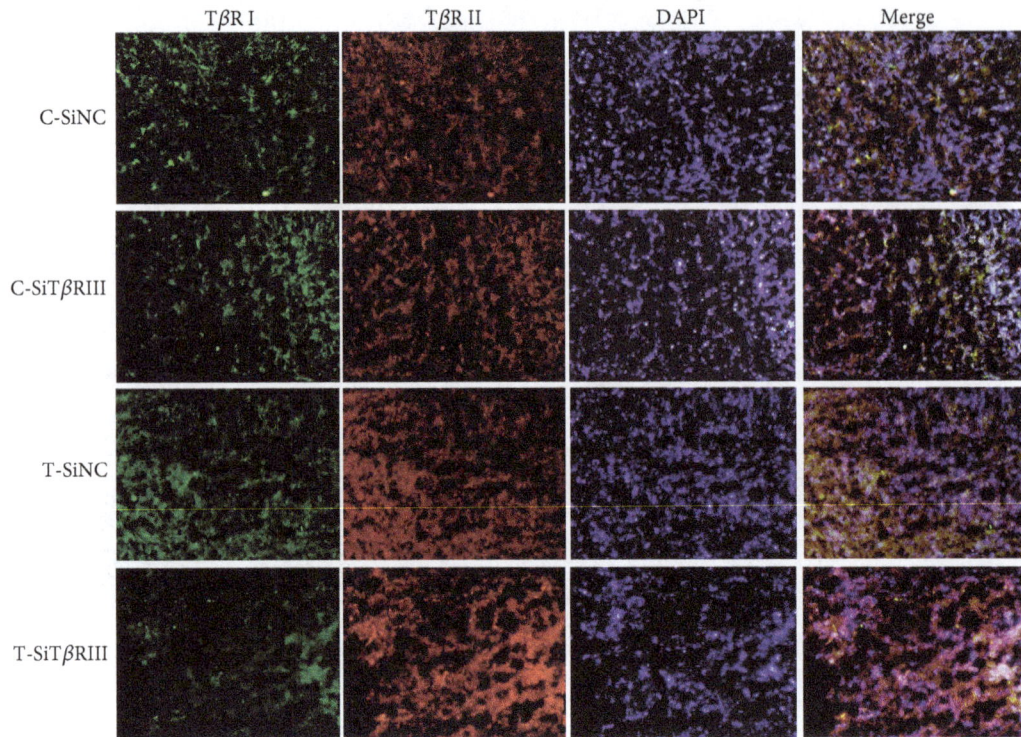

(a)

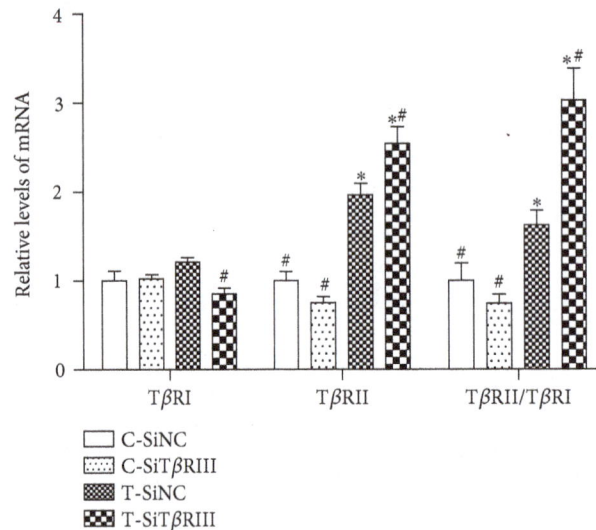

(b)

Figure 4: TβRIII RNAi increased the ratio of TβRII to TβRI. SiNC- or SiTβRIII-infected cells were cultured in control medium (C-SiNC group; C-SiTβRIII group) or chondrogenic medium containing TGF-β3 (T-SiNC group; T-SiTβRIII group) for 7days ($n = 3$). (a) The expression of TβRI and that of TβRII were visualized by immunofluorescence staining using anti-TβRI (green) and anti-TβRII (red) antibodies. Nuclei were counterstained using DAPI (blue). The far right panels show merged images. Scale bar = 20 μm. (b) mRNA expression of TβRI and TβRII and the ratio of TβRII to TβRI by real-time RT-PCR. *$P < 0.05$ versus C-SiNC group; #$P < 0.05$ versus T-SiNC group.

exerting effects on the ALK5/Smad2/3 pathway of the TGFβR3 gene proximal promoter. Three highly homologous isoforms of TGF-β in humans (TGF-β1, TGF-β2, and TGF-β3) share a similar receptor complex and signaling pathway [20]. Therefore, the mechanism underlying the suppression by TGF-β3 on TβRIII may be the same as that involved in TGF-β1-mediated downregulation of TβRIII.

In recent years, many studies have investigated the effects of altering the expression level of TβRIII and its roles on mediating cell migration, invasion, growth, and differentiation in several cell types, including cancer and epithelial cells [13, 20, 22, 23]. However, the regulatory roles of TβRIII in MSCs have not been explored. RNAi is a powerful tool for studying protein function [24]. Lentiviral vectors encoding

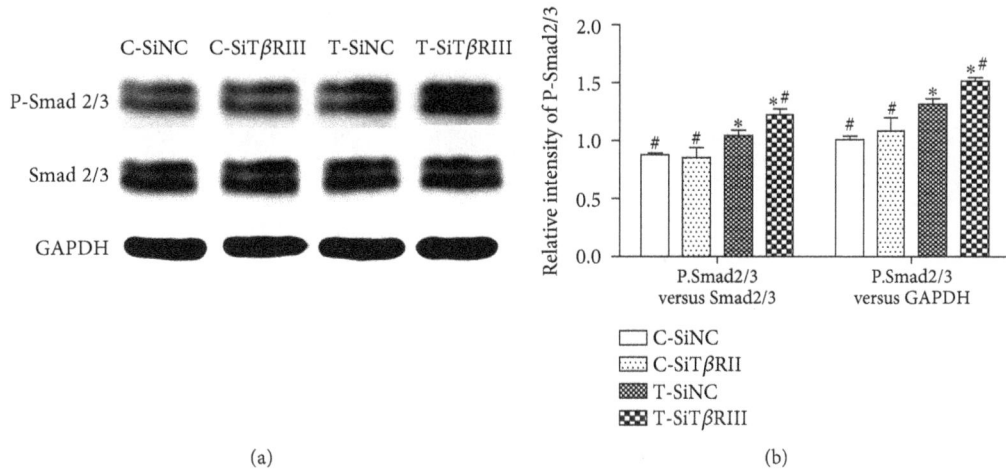

(a)

(b)

FIGURE 5: TβRIII RNAi strengthened TGF-β3-mediated Smad2/3 phosphorylation. SiNC- or SiTβRIII-infected cells were cultured in control medium (C-SiNC group; C-SiTβRIII group) or chondrogenic medium containing TGF-β3 (T-SiNC group; T-SiTβRIII group) and harvested after 24 h. (a) A Western blot of protein levels of P-Smad2/3, total Smad2/3, and GAPDH. (b) Quantification of protein levels of P-Smad2/3 normalized to total levels of Smad2/3 or GAPDH. Error bars represent the means $\pm$ SD, $n = 3$. $^{*}P < 0.05$ versus C-SiNC group; $^{\#}P < 0.05$ versus T-SiNC group.

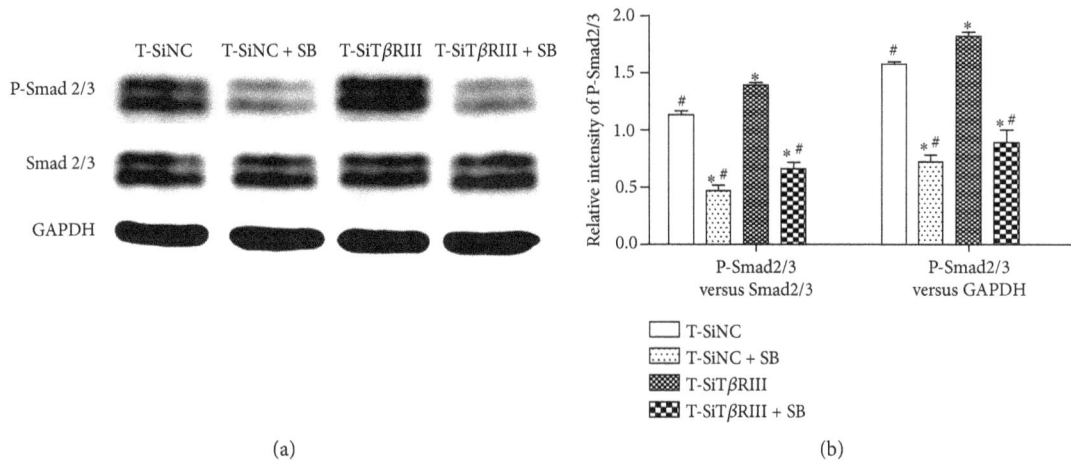

(a)

(b)

FIGURE 6: SB431542 blocked TβRIII RNAi-activated TGF-β3-mediated phosphorylation of Smad2/3. SiNC- or SiTβRIII-infected hMSCs were cultured in chondrogenic medium, supplemented with TGF-β3 (T-SiNC group or T-SiTβRIII group) and exposed to SB431542 treatment for 2 h before treatment with TGF-β3 (T-SiNC + SB group or T-SiTβRIII + SB group). Samples were harvested after 24 h. (a) Western blot of protein levels of P-Smad2/3, total Smad2/3, and GAPDH. (b) Quantification of protein levels of P-Smad2/3 normalized to total levels of Smad2/3 and GAPDH. Error bars represent the means $\pm$ SD, $n = 3$. $^{*}P < 0.05$ versus T-SiNC group, $^{\#}P < 0.05$ versus T-SiTβRIII group.

short hairpin RNAs (shRNAs) or microRNAs (miRNAs) can be used to specifically knock down target mRNAs [25]. Besides the ability to transfer vectors in primary and nondividing cells, the reverse-transcribed lentiviral vector is integrated in the genome, allowing stable expression of the gene or shRNA of interest [26]. We used GV248-based lentiviral vectors for delivery of shRNAs, precursors of TβRIII siRNA, into MSCs to suppress TβRIII gene expression. This vector coexpressed enhanced GFP, a reporter gene, permitting infected cells to be detected by fluorescence microscopy. Three days after infection with Lenti-siTβRIII or Lenti-NC, fluorescence microscopy images revealed efficient infection of MSCs with lentiviral vectors. The data also demonstrated

that the lentiviral vector-based shRNA vector effectively downregulated mRNA and protein expression of TβRIII. These data indicated that Lenti-siTβRIII MSCs could be used as a powerful tool for studying the effect of the siTβRIII gene on MSC chondrogenesis.

Our study is the first to demonstrate that TβRIII knockdown in MSCs enhanced TGF-β3-induced chondrogenic differentiation, indicating a role for TβRIII as a negative modulator of MSC chondrogenesis. Previous research reported that the functional impact of TβRIII on TGF-β ligand signaling was cell-type dependent [9]. Li et al. [13] demonstrated that transfection of TβRIII-containing plasmid DNA dramatically promoted a TGF-β1-induced

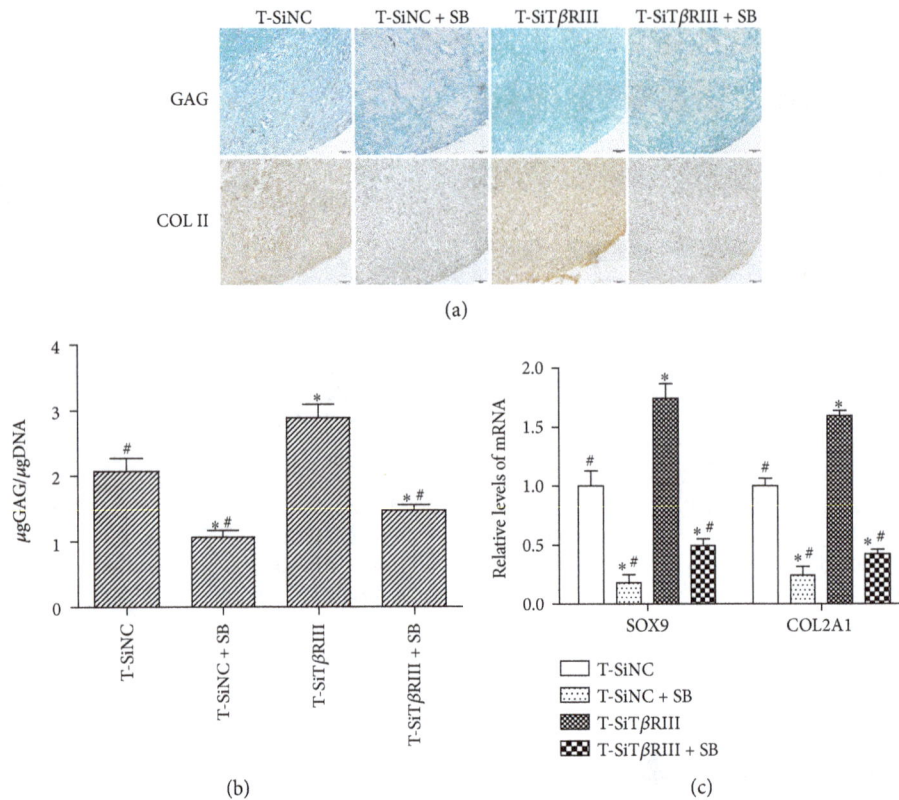

FIGURE 7: SB431542 inhibited TβRIIIRNAi-enhanced TGF-β3-induced chondrogenic differentiation of hMSCs. Cells from T-SiNC, T-SiNC + SB, T-SiTβRIII, and T-SiTβRIII + SB groups were cultured for 14 days. (a) Alcian blue staining for GAG expression and immunohistochemistry staining for COL II expression. $n = 3$, scale bar = 50 μm. (b) GAG content was quantitatively analyzed and normalized by DNA content. (c) mRNA levels of SOX9 and COL2A1 were measured by real-time PCR. Error bars represent the means ± SD, $n = 3$. *$P < 0.05$ versus T-SiNC group, #$P < 0.05$ versus T-SiTβRIII group.

decrease in cell viability, apoptosis, and cell arrest. On the other hand, Eickelberg et al. indicated that the expression of TβRIII in renal epithelial LLC-PK1 cells resulted in inhibition of TGF signaling [27]. They also suggested that TβRIII with larger proteoglycans negatively modulated TGF-β1-induced cellular responses, whereas TβRIII containing smaller proteoglycans enhances TGF-β1-induced cellular responses [27]. These results suggested that TβRIII in MSCs may contain larger proteoglycans.

TGF-βs (TGF-β1, TGF-β2, and TGF-β3, resp.) are small secreted signaling proteins, each of which signals through TβRI and TβRII. In contrast to TβRI and TβRII, TβRIII is a membrane-anchored nonsignaling receptor, and its function is to bind and concentrate TGF-β isoforms on the cell surface and promote the binding of TβRII and recruitment of TβRI [11]. Chen et al. [15] demonstrated that TβRI was recruited to form TβRIII/TβRII/TβRI ternary complexes that it had two forms: complex I and complex II. Complex I contained more TβRII than TβRI, underwent clathrin-mediated endocytosis, and transduced signals in endosomes. Complex II, which contained more TβRI than TβRII, underwent caveolae/lipid-raft-mediated endocytosis and rapid degradation. The formation of these complexes was regulated by the proteoglycan moiety of TβRIII and altered the expression of TβRII or TβRI [15]. Herein, we demonstrated that TβRIII RNAi decreased TβRI expression and increased

TβRII expression in the T-SiTβRIII group when MSCs were cultured with TGF-β3 as compared with the T-SiNC group (Figure 4). The data, combined with the findings of previous reports [15], indicated that TβRIII RNAi increased the ratio of TβRII to TβRI of the receptor complex and formed complex I, therefore enhancing TGF-β3 signaling in MSC chondrogenesis.

TGF-β signals predominantly bind to the ALK5 receptor (TβRI) and subsequently activate C-terminal Smad 2/3 phosphorylation. This signaling route stimulates the production of matrix components [19]. The present study also showed that TβRIII RNAi further enhanced the TGF-β3-activated downstream Smad2/3 signaling pathway (Figure 5). In addition, SB431542, a TβRI inhibitor, as well as dominant negative Smad2/3 specifically [28], significantly reversed TβRIII RNAi-mediated increases in TGF-β3-induced MSC chondrogenesis (Figures 6 and 7). These data indicated that TβRIII knockdown enhanced TGF-β3-induced MSC chondrogenesis via the Smad2/3 signaling pathway.

5. Conclusions

This study demonstrated that TGF-β3 inhibited the expression of TβRIII. TβRIII RNAi enhanced TGF-β3-induced chondrogenic differentiation of hMSCs by increasing the ratio of TβRII to TβRI in the receptor complex and further activating downstream Smad2/3 signaling. These findings contribute to the understanding of the molecular mechanisms that control chondrogenic differentiation of MSCs and provide a potential strategy (i.e., modification of MSCs by TβRIII knockdown for cell-based cartilage tissue engineering).

Authors' Contributions

Shuhui Zheng and Hang Zhou contributed equally to this work.

Acknowledgments

This research was supported by grants from the National Natural Science Foundation of China (nos. 81472039, 81772302, 816018988, and 1572091) and the Guangzhou Science and Technology Program key projects (201704020120).

References

[1] Y. Wang, M. Yuan, Q.-Y. Guo, S.-B. Lu, and J. Peng, "Mesenchymal stem cells for treating articular cartilage defects and osteoarthritis," *Cell Transplantation*, vol. 24, no. 9, pp. 1661–1678, 2015.

[2] S. W. Huh, A. A. Shetty, S. Ahmed, D. H. Lee, and S. J. Kim, "Autologous bone-marrow mesenchymal cell induced chondrogenesis (MCIC)," *Journal of Clinical Orthopaedics and Trauma*, vol. 7, no. 3, pp. 153–156, 2016.

[3] S. Yamasaki, H. Mera, M. Itokazu, Y. Hashimoto, and S. Wakitani, "Cartilage repair with autologous bone marrow mesenchymal stem cell transplantation: review of preclinical and clinical studies," *Cartilage*, vol. 5, no. 4, pp. 196–202, 2014.

[4] A. R. Tan and C. T. Hung, "Concise review: mesenchymal stem cells for functional cartilage tissue engineering: taking cues from chondrocyte-based constructs," *Stem Cells Translational Medicine*, vol. 6, no. 4, pp. 1295–1303, 2017.

[5] S. Yoshiya and A. Dhawan, "Cartilage repair techniques in the knee: stem cell therapies," *Current Reviews in Musculoskeletal Medicine*, vol. 8, no. 4, pp. 457–466, 2015.

[6] Q. O. Tang, K. Shakib, M. Heliotis et al., "TGF-β3: a potential biological therapy for enhancing chondrogenesis," *Expert Opinion on Biological Therapy*, vol. 9, no. 6, pp. 689–701, 2009.

[7] J. Nickel, P. ten Dijke, and T. D. Mueller, "TGF-β family co-receptor function and signaling," *Acta Biochimica et Biophysica Sinica*, vol. 50, no. 1, pp. 12–36, 2018.

[8] K. B. Marcu, L. M. G. de Kroon, R. Narcisi et al., "Activin receptor-like kinase receptors ALK5 and ALK1 are both required for TGFβ-induced chondrogenic differentiation of human bone marrow-derived mesenchymal stem cells," *PLoS One*, vol. 10, no. 12, article e0146124, 2015.

[9] M. Bilandzic and K. L. Stenvers, "Betaglycan: a multifunctional accessory," *Molecular and Cellular Endocrinology*, vol. 339, no. 1-2, pp. 180–189, 2011.

[10] F. López-Casillas, H. M. Payne, J. L. Andres, and J. Massagué, "Betaglycan can act as a dual modulator of TGF-beta access to signaling receptors: mapping of ligand binding and GAG attachment sites," *Journal of Cell Biology*, vol. 124, no. 4, pp. 557–568, 1994.

[11] M. M. Villarreal, S. K. Kim, L. Barron et al., "Binding properties of the transforming growth factor-β coreceptor betaglycan: proposed mechanism for potentiation of receptor complex assembly and signaling," *Biochemistry*, vol. 55, no. 49, pp. 6880–6896, 2016.

[12] S. McLean and G. M. Di Guglielmo, "TGFβ (transforming growth factor β) receptor type III directs clathrin-mediated endocytosis of TGFβ receptor types I and II," *Biochemical Journal*, vol. 429, no. 1, pp. 137–145, 2010.

[13] D. Li, D. Xu, Z. Lu, X. Dong, and X. Wang, "Overexpression of transforming growth factor type III receptor restores TGF-β1 sensitivity in human tongue squamous cell carcinoma cells," *Bioscience Reports*, vol. 35, no. 4, article e00243, 2015.

[14] K. Tazat, M. Hector-Greene, G. C. Blobe, and Y. I. Henis, "TβRIII independently binds type I and type II TGF-β receptors to inhibit TGF-β signaling," *Molecular Biology of the Cell*, vol. 26, no. 19, pp. 3535–3545, 2015.

[15] C.-L. Chen, S. S. Huang, and J. S. Huang, "Cellular heparan sulfate negatively modulates transforming growth factor-β₁(TGF-β₁) responsiveness in epithelial cells," *Journal of Biological Chemistry*, vol. 281, no. 17, pp. 11506–11514, 2006.

[16] J. Chen, Y. Wang, C. Chen et al., "Exogenous heparan sulfate enhances the TGF-β3-induced chondrogenesis in human mesenchymal stem cells by activating TGF-β/Smad signaling," *Stem Cells International*, vol. 2016, Article ID 1520136, 10 pages, 2016.

[17] C. Xu, Z. Zheng, L. Fang et al., "Phosphatidylserine enhances osteogenic differentiation in human mesenchymal stem cells via ERK signal pathways," *Materials Science and Engineering: C*, vol. 33, no. 3, pp. 1783–1788, 2013.

[18] L. Zhang, P. Su, C. Xu, J. Yang, W. Yu, and D. Huang, "Chondrogenic differentiation of human mesenchymal stem cells: a comparison between micromass and pellet culture systems," *Biotechnology Letters*, vol. 32, no. 9, pp. 1339–1346, 2010.

[19] A. van Caam, W. Madej, A. Garcia de Vinuesa et al., "TGFβ1-induced SMAD2/3 and SMAD1/5 phosphorylation are both ALK5-kinase-dependent in primary chondrocytes and mediated by TAK1 kinase activity," *Arthritis Research & Therapy*, vol. 19, no. 1, p. 112, 2017.

[20] S. E. N. Zhang, W.-Y. Sun, J.-J. Wu, Y.-J. Gu, and W. E. I. Wei, "Decreased expression of the type III TGF-β receptor enhances metastasis and invasion in hepatocellullar carcinoma progression," *Oncology Reports*, vol. 35, no. 4, pp. 2373–2381, 2016.

[21] N. Hempel, T. How, S. J. Cooper et al., "Expression of the type III TGF-β receptor is negatively regulated by TGF-β," *Carcinogenesis*, vol. 29, no. 5, pp. 905–912, 2008.

[22] D. Xu, D. U. O. Li, Z. Lu, X. Dong, and X. Wang, "Type III TGF-β receptor inhibits cell proliferation and migration in salivary glands adenoid cystic carcinoma by suppressing NF-κB signaling," *Oncology Reports*, vol. 35, no. 1, pp. 267–274, 2016.

[23] L. M. Jenkins, P. Singh, A. Varadaraj et al., "Altering the proteoglycan state of transforming growth factor β type III receptor (TβRIII)/Betaglycan modulates canonical Wnt/β-catenin signaling," *Journal of Biological Chemistry*, vol. 291, no. 49, pp. 25716–25728, 2016.

receptor (TβRIII)/Betaglycan modulates canonical Wnt/β-catenin signaling," *Journal of Biological Chemistry*, vol. 291, no. 49, pp. 25716–25728, 2016.

[24] L. Zhang, H.-j. Liu, T.-j. Li et al., "Lentiviral vector-mediated siRNA knockdown of SR-PSOX inhibits foam cell formation *in vitro*," *Acta Pharmacologica Sinica*, vol. 29, no. 7, pp. 847–852, 2008.

[25] Y. P. Liu, M. A. Vink, J. T. Westerink et al., "Titers of lentiviral vectors encoding shRNAs and miRNAs are reduced by different mechanisms that require distinct repair strategies," *RNA*, vol. 16, no. 7, pp. 1328–1339, 2010.

[26] C. Albrecht, S. Hosiner, B. Tichy, S. Aldrian, S. Hajdu, and S. Nürnberger, "Comparison of lentiviral packaging mixes and producer cell lines for RNAi applications," *Molecular Biotechnology*, vol. 57, no. 6, pp. 499–505, 2015.

[27] O. Eickelberg, M. Centrella, M. Reiss, M. Kashgarian, and R. G. Wells, "Betaglycan inhibits TGF-β signaling by preventing type I-type II receptor complex formation: glycosaminoglycan modifications alter betaglycan function," *Journal of Biological Chemistry*, vol. 277, no. 1, pp. 823–829, 2002.

[28] H. J. You, M. W. Bruinsma, T. How, J. H. Ostrander, and G. C. Blobe, "The type III TGF-β receptor signals through both Smad3 and the p38 MAP kinase pathways to contribute to inhibition of cell proliferation," *Carcinogenesis*, vol. 28, no. 12, pp. 2491–2500, 2007.

7

Intravenous Transplantation of Mesenchymal Stem Cells Reduces the Number of Infiltrated Ly6C$^+$ Cells but Enhances the Proportions Positive for BDNF, TNF-1α, and IL-1β in the Infarct Cortices of dMCAO Rats

Yunqian Guan,[1] Xiaobo Li,[2] Wenxiu Yu,[2] Zhaohui Liang,[2] Min Huang,[2] Renchao Zhao,[2] Chunsong Zhao,[1] Yao Liu,[2] Haiqiang Zou,[3] Yanli Hao,[4] and Zhiguo Chen ⓘ[1]

[1]Cell Therapy Center, Xuanwu Hospital, Capital Medical University, and Key Laboratory of Neurodegeneration, Ministry of Education, Beijing, China
[2]Department of Neurology, Northern Jiangsu People's Hospital, Clinical Medical School of Yangzhou University, Yangzhou, China
[3]Department of Neurology, The General Hospital of Guangzhou Military Command, Guangzhou, China
[4]Department of Anatomy, Guangzhou Medical University, Guangzhou, China

Correspondence should be addressed to Zhiguo Chen; chenzhiguo@gmail.com

Academic Editor: Jane Ru Choi

The resident microglial and infiltrating cells from peripheral circulation are involved in the pathological processes of ischemia stroke and may be regulated by mesenchymal stem/stromal cell (MSC) transplantation. The present study is aimed at differentiating the neurotrophic and inflammatory roles played by microglial vs. infiltrating circulation-derived cells in the acute phase in rat ischemic brains and explore the influences of intravenously infused allogeneic MSCs. The ischemic brain injury was induced by distal middle cerebral artery occlusion (dMCAO) in SD rats, with or without MSC infusion in the same day following dMCAO. Circulation-derived infiltrating cells in the brain were identified by Ly6C, a majority of which were monocytes/macrophages. Without MSC transplantation, among the infiltrated Ly6C$^+$ cells, some were positive for BDNF, IL-1β, or TNF-α. Following MSC infusion, the overall number of Ly6C$^+$ infiltrated cells was reduced by 50%. In contrast, the proportions of infiltrated Ly6C$^+$ cells coexpressing BDNF, IL-1β, or TNF-α were significantly enhanced. Interestingly, Ly6C$^+$ cells in the infarct area could produce either neurotrophic factor BDNF or inflammatory cytokines (IL-1β or TNF-α), but not both. This suggests that the Ly6C$^+$ cells may constitute heterogeneous populations which react differentially to the microenvironments in the infarct area. The changes in cellular composition in the infarct area may have contributed to the beneficial effect of MSC transplantation.

1. Introduction

Mesenchymal stem/stromal cells (MSCs) have a potential for treatment of neurological diseases, such as stroke. Bone marrow-derived MSCs (BM-MSCs) show merits in that they can be allogeneically or autologously transplanted without raising ethical or immunological problems.

The therapeutic mechanisms of intravenous MSC transplantation have been mainly ascribed to the neurotrophic and anti-inflammatory effects [1]. MSCs are capable of

secreting a lot of cytokines and eliciting the host to produce many kinds of neurotrophic factors, including brain-derived neurotrophic factor (BDNF) [2], glial cell-derived neurotrophic factor (GDNF) [3], and insulin growth factor-1 (IGF-1) [4].

Inflammatory responses in stroke, including immune cells, cytokines, and chemokines, are important for stroke development and recovery. Local microglial cells and periphery circulation-derived cells, such as monocytes/macrophages, are important participants in stroke-induced inflammation and can be both beneficial and detrimental after stroke injury. Despite extensive studies on microglia in stroke, the roles of periphery-derived cells during ischemic stroke have not been fully characterized [5, 6].

We have previously shown a rapid accumulation of ionized calcium binding adaptor molecule-1- (Iba-1-) positive microglia in the injured cerebral cortex two days after dMCAO in rats [7]. After intravenous MSC transplantation, the concentrations of neurotrophin BDNF and proinflammatory cytokines TNF-α and IL-1β are all increased [7]. It will be interesting to examine the respective contribution from microglial vs. infiltrated cells in production of BDNF, TNF-α, and IL-1β.

However, microglial and infiltrating monocytes/macrophages share many features. Iba-1 expression does not allow complete discrimination of resident microglia from infiltrated monocytes/macrophages. Other commonly used pan-markers for microglia, such as CD11b, isolectin (IB4), and F4/80, are not specific enough either [6]. CD45 alone is not sufficient because although infiltrated hematopoietic cells express high levels of CD45, activated microglia express low levels of CD45 too [8].

It is therefore important to find a marker that can differentiate microglia from infiltrated monocytes/macrophages in rats. Ly6C$^+$ cells represent circulation-derived monocytes/macrophages in mice and human [9, 10]. Whether the same holds true in rats is one of the questions that will be addressed in the current study.

One of the main therapeutic effects of MSCs after stroke is the neurotrophic effects [11]. Neurotrophins, such as BDNF, may be derived from the MSCs that have migrated into the brain, the endogenous neurons, and/or microglia/macrophages. BDNF is distributed in substantial amount in the ischemic core, peri-ischemic core cortex, ipsilateral striatum, and contralateral hemisphere [2, 12]. BDNF plays a crucial role in neuronal survival and plasticity, and its importance for stroke recovery has been demonstrated in Kurozumi's study. MSCs are transfected with BDNF, ciliary neurotrophic factor (CNTF), or neurotrophin 3 (NT3) vectors. Rats that undergo middle cerebral artery occlusion (MCAO) and receive MSC-BDNF exhibit significantly better functional recovery than do control stroke rats. MCAO rats that have received MSC-CNTF and MSC-NT3 do not show significant improvement vs. control stroke rats [13, 14].

We have previously found that in the ischemic brain, BDNF is expressed in NeuN-positive neurons and CD68-positive microglia/macrophages in the peri-infarct areas, but mainly by Iba-1-positive microglia in the infarct core [7]. Whether BDNF production can be derived from infiltrated cells and regulatable by MSC treatment is still unclear, and the current study will try to address these questions as well.

The other main therapeutic mechanism underlying MSC effect in stroke is the immunosuppressive effects, including downregulation of proinflammatory cytokines produced by microglia/macrophages [15]. Macrophage infiltration is normally thought to exacerbate focal inflammatory responses and further damage the brain by producing proinflammatory cytokines, such as TNF-α and IL-1β [16, 17]. As the most studied cytokines in adult stroke, IL-1β and TNF-α have been found to exacerbate brain damage by directly inducing neuronal injury and via consequent production of additional cytokines/chemokines and upregulation of adhesion molecules [18, 19]. Some groups found that IL-1β and TNF-α are expressed in largely segregated populations of CD11b$^+$CD45dim microglia and CD11b$^+$CD45high macrophages in mice [20].

In the current study, we will investigate whether neurotrophic factor BDNF and proinflammatory factors IL-1β and TNF-α are produced by infiltrated cells and how the production is regulated by MSC treatment.

2. Materials and Methods

2.1. Distal Middle Cerebral Artery Occlusion (dMCAO) Model, Peripheral Macrophage Depletion, and Cell Transplantation. The performance of allogeneic bone marrow MSC culture, cell transplantation, dMCAO model establishment, and behavioral tests have been described in our previous study [7]. In brief, 1×10^6 MSCs in 1 mL 0.9% saline were administered via intravenous injection one hour after ischemia. One mL of 0.9% saline was given to the ischemia vehicle group ($n = 10$ per group).

Intravenous administration of clodronate liposomes was widely used for depletion of the monocyte/macrophage population in blood circulation. Clodronate liposomes do not affect CNS-resident microglia because they cannot pass the blood-brain barrier (BBB). In this study, clodronate liposomes (Liposoma BV, Amsterdam, Netherlands) were intraperitoneally injected 1, 2, and 3 days before the dMCAO. The dose of clodronate liposomes was 50 mg/kg according to the manufacturer's instructions. PBS injection was used as a negative control [21, 22].

The SD rats used in this study were divided into three groups, "sham" controls (skull was opened but without arterial occlusion), "ischemia + vehicle" group (dMCAO models with saline injection), and "ischemia + MSC" group (dMCAO models with MSC infusion). Three time points, 3, 24, and 48 h post-ischemia, were chosen. Under each condition, 5–10 rats were included.

2.2. Immunohistochemistry. The rats were anesthetized and transcranially perfused with 0.9% saline, followed by cold 4% formaldehyde (PFA). The brains were removed, postfixed in 4% PFA for 24 h, and stored in 30% sucrose/PBS at 4°C. All brains were sectioned on vibrating microtome at 40 μm thickness. Free-floating sections across the entire brains were collected.

Immunohistochemistry and cell counting were performed as previously described [7]. In brief, floating brain sections were incubated in 0.3% Triton-100 PBS for 30 min and blocked with 2% donkey serum in PBS for 30 min at room temperature (RT). Sections were incubated overnight with Ly6C primary antibody (1:500 dilution, Santa Cruz Biotechnology, CA, USA). In the following day, sections were rinsed 3 × 15 minutes in TBS and incubated with FITC- or Cy3-conjugated secondary antibodies (1:300; Immune-Jackson Inc., CA, USA) for 2 h at RT. The sections were reblocked by 2% donkey serum in PBS for 30 min, then incubated with anti-CD45 (1:200 dilution, eBioscience, CA, USA), anti-CD68 (1:500 dilution, Chemicon, Temecula, CA, USA), biotin-conjugated anti-BDNF (1:500 dilution, R&D Systems, Minneapolis, USA), biotin-conjugated anti-TNF-α (1:500 dilution, R&D Systems, Minneapolis, USA), or biotin-conjugated anti-IL-1β antibodies (1:500 dilution, NeoBioscience Technology Co., Ltd, Shanghai, China). Other primary antibodies used included rat anti-rat Ly6C primary antibody (1:500 dilution, Santa Cruz Biotechnology, CA, USA), mouse anti-rat neutrophil elastase (1:500 dilution, Santa Cruz Biotechnology, CA, USA), and mouse anti-rat CD3 (1:500 dilution, NeoBioscience Technology Co., Ltd, Shanghai, China).

After being washed by PBS for 3 times, secondary antibodies were applied for 2 hours, followed by DAPI treatment for 20 min. Control reactions for antibody specificity were performed by omission of the primary antibodies. After being mounted onto slides, the positive cells were counted using a TCS SP5 II confocal laser scanning microscope (Leica, Wetzlar, Germany) at 200x magnification. The confocal settings, such as gain and offset, were designed to ensure that all pixels of all the selected sections were within the photomultiplier detection range. The setting was maintained to ensure all images were collected with the same parameters.

2.3. Cell Counting. In our experiments, the distribution of Ly6C, Iba-1, and BDNF was not restricted within the infarct area. For analysis, we counted the cells only in the cortical infarct areas.

The border zone between infarcted and healthy brain tissue is compartmentalized into an inner macrophage-rich part and a more peripheral zone dominated by reactive astrocytes [23, 24]. Based on this concept and the demarcation method of Gelosa et al. [25], we outlined the inner infarct boundary zone (IBZ) as within 400 μm to the boundary line between the normal and infarct areas. The counting region is a 1.6 mm $\times$ 0.8 mm rectangle (rectangle in Figure 1(i)), which is located in the infarct cortex area and adjacent to the inner IBZ.

The selection of sections for each rat was in accordance with Simsek and Duman [26]. For each section, the Ly6C-positive and Ly6C/BDNF-, Ly6C/TNF-α-, and Ly6C/IL-1β double-positive cells that were located in the counting region were counted as previously described [26, 27]. The numbers of neurotrophils (neurotrophil elastase$^+$) and T cells (CD3$^+$) coexpressing BDNF, TNF-α, and IL-1β were also counted. The number of labeled cells was calculated in 3 coronal sections from each rat, located between −2.0 mm and 2.0 mm to the bregma and expressed as the mean number of cells per view field (20x objective). The estimated cell numbers were determined using the method of Simsek and Duman [26]. All analyses were performed by investigators blinded to the sample identity and treatment groups.

2.4. Statistics. The data of cell counting were expressed as mean ± SEM. The comparisons were analyzed by one-way analysis of variance (one-way ANOVA) and Bonferroni-Dunnett corrections using SPSS 10.0. The level of significance of all comparisons was set at $p < 0.05$.

3. Results

The success of ischemia model generation was validated by HE staining. The mortality rates of animals following dMCAO for the sham control, "ischemia + vehicle," and "ischemia + MSCs" groups were 0, 16.7%, and 13.3%, respectively. There was no significant difference of mortality rates between the groups.

3.1. Ly6C$^+$ Cells at the Infarct Area in Rat Brains Are Circulation-Derived Cells. Accumulation of Ly6C$^+$ cells in the infarct area boundary zone (IBZ) was induced continuously over time following ischemia (Figures 1(a)–1(d)). The lineage identification is shown in Figures 1(e)–1(h), and the demarcation of inner IBZ and counting region was demonstrated in Figure 1(i).

Brain slices of naïve rats (no surgical operation, no dMCAO, and no MSC infusion) were stained, and no Ly6C$^+$ cells in the cerebral cortex was detected, suggesting that the Ly6C$^+$ cells observed in the dMCAO brains were derived from peripheral circulation (Figure S1A–D).

To further confirm the origin of Ly6C$^+$ cells in dMCAO brains, we deleted the monocytes/macrophages in the periphery by i.p. injection of clodronate liposomes, which cannot cross BBB and therefore do not affect brain-resident microglia. Two days after dMCAO, the number of Ly6C$^+$ cells in the cerebral cortex was reduced by 80–90% as compared with the sham group (Figure S1E–H).

In sham control rats, almost no Ly6C-expressing cells were found in the ischemia core cortex. Only after ischemia occurred did the Ly6C$^+$ cells emerge in the infarct boundary zone (Figure 1(a)). Three hours after ischemia, Ly6C$^+$ cells began to appear in the infarct area (Figure 1(b)). At 24 and 48 h, more and more Ly6C$^+$ cells accumulated around almost the entire cerebral ischemia core cortex and striatum and were distributed widely in the ischemic hemisphere (Figures 1(c) and 1(d)). In contrast, few Ly6C$^+$ cells were located in the ipsilateral cortex in the sham group 3, 24, and 48 h after ischemia.

At two days after the onset of ischemia, immunohistological examination showed strong expression of Ly6C in the infarct area (Figure 1(e)). The strong expression of CD45 (Figures 1(f)–1(h)) together with Ly6C reactivity confirmed that the cells were derived from periphery circulation.

3.2. Ly6C$^+$ Cells Represent a Population Partly Overlapping with Iba-1$^+$ Cells. To delineate the histological distribution and find out to what extent the two markers are overlapped, we performed double immunohistochemistry for Iba-1 and Ly6C.

A large portion of Ly6C$^+$ cells were found accumulated in the inner infarct boundary zone and in the infarct area (Figures 2(a)–2(d)) after ischemia induction. The distribution of Iba-1$^+$ cells was wider than that of Ly6C$^+$ cells. Plenty of Iba-1$^+$ cells were detected not only in the infarct area but also in the intact ipsilateral cortex (Figures 2(e)–2(h)),

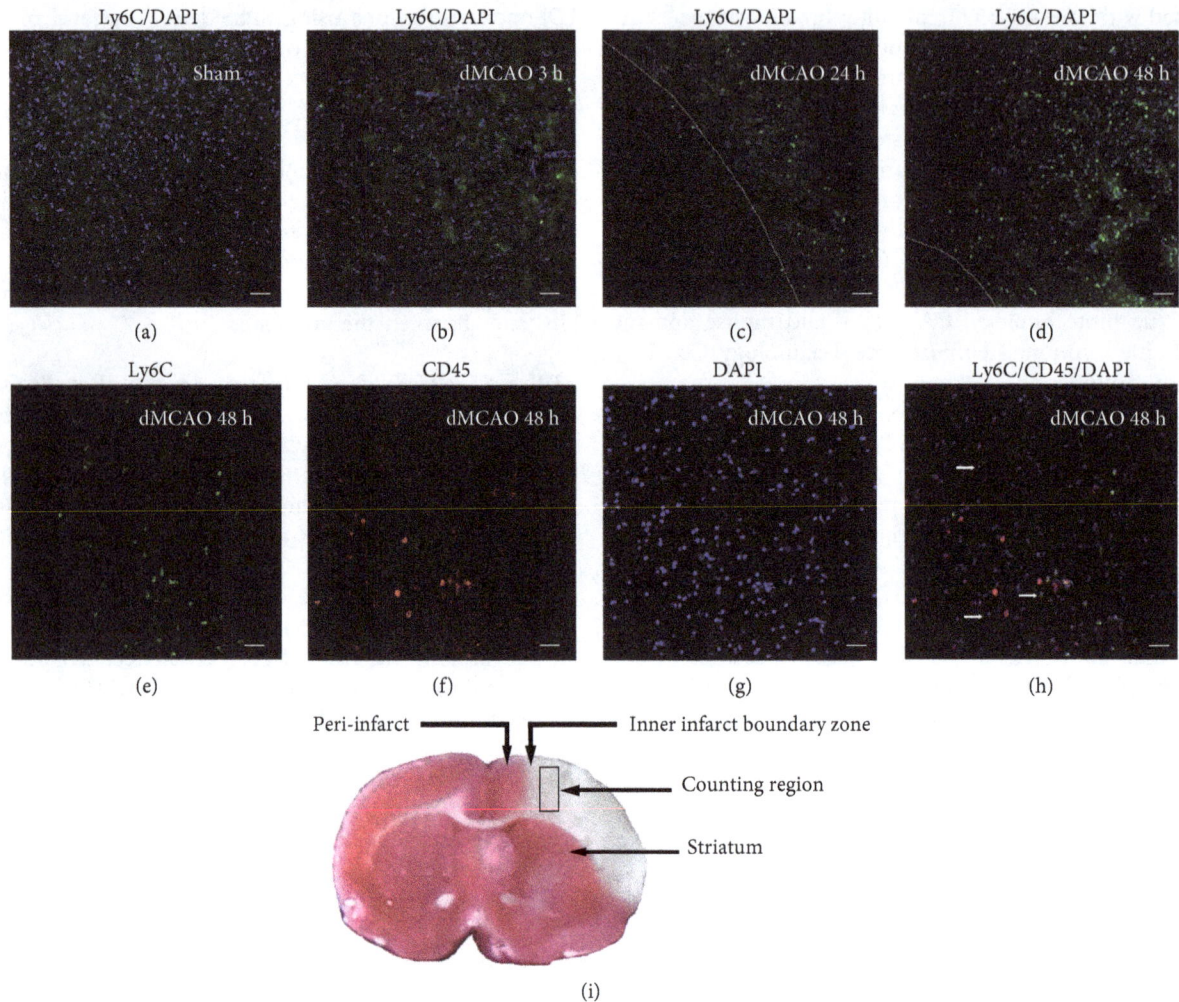

FIGURE 1: Ly6C$^+$ cells in the ischemic core cortex. The number of Ly6C$^+$ cells gradually increases at the IBZ of infarct dMCAO in rats. (a) Ly6C staining of the sham group. (b) Ly6C staining of the infarct area 3 h after the onset of ischemia. (c) 24 h. (d) 48 h. (e) Ly6C staining in the infarct area at 48 h. (f) CD45 staining in the same view field as (e). (g) DAPI nucleus staining. (h) Merged image of (e), (f), and (g), showing that Ly6C-positive cells are all CD45-positive. Arrow: double-labeled cells. (i) Cerebral infarct of the "ischemia + vehicle" group, as stained by triphenyltetrazolium chloride (TTC). Rectangle: the area where cell counting was performed. Dotted lines: the boundary of the infarct areas. Scale bar, 50 μm.

striatum, and corpus callosum (Figures 2(i)–2(l)) and even in the contralateral hemisphere. In the intact areas of both contra- and ipsilateral hemispheres, the majority of the Iba-1$^+$ cells were of magnified morphology, and in the infarct, the predominant morphology of Iba-1$^+$ cells was amoeboid-like round (Figures 2(d), 2(h), and 2(l)).

Only in the infarct cortex and the inner IBZ were a few Ly6C$^+$ cells reactive for Iba-1 (Figures 2(a)–2(d)). The percentage of double labeled Iba-1$^+$/Ly6C$^+$ cells in the infarct area and the inner IBZ was 30.18 ± 8.57% and 30.91 ± 15.56% among the Iba-1$^+$ cells, respectively (Figures 2(m) and 2(n)). Among the Ly6C$^+$ cells, about 25.35 ± 3.26% coexpressed Iba-1 in the infarct area and 24.68 ± 4.14% coexpressed Iba-1 in the IBZ. There was no significant difference between the numbers at the infarct area and the inner IBZ. After MSC transplantation, the overlapping percentage of Iba-1$^+$ and Ly6C$^+$ cells was not changed in the infarct area and inner IBZ.

In peri-infarct area (Figures 2(e)–2(h)), striatum, and corpus callosum (Figures 2(i)–2(l)), few Ly6C$^+$ cells were found, and they were negative for Iba-1 (Figures 2(o) and 2(p)).

When all of the Iba-1$^+$ cells, including the contra- and ipsilateral cortices, striatum, and corpus callosum, were taken into account, the overlapped proportion with Ly6C was less than 0.01% among the Iba-1$^+$ cells.

3.3. Ly6C$^+$ Cell Is One of the Major Contributors for BDNF Production.

We have shown that in the ipsilateral ischemia core cortex, Iba-1$^+$ cells are one of the main sources for the production of BDNF [7]. Other cell types, such as CD68$^+$ microglia, and NeuN$^+$ neurons, are partly responsible for production of BDNF, even after the induction of ischemia. But all of these cells together do not represent the entire BDNF$^+$ population. These results strongly suggest that there are other cell types as the source of BDNF in the infarct region.

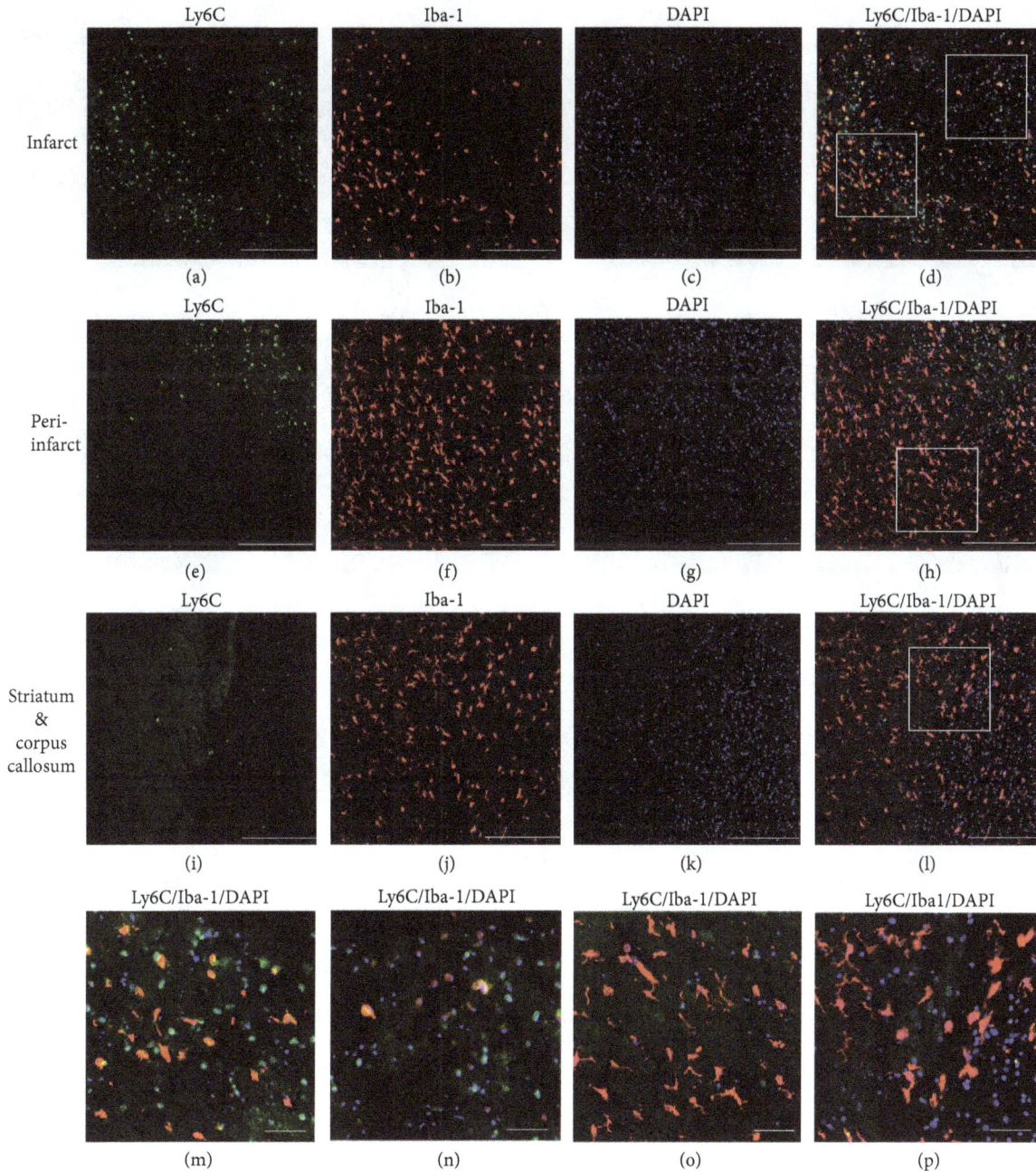

FIGURE 2: Few Ly6C$^+$ cells are double-stained with Iba-1 in the ischemia core cortex at day 2. (a–d) Distribution of Ly6C$^+$ and Iba-1$^+$ cells in the infarct areas. (e–h) Distribution of Ly6C$^+$ and Iba-1$^+$ cells in the peri-infarct area of the ipsilateral cortex. (i–l) Distribution of Ly6C$^+$ and Iba-1$^+$ cells in the ipsilateral striatum and corpus callosum. (a, e, i) Ly6C staining. (b, f, j) Iba-1. (c, g, k) DAPI nucleus staining. (d, h, l) Double-stained Ly6C$^+$/Iba-1$^+$ cells. (d) Ly6C$^+$/Iba-1$^+$ cells scattered in the infarct area (right square) and the inner infarct boundary zone (left square). (h) Very few Ly6C$^+$ cells were found in the ipsilateral peri-infarct area (to the left of the dashed line). (l) Very few Ly6C$^+$ cells were found in the ipsilateral striatum (to the left of the dashed line) and corpus callosum (to the right of the dashed line), and no double stained Ly6C$^+$/Iba-1$^+$ cells were spotted in the striatum or corpus callosum. Arrow: double-labeled cells. Scale bar, 50 μm. (m) (left square in (d)): in the inner infarct boundary zone, 30–40% of Ly6C$^+$ cells were Iba-1-positive. (n) (right square in (d)): in the infarct area, 20–30% of Ly6C$^+$ cells were Iba-1-positive. (o, p) (squares in (h) and (l)): very few or no double-stained Ly6C$^+$/Iba-1$^+$ cells was spotted in the striatum or corpus callosum. Scale bar: (a–l) 250 μm and (m–p) 50 μm.

We performed double immunohistochemistry for BDNF and Ly6C (Figure 3) and found that, two days after ischemia onset, BDNF expression was enhanced in infiltrating Ly6C$^+$ cells in the ischemia core cortex as compared with the sham control group, and only in the infarct area was BDNF staining found overlapped with Ly6C (Figures 3(a)–3(d)). The numbers of Ly6C$^+$ cells, BDNF single-positive cells, Ly6C$^+$/BDNF$^+$ double-positive cells were 93.8 ± 14.56, 40.2 ± 9.59, and 29.7 ± 6.18 per view field, respectively (Figure 3(k)).

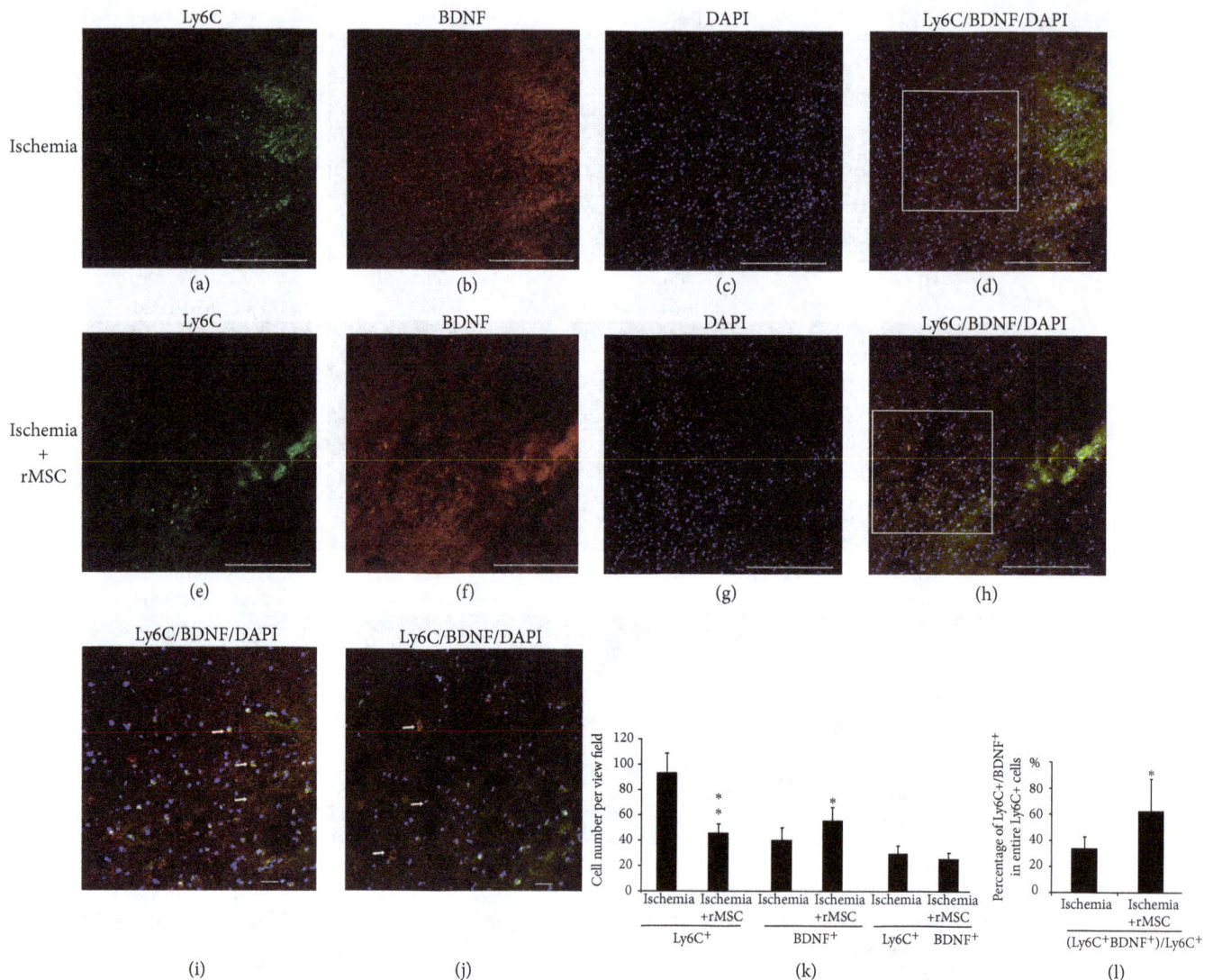

FIGURE 3: Ly6C$^+$ cells are one of the major contributors for BDNF production at day 2. (a–d) Distribution of Ly6C$^+$ and BDNF$^+$ cells in the infarct before MSC transplantation. (e–h) Distribution of Ly6C$^+$ and BDNF$^+$ cells in the infarct after MSC transplantation. (a, e) Ly6C staining. (b, f) BDNF. (c, g) DAPI nucleus staining. (d) Double-stained Ly6C$^+$/BDNF$^+$ cells scattered in the infarct area after dMCAO. (h) Ly6C$^+$/BDNF$^+$ cells 2 days after MSC transplantation. (i, j) Squares in (d) and (h). Ly6C$^+$ cell number was reduced in the infarct area 2 days after MSC transplantation, and the quantity and percentage of double-stained BDNF$^+$ Ly6C$^+$ cells were increased in these areas. (k) The cell counting results of Ly6C$^+$, BDNF$^+$, and Ly6C$^+$/BDNF$^+$ cells before and after MSC transplantation. (l) The percentage of Ly6C$^+$/BDNF$^+$ cells among Ly6C$^+$ cells was increased by MSC treatment. ($^*p < 0.05$ and $^{**}p < 0.01$, as compared with the ischemia vehicle group). Arrow: double-labeled cells. $n = 5$; scale bar: (a–h) 250 μm and (i, j) 50 μm.

MSC treatment reduced the quantity of Ly6C$^+$ cells that had infiltrated into the brain to 35.7 ± 7.04 per view field, but increased the number of BDNF$^+$ cells to 55.7 ± 10.10 (Figures 3(e)–3(k)). MSC transplantation did not change the number of Ly6C$^+$/BDNF$^+$ double-positive cells ($25.5 + 4.45$), but increased the proportion of Ly6C$^+$ cells coexpressing BDNF from $32.40 \pm 7.25\%$ before MSC treatment to $71.65 \pm 4.26\%$ after treatment (Figures 3(i), 3(j), and 3(l)).

We have previously reported that BDNF expression was enhanced in Iba-1$^+$ cells following ischemia [7]. Although around 25% of Ly6C$^+$ cells were also Iba-1-positive in the infarct area, the current study strongly suggested that Ly6C$^+$ cells may be another major contributor for BDNF

production since the proportion of Ly6C$^+$ cells coexpressing BDNF was dramatically enhanced to $71.65 \pm 4.26\%$ after MSC treatment.

3.4. Ly6C$^+$ Cells Positive for IL-1β Are Upregulated by MSC Treatment. We examined IL-1β reactivity in Ly6C$^+$ cells in the ischemia vehicle group (Figures 4(a)–4(d)) and in the ischemia + MSC group (Figures 4(e)–4(h)). The ischemia vehicle group showed a higher level of IL-1β compared to the sham control group (data not shown, $p < 0.01$), as evidenced by the increased number of IL-1β$^+$/Ly6C$^+$ cells in the infarct area.

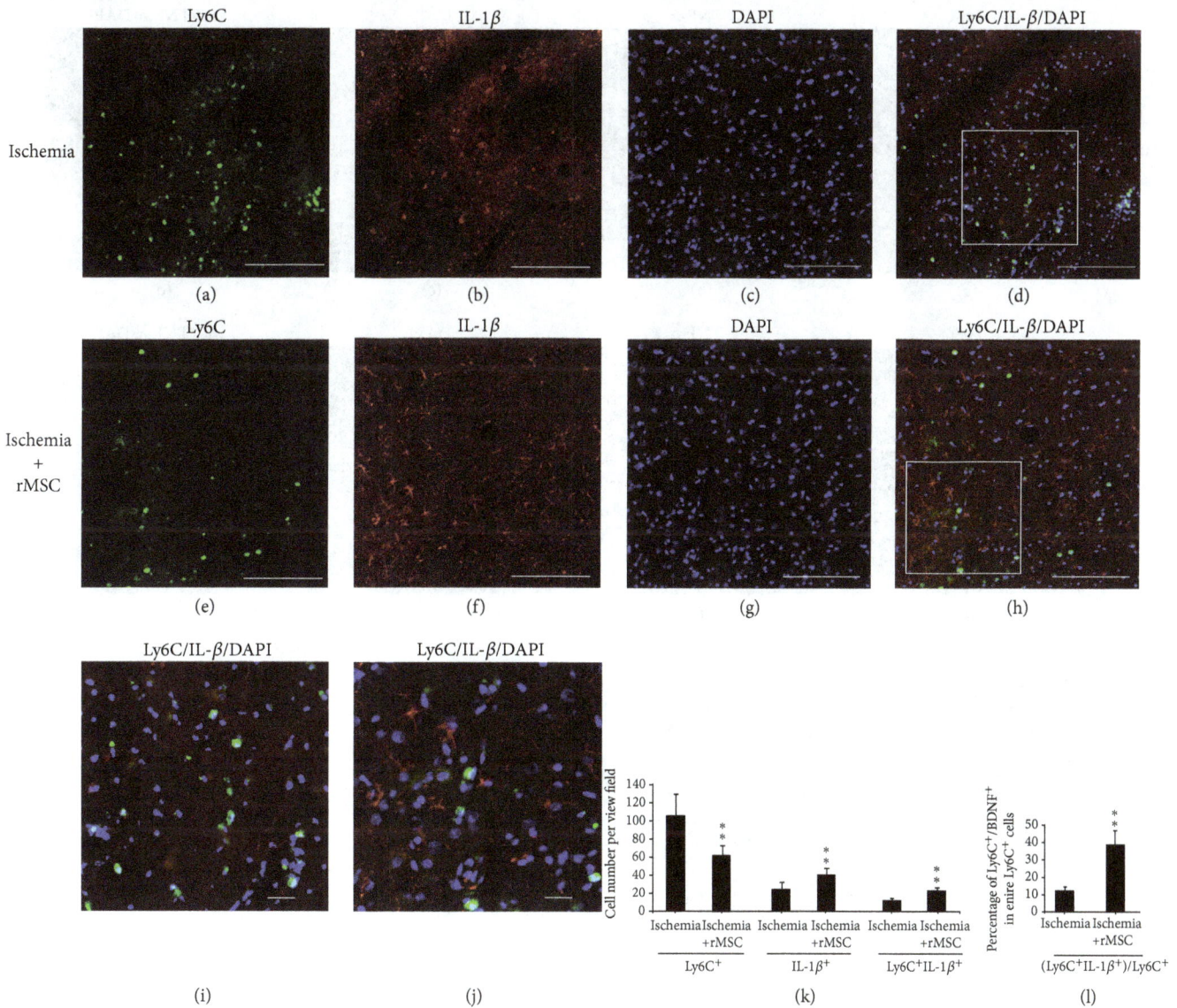

FIGURE 4: MSC treatment reduces the quantity of Ly6C$^+$ cells but increases the proportion that produces IL-1β at day 2. (a–d) Distribution of Ly6C$^+$ and IL-1β^+ cells in the infarct before MSC treatment. (e–h) Distribution of Ly6C$^+$ and IL-1β^+ cells in the infarct after MSC treatment. (a, e) Ly6C staining. (b, f) IL-1β staining. (c, g) DAPI nucleus staining. (d) Double-stained Ly6C$^+$/IL-1β^+ cells scattered in the infarct area 2 days after dMCAO. (h) Ly6C$^+$/IL-1β^+ cells in the infarct area 2 days after MSC transplantation. (i) The magnified image of the square in (d). (j) The magnified image of the square in (h). (k) Ly6C$^+$ cell number was reduced in the infarct area 2 days after MSC transplantation, but the quantity of IL-1β^+ cells and IL-1β^+/Ly6C$^+$ cells was increased in the infarct area. (l) The percentage of Ly6C/IL-1β double-positive cells among the whole Ly6C$^+$ cells was increased by MSC treatment. ($^*p < 0.05$ and $^{**}p < 0.01$, as compared with the ischemia vehicle group). Arrow: double-labeled cells. $n = 5$; scale bar: (a–h) 250 μm and (i, j) 50 μm.

MSC transplantation reduced the number of Ly6C$^+$ cells infiltrated into the brain but increased the number of IL-1β^+ cells from 24.75 ± 7.35 per view field before MSC transplantation to 41 ± 6.82 after transplantation ($p < 0.01$, Figure 4(k)). After all, the quantity of IL-1β^+/Ly6C$^+$ double-positive cells was increased by MSC treatment from 12.5 ± 2.18 to 23.75 ± 3.16 per view field ($p < 0.01$, Figure 4(k)). The percentage of IL-1β^+/Ly6C$^+$ double-positive cells in the entire Ly6C$^+$ cells was also increased by MSC treatment from 12.30 ± 2.03% to 38.62 ± 7.99% ($p < 0.01$, Figure 4(l)).

We have previously reported that IL-1β protein level was enhanced in the infarct area 48 h after MSC transplantation [7]. The results from the current study suggest that Ly6C$^+$ infiltrated cells in the brain may have contributed to this enhancement.

3.5. MSC Treatment Induces TNF-α Expression in Ly6C$^+$ Cells. It was previously reported that in mouse stroke models, microglia are the main producer of TNF-α while macrophages are of IL-1(b) [20]. We examined TNF-α reactivity in Ly6C$^+$ cells in the ischemia vehicle group and in the

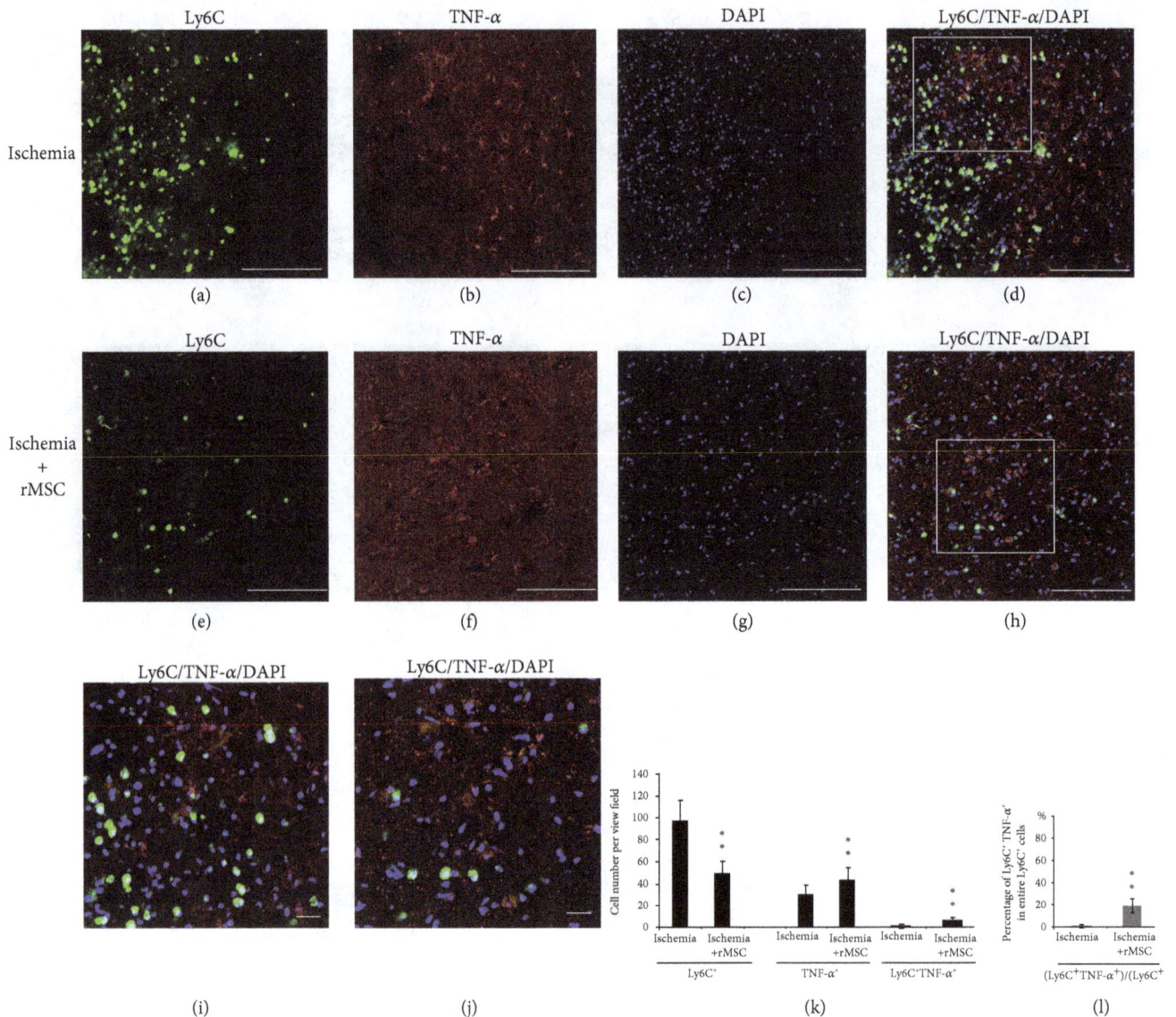

FIGURE 5: MSC increases the proportion of Ly6C$^+$ cells coexpressing TNF-α in the ischemia core of the cortex at day 2. (a–d) Distribution of Ly6C$^+$ and TNF-α^+ cells in the infarct area before MSC treatment. (e–h) Distribution of Ly6C$^+$ and TNF-α^+ cells in the infarct area after MSC treatment. (a, e) Ly6C staining. (b, f) TNF-α staining. (c, g) DAPI nucleus staining. (d) Double-stained Ly6C$^+$/TNF-α^+ cells scattered in the infarct area 2 days after dMCAO. (h) Ly6C$^+$/TNF-α^+ cells in the infarct area 2 days after MSC transplantation. (i) The magnified image of the square in (d). (j) The magnified image of the square in (h). (k) The quantities of Ly6C$^+$, TNF-α^+, and TNF-α^+/Ly6C$^+$ double-positive cells were increased in the infarct area. (l) The percentage of TNF-α^+/Ly6C$^+$ double-positive cells among the entire Ly6C$^+$ cells was increased by MSC treatment. ($^*p < 0.05$ and $^{**}p < 0.01$, as compared with the ischemia vehicle group). Arrow: double-labeled cells. $n = 5$; scale bar: (a–h) 250 μm, (i, j) 50 μm.

ischemia + MSC group. In the ischemia vehicle group (Figures 5(a)–5(d)), few TNF-α^+/Ly6C$^+$ double-positive cells were detected in the infarct area (Figures 5(d) and 5(i)). The numbers of TNF-α single-positive and TNF-α^+/Ly6C$^+$ double-positive cells were 31 ± 7.87 and 1.0 ± 1.73 per view field in the ischemia vehicle group, and the proportion of Ly6C$^+$ cells coexpressing TNF-α was 0.9 ± 1.2% (Figures 5(k) and 5(l)).

After MSC treatment, TNF-α expression was upregulated (Figures 5(e)–5(h)). The distribution of TNF-α^+/Ly6C$^+$ cells was still restricted within the infarct area and was not changed by MSC treatment (Figure 5(j)). The proportion of

Ly6C$^+$ cells coexpressing TNF-α was significantly increased (19.67 ± 6.54%) vs. the ischemia vehicle group (0.9 ± 2.2%, $p < 0.01$) (Figure 5(l)). Also, the number of TNF-α^+/Ly6C$^+$ double stained cells was enhanced to 7.5±0.87 per view field (Figure 5(k)).

3.6. Iba-1$^+$ Cells Are Not the Source of TNF-α or IL-1β Production in Rat Ischemia Brains and Cannot Be Induced by MSC Treatment. After the onset of ischemia in rats, in the contralateral hemisphere of the ischemia vehicle group, the Iba-1$^+$ cells with resting morphology were found in the intact cortex, striatum, and corpus callosum, but in these

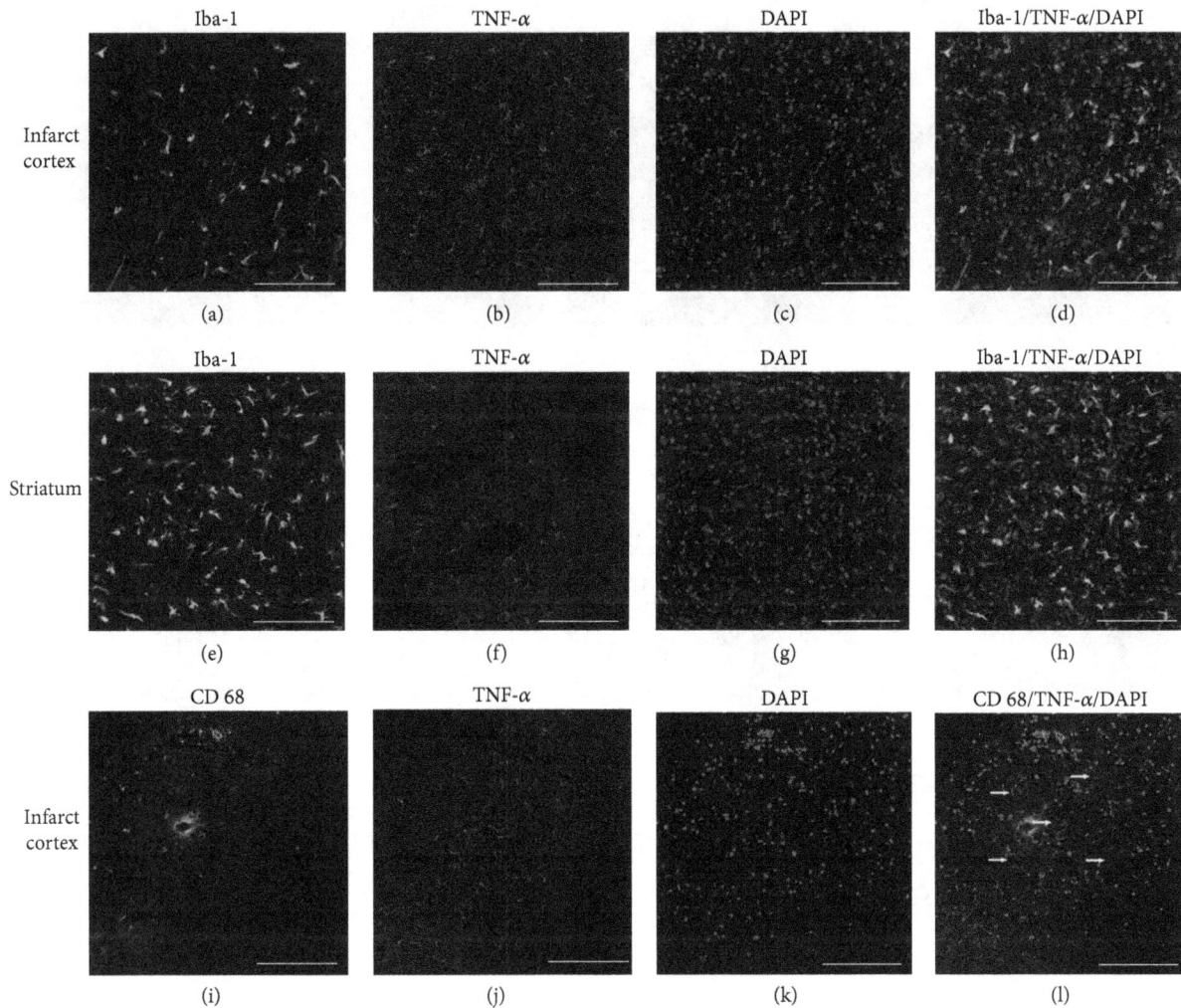

FIGURE 6: CD68$^+$ microglia but not Iba-1$^+$ cells express TNF-α in the ischemia ipsilateral hemisphere at day 2. (a–d) Distribution of Iba-1$^+$ and TNF-α^+ cells in the infarct areas after MSC transplantation. (e–h) Distribution of Iba-1$^+$ and TNF-α^+ cells in the striatum after MSC transplantation. (i–l) Distribution of CD68$^+$ and TNF-α^+ cells in the infarct areas after MSC transplantation. (a, e) Iba-1 staining. (i) CD68 staining. (b, f, j) TNF-α. (c, g, k) DAPI nucleus staining. (d) No double-stained Iba-1$^+$/TNF-α^+ cells were found in the infarct area after dMCAO. (h) No Iba-1+/TNF-α cells was found 2 days after MSC transplantation in the striatum. (l) Some CD68$^+$ cells in the infarct areas were positive for TNF-α. Arrow: double-labeled cells. Scale bar, 250 μm.

areas, TNF-α or IL-β reactivity was not detected (image not shown). In the ipsilateral hemisphere, Iba-1$^+$ microglia of both activated and resting forms were detected, but the resting phenotype existed in the infarct core cortex and intact striatum, whereas the active form was only found in the infarct core cortex.

In the infarct area, the spatial distribution of Iba-1 signals was correlated with those of TNF-α (Figures 6(a)–6(h)), although the two signals were never overlapped, whether in the infarct area (Figures 6(a)–6(d)) or the intact striatum and corpus callosum (Figures 6(e)–6(h)). Some CD68$^+$ cells in the infarct area (possibly activated microglia) were positive for TNF-α (Figures 6(i)–6(l)).

Similarly, the distribution of Iba-1$^+$ and IL-β^+ cells was spatially correlated but not overlapped (Figures 7(a)–7(h)). We have previously reported that the number of Iba-1$^+$ cells can be regulated by MSC infusion [7]. The current results indicated that in mild damage such as dMCAO, MSC treatment did not alter production levels of TNF-α or IL-β from Iba-1$^+$ cells. Iba-1$^+$ cells might not be the target of MSC regulation with respect to secretion of proinflammatory cytokines TNF-α and IL-β.

3.7. BDNF-Positive Cells Do Not Overlap with TNF-α- or IL-1β-Positive Cells.

Ischemia-induced accumulation of Ly6C$^+$ cells was localized in the ischemia core cortex and the surrounding areas, the same region where BDNF$^+$ cells resided. Here raises a question of whether BDNF and proinflammatory cytokines, such as TNF-α or IL-β, can be produced in the same cell positive for Ly6C.

We examined BDNF reactivity in TNF-α^+ and IL-β^+ cells (not restricted to macrophages) two days after stroke. No BDNF$^+$ cells were double labeled with TNF-α^+ or IL-β^+ cells in the brain, whether at the ischemia damaged areas or the intact areas (Figure 8).

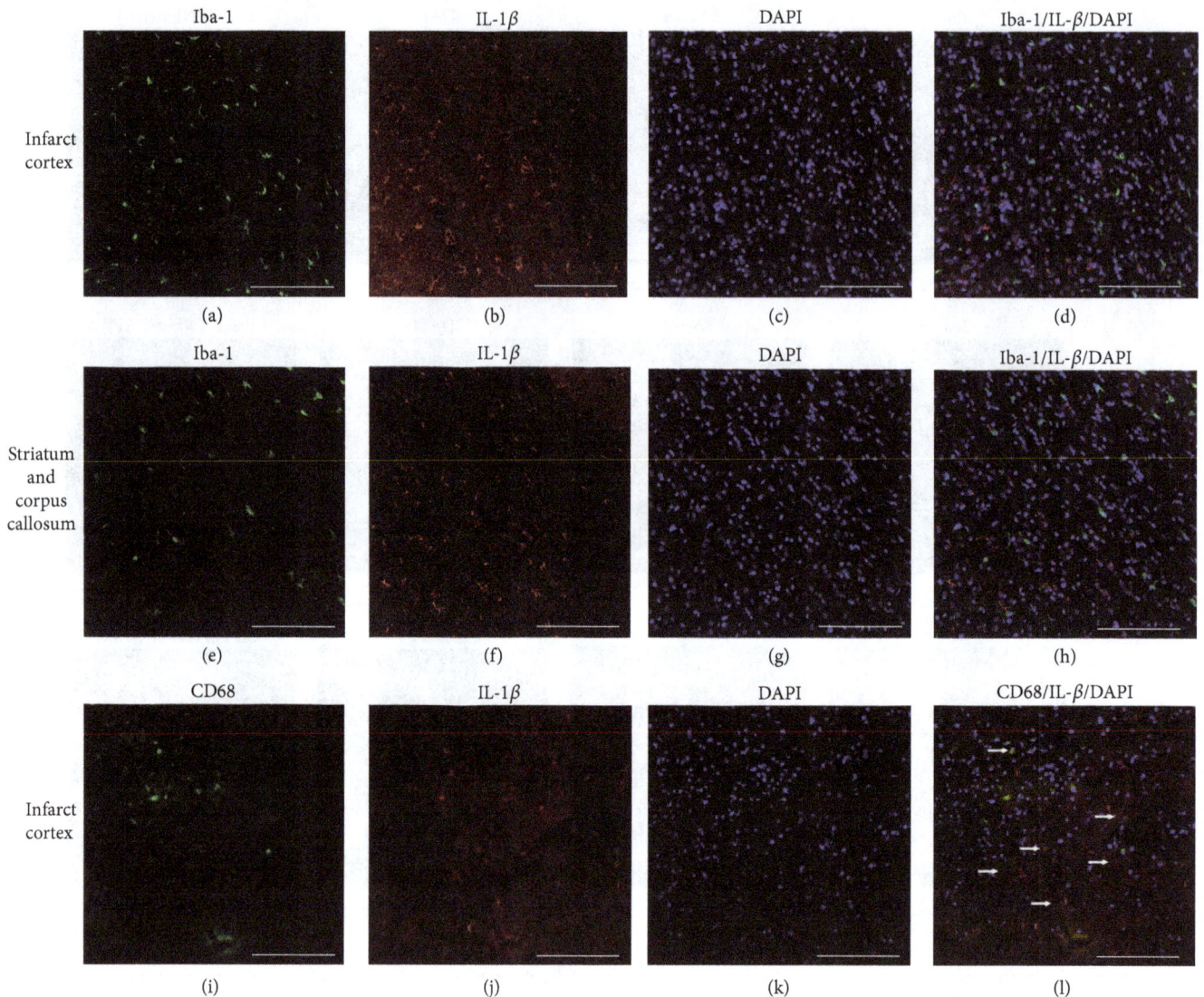

FIGURE 7: CD68$^+$ microglia but not Iba-1$^+$ cells express IL-β in the ischemic ipsilateral hemisphere at day 2. (a–d) Distribution of Iba-1$^+$ cells and IL-β^+ cells in the infarct areas after MSC transplantation. (e–h) Distribution of Iba-1$^+$ cells and IL-β^+ cells in the striatum after MSC transplantation. (i–l) Distribution of CD68$^+$ cells and IL-β^+ cells in the infarct areas after MSC transplantation. (a, e) Iba-1 staining. (i) CD68 staining. (b, f, j) IL-β. (c, g, k) DAPI nucleus staining. (d) No double-stained Iba-1$^+$/IL-β^+ cells were found in the infarct area after dMCAO. (h) No Iba-1$^+$/IL-β^+ cells were found 2 days after MSC transplantation in the striatum and corpus callosum after MSC transplantation. (i–l) Some CD68$^+$ cells were positive for IL-β. Arrow: double-labeled cells. Scale bar, 250 μm.

3.8. Ly6C$^+$ Cells Are Partly Positive for Neutrophil Antigen Neutrophil Elastase (NE) or T Cell Antigen CD3. We also tried to identify the cell populations that comprise the Ly6C$^+$ cells in the ischemic brain. Since most of the granulocytes are neutrophils in the blood of rats, we selected neutrophil elastase (NE), to identify neutrophils in the brain. Approximately 8.62 ± 2.62% of Ly6C$^+$ cells coexpressed NE in the infarct areas (Figure S2A–D). MSC transplantation did not change the proportion significantly (9.31 ± 2.45%).

We also examined the coexpression of Ly6C and T cell marker CD3. Around 15.21 ± 4.62% of Ly6C$^+$ cells in the infarct areas coexpressed CD3 (Figure S2E–H). MSC transplantation did not significantly change the proportion either (17.31 ± 5.45%).

Here raised another question—could these overlapping cells also contribute to the production of BDNF, TNF-α,

and IL-1β following dMCAO? We found that very few NE- or CD3-positive cells were double-stained with BDNF (<1%) (Figure S3A–H). In terms of IL-1β, it was expressed by nearly 2% NE$^+$ neutrophils and 3–5% CD3$^+$ T cells (Figure S4A–H). Only 1–2% NE$^+$ neutrophils and 2–4% CD3$^+$ T cells expressed TNF-α (Figure S5A–H).

The results suggest that it is probably the infiltrating monocytes/macrophages that are the major contributors for Ly6C$^+$ cells that coexpress BDNF, TNF-α, or IL-1β.

4. Discussion

In the acute and subacute phases, resident microglial activation [28] and infiltration of circulating leukocytes to the

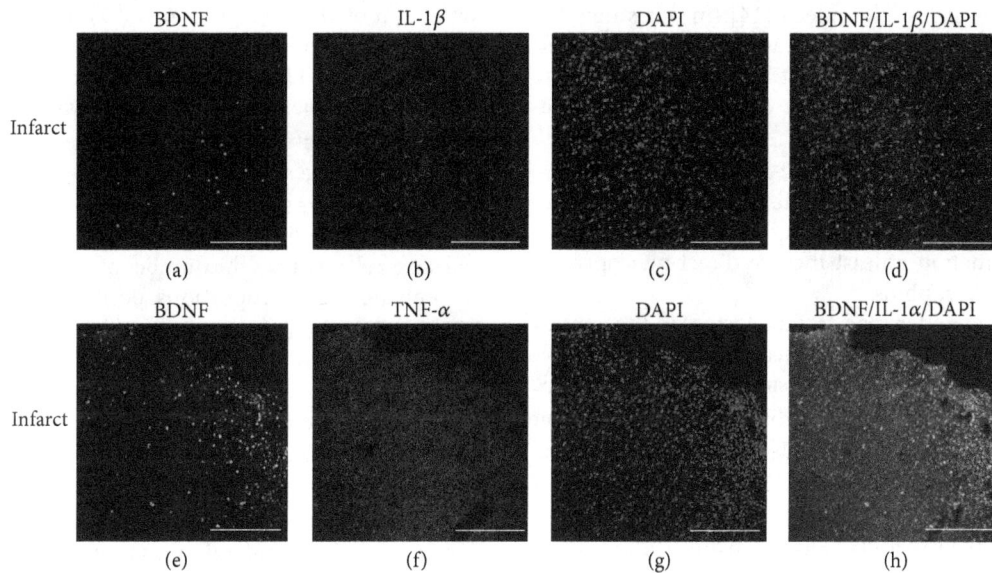

Figure 8: BDNF-producing cells do not overlap with TNF-α-or IL-1b-expressing cells at day 2. (a–d) Distribution of BDNF$^+$ cells and IL-β^+ cells in the infarct areas after MSC transplantation. (e–h) Distribution of BDNF$^+$ cells and TNF-α^+ cells in the infarct area after MSC transplantation. (a, e) BDNF staining. (b) IL-β. (f) TNF-α. (c, g) DAPI nucleus staining. (d) No double-stained BDNF$^+$/IL-β^+ cells were found in the infarct area after dMCAO. (h) No BDNF$^+$/TNF-α^+ cells were found 2 days after MSC transplantation in the striatum and corpus callosum after MSC transplantation. Scale bar, 250 μm.

ischemic brain [29] are the key features of the neuroimmunological responses to brain ischemia.

Previously, both microglia and infiltrated circulating leukocytes have been considered by many researchers to be harmful to the brain, since inhibition of some of these inflammatory responses improved the outcome in animal experiments. However, clinical trials aimed at inhibiting microglial activation or preventing leukocyte trafficking into the ischemic brain were unsuccessful [30]. It is nowadays accepted that the roles of inflammation in stroke are complicated in that they play both harmful and protective functions. This may be one reason why previous clinical trials of inhibiting immunological responses in stroke uniformly failed [30, 31].

Immune cells present in the healthy CNS and those recruited into stroke lesions are heterogeneous, including neutrophils, monocytes, macrophages, dendritic cells, T and B lymphocytes, and natural killer cells. Among these cells, monocytes/macrophages are important in the development of cerebral ischemia damages.

Given the importance of microglia and monocytes/macrophages in the stroke damage and that the marker "Iba-1" is normally expressed by both microglia and macrophages, it is important to identify a specific marker for infiltrated monocytes/macrophages in the ischemic brain.

Since Ly6C is widely used as the marker of mouse and human monocytes/macrophages, we selected Ly6C in this rat stroke study. Firstly, Ly6C$^+$ cells were not detected in brains of naïve rats and were only detected in brains of dMCAO rats. Secondly, depletion of peripheral immune cells by treatment with clodronate liposomes led to 80–90% reduction in the number of Ly6C$^+$ cells in dMCAO brains.

Together with the observation that Ly6C$^+$ cells were also CD45$^+$ in infarcted rat brains, it is suggested that Ly6C$^+$ cells in the brain represent circulation-derived infiltrated cells.

In ischemic brains, around 25% of Ly6C$^+$ cells were double-positive for Iba-1, and these double-stained cells were only detected inside the infarct areas. It is possible that some of the infiltrating Ly6C$^+$ immune cells may become Iba-1$^+$ over time.

CD68 is another important microglial marker. In our study, although, functionally, CD68$^+$ cells were a separated population from Iba-1$^+$ cells, morphologically, CD68$^+$ cells were part of Iba-1$^+$ cells (Figure S6). Less than 5% of Ly6C$^+$ cells were double-positive for CD68 (Figure S6), indicating that Ly6C$^+$ cells are mostly a different population than activated microglial cells.

Our results also suggest that Ly6C$^+$ cells in the ischemic brains were not purely monocytes/macrophages and included approximately 10% NE$^+$ neutrophils and 15% CD3$^+$ T cells. However, the infiltrated neutrophils and T cells did not produce BDNF, and only few of them (1–5%) were positive for TNF-α or IL-1β two days after dMCAO. Among the Ly6C$^+$ infiltrated cells, it is probably monocytes/macrophages that are the major contributors for production of BDNF, IL-1β, and TNF-α.

The spleen was reported to be a major reservoir of undifferentiated Ly6C$^+$ cells and proinflammatory cytokines that are readily mobilized during inflammatory processes, including stroke [5]. In this study, we found that dMCAO leads to infiltration of Ly6C$^+$ cells into the brain after stroke. It was reported that systemic administration of human umbilical cord blood progenitor cells (HUCBC) significantly reduces the number of macrophage/microglia in the injured brain and maintains the size of the spleen [14]. In our study, the number of infiltrated Ly6C$^+$ cells was significantly reduced after MSC infusion. The MSCs that had migrated into the spleen may be responsible for these effects by an immune-inhibitory mechanism [32].

On the other hand, inflammation can also be seen as part of a protective response indispensable for limiting stroke-induced brain damage and inducing repair. The beneficial effects of inflammation at least include direct neuroprotection through neurotrophins.

One of the best understood trophic factors in the context of stroke is BDNF, which promotes neurological recovery following middle cerebral artery occlusion [33]. BDNF can be produced by neurons through neuronal activity-dependent exocytosis. Our previous study showed that BDNF can also be secreted by Iba-1$^+$ microglia [7]. Now we have demonstrated that monocytes/macrophages are probably another important participant that mediates the neurotrophic effects after dMCAO. At 48 h after ischemia onset, nearly 32.40% of Ly6C$^+$ cells were BDNF-positive. Although MSC infusion reduced the total number of Ly6C$^+$ cells in the brain, MSC treatment nevertheless enhanced the total number of BDNF$^+$/Ly6C$^+$ cells and increased the percentage of BDNF-producing cells among the infiltrated monocytes/macrophages in the infarct area two days after ischemia onset.

In our previous study, we have shown that in the infarct areas, proinflammatory cytokines IL-1β and TNF-α levels are increased [7]. However, the cell types that have contributed to production of these two cytokines have not been carefully examined. In the current study, we looked mainly into monocytes/macrophages and microglia for cytokine production. Quantification of cells using secretory proteins such as cytokines and growth factors by immunostaining is challenging. Perhaps a better approach to overcome the limitation is quantifying the transcript as validation, which will be employed in our future studies.

In terms of IL-1β, 12.30 ± 2.03% of infiltrated Ly6C$^+$ cells were positive for IL-1β after ischemia, and MSC treatment increased the percentage to 38.62 ± 6.99%. MSC treatment also increased the numbers of IL-1β^+ and IL-1β^+/Ly6C$^+$ cells from 24.75 ± 7.35 and 12.5 ± 2.18 to 41.00 ± 6.82 and 23.75 ± 3.16 per view field, respectively.

Interestingly, very few Ly6C$^+$ cells expressed TNF-α before MSC transplantation (0.9 ± 1.0 per view field). After MSC treatment, although the quantity of Ly6C$^+$ cells decreased in the brain, the number of TNF-α^+/Ly6C$^+$ cells and its proportion among Ly6C$^+$ cells both increased.

Ritzel et al. have shown that, in mice, 72 h after a 90 min MCAO, monocytes/macrophages accumulated in the ischemic brain compared to sham controls. Microglia produce relatively higher levels of reactive oxygen species and TNF-α, whereas monocytes/macrophages are the predominant IL-1β producer [20]. Unexpectedly, in the current study, Iba-1$^+$ microglial cells did not express any significant level of TNF-α or IL-1β, whether in the infarct area, the intact cortex and striatum, or the corpus callosum. Some CD68$^+$ cells (possibly activated microglia in our study) were positive

for TNF-α or IL-1β (Figures 6 and 7). Ischemic damage and MSC transplantation after stroke did not induce the Iba-1$^+$ cells to produce TNF-α or IL-1β either. It seems that, in the current experimental setting and with respect to only microglia and monocytes/macrophages, infiltrated monocytes/macrophages, rather than microglia, are the predominant contributors for IL-1β and TNF-α production.

In our study, intravenous transplantation of mesenchymal stem cells reduces the number of infiltrated macrophages but enhances the proportions positive for BDNF, TNF-α, and IL-1β in the infarct cortices of dMCAO rats. The possible mechanisms may include, but may not be limited to, the following.

The majority of infused MSCs are trapped in the lung and spleen. Spleen is one of the organs that play an important role in the periphery after stroke. In the case of severe ischemia, the spleen contracts under the regulation of the hypothalamic-pituitary-adrenal axis and the sympathetic nervous system. This reduction in spleen size is associated with increased release of immune cells and proinflammatory cytokines into the blood, a greater extent of infiltration of leukocytes and monocytes, and a higher level of microglial activation in the brain. It seems that intravenous infusion of MSCs may suppress the "overactivated" inflammation and immune reaction in the spleen, reduce the influx of immune cells, prevent the exhaustion of immune capacities of spleen, and eventually avoid immunosuppression in stroke patients [34].

A noteworthy phenomenon was that only the Ly6C$^+$ cells located in the infarct area were positive for BDNF or proinflammatory cytokines IL-1β and TNF-α. The majority of Ly6C$^+$ cells surrounding the infarct area were negative for BDNF, TNF-α, and IL-1β. Two interesting aspects were implicated in this observation. First, after infusion, MSCs mostly accumulated at the peri-infarct areas too. The spatial correlation suggests that MSCs may have influenced the infiltrated cells through a paracrine and/or cell-cell contact mechanism. Second, Ly6C$^+$ cells in the infarct areas could be positive for either BDNF or proinflammatory cytokines (IL-1β and TNF-α), but not for both, whereas Ly6C$^+$ cells at the peri-infarct areas were mostly negative for all three. These results suggest that the infiltrated cells, including monocytes, may be intrinsically heterogeneous and can react differentially to different microenvironments. Microglia can be categorized into M1 and M2 subtypes, and the two subtypes can be switched in a certain context [34, 35]. Microglia originate from the hematopoietic lineage and are derived from the infiltrated monocytes during embryo development [21]. Like microglia, monocytes are possibly heterogeneous as well. Further efforts are warranted to identify the molecular cues in the infarct and peri-infarct areas that can induce infiltrated monocytes to assume different phenotypes. Once identified, these cues may offer a potential candidate for manipulating the functions of macrophages and improve the treatment of stroke.

Authors' Contributions

Yunqian Guan, Xiaobo Li, and Wenxiu Yu contributed equally to this work.

Acknowledgments

This work was supported by the Stem Cell and Translation National Key Project (2016YFA0101403), National Basic Research Program of China (2011CB965103), National Natural Science Foundation of China (81371377, 81661130160, 81422014, and 81561138004), Beijing Municipal Natural Science Foundation (7172055, 5142005), Beijing Talents Foundation (2017000021223TD03), Support Project of High-level Teachers in Beijing Municipal Universities in the Period of 13th Five–year Plan (CIT&TCD20180333), Beijing Medical System High Level Talent Award (2015-3-063), the Royal Society-Newton Advanced Fellowship (NA150482), Shandong Provincial Natural Science Foundation (2016ZDJS07A09), and Science and Technology project item in a social development area of Guangdong Province (2014A020212563).

Supplementary Materials

Supplementary Figure 1: Ly6C$^+$ cells in ischemic brains are derived from periphery circulation at day 2. Supplementary Figure 2: a small part of Ly6C$^+$ cells costained with neutrophil elastase and CD3 at day 2. Supplementary Figure 3: infiltrated neutrophils and T cells minimally contribute to BDNF production at day 2. Supplementary Figure 4: infiltrated neutrophils and T cells minimally contribute to IL-1β production at day 2. Supplementary Figure 5: infiltrated neutrophils and T cells minimally contribute to TNF-α production at day 2. Supplementary Figure 6: the overlapping of CD68$^+$ cells with Ly6C$^+$ and Iba-1$^+$ cells, respectively, at day 2. (*Supplementary Materials*)

References

[1] L. Crigler, R. C. Robey, A. Asawachaicharn, D. Gaupp, and D. G. Phinney, "Human mesenchymal stem cell subpopulations express a variety of neuro-regulatory molecules and promote neuronal cell survival and neuritogenesis," *Experimental Neurology*, vol. 198, no. 1, pp. 54–64, 2006.

[2] A. Chen, L.-J. Xiong, Y. Tong, and M. Mao, "The neuroprotective roles of BDNF in hypoxic ischemic brain injury," *Biomedical Reports*, vol. 1, no. 2, pp. 167–176, 2013.

[3] P. Kaengkan, S. E. Baek, J. Y. Kim et al., "Administration of mesenchymal stem cells and ziprasidone enhanced amelioration of ischemic brain damage in rats," *Molecules and Cells*, vol. 36, no. 6, pp. 534–541, 2013.

[4] L. Du, Y. Yu, H. Ma et al., "Hypoxia enhances protective effect of placental-derived mesenchymal stem cells on damaged intestinal epithelial cells by promoting secretion of insulin-like growth factor-1," *International Journal of Molecular Sciences*, vol. 15, no. 2, pp. 1983–2002, 2014.

[5] L. N. Zhou, S. C. Li, X. Y. Li, H. Ge, and H. M. Li, "Identification of differential protein-coding gene expressions in early phase lung adenocarcinoma," *Thoracic Cancer*, vol. 9, no. 2, pp. 234–240, 2018.

[6] L. Garcia-Bonilla, G. Faraco, J. Moore et al., "Spatio-temporal profile, phenotypic diversity, and fate of recruited monocytes into the post-ischemic brain," *Journal of Neuroinflammation*, vol. 13, no. 1, p. 285, 2016.

[7] A. Gupta, M. R. Capoor, T. Shende et al., "Comparative evaluation of galactomannan test with bronchoalveolar lavage and serum for the diagnosis of invasive aspergillosis in patients with hematological malignancies," *Journal of Laboratory Physicians*, vol. 9, no. 4, pp. 234–238, 2017.

[8] B. Haghshenas, Y. Nami, A. Almasi et al., "Isolation and characterization of probiotics from dairies," *Iranian Journal of Microbiology*, vol. 9, no. 4, pp. 234–243, 2017.

[9] H. X. Chu, H. A. Kim, S. Lee, B. R. S. Broughton, G. R. Drummond, and C. G. Sobey, "Evidence of CCR2-independent transmigration of Ly6C^{hi} monocytes into the brain after permanent cerebral ischemia in mice," *Brain Research*, vol. 1637, pp. 118–127, 2016.

[10] H. Lund, M. Pieber, and R. A. Harris, "Lessons learned about neurodegeneration from microglia and monocyte depletion studies," *Frontiers in Aging Neuroscience*, vol. 9, 2017.

[11] N. Karlupia, N. C. Manley, K. Prasad, R. Schäfer, and G. K. Steinberg, "Intraarterial transplantation of human umbilical cord blood mononuclear cells is more efficacious and safer compared with umbilical cord mesenchymal stromal cells in a rodent stroke model," *Stem Cell Research & Therapy*, vol. 5, no. 2, p. 45, 2014.

[12] G. Pajenda, D. Hercher, G. Márton et al., "Spatiotemporally limited BDNF and GDNF overexpression rescues motoneurons destined to die and induces elongative axon growth," *Experimental Neurology*, vol. 261, pp. 367–376, 2014.

[13] E. Kim, J. Yang, C. D. Beltran, and S. Cho, "Role of spleen-derived monocytes/macrophages in acute ischemic brain injury," *Journal of Cerebral Blood Flow & Metabolism*, vol. 34, no. 8, pp. 1411–1419, 2014.

[14] M. Vendrame, J. Cassady, J. Newcomb et al., "Infusion of human umbilical cord blood cells in a rat model of stroke dose-dependently rescues behavioral deficits and reduces infarct volume," *Stroke*, vol. 35, no. 10, pp. 2390–2395, 2004.

[15] G. Ren, L. Zhang, X. Zhao et al., "Mesenchymal stem cell-mediated immunosuppression occurs via concerted action of chemokines and nitric oxide," *Cell Stem Cell*, vol. 2, no. 2, pp. 141–150, 2008.

[16] O. B. Dimitrijevic, S. M. Stamatovic, R. F. Keep, and A. V. Andjelkovic, "Absence of the chemokine receptor CCR2 protects against cerebral ischemia/reperfusion injury in mice," *Stroke*, vol. 38, no. 4, pp. 1345–1353, 2007.

[17] Y. Chen, J. M. Hallenbeck, C. Ruetzler et al., "Overexpression of monocyte chemoattractant protein 1 in the brain exacerbates ischemic brain injury and is associated with recruitment of inflammatory cells," *Journal of Cerebral Blood Flow & Metabolism*, vol. 23, no. 6, pp. 748–755, 2016.

[18] S. M. Allan, P. J. Tyrrell, and N. J. Rothwell, "Interleukin-1 and neuronal injury," *Nature Reviews Immunology*, vol. 5, no. 8, pp. 629–640, 2005.

[19] B. H. Clausen, M. Degn, N. A. Martin et al., "Systemically administered anti-TNF therapy ameliorates functional outcomes after focal cerebral ischemia," *Journal of Neuroinflammation*, vol. 11, no. 1, p. 203, 2014.

[20] R. M. Ritzel, A. R. Patel, J. M. Grenier et al., "Functional differences between microglia and monocytes after ischemic stroke," *Journal of Neuroinflammation*, vol. 12, no. 1, p. 106, 2015.

[21] Y. Ma, Y. Li, L. Jiang et al., "Macrophage depletion reduced brain injury following middle cerebral artery occlusion in mice," *Journal of Neuroinflammation*, vol. 13, no. 1, p. 38, 2016.

[22] M. Gliem, A. K. Mausberg, J. I. Lee et al., "Macrophages prevent hemorrhagic infarct transformation in murine stroke models," *Annals of Neurology*, vol. 71, no. 6, pp. 743–752, 2012.

[23] M. Pekny and M. Nilsson, "Astrocyte activation and reactive gliosis," *Glia*, vol. 50, no. 4, pp. 427–434, 2005.

[24] M. Schroeter, K. Schiene, M. Kraemer et al., "Astroglial responses in photochemically induced focal ischemia of the rat cortex," *Experimental Brain Research*, vol. 106, no. 1, pp. 1–6, 1995.

[25] P. Gelosa, D. Lecca, M. Fumagalli et al., "Microglia is a key player in the reduction of stroke damage promoted by the new antithrombotic agent ticagrelor," *Journal of Cerebral Blood Flow & Metabolism*, vol. 34, no. 6, pp. 979–988, 2014.

[26] M. Simsek and R. Duman, "Investigation of effect of 1,8-cineole on antimicrobial activity of chlorhexidine gluconate," *Pharmacognosy Research*, vol. 9, no. 3, pp. 234–237, 2017.

[27] Z. Chen and T. D. Palmer, "Differential roles of TNFR1 and TNFR2 signaling in adult hippocampal neurogenesis," *Brain, Behavior, and Immunity*, vol. 30, pp. 45–53, 2013.

[28] T. Mabuchi, K. Kitagawa, T. Ohtsuki et al., "Contribution of microglia/macrophages to expansion of infarction and response of oligodendrocytes after focal cerebral ischemia in rats," *Stroke*, vol. 31, no. 7, pp. 1735–1743, 2000.

[29] C. Iadecola and J. Anrather, "The immunology of stroke: from mechanisms to translation," *Nature Medicine*, vol. 17, no. 7, pp. 796–808, 2011.

[30] Y. Fu, Q. Liu, J. Anrather, and F. D. Shi, "Immune interventions in stroke," *Nature Reviews Neurology*, vol. 11, no. 9, pp. 524–535, 2015.

[31] M. Gliem, M. Schwaninger, and S. Jander, "Protective features of peripheral monocytes/macrophages in stroke," *Biochimica et Biophysica Acta (BBA) - Molecular Basis of Disease*, vol. 1862, no. 3, pp. 329–338, 2016.

[32] S. A. Acosta, N. Tajiri, J. Hoover, Y. Kaneko, and C. V. Borlongan, "Intravenous bone marrow stem cell grafts preferentially migrate to spleen and abrogate chronic inflammation in stroke," *Stroke*, vol. 46, no. 9, pp. 2616–2627, 2015.

[33] S. Yousuf, F. Atif, I. Sayeed, J. Wang, and D. G. Stein, "Post-stroke infections exacerbate ischemic brain injury in middle-aged rats: immunomodulation and neuroprotection by progesterone," *Neuroscience*, vol. 239, pp. 92–102, 2013.

[34] Y. Guan, X. Ji, J. Chen, Y. Alex Zhang, and Z. Chen, "Mesenchymal stem cells for stroke therapy," in *Bone Marrow Stem Cell Therapy for Stroke*, K. Jin, X. Ji, and Q. Zhuge, Eds., pp. 107–132, Springer Singapore, Singapore, 2017.

[35] Y. Ohya, M. Osaki, S. Sakai et al., "A case of recurrent ischemic stroke due to intravascular lymphomatosis, undiagnosed by random skin biopsy and brain imaging," *Case Reports in Neurology*, vol. 9, no. 3, pp. 234–240, 2017.

8

Differential Proteomic Analysis Predicts Appropriate Applications for the Secretome of Adipose-Derived Mesenchymal Stem/Stromal Cells and Dermal Fibroblasts

Stefania Niada ⓘ,[1] Chiara Giannasi,[1,2] Alice Gualerzi,[3] Giuseppe Banfi,[1,4] and Anna Teresa Brini ⓘ[1,2]

[1]IRCCS Istituto Ortopedico Galeazzi, Milan, Italy
[2]Department of Biomedical, Surgical and Dental Sciences, Università degli Studi di Milano, Milan, Italy
[3]Laboratory of Nanomedicine and Clinical Biophotonics, IRCCS Fondazione Don Carlo Gnocchi, via Capecelatro 66, 20148 Milan, Italy
[4]Vita-Salute San Raffaele University, via Olgettina 58, 20132 Milan, Italy

Correspondence should be addressed to Stefania Niada; stefania.niada@unimi.it

Academic Editor: Huseyin Sumer

The adult stem cell secretome is currently under investigation as an alternative to cell-based therapy in regenerative medicine, thanks to the remarkable translational opportunity and the advantages in terms of handling and safety. In this perspective, we recently demonstrated the efficient performance of the adipose-derived mesenchymal stem/stromal cell (ASC) secretome in contrasting neuroinflammation in a murine model of diabetic neuropathy, where the administration of factors released by dermal fibroblasts (DFs) did not exert any effect. Up to now, the complex mixture of the constituents of the conditioned medium from ASCs has not been fully deepened, although its appropriate characterization is required in the perspective of a clinical use. Herein, we propose the differential proteomic approach for the identification of the players accounting for the functional effects of the cell secretome with the aim to unravel its appropriate applications. Out of 967 quantified proteins, 34 and 62 factors were found preponderantly or exclusively secreted by ASCs and DFs, respectively. This approach led to the recognition of distinct functions related to the conditioned medium of ASCs and DFs, with the former being involved in the regulation of neuronal death and apoptosis and the latter in bone metabolism and ossification. The proosteogenic effect of DF secretome was validated *in vitro* on human primary osteoblasts, providing a proof of concept of its osteoinductive potential. Besides discovering new applications of the cell type-specific secretome, the proposed strategy could allow the recognition of the cocktail of bioactive factors which might be responsible for the effects of conditioned media, thus providing a solid rationale to the implementation of a cell-free approach in several clinical scenarios involving tissue regeneration.

1. Introduction

Adult stem cell-based therapies have been proven effective in resolving a wide array of clinical questions, opening the way to their translation from preclinical models to medical practice. Up to date, 301 clinical trials explored or are currently investigating the safety and performance of mesenchymal stem/stromal cells (MSCs), a class of adult stem cells that can be conveniently harvested from several tissue sources (source: http://clinicaltrials.gov, applied filters: Active, not recruiting + Terminated + Completed as Recruitment Status, Interventional (Clinical Trial) as Study Type). Currently, the therapeutic effect of MSC administration has been tested for the treatment of numerous acute and chronic pathologies, spanning from cardiovascular disorders to musculoskeletal and immune diseases [1, 2]. In the last few years, it has become increasingly evident that the beneficial action exerted by MSCs in these heterogeneous clinical scenarios largely depends on paracrine mechanisms rather than being a direct consequence of cell engraftment [3–9]. The therapeutic potential of the secretome of these cells is currently under investigation, gathering growing consensus because of the remarkable translational ability of the cell-free approach that presents substantial advantages over cell therapy, especially in terms of handling and safety. In the context of tissue regeneration, the secretome of MSCs from bone marrow, adipose tissue, and Warton jelly has been proven effective in preclinical models of Parkinson's disease, spinal cord injury, and ischemic stroke [10, 11], while the one from human umbilical cord mesenchymal stem/stromal cells has been proven effective in ameliorating kidney damage and regenerating atrophied muscles [12, 13]. Moreover, the effects of conditioned medium (CM) from cultured MSCs have been largely explored in multiple biological processes linked to clinically significant events, such as wound healing [14, 15], inflammation blunting [16, 17], angiogenesis [18, 19], and neuropathic pain [8]. In this scenario, we recently demonstrated the therapeutic effect of the administration of the CM from adipose-derived stem/stromal cells (ASCs) in a mouse model of diabetes mellitus, providing a solid evidence of its efficiency in contrasting neuropathic pain, neuroinflammation, and peripheral immune activation [20]. Interestingly, we also established that the observed effects were specifically linked to the cell source, as the treatment with CM derived from dermal fibroblasts (DFs) did not counteract the monitored symptoms.

Considering the therapeutic potential of the cell secretome, we believe that an appropriate characterization is required in the perspective of a clinical use. Since it is widely accepted that the efficacy of the cell secretome is not linked to a single "ingredient" but depends on a cocktail of factors acting in synergy, we are currently characterizing the CM content, in terms of both soluble components and vesicular cargos, by multiple approaches. Recently, we demonstrated that the extracellular vesicles released by different MSCs (i.e., ASCs and MSCs from bone marrow) and DFs possess peculiar features that allow their discrimination through Raman spectroscopy with an accuracy of 93.7% [21]. In our previous *in vitro* and *in vivo* works, DFs were chosen as the term of comparison for MSCs as these cell populations present some common features, such as stromal localization, phenotypic profile, and multilineage differentiative capabilities. Nevertheless, MSCs and DFs differ for important characteristics, among which the distinct anti-inflammatory and angiogenic potential are particularly interesting in the perspective of their employment in the regenerative medicine field [22, 23]. Here, we compared the secretome from ASCs to the one from DFs through a differential proteomic approach, focusing on its potential to predict the action of CM deriving from distinct cell sources on different targets and pathological conditions. We examined the factors differentially expressed between the two populations that may be involved in the antineuroinflammatory properties of ASCs observed *in vivo*. Moreover, on the basis of the factors preponderantly released by dermal fibroblasts, we hypothesize a proosteogenic effect of CM-DFs that was validated *in vitro* with human primary osteoblasts.

2. Materials and Methods

Unless otherwise stated, reagents and chemicals were purchased from Sigma-Aldrich (Saint Louis, MO, USA).

2.1. Cell Culture. All the cell types used in this study were isolated from waste tissues of healthy donors undergoing plastic (abdominoplasty and liposuction) or orthopaedic surgery, after written consent and following the procedure PQ 7.5.125, version 4, dated 2015-01-22, approved by the IRCCS Galeazzi Orthopaedic Institute. ASCs were isolated from the subcutaneous adipose tissue of 3 female donors (age range: 26–65 y/o) while DFs were isolated from the deepidermised dermis of 3 female patients (age range: 26–46 y/o). Cells were isolated following previously described protocols [21]. Briefly, ASCs were isolated from adipose tissue samples following digestion with 0.75 mg/ml type I collagenase (250 U/mg, Worthington Biochemical Corporation, Lakewood, NJ, USA) and filtering of the stromal vascular fraction. DFs were obtained from fragmented dermis after digestion with 0.1% type I collagenase. Osteoblasts were isolated from the cancellous bone of a female patient (66 y/o) undergoing total hip replacement surgery. Briefly, bone fragments were excised and minced with a scalpel, washed several times in phosphate buffered saline (PBS), and vortexed at high speed in order to remove residual adipose and/or hematopoietic tissue. Bone chips were then plated in petri dishes until cell outgrowth. All cell types were maintained in a humidified atmosphere at 37°C, 5% CO_2 in complete culture medium (DMEM, 2 mM L-glutamine, 50 U/ml penicillin, 50 μg/ml streptomycin) added with 10% FBS (EuroClone, Milan, Italy). The medium was replaced every other day and, at 70–80% confluence, cells were detached with 0.5% trypsin/0.2% EDTA, plated at a density of 10,000 cells/cm^2 for ASCs and OBs, 5000 cells/cm^2 for DFs, and expanded.

2.2. Conditioned-Media Production. Conditioned medium was prepared as previously described [20]. Once at 80–90% confluence, cells at the 4th passage were washed twice with PBS, kept for one hour in serum-free, phenol-free complete DMEM, and cultured in the same starving conditions for 72 hours. Conditioned media were then centrifuged at 2500g for 15 minutes to remove cell debris and concentrated using Amicon® Ultra-15 centrifugal filter columns with a 3 kDa molecular weight cutoff (Merck Millipore, Burlington, MA, USA). Protein concentration was measured by a Bradford assay (Bio-Rad Laboratories, Hercules, CA, USA).

2.3. nLC-MS/MS Analysis and Bioinformatics. Conditioned media samples were delivered to ProMiFa (Protein Microsequencing Facility, San Raffaele Scientific Institute, Milan, Italy) to perform nLC-MS/MS analysis. 20 μg of total proteins from each sample were in-solution digested using the Filter Aided Sample Preparation (FASP) protocol as reported in literature [24]. Aliquots of the samples containing tryptic peptides were desalted using StageTip C18 (Thermo Fisher Scientific, Waltham, MA, USA) and analysed by nLC-MS/MS using a Q-Exactive mass spectrometer (Thermo Fisher Scientific) equipped with a nanoelectrospray ion source (Proxeon Biosystems, Odense, Denmark) and a nUPLC Easy-nLC 1000 (Proxeon Biosystems). Peptide separations occurred on a homemade ($75\,\mu m$ i.d., 12 cm long) reverse phase silica capillary column, packed with $1.9\,\mu m$ ReproSil-Pur 120 C18-AQ (Dr. Maisch GmbH, Germany). A gradient of eluents A (distilled water with 0.1% v/v formic acid) and B (acetonitrile with 0.1% v/v formic acid) was used to achieve separation (300 nl/min flow rate), from 2% B to 40% B in 88 minutes. Full-scan spectra were acquired with the lock-mass option, resolution set to 70,000 and mass range from m/z 300 to 2000 Da. The ten most intense doubly- and triply-charged ions were selected and fragmented. All MS/MS samples were analysed using the Mascot (version 2.6, Matrix Science) search engine to search the human_proteome 20171122 (93,786 sequences; 37,178,108 residues). Searches were performed with the following settings: trypsin as proteolytic enzyme; 2 missed cleavages allowed; carbamidomethylation on cysteine as fixed modification; protein N-terminus-acetylation, methionine oxidation as variable modifications; and mass tolerance was set to 5 ppm and to 0.02 Da for precursor and fragment ions, respectively. To quantify proteins, the raw data were loaded into the MaxQuant software version 1.5.2.8 [25]. Label-free protein quantification was based on the intensities of precursors. The experiments were performed in technical triplicates. The complete dataset of identified and quantified proteins, as obtained by proteomic analysis, was subjected to Student's t-test in order to define significantly differently expressed proteins with a p value < 0.05, followed by hierarchical clustering analysis, using MeV software v. 4_9_0 [26].

2.4. In Vitro Functional Analysis of CM-ASCs and CM-DFs

2.4.1. Cell Viability. 3×10^3 osteoblasts/cm^2 were plated in triplicate on 96-well plates and maintained in culture for 16 days in complete culture medium. At days 2, 4, 7, 9, 11, and 14, cells were treated with CM deriving from 10,000 ASCs or DFs (recipient to donor cell ratio 1 : 10) and viability/proliferation was monitored through time as previously described [27]. Briefly, at each time point the culture media were replaced with the addition of 10% alamarBlue® (Thermo Fisher Scientific, Waltham, MA, USA) and cells were incubated for 3.5 hours at 37°C in the dark. $100\,\mu l$ of supernatant was then transferred to black-bottom 96-well plates and fluorescence (540 nm excitation λ, 600 nm emission λ) was read with a Wallac Victor 2 plate reader (PerkinElmer, Waltham, MA, USA). At the end of the experiment, cells were fixed and stained by Diff-Quik, following standard protocol (Medion Diagnostics, Miami, FL, USA). Statistical analysis was performed by two-way ANOVA and Bonferroni's multiple comparison test using GraphPad Prism 5 Software (San Diego, CA, USA).

2.4.2. Real-Time PCR. OBs were plated at a density of 6000 cells/cm^2 and cultured in standard conditions until confluence. Then, cells were treated with conditioned medium deriving from 120,000 ASCs or DFs (recipient to donor cell ratio 1 : 5). After 24 hours, the expression of osteogenic marker genes (RUNX2, SPP1, and COLL I) and of VEGF (recently identified as a fundamental factor involved in bone

repair and regeneration [28]) was assessed by real-time polymerase chain reaction (RT-PCR, StepOne Plus, Life Technologies, Carlsbad, CA, USA) [29]. Briefly, total RNA was purified using an RNeasy Mini Kit (Qiagen, Hilden, Germany). cDNA was obtained by a high-capacity cDNA reverse transcription kit and amplified by Single Tube TaqMan® Gene Expression Assays (RUNX2: hs00231692_m1, SPP1: hs00959010_m1, VEGF: hs00959010_m1, and COLL I: hs01076777_m1) (Applied Biosystems, Foster City, CA, USA). Data were normalized on ACTB (Hs01060665_g1) and the relative quantification was determined using the delta delta CT ($\Delta\Delta$CT) method.

2.4.3. Western Blot. OBs were seeded at a density of 8000 cells/cm^2 and cultured in standard conditions until confluence. Cells were treated with conditioned medium deriving from 400,000 ASCs or DFs (recipient to donor cell ratio 1 : 5) for 72 hours. Cells were then lysed in 65 mM Tris-HCl, pH 6.8, with 2% sodium dodecyl sulfate (SDS) supplemented with protease-inhibitor cocktail. $15\,\mu g$ of whole cell lysates, quantified by BCA Protein Assay (Thermo Fisher Scientific), were resolved into 8% SDS-PAGE and transferred to nitrocellulose membranes (GE Healthcare, Little Chalfont, UK). Membranes were probed overnight with either rabbit polyclonal antibody raised against osteopontin (OPN; Abcam, Cambridge, UK) or mouse monoclonal antibody raised against SPARC (Santa Cruz Biotechnology, Dallas, TX, USA). Goat polyclonal anti-GAPDH antibody (Santa Cruz Biotechnology, Dallas, TX, USA) was employed as a housekeeping protein. Proteins of interest were detected after 45 minutes of incubation with appropriate HRP-conjugated secondary antibodies (Santa Cruz Biotechnology, Dallas, TX, USA) using LiteAblot® Turbo Extra-Sensitive Chemiluminescent Substrate (EuroClone, Milan, Italy). Images were acquired through ChemiDoc Imaging System™ and analysed through Image Lab™ software (Bio-Rad Laboratories, Hercules, CA, USA).

3. Results

3.1. Differential Secretome Analysis. We performed a nLC-MS/MS analysis to identify differentially secreted proteins between ASCs and DFs. Three conditioned media of each cell type were analysed. 1208 proteins were identified, 976 of which were quantified. Following a hierarchical clustering approach, we identified two groups of factors that were differently secreted among ASCs and DFs (Figure 1(a)). The results showed that 15 proteins were uniquely or preponderantly present in CM-ASCs, while 21 were present in those from DFs. Using this list as input in the STRING platform [30], it resulted in the majority of differently secreted proteins in both groups (9 for ASCs—FDR: 0.00433 and 15 for DFs—FDR: $4.66e-07$) being associated to extracellular exosomes. No relevant functional pathway was associated to these proteins, even though DF-specific factors appeared to be involved in sugar metabolism (monosaccharide biosynthetic process—FDR: $3.47e-05$, xylulose biosynthetic process—FDR: 0.00461, and nonoxidative branch of pentose-phosphate shunt—FDR: 0.023).

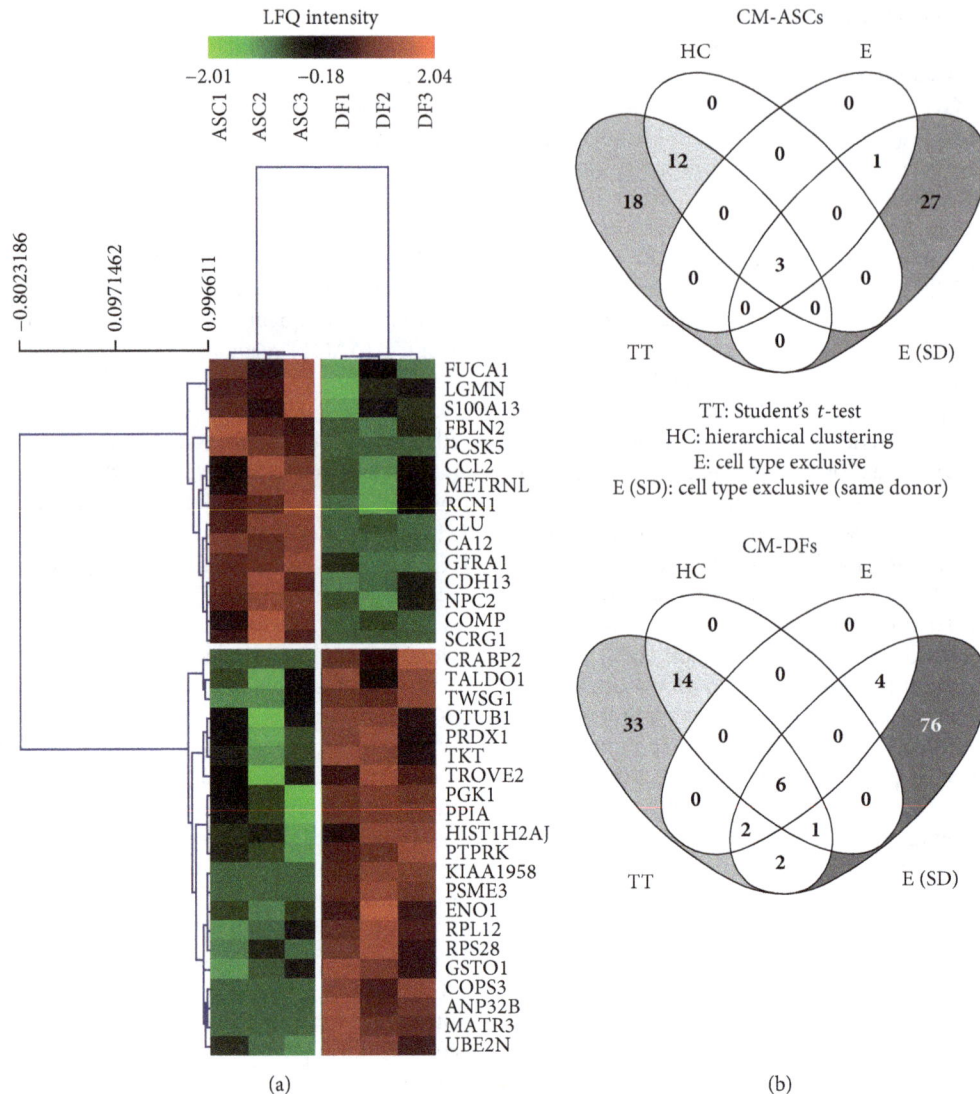

(a)

(b)

FIGURE 1: Differential proteome analysis of CM-ASCs and CM-DFs. (a) Hierarchical clustering criteria identify 15 proteins preponderantly secreted by ASCs ($n = 3$) and 21 factors predominantly released by DFs ($n = 3$). The color scale represents the label-free quantification (LFQ) of the relative amount of proteins in the biological samples. (b) Venn diagrams (http://bioinfogp.cnb.csic.es/tools/venny) representing the number of differentially expressed proteins identified by distinct statistical analyses (Student's t test alone (TT) or followed by hierarchical clustering (HC)) and discrimination criteria (factors uniquely present in the CM of one cell type considering all samples (E) or considering only ASCs and DFs harvested from the same donor (E (SD))).

Despite that no link to reported pathways was identified for the 15 ASC-specific proteins, several of them have a known immune function (S100 A13 protein, CCL2, LGMN, FUCA1, and METRNL) and/or are involved in neuron death and apoptosis (CCL2, CLU, LGMN, and PCSK5). To widen our analysis and deepen our understanding of the differentially secreted proteins, we applied different criteria. At first, we manually checked the data to identify factors exclusively secreted by either ASCs or DFs. Among the proteins released exclusively by one cell type (4 and 12 for ASCs and DFs, resp.), some factors were not identified through the previous clustering (1 for ASCs and 6 for DFs) (Figure 1(b)). Moreover, applying Student's t test with no further correction, we identified additional factors differentially secreted from ASCs ($n = 18$) and DFs ($n = 35$). Finally, we compared the

CM of same-donor ASCs and DFs and the factors released uniquely by one population were manually selected. These data confirmed that the two cell types peculiarly release a multitude of different factors (31 ASC-specific proteins and 91 DF-specific proteins), regardless of the donor features. However, since many proteins were solely selected with this criterion (Figure 1(b)), they were not included in further analyses. Considering the Student's t test results combined with cell type-exclusive data, we obtained novel and more comprehensive lists accounting for 34 (Figure 2) and 62 (Figure 3) factors differentially or exclusively secreted by ASCs and DFs, respectively.

These multiple proteins were run in a novel STRING analysis. Functional enrichment confirmed that the conditioned media of the two cell types contained many different

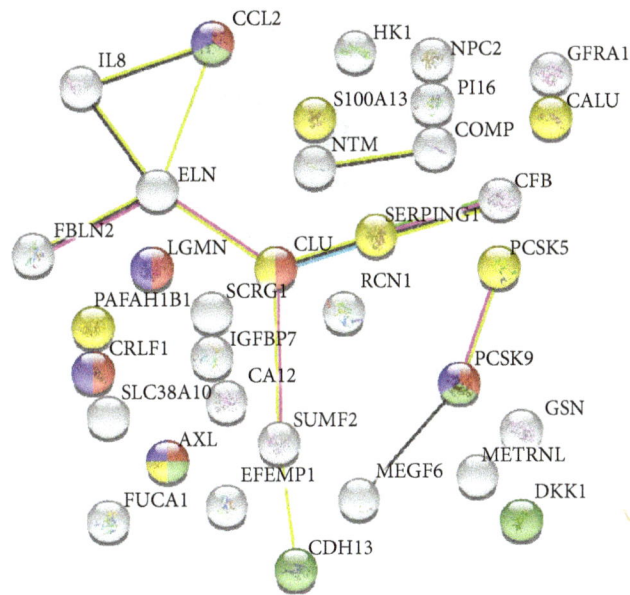

Pathway ID number	Pathway description	Observed gene count	False discovery rate	Matching proteins in your network (labels)
GO.0048731	System development	17	0.0213	CALU,CCL2, CDH13, CLU, CRLF1, DKK1, EFEMP1, GFRA1, GSN,IL8, NTM, PAFAH1B1, PCSK5, PCSK9, RCN1, SCRG1, SLC38A10
GO.1901214	Regulation of neuron death	6	0.0213	AXL, CCL2, CLU, CRLF1, LGMN, PCSK9
GO.0030100	Regulation of endocytosis	5	0.0346	AXL, CCL2, CDH13, DKK1, PCSK9
GO.0032940	Secretion by cell	7	0.0346	AXL, CALU, CLU, PAFAH1B1, PCSK5, S100A13, SERPING1
GO.0043523	Regulation of neuron apoptotic process	5	0.0346	AXL, CCL 2, CRLF1, LGMN, PCSK9
GO.0007275	Multicellular organismal development	17	0.0422	CALU, CCL2, CDH13, CLU, CRLF1, DKK1, EFEMP1, GFRA1, GSN, IL8, NTM, PAFAH1B1, PCSK5, PCSK9, RCN1, SCRG1, SLC38A10
GO.0044767	Single-organism developmental process	18	0.0422	CALU, CCL2, CDH13, CLU, CRLF1, DKK1, EFEMP1, GFRA1, IL8, METRNL, NTM, PAFAH1B1, PCSK5, PCSK9, RCN1, SCRG1, SERPING1, SLC38A10

FIGURE 2: STRING analysis uncovering protein-protein interactions and biological processes associated to the 34 proteins solely or preponderantly secreted by ASCs.

proteins associated to extracellular vesicles (17 proteins for ASCs—FDR: $3.55e-05$ and 34 proteins for DF—FDR: $7.84e-13$). Moreover, it reinforced the previous observation that CM-DFs contain proteins involved in metabolic processes (Figure 3) and suggested that in CM-ASCs there are different factors regulating endocytosis and cell secretion (Figure 2). Regeneration functions associated to cell type-specific factors were also identified. In particular, the regulation of neuron death and of neuronal apoptotic properties were among the first 5 results regarding biological processes associated to ASC factors (Figure 2), consistently with our preclinical data on neuropathic pain [20]. Differently, beside sugar metabolism, several DF factors appeared to have a role in ossification and/or bone metabolism (HNRNPC, MRC2, RBMX, RRBP1, TNC, and TWSG1, Figure 3). In order to validate this last observation, we performed functional tests on osteoblasts isolated from a human bone specimen.

3.2. Effects of ASC and DF Secretome on Human Primary Osteoblasts. As a proof of concept, the involvement of

DF-specific factors in bone metabolism/ossification was validated by testing the effects of the secretome of same-donor (46 y/o female donor) ASCs and DFs, on cultured human primary osteoblasts. At first, we investigated the influence of CM treatments on osteoblast viability over a period of two weeks (Figure 4(a)). While the effect of CM-ASCs was almost undetectable, CM-DFs strongly stimulated osteoblast viability through time and the lag phase observed between days 7 and 9 in other groups was avoided. At day 14, we observed a larger number of osteoblasts treated with CM-DFs with respect to other groups (Figure 4(a), microphotographs), demonstrating that this treatment favored cell proliferation rather than enhancing cell metabolism. Then, the short-term effect of the secretome on gene expression was investigated (Figure 4(b)). After 24 hours of treatment, the levels of *RUNX2*, *SPP1*, and *VEGF* mRNA resulted in an enhancement by CM-DFs (fold change of 4.1 for *RUNX2* and 5.2 for both *SPP1* and *VEGF*), thus supporting our hypothesis of a proosteoblastic action of CM-DFs. By contrast, CM-ASCs reduced the expression of these genes of

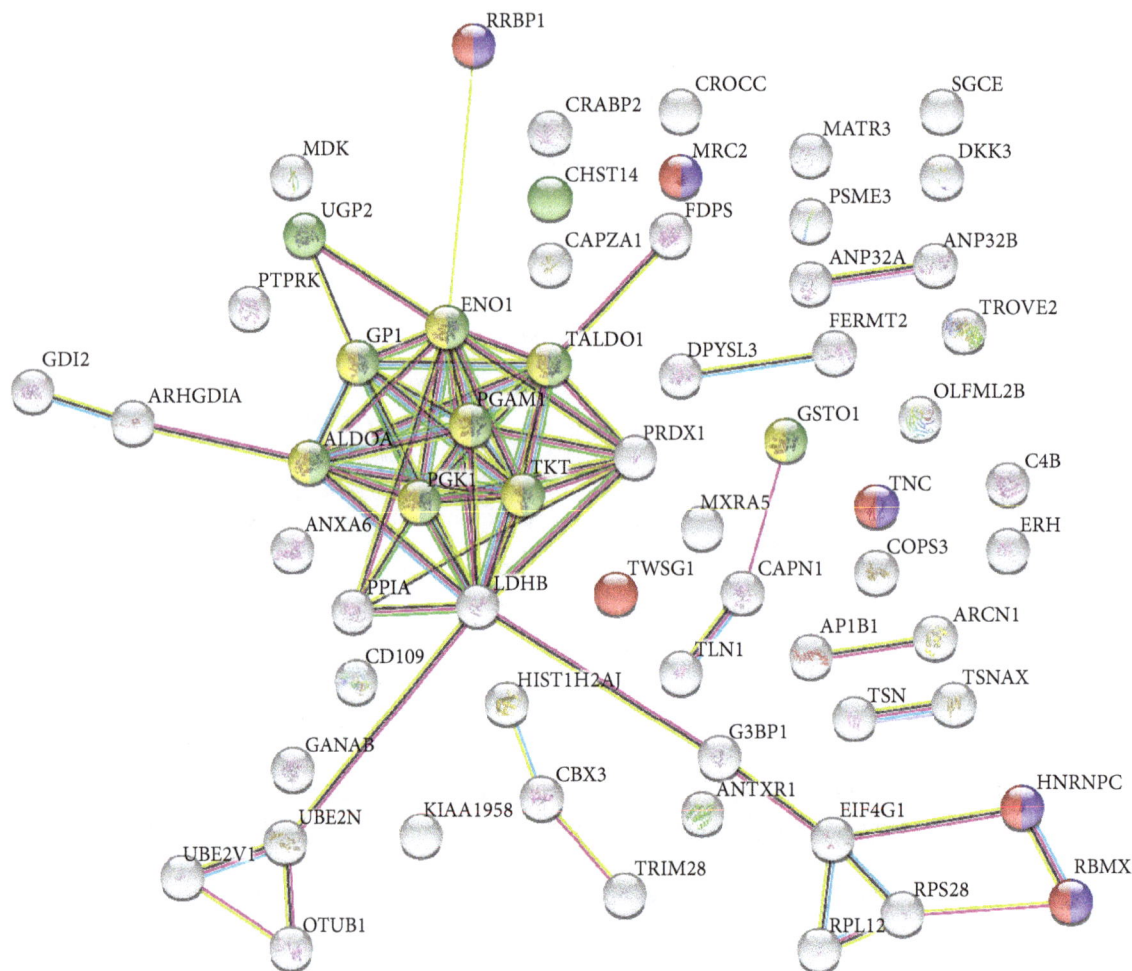

Pathway ID number	Pathway description	Observed gene count	False discovery rate	Matching proteins in your network (labels)
GO.0016051	Carbohydrate biosynthetic process	10	3.19E-08	ALDOA, CHST14, ENO1, GPI, GSTO1, PGAM1, PGK1, TALDO1, TKT, UGP2
GO.0046364	Monosaccharide biosynthetic process	8	3.89E-08	ALDOA, ENO1, GPI, GSTO1, PGAM1, PGK1, TALDO1, TKT
Other metabolic processes: GO.0046496, GO.0019674, GO.0061621, GO.0006090, GO.0006094, GO.0005996, GO.0006006, GO.0009117, GO.0044723, GO.0005999, GO.0006091				
GO.0001649	Osteoblast differentiation	5	0.00831	HNRNPC, MRC2, RBMX, RRBP1, TNC
GO.0006282	Regulation of DNA repair	4	0.0131	OTUB1, TRIM28, UBE2N, UBE2V1
GO.0046184	Aldehyde biosynthetic process	2	0.0166	GPI, TKT
GO.0032787	Monocarboxylic acid metabolic process	8	0.0168	ALDOA, CHST14, CRABP2, ENO1, GPI, PGAM1, PGK1, UGP2
GO.0005975	Carbohydrate metabolic process	10	0.0183	ALDOA, ENO1, GANAB, GPI, LDHB, PGAM1, PGK1, TALDO1, TKT, UGP2
GO.0001503	Ossification	6	0.0243	HNRNPC, MRC2, RBMX, RRBP1, TNC, TWSG1
GO.0009052	Pentose-phosphate shunt, nonoxidative branch	2	0.0243	TALDO1, TKT
GO.0055086	Nucleobase-containing small-molecule metabolic process	8	0.0243	ALDOA, ENO1, GPI, LDHB, PGAM1, PGK1, TKT, UGP2
GO.0055114	Oxidation-reduction process	11	0.0243	ALDOA, ENO1, GPI, GSTO1, LDHB, PGAM1, PGK1, PRDX1, TALDO1, TKT, UGP2

FIGURE 3: STRING analysis uncovering protein-protein interactions and biological processes associated to the 62 proteins solely or preponderantly secreted by DFs.

$$y = 2745.7e^{0.135x}$$
$$y = 2343.6e^{0.1509x}$$
$$y = 1797.6e^{0.1831x}$$

(a)

(b)

(c)

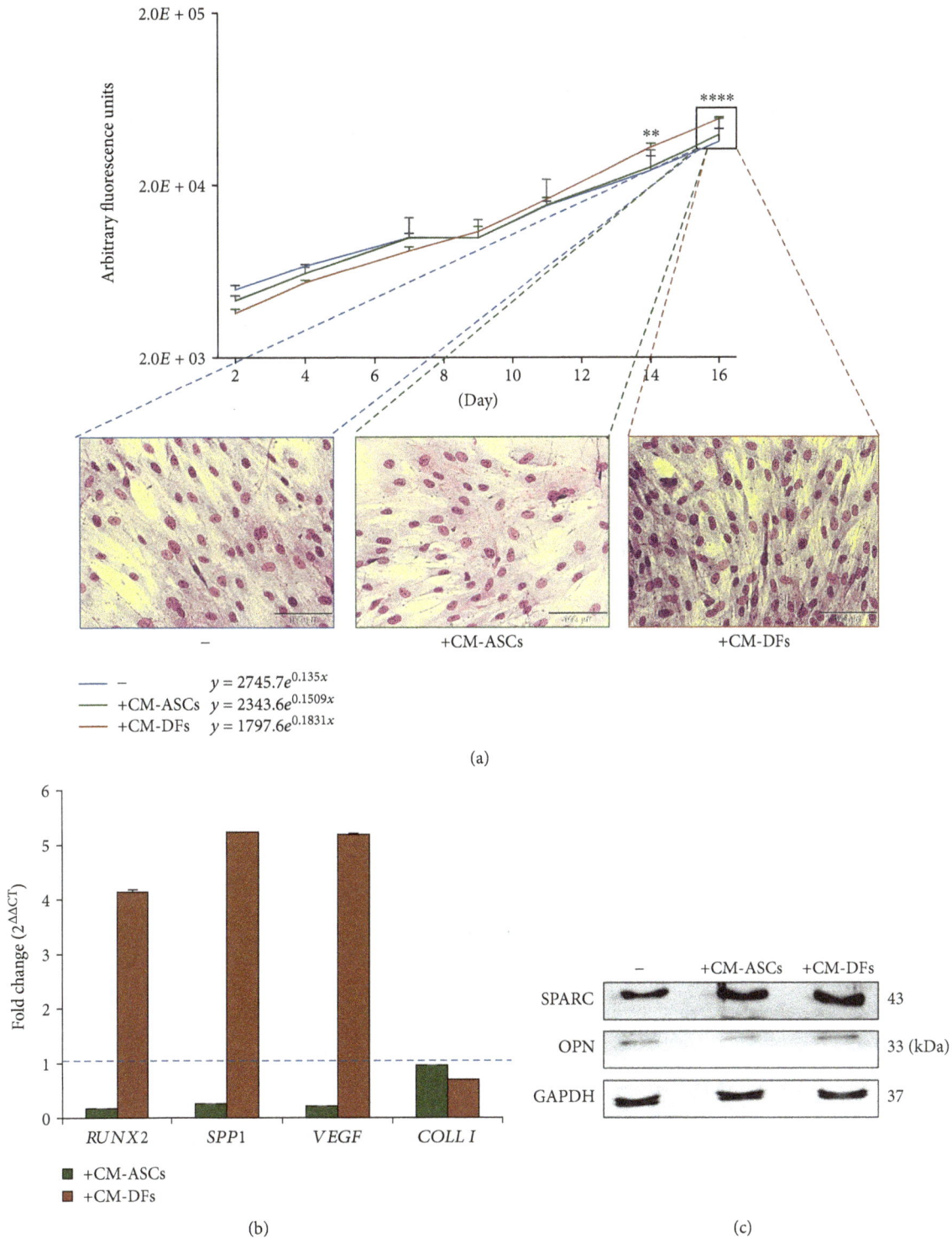

FIGURE 4: *In vitro* effect of CM-ASCs and CM-DFs on osteoblasts. (a) Semilog graph representing osteoblast viability assessment at different time points of untreated cells (blue line), cells treated with CM-ASCs (green line), or cells treated with CM-DFs (orange line). The equations of the exponential functions describing osteoblast growth in the different conditions are shown. Data represents the mean ± SD of 3 replicates (difference versus untreated $^{**}p < 0.01$ and $^{****}p < 0.0001$). Microphotographs are representative of cell confluence for each group at the final time point. Scale bars = 100 μm. (b) Relative expression of important osteoblast genes after 24 hours of treatment with CM-ASCs (green bars) or CM-DFs (orange bars) in respect to untreated cells, by RT-PCR. The mRNA levels of Runt-related transcription factor 2 (*RUNX2*), osteopontin (*SPP1*), vascular endothelial growth factor (*VEGF*), and type I collagen (*COLL I*) are represented in relation to β-actin, here used as a internal control. Data are shown as mean ± SD of technical duplicates. (c) Protein expression of extracellular matrix components by osteoblasts treated with CM-ASCs or CM-DFs for 72 hours. Western blot analysis of osteonectin (SPARC) and osteopontin (OPN) expression following the treatments. Bands were quantified by densitometry and normalized on GAPDH.

about 4 times while *COLL I* expression was slightly diminished by both treatments. Finally, we investigated the effect of a longer CM treatment (72 hours) on the intracellular protein levels of SPARC and OPN (Figure 4(c)), two important extracellular matrix components. The stimulating effect of CM-DFs on osteoblasts was confirmed by a +123% increase in SPARC expression with respect to untreated cells. However, a slightly minor upregulation of SPARC was also induced by CM-ASCs. In addition, a little increase (+29%) in the naïve 33 kDa form of OPN [31] was also ascribable to the DF secretome only. Nevertheless, this effect was not maintained for all the protein isoforms subject to posttranslational modifications (data not shown).

4. Discussion

In light of the fact that conditioned media could be used in the future as biotechnological products for regenerative medicine, it is essential to carry out their characterization before proceeding to clinics. Here, we have implemented differential proteomics to investigate the secretome of ASCs and DFs, focusing on the potential applications in the regenerative medicine field. We applied different criteria to select proteins that were differentially or exclusively released by one cell type and we came up with 34 and 62 factors uniquely or prevalently secreted by ASCs and DFs, respectively. The STRING analysis of these factors led to the recognition of distinct functions related to the CM of ASCs and DFs which are consistent with previous findings on ASC-CM neuroprotective effects [20, 32–34] and with our current results on DF secretome osteoinductive properties (Figure 4). Several proteins released more abundantly or exclusively by ASCs, namely AXL, CCL2, CLU, CRLF1, LGMN, and PCSK9, were found to be significantly associated with the regulation of neuronal death and apoptosis. These bioactive factors might contribute to the modulation of neuroinflammation exerted by CM-ASCs in our preclinical models of neuropathic pain [20, 35] by activating different mechanisms. AXL is a receptor tyrosine kinase which regulates the innate immune system activation [36] and controls the phagocytosis of dead neurons. Even though this protein is probably released by ASCs through exosomes (STRING, Exocarta), it still needs to be shown whether it is transferred to recipient cells. Chemokine (C-C motif) Ligand 2 (CCL2) is a pleiotropic chemokine with an important role in neurogenesis exerted by promoting glial cell proliferation and growth, inducing stem cell migration into sites of damage, and directing differentiation of precursor cells into neurons, astrocytes, and oligodendrocytes [37]. Clusterin (CLU) is a stress-induced chaperone involved in neuronal protection [38]. Its levels are increased in multiple degenerative conditions [39] and following traumatic brain injury [40]. CLU modulates neuroinflammation also thanks to its capacity to suppress complement activation. Legumain (LGMN) is a cysteine protease which regulates the development of immune response and tolerance by playing a key role in the processing of antigens [41]. Among its functions, the involvement in the axonal regeneration following spinal cord injury in zebrafish is particularly intriguing [42]. Finally, the soluble receptor

Cytokine Receptor-Like Factor 1 (CRLF1) and the secreted protease Proprotein Convertase Subtilisin/Kexin type 9 (PCSK9) may contribute to neuroprotection due to their activity in promoting neuronal cell survival [43] and in regulating neuronal apoptosis [44], respectively. In addition, two factors specifically released only by ASCs could contribute to the therapeutic action of their CM. Indeed, similarly to CCL2, CXCL8/IL-8 is known to possess neuroprotective features [37]. Furthermore, Scrapie Responsive Gene 1 (SCRG1), which is a positive regulator of stem cell self-renewal, migration, and differentiation potential [45], has been recently proposed as an inhibitor of the infiltration of monocytes, dendritic cells, natural killer cells, and chronically activated T lymphocytes [46]. Other proteins with a known immune function were highlighted by the hierarchical clustering analysis. Among them, Alpha-L-Fucosidase 1 (FUCA1) exerts immunoregulatory actions [47], Meteorin-like protein (METRL) stimulates the expression of anti-inflammatory cytokines [48], and S100 calcium-binding protein A13 (S100A13) acts as a regulator of macrophage inflammation [49]. Our hypothesis is that all these proteins concur in the conversion of the proinflammatory/neurodestructive environment observed in diabetic mice into an anti-inflammatory/neuroprotective one [20]. Further investigations with CM previously deprived of specific factors could confirm their involvement in the neuroinflammation blunting. In any case, our unbiased approach allowed us to identify neuroprotection as one of the main functions of the ASC secretome. The modulation of neurodegenerative and neuroinflammatory diseases by the release of neurotrophic and immunomodulative molecules is well documented not only for ASCs but also for other MSCs [10, 33] and it explains the multitude of applications for MSCs and their conditioned media in these contexts [20, 32, 35, 50, 51].

On the other hand, the analysis of the factors preponderantly or specifically released by DFs produced unexpected outcomes. CM-DFs resulted particularly enriched in proteins involved in sugar metabolism and further investigations should aim at deciphering whether these factors might be involved in the production of glycosaminoglycans and/or in other metabolic processes. Of note, several proteins, which are involved in bone metabolism and ossification (HNRNPC, MRC2, RBMX, RRBP1, TNC, and TWSG1), were also highlighted. Among them, Tenascin C (TNC) is an extracellular matrix glycoprotein implicated in osteoblastic differentiation and mineralization within the bone, probably acting as a mediator of TGF-β-induced new bone formation [52]. C-type mannose receptor 2 (MRC2, also known as ENDO180, CD280, or uPARAP) plays a supporting role in bone development being involved in collagen trafficking and deposition [53]. Another factor involved in collagen turnover, particularly in its biosynthesis, is Ribosome-Binding Protein 1 (RRBP1, also known as p180). All these proteins, together with RBMX (RNA-Binding Motif Protein, X-Linked) and HNRNPC (Heterogeneous Nuclear Ribonucleoproteins C1/C2), have been reported to be significantly upregulated during the osteogenic differentiation of MSCs [54], suggesting their role in osteogenesis. Finally, the secreted protein Twisted Gastrulation Homolog 1 (TWSG1) is known to bind bone morphogenetic proteins and to influence osteoblast maturation, even though with contrasting effects [55, 56]. Interestingly, it also inhibits osteoclastogenesis [57], supporting a primary role as a bone-building effector. Since up to now the CM-DF osteoinductive potential has never been reported, we performed a functional *in vitro* test which provided evidence of the proosteogenic function predicted from the proteomic analysis. In this study, CM-DFs switched from a term of comparison, convenient to point out the specific effectors contained in CM-ASCs, to an interesting source of bioactive factors. With our results, we do not want to minimize the proosteogenic potential of the MSC secretome, which has been already documented especially for BMSCs [58], but to suggest novel applications for DFs. In fairness, the potential use of these cells in supporting tissue regeneration has been largely investigated, mainly considering their ability to synthesize and deposit extracellular matrices and release bioactive molecules [59]. Further investigations will be focused on assessing the effects of the DF secretome and/or of its single components on other cell types.

Interestingly, most of the factors differentially released by ASCs and DFs are contained in extracellular vesicles, but only half of the proteins involved in the regenerative functions are released as vesicular cargos (STRING). This remark is consistent with recent observations of a major effect exerted by the whole conditioned medium compared to the exosomes only [60] (our unpublished observations). Further studies investigating this issue are strongly recommended before choosing the proper cell product to be used in specific applications.

5. Conclusions

This study provides evidence that the differential proteomic analysis constitutes a useful tool to determine the proper therapeutic target of conditioned media derived from different cell types. Our data reinforced previous observations on the neuroprotective action of the ASC secretome by pointing out specific factors involved in this process and identifying an unexpected proosteogenic aptitude of CM-DFs. This method might be applied to identify the bioactive factors which are released by different cells and are responsible for the biological effect of their conditioned media. At last, a proper validation of specific CM factors could pave the way for the future production of artificial cocktails of bioactive molecules (a novel biological medical product) to be used in different regenerative medicine applications.

Authors' Contributions

Stefania Niada and Chiara Giannasi contributed equally this work.

Acknowledgments

This study was funded by the Italian Ministry of Health (Ricerca Corrente L1027 and L4097, IRCCS Galeazzi Ortho-paedic Institute) and the Department of Biomedical, Surgical, and Dental Sciences, University of Milan (Grant no. PSR2015-1716ABRIN_M). The authors would like to thank Dr. Giovanni Lombardi for providing the antibody raised against osteopontin used for the Western blot analysis.

References

[1] S. Wang, X. Qu, and R. C. Zhao, "Clinical applications of mesenchymal stem cells," *Journal of Hematology & Oncology*, vol. 5, no. 1, p. 19, 2012.

[2] T. Squillaro, G. Peluso, and U. Galderisi, "Clinical trials with mesenchymal stem cells: an update," *Cell Transplantation*, vol. 25, no. 5, pp. 829–848, 2016.

[3] M. Gnecchi, Z. Zhang, A. Ni, and V. J. Dzau, "Paracrine mechanisms in adult stem cell signaling and therapy," *Circulation Research*, vol. 103, no. 11, pp. 1204–1219, 2008.

[4] A. J. Braga Osorio Gomes Salgado, R. I. L. Goncalves Reis, N. J. C. Sousa et al., "Adipose tissue derived stem cells secretome: soluble factors and their roles in regenerative medicine," *Current Stem Cell Research & Therapy*, vol. 5, no. 2, pp. 103–110, 2010.

[5] M. Z. Ratajczak, M. Kucia, T. Jadczyk et al., "Pivotal role of paracrine effects in stem cell therapies in regenerative medicine: can we translate stem cell-secreted paracrine factors and microvesicles into better therapeutic strategies?," *Leukemia*, vol. 26, no. 6, pp. 1166–1173, 2012.

[6] S. Bruno, M. C. Deregibus, and G. Camussi, "The secretome of mesenchymal stromal cells: role of extracellular vesicles in immunomodulation," *Immunology Letters*, vol. 168, no. 2, pp. 154–158, 2015.

[7] A. J. Salgado, J. C. Sousa, B. M. Costa et al., "Mesenchymal stem cells secretome as a modulator of the neurogenic niche: basic insights and therapeutic opportunities," *Frontiers in Cellular Neuroscience*, vol. 9, p. 294, 2015.

[8] K. B. Gama, D. S. Santos, A. F. Evangelista et al., "Conditioned medium of bone marrow-derived mesenchymal stromal cells as a therapeutic approach to neuropathic pain: a preclinical evaluation," *Stem Cells International*, vol. 2018, Article ID 8179013, 12 pages, 2018.

[9] M. C. Ciuffreda, G. Malpasso, C. Chokoza et al., "Synthetic extracellular matrix mimic hydrogel improves efficacy of mesenchymal stromal cell therapy for ischemic cardiomyopathy," *Acta Biomaterialia*, vol. 70, pp. 71–83, 2018.

[10] F. G. Teixeira, M. M. Carvalho, N. Sousa, and A. J. Salgado, "Mesenchymal stem cells secretome: a new paradigm for central nervous system regeneration?," *Cellular and Molecular Life Sciences*, vol. 70, no. 20, pp. 3871–3882, 2013.

[11] D. Cizkova, V. Cubinkova, T. Smolek et al., "Localized intrathecal delivery of mesenchymal stromal cells conditioned medium improves functional recovery in a rat model of spinal cord injury," *International Journal of Molecular Sciences*, vol. 19, no. 3, 2018.

[12] V. B. R. Konala, M. K. Mamidi, R. Bhonde, A. K. Das, R. Pochampally, and R. Pal, "The current landscape of the mesenchymal stromal cell secretome: a new paradigm for cell-free regeneration," *Cytotherapy*, vol. 18, no. 1, pp. 13–24, 2016.

[13] M. J. Kim, Z. H. Kim, S. M. Kim, and Y. S. Choi, "Conditioned medium derived from umbilical cord mesenchymal stem cells regenerates atrophied muscles," *Tissue & Cell*, vol. 48, no. 5, pp. 533–543, 2016.

[14] M. N. Walter, K. T. Wright, H. R. Fuller, S. MacNeil, and W. E. Johnson, "Mesenchymal stem cell-conditioned medium accelerates skin wound healing: an *in vitro* study of fibroblast and keratinocyte scratch assays," *Experimental Cell Research*, vol. 316, no. 7, pp. 1271–1281, 2010.

[15] M. Li, F. Luan, Y. Zhao et al., "Mesenchymal stem cell-conditioned medium accelerates wound healing with fewer scars," *International Wound Journal*, vol. 14, no. 1, pp. 64–73, 2017.

[16] A. G. Kay, G. Long, G. Tyler et al., "Mesenchymal stem cell-conditioned medium reduces disease severity and immune responses in inflammatory arthritis," *Scientific Reports*, vol. 7, no. 1, article 18019, 2017.

[17] F. Yousefi, M. Ebtekar, S. Soudi, M. Soleimani, and S. M. Hashemi, "*In vivo* immunomodulatory effects of adipose-derived mesenchymal stem cells conditioned medium in experimental autoimmune encephalomyelitis," *Immunology Letters*, vol. 172, pp. 94–105, 2016.

[18] L. Timmers, S. K. Lim, I. E. Hoefer et al., "Human mesenchymal stem cell-conditioned medium improves cardiac function following myocardial infarction," *Stem Cell Research*, vol. 6, no. 3, pp. 206–214, 2011.

[19] P. Danieli, G. Malpasso, M. C. Ciuffreda et al., "Conditioned medium from human amniotic mesenchymal stromal cells limits infarct size and enhances angiogenesis," *Stem Cells Translational Medicine*, vol. 4, no. 5, pp. 448–458, 2015.

[20] A. T. Brini, G. Amodeo, L. M. Ferreira et al., "Therapeutic effect of human adipose-derived stem cells and their secretome in experimental diabetic pain," *Scientific Reports*, vol. 7, no. 1, p. 9904, 2017.

[21] A. Gualerzi, S. Niada, C. Giannasi et al., "Raman spectroscopy uncovers biochemical tissue-related features of extracellular vesicles from mesenchymal stromal cells," *Scientific Reports*, vol. 7, no. 1, p. 9820, 2017.

[22] A. Blasi, C. Martino, L. Balducci et al., "Dermal fibroblasts display similar phenotypic and differentiation capacity to fat-derived mesenchymal stem cells, but differ in anti-inflammatory and angiogenic potential," *Vascular Cell*, vol. 3, no. 1, p. 5, 2011.

[23] C. A. Brohem, C. M. de Carvalho, C. L. Radoski et al., "Comparison between fibroblasts and mesenchymal stem cells derived from dermal and adipose tissue," *International Journal of Cosmetic Science*, vol. 35, no. 5, pp. 448–457, 2013.

[24] J. R. Wisniewski, A. Zougman, N. Nagaraj, and M. Mann, "Universal sample preparation method for proteome analysis," *Nature Methods*, vol. 6, no. 5, pp. 359–362, 2009.

[25] J. Cox, N. Neuhauser, A. Michalski, R. A. Scheltema, J. V. Olsen, and M. Mann, "Andromeda: a peptide search engine integrated into the MaxQuant environment," *Journal of Proteome Research*, vol. 10, no. 4, pp. 1794–1805, 2011.

[26] A. I. Saeed, V. Sharov, J. White et al., "TM4: a free, open-source system for microarray data management and analysis," *BioTechniques*, vol. 34, no. 2, pp. 374–378, 2003.

[27] C. Giannasi, G. Pagni, C. Polenghi et al., "Impact of dental implant surface modifications on adhesion and proliferation of primary human gingival keratinocytes and progenitor cells," *The International Journal of Periodontics & Restorative Dentistry*, vol. 38, no. 1, pp. 127–135, 2018.

[28] K. Hu and B. R. Olsen, "Osteoblast-derived VEGF regulates osteoblast differentiation and bone formation during bone repair," *The Journal of Clinical Investigation*, vol. 126, no. 2, pp. 509–526, 2016.

[29] S. Niada, C. Giannasi, L. M. J. Ferreira, A. Milani, E. Arrigoni, and A. T. Brini, "17β-Estradiol differently affects osteogenic differentiation of mesenchymal stem/stromal cells from adipose tissue and bone marrow," *Differentiation*, vol. 92, no. 5, pp. 291–297, 2016.

[30] D. Szklarczyk, J. H. Morris, H. Cook et al., "The STRING database in 2017: quality-controlled protein-protein association networks, made broadly accessible," *Nucleic Acids Research*, vol. 45, no. D1, pp. D362–d368, 2017.

[31] T. E. Kruger, A. H. Miller, A. K. Godwin, and J. Wang, "Bone sialoprotein and osteopontin in bone metastasis of osteotropic cancers," *Critical Reviews in Oncology/Hematology*, vol. 89, no. 2, pp. 330–341, 2014.

[32] C. V. Fontanilla, H. Gu, Q. Liu et al., "Adipose-derived stem cell conditioned media extends survival time of a mouse model of amyotrophic lateral sclerosis," *Scientific Reports*, vol. 5, no. 1, article 16953, 2015.

[33] A. O. Pires, B. Mendes-Pinheiro, F. G. Teixeira et al., "Unveiling the differences of secretome of human bone marrow mesenchymal stem cells, adipose tissue-derived stem cells, and human umbilical cord perivascular cells: a proteomic analysis," *Stem Cells and Development*, vol. 25, no. 14, pp. 1073–1083, 2016.

[34] G. Marfia, S. E. Navone, L. A. Hadi et al., "The adipose mesenchymal stem cell secretome inhibits inflammatory responses of microglia: evidence for an involvement of sphingosine-1-phosphate signalling," *Stem Cells and Development*, vol. 25, no. 14, pp. 1095–1107, 2016.

[35] P. Sacerdote, S. Niada, S. Franchi et al., "Systemic administration of human adipose-derived stem cells reverts nociceptive hypersensitivity in an experimental model of neuropathy," *Stem Cells and Development*, vol. 22, no. 8, pp. 1252–1263, 2013.

[36] G. Lemke and C. V. Rothlin, "Immunobiology of the TAM receptors," *Nature Reviews Immunology*, vol. 8, no. 5, pp. 327–336, 2008.

[37] B. D. Semple, T. Kossmann, and M. C. Morganti-Kossmann, "Role of chemokines in CNS health and pathology: a focus on the CCL2/CCR2 and CXCL8/CXCR2 networks," *Journal of Cerebral Blood Flow and Metabolism*, vol. 30, no. 3, pp. 459–473, 2010.

[38] J. M. Gregory, D. R. Whiten, R. A. Brown et al., "Clusterin protects neurons against intracellular proteotoxicity," *Acta Neuropathologica Communications*, vol. 5, no. 1, p. 81, 2017.

[39] J. T. Yu and L. Tan, "The role of clusterin in Alzheimer's disease: pathways, pathogenesis, and therapy," *Molecular Neurobiology*, vol. 45, no. 2, pp. 314–326, 2012.

[40] C. Troakes, R. Smyth, F. Noor et al., "Clusterin expression is upregulated following acute head injury and localizes to astrocytes in old head injury," *Neuropathology*, vol. 37, no. 1, pp. 12–24, 2017.

[41] E. Dall and H. Brandstetter, "Structure and function of legumain in health and disease," *Biochimie*, vol. 122, pp. 126–150, 2016.

[42] L. Ma, Y. Q. Shen, H. P. Khatri, and M. Schachner, "The asparaginyl endopeptidase legumain is essential for functional recovery after spinal cord injury in adult zebrafish," *PLoS One*, vol. 9, no. 4, article e95098, 2014.

[43] G. C. A. Elson, E. Lelièvre, C. Guillet et al., "CLF associates with CLC to form a functional heteromeric ligand for the CNTF receptor complex," *Nature Neuroscience*, vol. 3, no. 9, pp. 867–872, 2000.

[44] Q. Wu, Z. H. Tang, J. Peng et al., "The dual behavior of PCSK9 in the regulation of apoptosis is crucial in Alzheimer's disease progression (review)," *Biomedical Reports*, vol. 2, no. 2, pp. 167–171, 2014.

[45] E. Aomatsu, N. Takahashi, S. Sawada et al., "Novel SCRG1/ BST1 axis regulates self-renewal, migration, and osteogenic differentiation potential in mesenchymal stem cells," *Scientific Reports*, vol. 4, no. 1, article 3652, 2014.

[46] M. Inoue, J. Yamada, E. Aomatsu-Kikuchi et al., "SCRG1 suppresses LPS-induced CCL22 production through ERK1/2 activation in mouse macrophage Raw264.7 cells," *Molecular Medicine Reports*, vol. 15, no. 6, pp. 4069–4076, 2017.

[47] S. Ali, Y. Jenkins, M. Kirkley et al., "Leukocyte extravasation: an immunoregulatory role for alpha-L-fucosidase?," *Journal of Immunology*, vol. 181, no. 4, pp. 2407–2413, 2008.

[48] R. R. Rao, J. Z. Long, J. P. White et al., "Meteorin-like is a hormone that regulates immune-adipose interactions to increase beige fat thermogenesis," *Cell*, vol. 157, no. 6, pp. 1279–1291, 2014.

[49] C. Xia, Z. Braunstein, A. C. Toomey, J. Zhong, and X. Rao, "S100 proteins as an important regulator of macrophage inflammation," *Frontiers in Immunology*, vol. 8, article 1908, 2018.

[50] R. Volkman and D. Offen, "Concise review: mesenchymal stem cells in neurodegenerative diseases," *Stem Cells*, vol. 35, no. 8, pp. 1867–1880, 2017.

[51] F. G. Teixeira, M. M. Carvalho, K. M. Panchalingam et al., "Impact of the secretome of human mesenchymal stem cells on brain structure and animal behavior in a rat model of Parkinson's disease," *Stem Cells Translational Medicine*, vol. 6, no. 2, pp. 634–646, 2017.

[52] L. De Laporte, J. J. Rice, F. Tortelli, and J. A. Hubbell, "Tenascin C promiscuously binds growth factors via its fifth fibronectin type III-like domain," *PLoS One*, vol. 8, no. 4, article e62076, 2013.

[53] M. P. Caley, G. Kogianni, A. Adamarek et al., "TGFβ_1-Endo180-dependent collagen deposition is dysregulated at the tumour-stromal interface in bone metastasis," *The Journal of Pathology*, vol. 226, no. 5, pp. 775–783, 2012.

[54] L. J. Foster, P. A. Zeemann, C. Li, M. Mann, O. N. Jensen, and M. Kassem, "Differential expression profiling of membrane proteins by quantitative proteomics in a human mesenchymal stem cell line undergoing osteoblast differentiation," *Stem Cells*, vol. 23, no. 9, pp. 1367–1377, 2005.

[55] C. Chang, D. A. Holtzman, S. Chau et al., "Twisted gastrulation can function as a BMP antagonist," *Nature*, vol. 410, no. 6827, pp. 483–487, 2001.

[56] M. Oelgeschlager, J. Larrain, D. Geissert, and E. M. De Robertis, "The evolutionarily conserved BMP-binding protein Twisted gastrulation promotes BMP signalling," *Nature*, vol. 405, no. 6788, pp. 757–763, 2000.

[57] R. Huntley, J. Davydova, A. Petryk et al., "The function of twisted gastrulation in regulating osteoclast differentiation is dependent on BMP binding," *Journal of Cellular Biochemistry*, vol. 116, no. 10, pp. 2239–2246, 2015.

[58] H. R. Hofer and R. S. Tuan, "Secreted trophic factors of mesenchymal stem cells support neurovascular and musculoskeletal therapies," *Stem Cell Research & Therapy*, vol. 7, no. 1, p. 131, 2016.

[59] R. Costa-Almeida, R. Soares, and P. L. Granja, "Fibroblasts as maestros orchestrating tissue regeneration," *Journal of Tissue Engineering and Regenerative Medicine*, vol. 12, no. 1, pp. 240–251, 2018.

[60] Y. Qin, L. Wang, Z. Gao, G. Chen, and C. Zhang, "Bone marrow stromal/stem cell-derived extracellular vesicles regulate osteoblast activity and differentiation in vitro and promote bone regeneration in vivo," *Scientific Reports*, vol. 6, no. 1, article 21961, 2016.

9

Optimizing Osteogenic Differentiation of Ovine Adipose-Derived Stem Cells by Osteogenic Induction Medium and FGFb, BMP2, or NELL1 In Vitro

Emil Østergaard Nielsen ⓘ,[1] Li Chen ⓘ,[2] Jonas Overgaard Hansen ⓘ,[1] Matilda Degn ⓘ,[3] Søren Overgaard,[1] and Ming Ding ⓘ[1]

[1]Orthopaedic Research Laboratory, Department of Orthopaedic Surgery and Traumatology, Odense University Hospital, Department of Clinical Research, University of Southern Denmark, Sdr. Boulevard 29, 5000 Odense, Denmark
[2]Department of Endocrinology and Metabolism, Molecular Endocrinology Laboratory (KMEB), Odense University Hospital, University of Southern Denmark, J. B. Winsløws Vej 25.1, 5000 Odense, Denmark
[3]Department of Pediatrics and Adolescent Medicine, University of Copenhagen, Rigshospitalet, Blegdamsvej 9, 2100 Copenhagen, Denmark

Correspondence should be addressed to Emil Østergaard Nielsen; emilnielsen90@gmail.com, Li Chen; lchen@health.sdu.dk, and Ming Ding; ming.ding@rsyd.dk

Academic Editor: Jun Liu

Although adipose-derived stromal cells (ADSCs) have been a major focus as an alternative to autologous bone graft in orthopedic surgery, bone formation potential of ADSCs is not well known and cytokines as osteogenic inducers on ADSCs are being investigated. This study aimed at isolating ADSCs from ovine adipose tissue (AT) and optimizing osteogenic differentiation of ovine ADSCs (oADSC) by culture medium and growth factors. Four AT samples were harvested from two female ovine (Texel/Gotland breed), and oADSCs were isolated and analyzed by flow cytometry for surface markers CD29, CD44, CD31, and CD45. Osteogenic differentiation was made in vitro by seeding oADSCs in osteogenic induction medium (OIM) containing fibroblast growth factor basic (FGFb), bone morphogenetic protein 2 (BMP2), or NEL-like molecule 1 (NELL1) in 4 different dosages (1, 10, 50, and 100 ng/ml, respectively). Basic medium (DMEM) was used as control. Analysis was made after 14 days by Alizarin red staining (ARS) and quantification. This study successfully harvested AT from ovine and verified isolated cells for minimal criteria for adipose stromal cells which suggests a feasible method for isolation of oADSCs. OIM showed significantly higher ARS to basic medium, and FGFb 10 ng/ml revealed significantly higher ARS to OIM alone after 14 days.

1. Introduction

Several conditions such as trauma, tumor, infection, and surgical procedure can cause larger bone defects. Due to the lack of easily accessible new bone formation materials, patients with these problems can be faced with major clinical challenges that affect treatment. Autograft primarily harvested from the iliac crest of the same patient is the gold standard as new bone formation material. Autograft bears the fundamental characteristics for new bone formation: osteogenesis,

osteoinduction, and osteoconduction [1]. Nonetheless, harvesting autograft has its disadvantages and complication frequency of between 8.5% and 20% has been reported. Complications from harvesting this material include infections, chronic pain, blood loss, and fractures from the donor site [2], and an important limitation is the restricted amount of autograft available for harvesting [3].

Mesenchymal stromal cells (MSC) as progenitor cells have been investigated regarding their capability to generate new bone tissue. These cells have displayed promising results and have the potential to replace autograft because of its good proliferation and osteogenic properties [4]. The most investigated MSC is the bone marrow-derived multipotent mesenchymal stromal cells (BMSCs) which have shown the most interesting results regarding new bone formation in vivo [5]. BMSCs are already being tested in preclinical [6] and clinical studies [7]. The disadvantages of this method are a low concentration of MSC in bone marrow aspirate, discomfort, and morbidity for the patient [8].

Adipose-derived stromal cells (ADSCs) have been investigated because they have the same properties as BMSCs. Easy access to the adipose tissue (AT) as well as the amount of this tissue in the human body together with high stem cell (SC) counts makes it an interesting area to explore [9]; moreover, ADSCs are easier to harvest when compared to BMSCs and have a lower risk of complications [8, 10]. It is important to ensure that your data is translatable to other studies; therefore, a minimal criteria for adipose stromal cells (ASCs) proposed by the Federation for Adipose Therapeutics (IFATS) and the International Society for Cellular Therapy (ISCT) was made by Bourin et al. [11].

Preclinical trials in large animals with ADSCs are necessary to obtain morphological and biomechanical information on bone repair before clinical trials [12]. Our recent study comparing cells derived from ovine bone marrow (BM) and cells from ovine AT revealed that the BM has superior ability to form new bone in vivo compared to AT in a severe combined immunodeficiency mouse (SCID) model [13] which is in line with recent studies comparing BMSCs and ADSCs [14–17]. Although new bone formation was seen in both AT and BM groups, the quantitative histomorphometry showed that the bone formation in the AT groups was 10-fold lower than in the BM groups [13].

Many factors may influence bone formation, and a key factor might be the osteogenic differentiation and commitment to osteogenic lineage. As summarized below, several known growth factor cytokines have been tried for osteogenic differentiation both in vitro and in vivo. To our knowledge, no studies have compared more than two growth factors on ADSCs in vitro and later in vivo.

Recombinant human fibroblast growth factor basic/2 (FGFb) has been shown to have positive osteogenic effects on human BMSCs and human ADMSCs by enhancing osteogenic differentiation in vitro and bone osteoid area in vivo [15]. Little is known about FGFb and its influence on ovine bone formation [18]. No studies have tested FGFb on any kind of ovine progenitor cells although FGFb has shown better bone formation in smaller animal models [19].

Bone morphogenetic proteins belong to the transforming growth factor-β family which is the best investigated enhancer of bone genesis. Recombinant human bone morphogenetic protein 2 (BMP2) has been widely studied and has been indicated to have great potential in bone formation in vitro and in vivo [20, 21]. Today, it is also used in clinical applications [22]. BMP2 has been shown to enhance results on human ADSC osteoblastic phenotype [21, 23] and in ovine ADSCs (oADSCs) in nonunion of the tibia [12]. BMP2 has also been shown a dose-dependent adipogenesis activation through peroxisome proliferator-activated

receptor γ (PPARγ) [24]. The effect of BMP2 in vivo is not well known and is probably highly dependent on the environment of applications suggested by Kim and Choe [25].

Recombinant human NEL-like molecule 1 (NELL1) is a secretory glycoprotein first discovered through its association with craniosynostosis (CS) in children [26]. Transgenic mice overexpressing NELL1 have also shown an association with CS [27], and mice with a deficiency of the of NELL1 gene have shown defects in calvaria and long bone volume which suggests that NELL1 may have an important role in bone development [28, 29]. The direct cellular role of NELL1 is not well known but is believed to have a downstream Runt-related transcription factor-2 (Runx2) activation separated from BMP2's signaling pathway [30]. It has been shown that NELL1 downregulates the expression of PPARγ and has an antiadipose pathway regulation; thus, a combination of NELL1 and BMP2 may lead to enhanced osteogenesis and have antiadipose tissue regulation [31]. NELL1 has been shown to boost the bone formation in osteoporotic ovine in the surrounding tissue of administration which suggests that the human version of the protein has a similar role in ovine [29].

This study investigates osteogenic differentiation on oADSCs by optimizing bone engineering (harvesting, seeding, and culturing) in vitro. We use Alizarin red staining (ARS) for calcium deposit in the extracellular matrix (ECM) of oADSCs which is believed to have high sensitivity for osteogenic differentiation [32, 33]. These results may possibly lead to more promising use of ADSCs in today's preclinic and clinic.

The primary aim of the study is to isolate oADSCs and verify for minimal criteria for ASCs. The secondary aim is to optimize the conditions for oADSC osteogenic differentiation by medium and growth factors.

We hypothesize that adding more bioactive factors to growth medium will improve the commitment to osteogenic differentiation of oADSCs which may significantly enhance the commitment to osteogenic lineage.

2. Method and Materials

2.1. Isolation and Expansion of Stem Cells from Adipose Tissue. Surgical procedures were performed at the Biomedical Laboratory at the University of Southern Denmark. A total of $n = 4$ AT extractions were made on 2 experimental female sheep (Texel/Gotland breed, 2–4 years of age) lateral to the vertebra on both sides (average sample weight of 6.58 g) under local anesthesia with 5 ml of lidocaine s.c. (Amgros, Copenhagen, Denmark), systemic Rompun (1.0–1.2 ml Vet, Bayer, Germany), and Temgesic (0.6–0.7 ml, Reckitt Benckiser, Hull, UK).

After scalpel incision, the sample was placed directly in falcon tubes with 5 ml of preheated (37°C) Dulbecco's phosphate-buffered saline (PBS, Gibco, cat. no. 14040-091, Roskilde, Denmark) with 10% bovine serum albumin (BSA; Sigma Aldrich, Denmark) and 1% penicillin/streptomycin (P/S; Sigma Aldrich). The oADSCs were obtained according to Gimble [34]. Samples were immediately taken to the cell culture lab where they were put into petri dishes and washed with PBS and 1% P/S. The samples were then put in falcon tubes, and 200 units/ml collagenase type I (Thermo Fisher, cat. no. 17018-029, Denmark) were added to them (10% BSA, 1% P/S in scale 1 : 1 (volume : weight)). Afterwards, the tubes were placed in a 37°C water bath for 60 min with shaking after which they were centrifuged at 300g for 5 minutes. This was followed by the careful aspiration of the adipocyte layer and liquid to isolate stromal vascular fraction (SVF) pellets. 1 : 10 erythrocyte lysis buffer (ELB, BD, cat. no. 555899, Denmark) in sterile water was then added and incubated at room temperature (RT) for 10 minutes. After incubation, cells were filtered through 100 μm filter to get rid of cell debris.

The harvested cells were centrifuged at 300g for 5 minutes after which the supernatant was discarded and the SVF pellets resolved in Dulbecco's modified eagle's medium/nutrient F-12/GlutaMax (DMEM, cat. no. 31331-028, Gibco) with 10% fetal bovine serum (FBS, Gibco, cat. no. 10270-098) and 1% P/S (hereafter referred to as *basic medium*). Cells were then mixed by pipet and counted by hemocytometer after which they were seeded in T75-150 flasks in basic medium dependent on SVF isolation yield and cultured in incubator 37°C with 5% CO_2 for 6–9 days before cell attachment was observed. Medium was then changed to wash away nonadherent cells, and the remaining cells were expanded until 60–85% confluence was reached. Trypsin/ethylenediaminetetraacetic acid (EDTA, Sigma Aldrich) was used to transfer cells for future further culturing.

2.2. Colonizing Forming Unit (CFU) Assay. CFU assays were made on SVF samples to measure proportion of ADSCs in the SVF isolation [35]. From sample one, $1 \cdot 10^5$ cells from SVF were seeded in a T75 flask. These cells were cultured for 7 days and analysed after standard protocol. In brief, cells were washed twice with PBS, fixed by 4% paraformaldehyde (PFA), washed in PBS, stained with 0.5% crystal violet methanol for 30 minutes, and finally washed with water to remove nonspecific staining. CFU were counted positive if more than 50 cells in a colony were observed. Due to the high number of CFU in the first sample, later SVF samples were seeded in lower numbers ($1 \cdot 10^4$ and $1 \cdot 10^3$ cells per T75 flask) for 12 days to make counting easier (Figure 1) and more reliable like the original protocol by Castro-Malaspina et al. [36].

2.3. Flow Cytometry (FC) Analysis. ADSCs from passage 1 (P1) were cryopreserved by standard protocol in 10% dimethyl sulfoxide (DSMO, Sigma Aldrich, cat. no. C6295) and kept at −80°C. After thawing, the cells were grown one passage. P2 cells were harvested and analysed for the expression of surface antigens by staining with CD29-APC (BioLegend, cat. no. 303007, clone TS2/16), CD45-PE (Bio-Rad, cat. no. MCA2220PE, clone 1.11.32), CD44-FITC (Bio-Rad, cat. no. MCA2219F, clone 25.32), or CD31-FITC (Bio-Rad, cat. no. MCA1097F, clone CO.3E1D4) for FC analysis on a FACSVerse (BD Biosciences). Corresponding isotype antibodies from BD Pharmingen were used as negative controls. In brief, cells were detached by EDTA, washed with PBS, counted, and stained with fixable viability dye eFluor 506

(eBioscience, cat. no. 65-0866-14) to show live/dead cells. The cells were subsequently fixed by cytoperm/cytofix (BD, cat. no. 51-2090KZ). $5 \cdot 10^5$ cells in each sample were washed with PBS and stained with relevant antibodies for 30 min at 4°C in the dark. The cells were stained for CD45 and CD29 in addition to either CD44-FITC or CD31-FITC, and another tube was stained with the isotype controls. 5–10 μl antibody solution per 200 μl cell suspension was used according to the manufacturer's recommendations.

2.4. Osteogenic Differentiation. oADSCs from P1 were resuspended in basic medium and counted. 4,000 cells/cm^2 were seeded in 4 flat-bottom 24-well plate with no coating (DACOS, Denmark), and 1 ml basic medium was added to each well. After 24 hours in a 37°C incubator, the 5% CO_2 medium was replaced with six different growth mediums. Each of the four plates had a different dosage (100 ng/ml, 50 ng/ml, 10 ng/ml, and 1 ng/ml) of growth factors:

(1) Basic medium (control)

(2) Basic medium with osteogenic induction medium (OIM) consisting of L-ascorbic 0.2 mM (Wako, cat. no. 013-12061, USA), dexamethasone $1 \cdot 10^{-8}$ M (Sigma, cat. no. D4902), and NaH_2PO_4 3 mM

(3) Basic medium, OIM, and rhFGF-basic (FGFb) (R&D, cat. no. 233-FB-025, Minneapolis, USA)

(4) Basic medium, OIM, and rhBMP2 (BMP2) (R&D, cat. no. 355-BEC-010, Minneapolis, USA)

(5) Basic medium, OIM, and rhNELL1 (NELL1) (R&D, cat. no. 5487-NL-050, Minneapolis, USA)

(6) Basic medium, OIM, rhBMP2, and rhNELL1

In each well, the medium was changed every 48–72 hours for 14 days. Medium was freshly prepared each time to minimise protein decay, and growth factors were added just before use. Technical triplicates were made in all groups.

2.5. Alizarin Red Staining and Quantification. After 14 days of osteogenic differentiation, medium was removed, and cells were both washed by PBS and fixed by 70% ethanol for 1 hour at −20°C. Afterwards, the cells were briefly washed in dH_2O. 40 mM Alizarin red (Sigma Aldrich, cat. no. A-5533) pH was adjusted to 4.1-4.2 and was added and placed under rotation for 10 minutes. Dye was removed and washed by dH_2O twice. PBS was added and placed under rotation for 5 minutes to wash away nonspecific stains. Pictures of stained layers were taken by scanner and pictured in an inverted microscope (Olympus, data not shown). For quantification of staining, 300 μl of 10% (v/v) hexadecylpyridinium chloride monohydrate (CC, Sigma Aldrich, cat. no. 6004-24-06) was added to each well and placed at RT for 30 minutes shaking. Dye was removed from stain, and colour changes were seen in CC solution. 100 μl/well solutions were transferred to a new 96-well plate and detected by spectrometry at 570 nm with FLUOstar Omega (BMG LABTECH, Offenburg, DE).

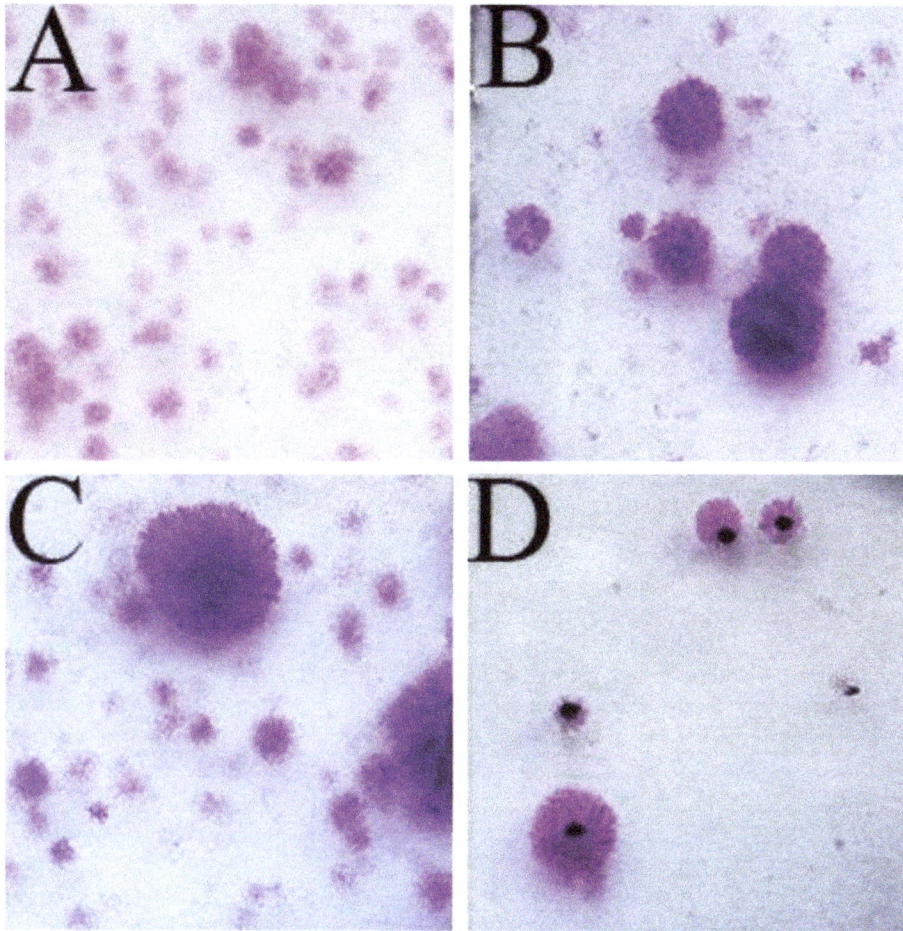

FIGURE 1: Part of the colonizing forming unit assay made by the crystal violet methanol after seeding SVF cells in T75 flasks. (A) Seeding of $1 \cdot 10^5$ SVF cells from sample 1 for 7 days. (B) Seeding of $1 \cdot 10^4$ SVF cells from sample 2 for 12 days. (C) Seeding of $1 \cdot 10^4$ SVF cells from sample 3 for 12 days. (D) Seeding of $1 \cdot 10^3$ SVF cells from sample 2 for 12 days. Low density of CFU is seen, and black dots form counting.

2.6. Morphological Examination of Cell Sheet and Histology. oADSCs from P1 were seeded (4000 cells/cm^2 concentration) in a T75 flask and OIM as previously described. Cells were cultured for 14 days before the cell sheet was removed by cell scraper and washed two times in PBS and fixed in 4% paraformaldehyde. Paraffin-embedded histological analysis was made by section cuts to the cell sheet to a thickness of 4 μm, deparaffinized, rehydrated, and stained with hematoxylin and eosin (H&E; DAKO-Aldrich, Denmark). Visualization pictures of cell sheet were captured with stereological software (newCAST™, Visiopharm, Denmark).

2.7. Statistical Analysis of Alizarin Red Quantification. Statistical analyses were performed using GraphPad Prism (version 7.03 software, La Jolla, CA). For normality, the Shapiro-Wilk test was performed. As data follow Gaussian distribution, ANOVA was made comparing the 4 test groups to the basic medium and OIM groups. Welch *t*-test was made comparing each group to the basic medium pairwise and OIM groups to reduce the risk of type I errors. Statistically significant values were defined as $p < 0.05$. Data is presented as the mean and standard deviation (SD).

3. Results

3.1. Characterization of oADSCs. The cells isolated from adipose tissue were plastic-adherent and had an average of 3.1% (range: 2.4%–3.9%) cells forming colonies from the isolated SVF after 12 days. No significant difference was seen between seeding density groups of $1 \cdot 10^4$ cells and $1 \cdot 10^3$ cells. Seeding density group of $1 \cdot 10^5$ cells was left out due to overcolonization and impossible reliable counting. The average of 3.1% from the two lower seeding groups met the minimal criteria of more than 1% CFU proposed by Bourin et al. [11]. Seeding density of $1 \cdot 10^3$ cells in T75 flask was most reliable for counting and therefore appropriate for use onwards.

The ASC immunophenotype was confirmed as 99% of the gated live cells were positive for the surface markers CD29 and CD44 (two typical ASC surface markers) and less than 0.5% positive to CD31 (endothelial cells) and CD45 (leukocytes) (Figure 2). The cell culture thus met the minimal criteria for ASCs by having more than 80% CD29- and CD44-positive cells and less than 2% CD31- and CD45-positive cells.

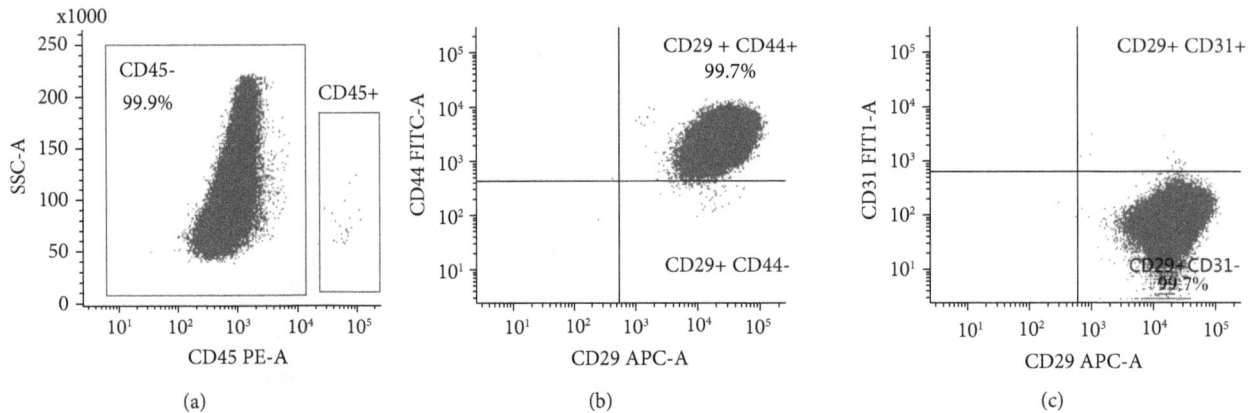

FIGURE 2: Immunophenotype of cells isolated from SVF conducted to be oADSCs. A gating of cells was based on FSC and SSC criteria, and the cells were subgated to only include single cells and only live cells were measured by fixable viability dye eFluor 506 staining and used subsequent analysis (data not shown). (a) CD45-negative cells were subgated to analyze the expression of (b) CD44 and CD29 and (c) CD31 and CD29. All quadrants were placed based on the isotype controls.

Table 1 summarizes the minimal criteria set for immunophenotypic characterization of ASCs: a minimum of two positive and two negative surface markers as determined by Bourin et al. The flow cytometry of at least 250,000 cells analyzed in each sample shows that the cells express CD29 and CD44 but not CD31 and CD45.

3.2. Osteogenic Differentiation Optimization.

Results from 14-day growth tests in different osteogenic mediums were visualized by Alizarin red staining (ARS). Representative stains from each triplicate group are presented in Figure 3. During growth period, cell sheet was formed in the OIM groups. Detachment of cell sheet from well bottom was seen in most groups after 7–9 days (data not shown). Cell sheet folding in orb-formation and new colonization of well bottom was observed during the rest of the growth period visualized in Figure 3. No folding was seen in the FGFb 10 ng/ml group, and a better visualized ARS was observed after 14 days.

Significantly higher mineralization from quantification of ARS was seen among (12/17) groups containing only OIM or including growth factors compared to basic medium alone. (Only FGFb 10 ng/ml had significantly higher mineralization compared to OIM alone marked by the symbols **.) This was not evident in higher concentrations of FGFb (Figure 4). No significant dose response was observed when stimulated with FGFb, BMP2, NELL1, and a combination of BMP2 and NELL1.

4. Discussion

This current study showed that it is possible to isolate and verify oADSCs from ovine AT and optimize commitment to osteogenic differentiation with OIM when compared to standard growth medium after 14 days in vitro. Significant differentiation was shown to occur by adding FGFb to the OIM; however, this differentiation was not shown to be significantly affected by BMP2, NELL1, and a combination of BMP2 and NELL1. This supports our hypothesis that adding some bioactive factors to normal growth medium may

TABLE 1: Immunophenotypic characterization.

Surface marker	ASCs criteria	Results from flow cytometry
CD29	Positive X > 80%	99.97% positive
CD44	Positive X > 80%	99.74% positive
CD45	Negative X < 2%	0.01% positive
CD31	Negative X < 2%	0.26% positive

significantly improve osteogenic differentiation and commitment to osteogenic lineage which may lead to an improved novo bone formation for later testing in vivo.

We aimed to harvest AT and isolate oADSCs from ovine and verify according to the minimal criteria for ASCs proposed by Bourin et al. [11]. Due to the low amount of available anti-ovine antibodies, only 3 primary anti-ovine were available. Anti-human CD29 (clone TS2/16) was used based on results from a basic local alignment search tool (BLAST) in the NCBI GenBank that showed sequence identity to the ovine form of integrin beta and had previously been used with success as antibody by Sanjurjo-Rodríguez et al. [37]. Both in terms of CFU assay and immunophenotypic characterization, this study succeeded in fulfilling the minimal criteria for ASCs isolated from ovine AT and proposes a feasible method for isolation of oADSCs from the lateral back of ovine.

A secondary aim of this study was to optimize the conditions for osteogenic differentiation and thereby select a better candidate for later examination in vivo. ARS and quantification were used to evaluate optimization by OIM and growth factors. We were able to show higher ARS and quantification after 14 days of culture in 12 out of 17 groups containing OIM (Figure 4) when compared to basic medium. The basic medium group represents our control cells, and the oADSCs in this group were treated as earlier cultures in vitro before implantation in vivo as was done in our previous study [13]. The OIM with FGFb 10 ng/ml showed significantly higher quantification than OIM alone. Both the results with OIM alone and FGFb 10 ng/ml suggested a stronger

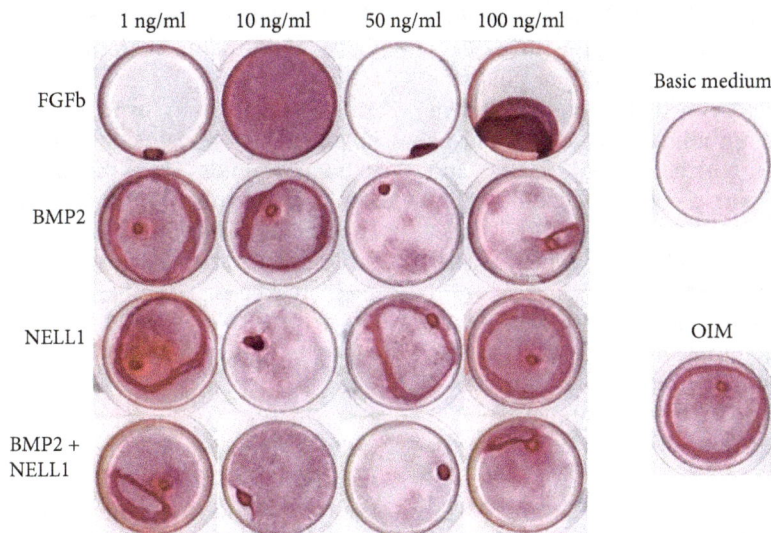

FIGURE 3: Alizarin red staining of oADSCs after a 14-day growth period in different growth mediums. Triplicates were made in all groups, and the most representative well from each group was chosen for the figure. The 4×4 square table is rhFGFb, rhBMP2, rhNELL1, and rhBMP2 plus rhNELL1 in different dosages with osteogenic induction medium (OIM). On the right the two controls: basic medium alone and OIM alone.

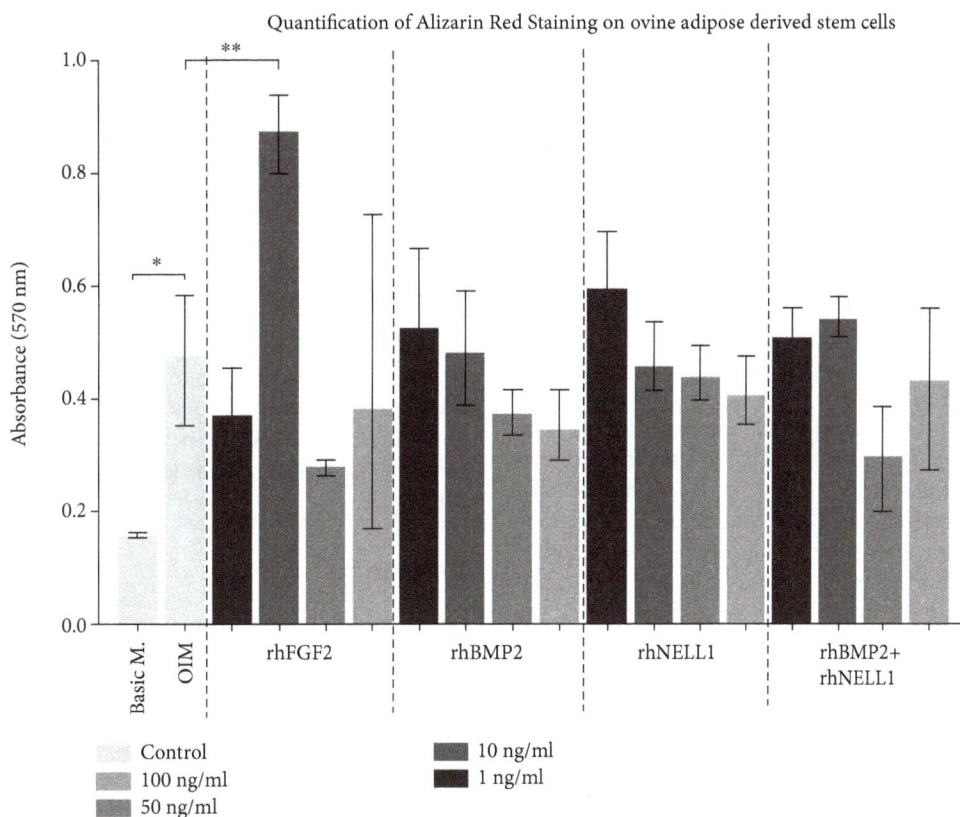

FIGURE 4: Quantification of the Alizarin red staining was made by hexadecylpyridinium chloride monohydrate (CC) after visualization. All wells were subtracted background from an average of 3 wells of 100 μl CC. Unpaired ANOVA was made on the mean values with SD of all wells and compared with Basic M. (basic medium) and OIM alone by Welch t-test. ∗ indicates statistical significance ($p < 0.05$) between basic medium and OIM group. ∗∗ indicates statistical significance ($p < 0.05$) to OIM in a nonpaired t-test between the two control groups.

commitment to osteogenic cell lineage. To our knowledge, this study is the first to test FGFb on oADSC for osteogenic differentiation in vitro.

Cell sheet was formed in all groups that included OIM, and cell sheet detachment from well bottom and folding in orb formation was observed in 48 out of 51 wells. This may have limited visualization and might have also limited the quantification results due to poor cell growth the days after folding and cell necrosis. As a result of this, the precision regarding individual growth factors in different concentrations may be compromised and may not be included in the context of whether FGFb, BMP2, and NELL1 will boost commitment to osteogenic differentiation and thereby osteogenic lineage or not. Cell sheet formation is a response to L-ascorbic acid which makes cells deposit more collagen and thereby makes ECM [38]. ECM is considered a great carrier for mesenchymal stem cells [39] and causes problems when analysed by ARS due to in-between binding strength of the oADSCs compared to the plastic-adhered binding strength of the cells to well bottom. Nutrient necrosis of OIM for unknown reasons may also be a possibility for cell detachment. A visualization of the cell sheet was added as supplementary data, and a thick sheet with many cells in several layers surrounded by ECM is illustrated in Supplementary Figure 5. Recent steps toward optimizing ADSC sheet in canine in vitro were done by Kim et al. [40]. In a new study comparing ADMSC and ADMSC sheets, both groups included scaffolds in critical size defect dog model and showed significantly higher new bone formation after 12 weeks in the ADMSC sheet group [41]. The cell sheet folding may have limited the analysis of potential osteogenic lineage inducers of oADSCs, but it may propose a solution for controlling cells in future tissue engineering at focal region when implanted in critical size defects or in subcutaneous ectopic mice models.

In terms of immunophenotypic characterization, a clear limitation is the lack of more cross-reactive or primary antibodies for ovine to verify cells as adipose-derived mesenchymal stromal cells. This makes comparison between individual studies more difficult which is a problem summarized by Khan et al. [42].

A limitation to this study is the use of ARS as solo evaluation. Alkaline phosphatase activity has been shown to not express gen activity on ovine by Kalaszczynska et al. [43]. Preosteogenic markers like RUNX2, osteocalcin, type I collagen, and bone sialoprotein may be other options. Whether higher results at given time points yield more novo bone formation in vivo is unknown as many factors may influence the process from in vitro culture to in vivo bone formation [44]. In vivo experiments on small and large animal models must be done to show significant optimization.

Future in vivo investigations using small and large animals may be based on the optimal outcome from the current study and the cell sheet formation induced by OIM. Cell sheet may propose a solution for cell control with scaffold at focal region in animal models. The OIM may also have committed the oADSCs to osteogenic lineage. A hypothesis could be that changing from fetal bovine (FBS) to ovine serum may further optimize osteogenic differentiation of oADSCs.

We hypothesize that significantly more novo bone formation may be seen in vivo. This may lead to a more closely related human clinical relevance and can possibly make ASCs useful for future tissue engineering in clinical settings [45].

Whether results from in vitro can be translated into in vivo models remains to be seen. Sample sizes and changes to human samples along the way must be done to make these results translatable into the human clinical setting. To our knowledge, only limited research on osteogenic capacity between human and ovine has been investigated and differences may be expected [43].

5. Conclusion

This study successfully harvested AT from ovine and was verified for minimal criteria for ASCs which enables us to suggest that this is a feasible method for isolation of oADSCs. We were able to show significant effect of 10 ng/ml rhFGFb and OIM alone compared to basic growth medium but were not able to show dosage response with rhFGFb on osteogenic differentiation and commitment to osteogenic lineage. rhBMP2 and rhNELL1 added to OIM had no effect on osteogenic differentiation and commitment to osteogenic lineage based on ARS and quantification.

Acknowledgments

The authors would like to thank laboratory technicians Gitte Reinberg and Kira Joensen for their assistance. We would also like to thank Bonkolab (Paediatric Oncology Research Laboratory, Rigshospitalet) and Kate Lykke Lambertsen (Department of Neurobiology Research) for their help with immunophenotypic characterization as well as the staff at the Biomedical Laboratory for handling and taking care of the animals.

The authors would like to express sincere gratitude towards the Danish Council for Independent Research, Medical Sciences (DFF– 4004-00256, MD) for funding this study and Odense University Hospital's pregraduated pool for scholarship to Emil Østergaard Nielsen during the project.

References

[1] T. J. Cypher and J. P. Grossman, "Biological principles of bone graft healing," *The Journal of Foot and Ankle Surgery*, vol. 35, no. 5, pp. 413–417, 1996.

[2] P. V. Giannoudis, H. Dinopoulos, and E. Tsiridis, "Bone substitutes: an update," *Injury*, vol. 36, no. 3, pp. S20–S27, 2005.

[3] C. Myeroff and M. Archdeacon, "Autogenous bone graft: donor sites and techniques," *The Journal of Bone and Joint Surgery-American Volume*, vol. 93, no. 23, pp. 2227–2236, 2011.

[4] B.-J. Kang, H.-H. Ryu, S. S. Park et al., "Comparing the osteogenic potential of canine mesenchymal stem cells derived from adipose tissues, bone marrow, umbilical cord blood, and Wharton's jelly for treating bone defects," *Journal of Veterinary Science*, vol. 13, no. 3, pp. 299–310, 2012.

[5] P. Mattar and K. Bieback, "Comparing the immunomodulatory properties of bone marrow, adipose tissue, and birth-

associated tissue mesenchymal stromal cells," *Frontiers in Immunology*, vol. 6, 2015.

[6] M. Peric, I. Dumic-Cule, D. Grcevic et al., "The rational use of animal models in the evaluation of novel bone regenerative therapies," *Bone*, vol. 70, pp. 73–86, 2015.

[7] H. Song, L. Tao, F. Wang et al., "Effect of bone mesenchymal stem cells transplantation on the micro-environment of early osteonecrosis of the femoral head," *International Journal of Clinical and Experimental Pathology*, vol. 8, no. 11, pp. 14528–14534, 2015.

[8] H.-T. Liao and C.-T. Chen, "Osteogenic potential: comparison between bone marrow and adipose-derived mesenchymal stem cells," *World Journal of Stem Cells*, vol. 6, no. 3, pp. 288–295, 2014.

[9] L. Aust, B. Devlin, S. J. Foster et al., "Yield of human adipose-derived adult stem cells from liposuction aspirates," *Cytotherapy*, vol. 6, no. 1, pp. 7–14, 2004.

[10] O. Hayashi, Y. Katsube, M. Hirose, H. Ohgushi, and H. Ito, "Comparison of osteogenic ability of rat mesenchymal stem cells from bone marrow, periosteum, and adipose tissue," *Calcified Tissue International*, vol. 82, no. 3, pp. 238–247, 2008.

[11] P. Bourin, B. A. Bunnell, L. Casteilla et al., "Stromal cells from the adipose tissue-derived stromal vascular fraction and culture expanded adipose tissue-derived stromal/stem cells: a joint statement of the International Federation for Adipose Therapeutics and Science (IFATS) and the International Society for Cellular Therapy (ISCT)," *Cytotherapy*, vol. 15, no. 6, pp. 641–648, 2013.

[12] A. A. Hernandez-Hurtado, G. Borrego-Soto, I. A. Marino-Martinez et al., "Implant composed of demineralized bone and mesenchymal stem cells genetically modified with AdBMP2/AdBMP7 for the regeneration of bone fractures in *Ovis aries*," *Stem Cells International*, vol. 2016, Article ID 7403890, 12 pages, 2016.

[13] K. Kjærgaard, C. H. Dreyer, N. Ditzel et al., "Bone formation by sheep stem cells in an ectopic mouse model: comparison of adipose and bone marrow derived cells and identification of donor-derived bone by antibody staining," *Stem Cells International*, vol. 2016, Article ID 3846971, 10 pages, 2016.

[14] Y. Liu, T. Chen, F. Du et al., "Single-layer graphene enhances the osteogenic differentiation of human mesenchymal stem cells in vitro and in vivo," *Journal of Biomedical Nanotechnology*, vol. 12, no. 6, pp. 1270–1284, 2016.

[15] S. Lim, H. Cho, E. Lee et al., "Osteogenic stimulation of human adipose-derived stem cells by pre-treatment with fibroblast growth factor 2," *Cell and Tissue Research*, vol. 364, no. 1, pp. 137–147, 2016.

[16] F. Saxer, A. Scherberich, A. Todorov et al., "Implantation of stromal vascular fraction progenitors at bone fracture sites: from a rat model to a first-in-man study," *Stem Cells*, vol. 34, no. 12, pp. 2956–2966, 2016.

[17] E. M. Fennema, L. A. H. Tchang, H. Yuan et al., "Ectopic bone formation by aggregated mesenchymal stem cells from bone marrow and adipose tissue: a comparative study," *Journal of Tissue Engineering and Regenerative Medicine*, vol. 12, no. 1, pp. e150–e158, 2017.

[18] U. Maus, S. Andereya, J. A. K. Ohnsorge, S. Gravius, C. H. Siebert, and C. Niedhart, "A bFGF/TCP-composite inhibits bone formation in a sheep model," *Journal of Biomedical Materials Research Part B: Applied Biomaterials*, vol. 85B, no. 1, pp. 87–92, 2008.

[19] K. Keiichi, K. Mitsunobu, S. Masafumi, D. Yutaka, and S. Toshiaki, "Induction of new bone by basic FGF-loaded porous carbonate apatite implants in femur defects in rats," *Clinical Oral Implants Research*, vol. 20, no. 6, pp. 560–565, 2009.

[20] A. W. James, J. N. Zara, X. Zhang et al., "Perivascular stem cells: a prospectively purified mesenchymal stem cell population for bone tissue engineering," *Stem Cells Translational Medicine*, vol. 1, no. 6, pp. 510–519, 2012.

[21] S. Vanhatupa, M. Ojansivu, R. Autio, M. Juntunen, and S. Miettinen, "Bone morphogenetic protein-2 induces donor-dependent osteogenic and adipogenic differentiation in human adipose stem cells," *Stem Cells Translational Medicine*, vol. 4, no. 12, pp. 1391–1402, 2015.

[22] K. Mesimäki, B. Lindroos, J. Törnwall et al., "Novel maxillary reconstruction with ectopic bone formation by GMP adipose stem cells," *International Journal of Oral and Maxillofacial Surgery*, vol. 38, no. 3, pp. 201–209, 2009.

[23] J. L. Dragoo, J. Y. Choi, J. R. Lieberman et al., "Bone induction by BMP-2 transduced stem cells derived from human fat," *Journal of Orthopaedic Research*, vol. 21, no. 4, pp. 622–629, 2003.

[24] J.-C. Park, J. C. Kim, B.-K. Kim et al., "Dose- and time-dependent effects of recombinant human bone morphogenetic protein-2 on the osteogenic and adipogenic potentials of alveolar bone-derived stromal cells," *Journal of Periodontal Research*, vol. 47, no. 5, pp. 645–654, 2012.

[25] M.-J. Kim and S. Choe, "BMPs and their clinical potentials," *BMB Reports*, vol. 44, no. 10, pp. 619–634, 2011.

[26] K. Ting, H. Vastardis, J. B. Mulliken et al., "Human NELL-1 expressed in unilateral coronal synostosis," *Journal of Bone and Mineral Research*, vol. 14, no. 1, pp. 80–89, 1999.

[27] X. Zhang, S.'i. Kuroda, D. Carpenter et al., "Craniosynostosis in transgenic mice overexpressing Nell-1," *Journal of Clinical Investigation*, vol. 110, no. 6, pp. 861–870, 2002.

[28] J. Desai, M. E. Shannon, M. D. Johnson et al., "Nell1-deficient mice have reduced expression of extracellular matrix proteins causing cranial and vertebral defects," *Human Molecular Genetics*, vol. 15, no. 8, pp. 1329–1341, 2006.

[29] A. W. James, J. Shen, X. Zhang et al., "NELL-1 in the treatment of osteoporotic bone loss," *Nature Communications*, vol. 6, no. 1, article 7362, 2015.

[30] X. Zhang, K. Ting, C. M. Bessette et al., "Nell-1, a key functional mediator of Runx 2, partially rescues calvarial defects in Runx 2+/− mice," *Journal of Bone and Mineral Research*, vol. 26, no. 4, pp. 777–791, 2011.

[31] Y. Liu, C. Chen, H. He et al., "Lentiviral-mediated gene transfer into human adipose-derived stem cells: role of NELL1 versus BMP2 in osteogenesis and adipogenesis in vitro," *Acta Biochimica et Biophysica Sinica*, vol. 44, no. 10, pp. 856–865, 2012.

[32] H. Puchtler, S. N. Meloan, and M. S. Terry, "On the history and mechanism of alizarin and alizarin red s stains for calcium," *Journal of Histochemistry & Cytochemistry*, vol. 17, no. 2, pp. 110–124, 2016.

[33] C. M. Stanford, P. A. Jacobson, E. D. Eanes, L. A. Lembke, and R. J. Midura, "Rapidly forming apatitic mineral in an osteoblastic cell line (UMR 10601 BSP)," *Journal of Biological Chemistry*, vol. 270, no. 16, pp. 9420–9428, 1995.

[34] J. M. Gimble, *Adipose-Derived Stem Cells: Methods and Protocols*, Springer, 2011.

[35] T. E. Patterson, K. Kumagai, L. Griffith, and G. F. Muschler, "Cellular strategies for enhancement of fracture repair," *The Journal of Bone and Joint Surgery-American Volume*, vol. 90, Supplement 1, pp. 111–119, 2008.

[36] H. Castro-Malaspina, R. E. Gay, G. Resnick et al., "Characterization of human bone marrow fibroblast colony-forming cells (CFU-F) and their progeny," *Blood*, vol. 56, no. 2, pp. 289–301, 1980.

[37] C. Sanjurjo-Rodríguez, R. Castro-Viñuelas, T. Hermida-Gómez et al., "Ovine mesenchymal stromal cells: morphologic, phenotypic and functional characterization for osteochondral tissue engineering," *PLoS One*, vol. 12, no. 1, article e0171231, 2017.

[38] X. Fang, H. Murakami, S. Demura et al., "A novel method to apply osteogenic potential of adipose derived stem cells in orthopaedic surgery," *PLoS One*, vol. 9, no. 2, article e88874, 2014.

[39] A. K. Kundu and A. J. Putnam, "Vitronectin and collagen I differentially regulate osteogenesis in mesenchymal stem cells," *Biochemical and Biophysical Research Communications*, vol. 347, no. 1, pp. 347–357, 2006.

[40] A. Y. Kim, Y. Kim, S. H. Lee, Y. Yoon, W.-H. Kim, and O.-K. Kweon, "Effect of gelatin on osteogenic cell sheet formation using canine adipose-derived mesenchymal stem cells," *Cell Transplantation*, vol. 26, no. 1, pp. 115–123, 2017.

[41] Y. Kim, S. H. Lee, B. Kang, W. H. Kim, H. Yun, and O. Kweon, "Comparison of osteogenesis between adipose-derived mesenchymal stem cells and their sheets on poly-ε-caprolactone/β-tricalcium phosphate composite scaffolds in canine bone defects," *Stem Cells International*, vol. 2016, 10 pages, 2016.

[42] M. R. Khan, A. Chandrashekran, R. K. W. Smith, and J. Dudhia, "Immunophenotypic characterization of ovine mesenchymal stem cells," *Cytometry Part A*, vol. 89, no. 5, pp. 443–450, 2016.

[43] I. Kalaszczynska, S. Ruminski, A. E. Platek et al., "Substantial differences between human and ovine mesenchymal stem cells in response to osteogenic media: how to explain and how to manage?," *BioResearch Open Access*, vol. 2, no. 5, pp. 356–363, 2013.

[44] J.-S. Lee, J.-M. Lee, and G.-I. Im, "Electroporation-mediated transfer of Runx 2 and osterix genes to enhance osteogenesis of adipose stem cells," *Biomaterials*, vol. 32, no. 3, pp. 760–768, 2011.

[45] M. Barba, G. Di Taranto, and W. Lattanzi, "Adipose-derived stem cell therapies for bone regeneration," *Expert Opinion on Biological Therapy*, vol. 17, no. 6, pp. 677–689, 2017.

10

Combining PLGA Scaffold and MSCs for Brain Tissue Engineering: A Potential Tool for Treatment of Brain Injury

Ling Zhou,[1] Jiangyi Tu,[2] Guangbi Fang,[2] Li Deng,[2,3] Xiaoqing Gao ⓘ,[2,3] Kan Guo,[3] Jiming Kong,[4] Jing Lv,[3] Weikang Guan,[3] and Chaoxian Yang ⓘ [2,3]

[1]Department of Endocrinology, The Affiliated Hospital, Southwest Medical University, Taiping Street, Luzhou 646000, China
[2]Department of Anatomy, Southwest Medical University, Zhongshan Road, Luzhou 646000, China
[3]Department of Neurobiology, Preclinical Medicine Research Center, Southwest Medical University, Zhongshan Road, Luzhou 646000, China
[4]Department of Human Anatomy and Cell Science, College of Medicine, University of Manitoba, Winnipeg, MB, Canada

Correspondence should be addressed to Chaoxian Yang; lyycx@foxmail.com

Academic Editor: Andrzej Lange

Nerve tissue engineering is an important strategy for the treatment of brain injuries. Mesenchymal stem cell (MSC) transplantation has been proven to be able to promote repair and functional recovery of brain damage, and poly (lactic-co-glycolic acid) (PLGA) has also been found to have the capability of bearing cells. In the present study, to observe the ability of PLGA scaffold in supporting the adherent growth of MSCs and neurons in vivo and vitro and to assess the effects of PLGA scaffold on proliferation and neural differentiation of MSCs, this study undertakes the following steps. First, MSCs and neurons were cultured and labeled with green fluorescent protein (GFP) or otherwise identified and the PLGA scaffold was synthesized. Next, MSCs and neurons were inoculated on PLGA scaffolds and their adhesion rates were investigated and the proliferation of MSCs was evaluated by using MTT assay. After MSCs were induced by a neural induction medium, the morphological change and neural differentiation of MSCs were detected using scanning electron microscopy (SEM) and immunocytochemistry, respectively. Finally, cell migration and adhesion in the PLGA scaffold in vivo were examined by immunohistochemistry, nuclear staining, and SEM. The experimental results demonstrated that PLGA did not interfere with the proliferation and neural differentiation of MSCs and that MSCs and neuron could grow and migrate in PLGA scaffold. These data suggest that the MSC-PLGA complex may be used as tissue engineering material for brain injuries.

1. Introduction

In recent years, the development of tissue engineering has provided a new strategy for the repair of tissue injuries. The core of tissue engineering is to construct new tissue substitutes composed of biological materials and cells for promoting the recovery and maintenance of biological functions [1, 2]. Biological materials not only offer three-dimensional space for cell adhesion, growth, and migration but also form adjustable microenvironments for the nutrition obtainment and waste excretion of cells [3]. Biological materials used for neural tissue engineering can be mainly divided into 5 categories: artificial synthetic nonbiodegradable materials, nondegradable composite ducts, natural biological materials, biodegradable composites, and biodegradable polymer materials.

Poly (lactic-co-glycolic acid) (PLGA) is one biodegradable polymer material and the degradation time of PLGA can be adjusted simply by altering the ratio of lactic acid and glycolic acid in its copolymer for particular applications. PLGA with a ratio of 75:25 of PLA:PGA showed great stability in body fluids (pH 7.2) with an optimum degradation rate (9% to 12% or so), and axons could regenerate into the implanted PLGA scaffolds in rats subjected to thoracic spinal cord transection injury [4]. Mesenchymal stem cells (MSCs) could differentiate into neuron-like cells under

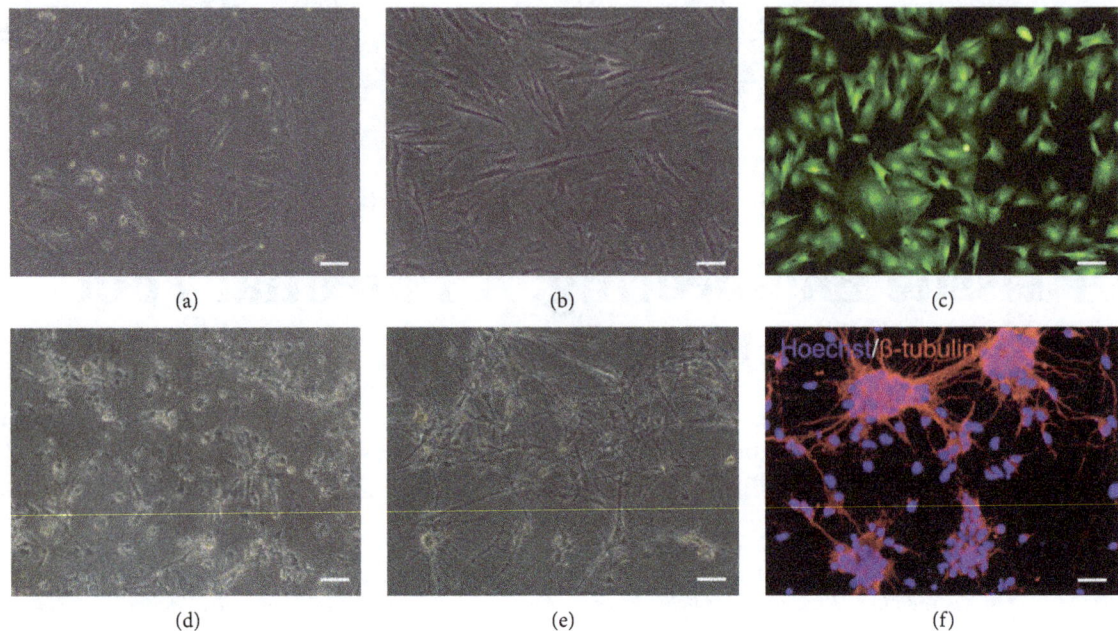

FIGURE 1: Morphologic characteristics of MSCs and neurons. (a) The primary MSCs were cultured for 4 days. (b) The 3rd-passage MSCs were cultured for 2 days. (c) The MSCs infected with adenovirus for 2 days were lighted green fluorescence. The primary neurons were cultured for (d) 3 days and (e) 7days. (f) The identification of neurons by immunostaining with β-tubulin. Bar = 50 μm.

specific culture conditions and had some electrophysiological properties of neurons [5–7], which makes them a kind of seed cells for the treatment of nerve tissue injuries. The aim of this study is to evaluate whether the MSC-PLGA scaffold complex is a potential tool for the treatment of brain injuries.

2. Materials and Methods

2.1. Preparation and Labeling of MSCs. Two-month-old adult and 1-day-old newborn Sprague Dawley (SD) rats (Animal House Center, Southwest Medical University) were used in this study. The procedure to use the animals was in accordance with the Guidance Suggestions for the Care and Use of Laboratory Animals formulated by the Ministry of Science and Technology of China. Bone marrow was obtained from femoral marrow cavities of 2-month-old rats. The MSCs were isolated and purified from bone marrow by density gradient centrifugation and adherent culture methods, and they were cultured by using alpha-minimum essential medium (α-MEM) (HyClone) supplemented with 10% FBS, 100 U/ml penicillin, and 100 mg/ml streptomycin (Gibco). When the cultured cells became confluent, they were resuspended and subcultured.

To facilitate the observation of the growth and migration of MSCs in the PLGA scaffold or a brain, MSCs were labeled with green fluorescent protein (GFP) as previously described [8]. Briefly, we amplified the previously frozen adenovirus (pAdEasy-1-pAdTrack cytomegalovirus) that contained the GFP gene. When the third passage MSCs grew to 70–80% confluence, the adenovirus solution was added, which was followed by incubation for 2 days in an incubator (37°C, 5% CO2), and MSCs showed green

fluorescence under fluorescent microscopy. Then the cells were harvested for follow-up experiments.

2.2. Preparation and Identification of Neurons. Cortical neurons were prepared from 1-day-old newborn rats as previously described [9]. Newborn rats were decapitated, and cerebral cortexes were transferred to PBS. After the removal of the meninges and blood vessels, tissues were cut into small pieces, followed by incubation in 0.25% trypsin-EDTA solution (Beyotime) at 37°C for 20 minutes. Then LG-DMEM with 20% fetal bovine serum was added to terminate the incubation. After centrifugation at 800 rpm for 10 minutes, the cells were collected for follow-up experiments.

Cortical neurons were dispersed with a neuronal medium (Sciencell) with 1% (vol/vol) neuronal growth supplement (Sciencell), and then they were seeded at a density of 5×10^5/ml onto coverslips precoated with poly-L-lysine in 6-well plates (Corning). The medium was replaced once every 3 days, and after 7 days, the cells were fixed with 4% formaldehyde and used for the identification of neurons by immunocytochemistry.

2.3. Fabrication of PLGA Scaffold. The PLGA was synthesized by the room temperature molding/particle leaching method as previous described [8]. In short, 75% lactic acid and 25% glycolic acid were dissolved in dichloromethane and blended with sieved sodium chloride particles ranging from 80 to 120 μm. The mixture was poured in molds to form discs (5 cm × 5 cm × 0.2 cm). After molding for 24 hours under pressure, the discs were taken out and immersed in deionized water to release the sodium

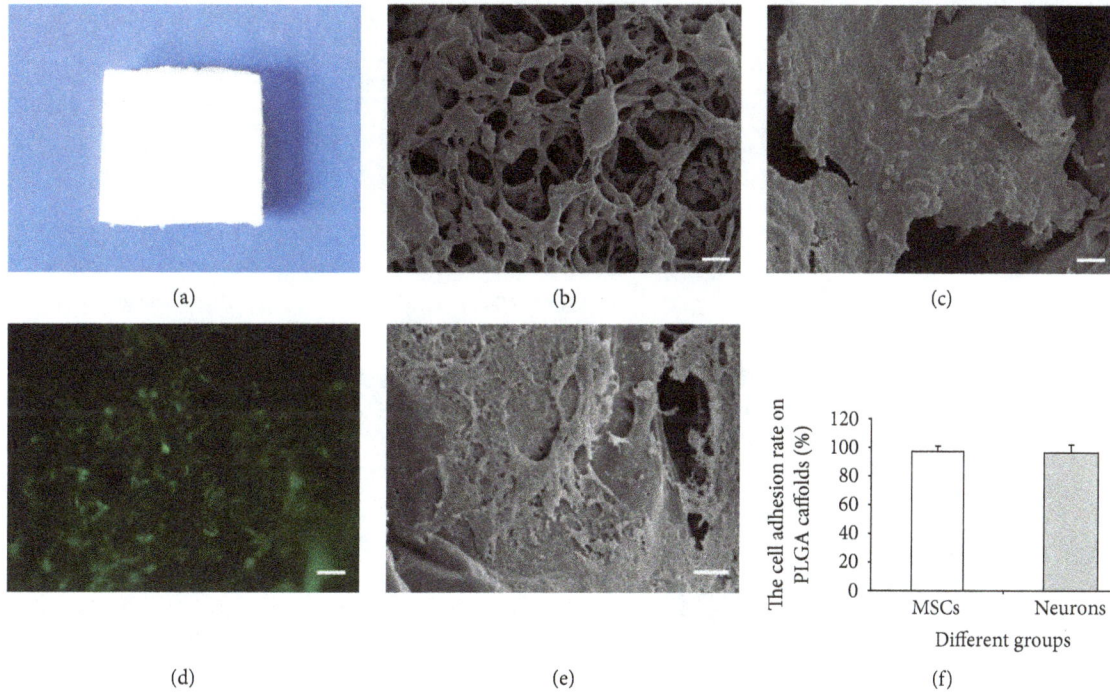

FIGURE 2: PLGA scaffold and cell adhesion. (a) PLGA scaffold. (b) SEM imaging of the PLGA scaffold. Bar = 100 μm. (c) SEM imaging of the neurons on the PLGA scaffold. Bar = 10 μm. (d) MSCs planted on the PLGA scaffold were lighted green fluorescence. Bar = 50 μm. (e) SEM imaging of MSCs on the PLGA scaffold. Bar = 10 μm. (f) The adhesion rates of MSCs and neurons on the PLGA scaffold.

chloride particles and the scaffolds were desiccated and kept in a vacuum plastic bag before use.

2.4. Cell Adhesion on PLGA Scaffold. The PLGA scaffold was cut into pieces (1 cm × 1 cm × 0.2 cm). The latter were dipped in 75% alcohol for 2 hours and then washed 3 times with sterile water and dried in clean bench; after that, the sterile PLGA scaffolds were placed in a 24-well culture plate. MSCs and neurons were seeded on the scaffolds at a density of 1×10^5 cells per scaffold in the corresponding medium under standard cell culture conditions. After 3 days, the culture mediums were removed and the cells on the scaffolds and wells were collected by trypsin digestion and counted as n_{PLGA} and n_{well}, respectively. The adhesion rates of MSCs and neurons on scaffolds were calculated as follows:

$$r = \frac{n_{PLGA}}{n_{PLGA} + n_{well}} \times 100\%. \quad (1)$$

2.5. MTT Assay. The effect of the PLGA on the proliferation of MSCs in vitro was assessed by using 3-(4,5-dimethyl-thiazol-2-yl)-2,5-diphenyl tetrazolium bromide (MTT) assay based on the instruction manual of the MTT Cell Proliferation and Cytotoxicity Assay Kit (Beyotime). Briefly, MSCs were seeded on PLGA scaffolds at a seeding concentration of 1×10^5 cells per scaffold (1 cm × 1 cm × 0.2 cm) per well of the 24-well culture plate and cultured for 48 hours. The control group was identically processed, except that the PLGA scaffolds were omitted. The culture medium was replaced with fresh medium for 24 hours. Then the MTT reaction solution was added to each well, and next, the plate was incubated for 4 hours at 37°C. After the mediums of all

wells were removed, formazan dissolving solution was added into each well and incubated at 37°C for 4 hours. The supernatants of all wells were transferred into a 96-well culture plate, and the absorbance of each well was measured at 570 nm by a microplate reader.

2.6. Neuronal Induction of MSCs. MSCs were seeded on coverslips and PLGA scaffolds in a 24-well culture plate in α-MEM supplemented with 10% FBS (HyClone). After 3 days, the medium was replaced with a preinduction solution composed of α-MEM with 10% FBS and 1 mmol/l β-mercaptoethanol (β-ME) for 24 hours. This was followed by a neuronal induction medium that consisted of α-MEM with 1 mmol/l β-ME, 2% dimethyl sulfoxide (DMSO), and 1 μmol/l all-trans retinoic acid (RA) (Sigma) for 6 hours. Five coverslips and 5 PLGA scaffolds were fixed with 4% paraformaldehyde (PFA) in phosphate-buffered saline, and the scaffolds were cut into 15 μm sections. The coverslips and sections were used to observe the effect of the PLGA scaffold on the differentiation of MSCs via immunocytochemistry. Five scaffolds were applied for transplantation and 5 scaffolds fixed with 4% glutaraldehyde were utilized for scanning electron microscopy (SEM).

2.7. PLGA Scaffold Transplantation. The traumatic brain injury (TBI) model was generated as previously described [10]. In brief, a 2-month-old rat was anesthetized with 1% pentobarbital sodium (40 mg/kg) via intraperitoneal administration and then fixed on a stereotaxic frame (Stoelting) in the prone position. Following the scalp incision, a piece of right parietal bone was removed by drilling. A dual incision

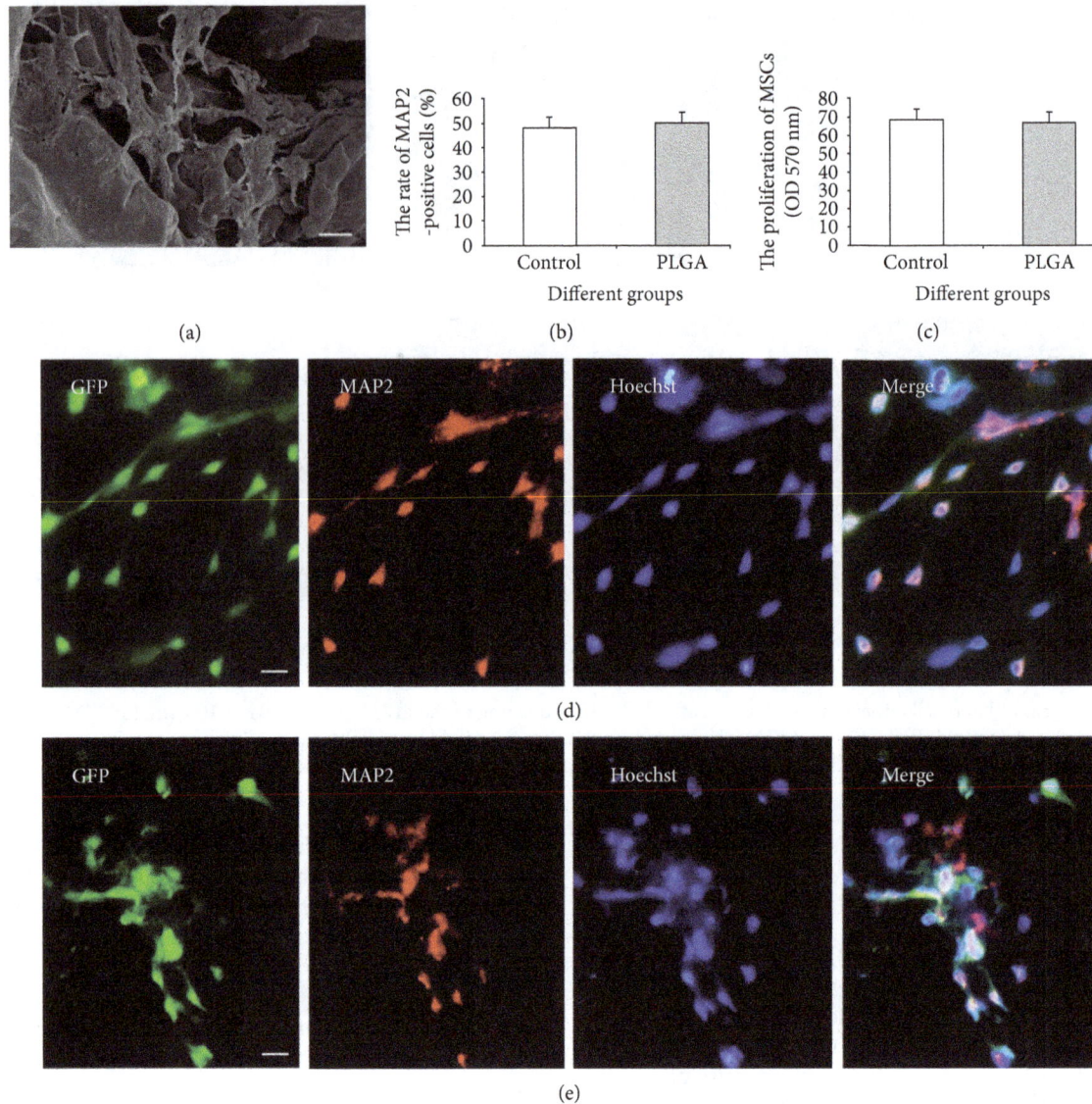

(a)   (b)   (c)

(d)

(e)

FIGURE 3: The effect of the PLGA scaffold on the differentiation and proliferation of MSCs in vitro. (a) SEM imaging of induced MSCs planted on the PLGA scaffold. Bar = 10 μm. (b) The rate of MAP2-positive cells among the MSCs after neural induction. (c) The proliferation of MSCs on the coverslip and PLGA scaffold. The control group (d) and the PLGA scaffold group (e): green fluorescence showed MSCs in vitro. Neurons (MAP2 positive) were stained with red fluorescence. Yellow fluorescence showed the colocalization of green and red, thus indicating the differentiation of MSCs. Bar =50 μm.

was made to expose the forebrain, and a defect area (3 mm × 3 mm × 2 mm) was created with a scalpel in the brain. The PLGA scaffold or MSC-PLGA scaffold complex was inserted in the brain, and the wound was sutured. On day 14 after TBI, rats (5/group) were killed by deep anesthesia and their brains were removed and then PLGA scaffolds and MSC-PLGA scaffold complex were taken for SEM. The other rats were perfused transcardially with 0.9% saline followed by ice-cold 4% PFA. The brains were taken out and postfixed in 4% PFA for 24 h. Then they were dehydrated with 30% sucrose solution, embedded in tissue-freezing medium, and cut into serial coronal sections (15 μm thickness) with a freezing microtome (Leica) for nuclear staining and immunohistochemical staining.

2.8. Scanning Electron Microscopy. Scanning electron microscopy (S-3400N, Hitachi, Japan) was used to observe the characteristics of the PLGA scaffold and the morphologies of the cells attached to it. Prior to imaging, cells that were cultured or grown on the scaffolds were fixed with 4% glutaraldehyde and dehydrated through a graded acetone series and then sputter coated with gold. Samples were examined at an accelerating voltage of 10 kV.

2.9. Immunohistochemistry. The slides of cells or frozen sections were treated with 0.3% Triton X-100 and then blocked with 8% goat serum. After being incubated with primary antibodies including β-tubulin (1 : 100 dilution, Abcam), microtubule-associated protein-2 (MAP2) (1 : 100 dilution,

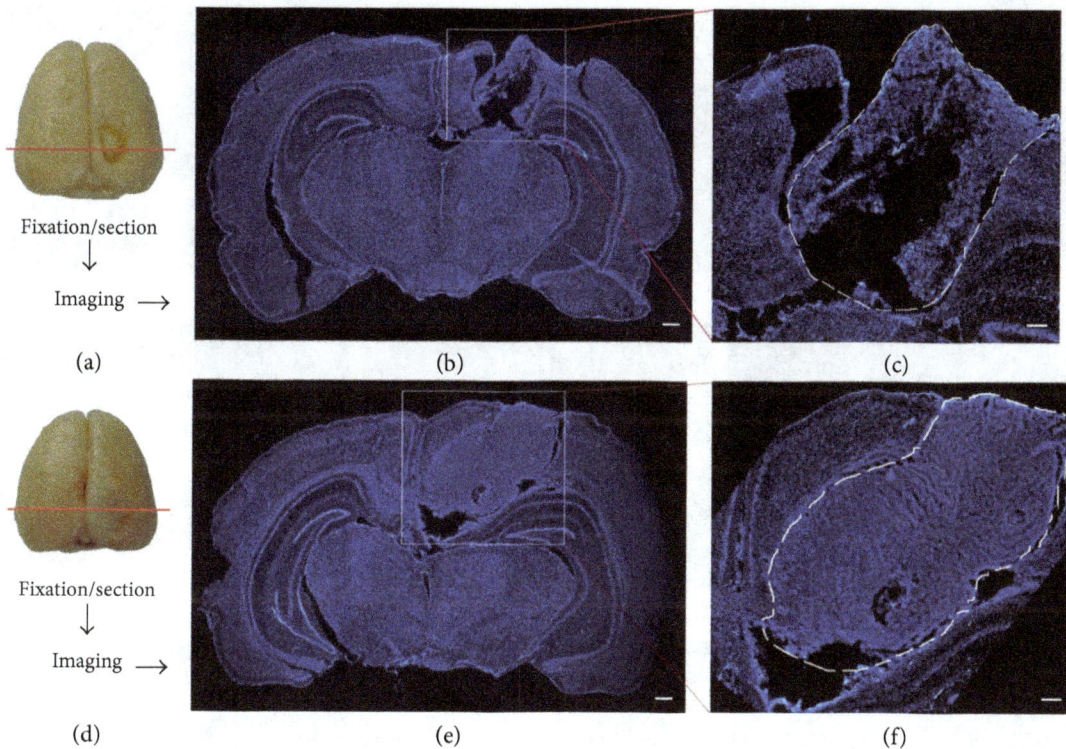

FIGURE 4: The structural change of the PLGA scaffold in brains with TBI. (a) Procedure to observe PLGA scaffold in the brain with TBI. (b) Nuclear staining shows the planted PLGA scaffold in the brain. Bar = 500 μm. (c) The magnifying picture of the square frame in (b). The PLGA scaffold in the outlined region (dashed line). Bar = 200 μm. (d) Procedure to observe the MSC-PLGA scaffold complex in the brain with TBI. (e) Nuclear staining shows the planted MSC-PLGA scaffold complex in the brain. Bar = 500 μm. (f) The magnified picture of the square frame in (e). The MSC-PLGA scaffold complex in the outlined region (dashed line). Bar = 200 μm.

Abcam), or glial fibrillary acidic protein (GFAP) (1 : 200 dilution, Sigma) overnight at 4°C, the samples were treated with anti-rabbit/mouse IgG (Alexa Fluor® 488/Fluor 594 Conjugate) (1200 dilution; Cell Signaling Technology) for 30 min at 37°C and then stained with Hoechst dye. Negative controls were identically processed, except that the primary antibodies were omitted.

2.10. Statistical Analysis. All cell experiments in vitro were repeated three times and the analyses were performed using the SPSS 18.0 software for Windows. The data are presented as the means ± standard error (SE), and the statistical comparisons were performed using one-way ANOVA. A P value < 0.05 was considered statistically significant.

3. Results

3.1. Morphologic Characteristics of Cultured Cells. The primary MSCs began to adhere within 12 hours and presented round, polygon, or spindle shapes after 3-4 days (Figure 1(a)). The 3rd passage of MSCs displayed obvious uniformity (Figure 1(b)), and they were infected by the adenovirus-lighted green fluorescence under fluorescence microscope (Figure 1(c)). The primary cortical neurons showed fewer and shorter protuberances within 3 days (Figure 1(d)). Then many neurites appeared, which formed many neural networks on the seventh day (Figure 1(e)),

and presented positive β-tubulin staining via immunocyto-chemistry (Figure 1(f)).

3.2. Attachment of MSCs and Neurons on PLGA Scaffolds. The volume of porosity of the PLGA scaffold approached 90% by using the liquid replacement approach, and the interior pores of the PLGA scaffold that were directly visualized by SEM were intercommunicated (Figures 2(a) and 2(b)). After culturing of the MSCs and neurons for 5 days, a large number of cells were found adhered and extended on the surface of the PLGA scaffold and the cells were flat and connected to each other (Figures 2(c)–2(e)). On the 3rd day after inoculation, the adhesion rates of MSCs and neurons on the PLGA scaffold were 97.4% and 96.5%, respectively, and there was no significant difference between the two groups (Figure 2(f)).

3.3. The Effect of PLGA Scaffold on Differentiation and Proliferation of MSCs In Vitro. After induction, the MSCs presented neuron-like morphology with swollen cell bodies and long thin processes, and intercellular boundaries became manifested (Figure 3(a)). The induced MSCs could express the marker of neurons (MAP2), and the rate of both MAP2$^+$ MSCs in the PLGA scaffold group was not significantly different compared with that in the control group (Figures 3(b), 3(d), and 3(e)). Furthermore, MTT assay was used to evaluate the proliferation of the MSCs cultured on the PLGA scaffold and the MSCs showed similar

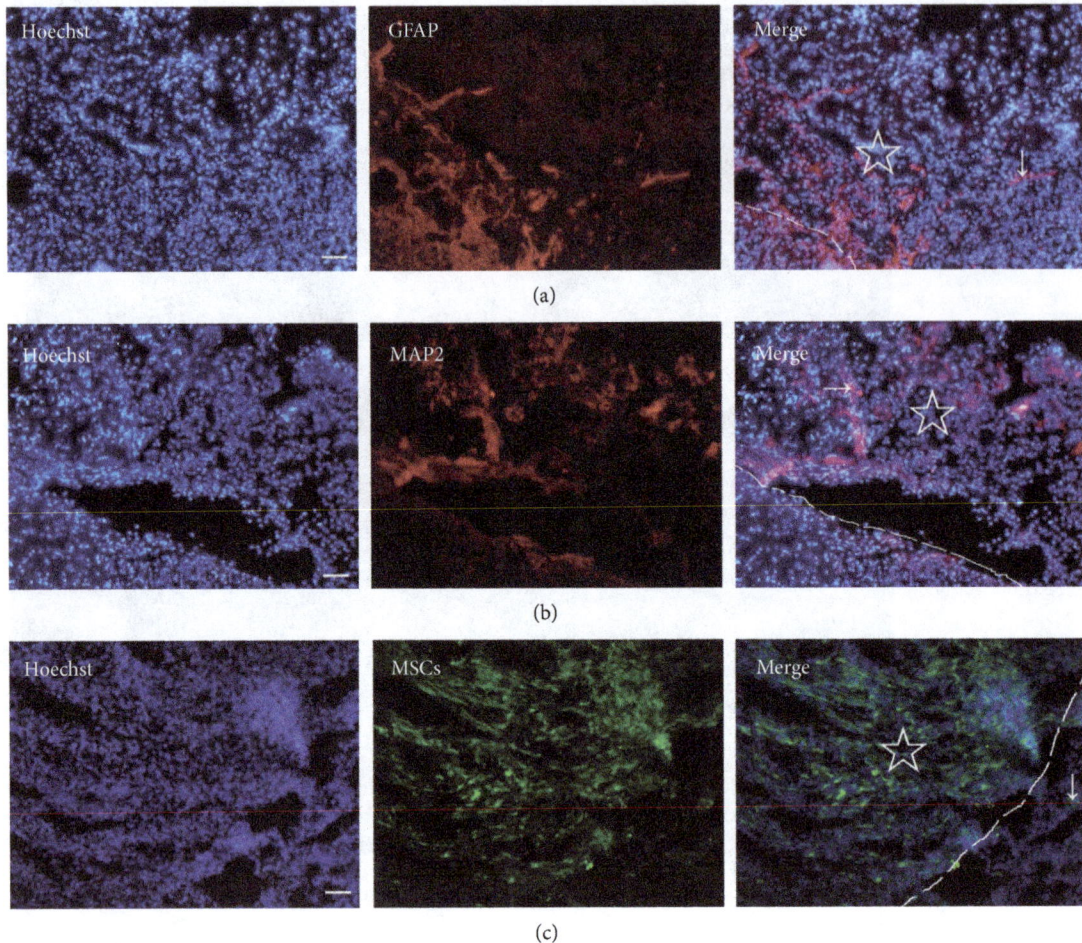

FIGURE 5: Cell migrations in the PLGA scaffold in the brain with TBI. (a) Astrocytes (arrow) stained with anti-GFAP (red) migrated in the PLGA scaffold. (b) Neurons (arrow) stained with anti-MAP2 (red) migrated in the PLGA scaffold. (c) MSCs (green, arrow) migrated out of the MSC-PLGA scaffold complex. "☆" shows the PLGA scaffold or the MSC-PLGA scaffold complex in the brain, and the dashed line indicates the boundary of the scaffold. Bar = 50 μm.

absorbance in the PLGA and control groups after incubation for 7 days ($P < 0.05$) (Figure 3(c)). These results suggest that the PLGA scaffold did not interfere with the proliferation and neuronal differentiation of MSCs in vitro.

3.4. The Structure of PLGA In Vivo. The structure of the PLGA in brains was assessed by morphological observation with nuclear staining at 14 days after TBI. Under a microscope, the tissue organization of the transplanted PLGA scaffold was distinctive between the PLGA scaffold group (Figures 4(a)–4(c)) and the MSC-PLGA scaffold group (Figures 4(d)–4(f)). In the former, the tissue structure was looser and the interstitial space was larger, while a more compact structure and smaller spaces could be observed in the latter.

3.5. Cell Migration and Adhesion in PLGA Scaffold In Vivo. After the transplantation of the PLGA scaffold into the brain at 14 days after TBI, some cells migrated into the PLGA, including glial cells (Figure 5(a)) and neurons (Figure 5(b)). When the MSC-PLGA scaffold complex was implanted in

the brain, the MSCs could migrate out to the adjacent brain area (Figure 5(c)). In addition, we found that cells could adhere better on the MSC-PLGA scaffold complex than the PLGA scaffold (Figures 6(a) and 6(b)). The results suggest that the PLGA-mixed MSCs are more beneficial to cell adhesion and migration, and thus, the combination of the brain tissue and scaffold is closer.

4. Discussion

Compatibility between the biomaterial scaffold and seed cells is a core issue to construct engineered tissues and organs. The biomaterial scaffold as the cell carrier and exogenous graft should have a positive effect or no palpable side effect on cell growth and differentiation, and it should be accompanied by good biocompatibility and easy degradation in vivo after implantation [11, 12]. PLGA has been served as a drug carrier because of its biocompatibility and biodegradation [13, 14]. Seed cells derived from autologous tissue used to construct engineered tissue are the preferable choice. MSCs have received extensive attention because they can be obtained

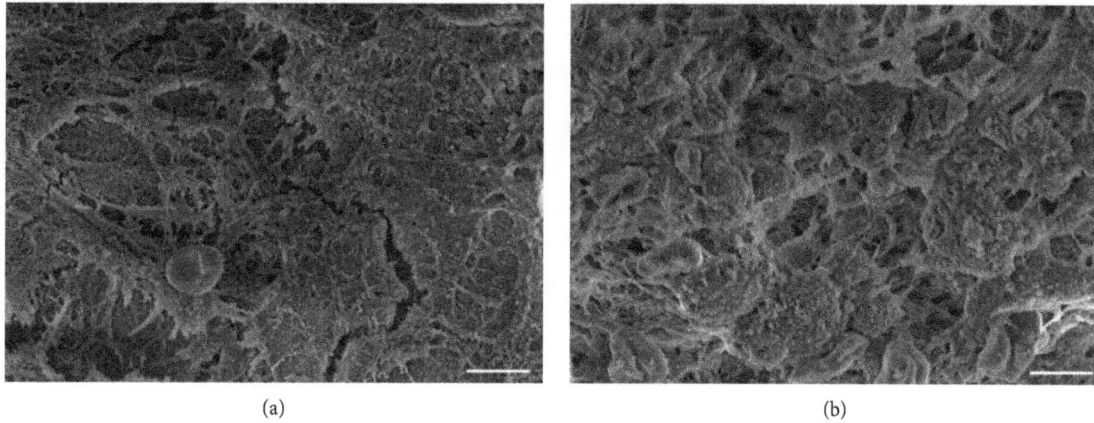

(a)

(b)

FIGURE 6: Cells' adhesion on the PLGA scaffold in the brain with TBI. (a) SEM imaging of cells' adhesion on the PLGA scaffold. (b) SEM imaging of cells' adhesion on the MSC-PLGA scaffold complex. Bar = 5 μm.

from autologous tissue and they were easily isolated, expanded in vitro, and further induced to differentiate into neuronal cells, adipocytes, osteoblasts, myocytes, and other cell types [15–18]. In this study, we found that PLGA did not interfere with the proliferation and neural differentiation of MSCs.

Cell adhesion and migration properties will influence the proliferation, differentiation, and function of cells [19, 20]. To achieve the function of the cell scaffold, the cell carrier should ensure good adhesion, growth, and reproduction of seed cells and host cells. In the present work, the advantages show that PLGA scaffolds are capable of supporting 3D growth for MSCs and neurons in vivo and in vitro and neural-induced MSCs can still adhere to the PLGA scaffold. Previous studies have shown that MSCs can secrete various extracellular matrixes, neurotrophic factors, and cell adhesion factors [21, 22] and the transplantation of MSCs can promote the repair of central nervous system injuries [23, 24]. We found that the transplantation of the MSC-PLGA complex made the impaired brain more complete than that of the simple PLGA scaffold. In summary, our results suggested that MSC-PLGA may be used as suitable graft for nerve tissue engineering, but its biological properties in vivo merit further study.

Authors' Contributions

Ling Zhou and Jiangyi Tu contributed equally to the article.

Acknowledgments

This work is supported by Research Project of Science Foundation of Sichuan Province Educational Commission of China (18ZA0516) and the joint research project of the Department of Science and Technology of Sichuan Province and Luzhou Municipal People's Government and Luzhou Medical College (14JC0140). The authors thank Yansheng Liao for the suggestion on experimental methods.

References

[1] E. Avolio, V. V. Alvino, M. T. Ghorbel, and P. Campagnolo, "Perivascular cells and tissue engineering: current applications and untapped potential," *Pharmacology & Therapeutics*, vol. 171, no. 171, pp. 83–92, 2017.

[2] R. Kurimoto, K. Kanie, K. Uto et al., "Combinational effects of polymer viscoelasticity and immobilized peptides on cell adhesion to cell-selective scaffolds," *Analytical Sciences*, vol. 32, no. 11, pp. 1195–1202, 2016.

[3] A. Haider, K. C. Gupta, and I. K. Kang, "Morphological effects of HA on the cell compatibility of electrospun HA/PLGA composite nanofiber scaffolds," *BioMed Research International*, vol. 2014, Article ID 308306, 11 pages, 2014.

[4] B. K. Chen, A. M. Knight, G. C. W. de Ruiter et al., "Axon regeneration through scaffold into distal spinal cord after transection," *Journal of Neurotrauma*, vol. 26, no. 10, pp. 1759–1771, 2009.

[5] J. L. Munoz, S. J. Greco, S. A. Patel et al., "Feline bone marrow-derived mesenchymal stromal cells (MSCs) show similar phenotype and functions with regards to neuronal differentiation as human MSCs," *Differentiation*, vol. 84, no. 2, pp. 214–222, 2012.

[6] Y. Zeng, M. Rong, Y. Liu et al., "Electrophysiological characterisation of human umbilical cord blood-derived mesenchymal stem cells induced by olfactory ensheathing cell-conditioned medium," *Neurochemical Research*, vol. 38, no. 12, pp. 2483–2489, 2013.

[7] K. J. Cho, K. A. Trzaska, S. J. Greco et al., "Neurons derived from human mesenchymal stem cells show synaptic transmission and can be induced to produce the neurotransmitter substance P by interleukin-1α," *Stem Cells*, vol. 23, no. 3, pp. 383–391, 2005.

[8] Y. S. Liao, L. Deng, X. Q. Gao, and C. X. Yang, "Three-dimensional culture and neural differentiation of bone marrow mesenchymal stem cells on PLGA scaffolds," in *Proceedings of the 2015 International Conference (2015 International Conference on Medicine and Biopharmaceutical), vol. 15-16, pp. 54–62, Guangzhou, China, 2015.

[9] C. Yang, L. Zhou, X. Gao et al., "Neuroprotective effects of bone marrow stem cells overexpressing glial cell line-derived

neurotrophic factor on rats with intracerebral hemorrhage and neurons exposed to hypoxia/reoxygenation," *Neurosurgery*, vol. 68, no. 3, pp. 691–704, 2011.

[10] W. Shi, C. J. Huang, X. D. Xu et al., "Transplantation of RADA16-BDNF peptide scaffold with human umbilical cord mesenchymal stem cells forced with CXCR4 and activated astrocytes for repair of traumatic brain injury," *Acta Biomater*, vol. 45, pp. 247–261, 2016.

[11] R. J. O'Keefe and J. Mao, "Bone tissue engineering and regeneration: from discovery to the clinic—an overview," *Tissue Engineering Part B: Reviews*, vol. 17, no. 6, pp. 389–392, 2011.

[12] X. Miao, D. M. Tan, J. Li, Y. Xiao, and R. Crawford, "Mechanical and biological properties of hydroxyapatite/tricalcium phosphate scaffolds coated with poly (lactic-co-glycolic acid)," *Acta Biomaterialia*, vol. 4, no. 3, pp. 638–645, 2008.

[13] B.-S. Lee, C.-C. Lee, Y.-P. Wang et al., "Controlled-release of tetracycline and lovastatin by poly(D,L-lactide-co-glycolide acid)-chitosan nanoparticles enhances periodontal regeneration in dogs," *International Journal of Nanomedicine*, vol. 11, pp. 285–297, 2016.

[14] C. Fornaguera, A. Dols-Perez, G. Calderó, M. J. García-Celma, J. Camarasa, and C. Solans, "PLGA nanoparticles prepared by nano-emulsion templating using low-energy methods as efficient nanocarriers for drug delivery across the blood-brain barrier," *Journal of Controlled Release*, vol. 211, pp. 134–143, 2015.

[15] R. Shokohi, M. Nabiuni, S. Irian, and J. A. Miyan, "In vitro effects of wistar rat prenatal and postnatal cerebrospinal fluid on neural differentiation and proliferation of mesenchymal stromal cells derived from bone marrow," *Cell Journal*, vol. 19, no. 4, pp. 537–544, 2018.

[16] J. Stachecka, A. Walczak, B. Kociucka, B. Ruszczycki, G. Wilczyński, and I. Szczerbal, "Nuclear organization during in vitro differentiation of porcine mesenchymal stem cells (MSCs) into adipocytes," *Histochemistry and Cell Biology*, vol. 149, no. 2, pp. 113–126, 2018.

[17] A. Nemoto, N. Chosa, S. Kyakumoto et al., "Water-soluble factors eluated from surface pre-reacted glass-ionomer filler promote osteoblastic differentiation of human mesenchymal stem cells," *Molecular Medicine Reports*, vol. 17, no. 3, pp. 3448–3454, 2018.

[18] S. Khajeniazi, M. Solati, Y. Yazdani, M. Soleimani, and A. Kianmehr, "Synergistic induction of cardiomyocyte differentiation from human bone marrow mesenchymal stem cells by interleukin 1β and 5-azacytidine," *Biological Chemistry*, vol. 397, no. 12, pp. 1355–1364, 2016.

[19] K. Anselme, "Osteoblast adhesion on biomaterials," *Biomaterials*, vol. 21, no. 7, pp. 667–681, 2000.

[20] N. Zhang and D. H. Kohn, "Using polymeric materials to control stem cell behavior for tissue regeneration," *Birth Defects Research, Part C Embryo Today*, vol. 96, no. 1, pp. 63–81, 2012.

[21] U. T. Arasu, R. Kärnä, K. Härkönen et al., "Human mesenchymal stem cells secrete hyaluronan-coated extracellular vesicles," *Matrix Biology*, vol. 64, pp. 54–68, 2017.

[22] L. Junyi, L. Na, and J. Yan, "Mesenchymal stem cells secrete brain-derived neurotrophic factor and promote retinal ganglion cell survival after traumatic optic neuropathy," *The Journal of Craniofacial Surgery*, vol. 26, no. 2, pp. 548–552, 2015.

[23] J. Qu and H. Zhang, "Roles of mesenchymal stem cells in spinal cord injury," *Stem Cells International*, vol. 2017, Article ID 5251313, 12 pages, 2017.

[24] D. Chen, W. Fu, W. Zhuang, C. Lv, F. Li, and X. Wang, "Therapeutic effects of intranigral transplantation of mesenchymal stem cells in rat models of Parkinson's disease," *Journal of Neuroscience Research*, vol. 95, no. 3, pp. 907–917, 2017.

11

The Myc/Max/Mxd Network is a Target of Mutated Flt3 Signaling in Hematopoietic Stem Cells in Flt3-ITD-Induced Myeloproliferative Disease

Farhan Basit,[1,2] **Maria Andersson,**[1] **and Anne Hultquist** ⓘ[1]

[1]*Hematopoietic Stem Cell Laboratory, Lund Stem Cell Center, Lund University, Klinikgatan 26, 221 84 Lund, Sweden*
[2]*Department of Tumor Immunology, Radboud Institute for Molecular Life Sciences, Radboudumc, Nijmegen, Netherlands*

Correspondence should be addressed to Anne Hultquist; anne.hultquist@med.lu.se

Academic Editor: Roberta Fusco

Acute myeloid leukemia (AML) has poor prognosis due to various mutations, e.g., in the FLT3 gene. Therefore, it is important to identify pathways regulated by the activated Flt3 receptor for the discovery of new therapeutic targets. The Myc network of oncogenes and tumor suppressor genes is involved in mechanisms regulating proliferation and survival of cells, including that of the hematopoietic system. In this study, we evaluated the expression of the *Myc* oncogenes and *Mxd* antagonists in hematopoietic stem cell and myeloid progenitor populations in the Flt3-ITD-knockin myeloproliferative mouse model. Our data shows that the expression of Myc network genes is changed in Flt3-ITD mice compared with the wild type. *Mycn* is increased in multipotent progenitors and in the pre-GM compartment of myeloid progenitors in the ITD mice while the expression of several genes in the tumor suppressor *Mxd* family, including *Mxd1*, *Mxd2*, and *Mxd4*, is concomitantly downregulated, as well as the expression of the Mxd-related gene *Mnt* and the transcriptional activator *Miz-1*. LSKCD150⁺CD48⁻ hematopoietic long-term stem cells are decreased in the Flt3-ITD cells while multipotent progenitors are increased. Of note, PKC412-mediated inhibition of Flt3-ITD signaling results in downregulation of *cMyc* and upregulation of the Myc antagonists *Mxd1*, *Mxd2*, and *Mxd4*. Our data provides new mechanistic insights into downstream alterations upon aberrant Flt3 signaling and rationale for combination therapies for tyrosine kinase inhibitors with Myc antagonists in treating AML.

1. Introduction

Acute myeloid leukemia (AML), despite aggressive treatment regimes, has a poor prognosis, and cure is difficult to attain. Mutations in the tyrosine kinase receptor Flt3, including internal tandem duplication (ITD) mutations and tyrosine kinase domain (TKD) mutations, are the most common changes in AML, which constitutively activate the Flt3 receptor [1]. Flt3 regulates growth and survival of myeloid progenitor cells; therefore, mutations in *FLT3* effectively abrogate growth-regulating controls [2]. Interestingly, mutations in *FLT3* are correlated with shorter progression-free survival and overall survival [3, 4].

Treatment strategies aimed at inhibiting the activated Flt3-ITD receptor have been evaluated in clinical trials; however, the use of Flt3-ITD inhibitors as single agents resulted in poor clinical outcome due to emergence of drug-resistant cells [5]. This underscores the need to develop combination treatment strategies [6]. Therefore, it is important to identify pathways regulated by the activated Flt3 receptor for the development of new treatment targets. Several pathways have been implicated downstream of the mutated Flt3 receptor in leukemias, including the Wnt pathway and the JAK/STAT pathway [7, 8].

Interestingly, the *MYC* oncogenes have been implicated downstream of Flt3-ITD signaling [9]. The *MYC* family genes, including *MYC*, *MYCN*, and *MYCL1*, are proto-oncogenes and known to be overexpressed or mutated in a plethora of different tumors, including that of the hematopoietic system [10, 11]. The MYC proteins function as transcription factors and bind to specific E-box DNA sequences, in promoters of target genes by heterodimerizing with their partner MAX [12]. However, Myc also regulates genes independent of DNA binding via Miz-1 protein [13]. Intriguingly, bone marrow-specific overexpression of Mycn results in rapid development of acute myeloid leukemia [14]. Furthermore, Myc has also been shown to induce myeloid myeloproliferative disease, even though mutations in myeloid neoplasias are not common [15]. The Mxd family of proteins also heterodimerizes with Max and binds to the common E-box sequences and generally works in an antagonistic way towards Myc [12].

Importantly, several reports have implicated Myc as a downstream target of Flt3-ITD signaling. To this end, it was shown that Flt3-ITD regulates cMyc via Wnt signaling [8]. Additionally, Flt3-ITD inhibits Foxo3a [16], which in turn suppresses the Myc antagonist Mxi-1 (Mxd2) to increase Myc activity [17]. Interestingly, studies of Myc function in hematopoietic stem cells have implicated Myc in pushing the HSCs out of the niche and into a proliferative progenitor state [18]. Given that both Flt3 and Myc regulate HSCs' self-renewal and differentiation, evaluating the interplay between Flt3-ITD signaling and Myc molecules may represent therapeutic targets for AML therapy.

In this study, we investigated the Myc network genes in different subpopulations in the bone marrow, including myeloid progenitors and stem cell populations, in the Flt3-ITD myeloproliferative mouse model [19]. Here, we report that the expression of the Myc network genes is changed in the Flt3-ITD mouse model, mainly with upregulation of the *Myc* genes and concomitant downregulation of the Myc antagonists, the *Mxd* genes, in different hematopoietic stem and progenitor cell subpopulations, as well as downregulation of the Mxd-related gene *Mnt* and the transcriptional activator *Miz-1*. Moreover, PKC412-mediated inhibition of Flt3-ITD signaling results in downregulation of *c-Myc* and upregulation of the Myc antagonists *Mxd1*, *Mxd2/Mxi1*, and *Mxd4*.

2. Materials and Methods

2.1. Cell Culture and PKC412 Inhibitor. MV4-11 cells were cultured in IMDM medium (Sigma-Aldrich) supplemented with 20% FCS, 1% L-glutamine, and 1% penicillin/streptomycin. Cells were constantly maintained at 37°C in 5% CO_2. The Flt3-ITD phosphokinase inhibitor was added to cell cultures of MV4-11 cells in 2 different concentrations for 15 minutes before the cells were harvested for mRNA extraction (0.1 mM and 1 mM) (LC Laboratories, Woburn, MA, USA).

2.2. Mice. Flt3-ITD-knockin mice on C57BL/6 background were previously described [19]. WT (Flt3$^{+/+}$) C57BL/6 littermate mice were used as WT controls. All experiments were approved by the Ethical Committee at Lund University.

2.3. Fluorescent Antibodies and Immunomagnetic Beads Used for FACS Analysis and Sorting. Antibodies used for cell surface staining were as follows: CD11b/Mac1 (M1/70), CD4

(H129.19), CD8a (53–6.7), B220/CD45 (RA3–6B2), CD5 (Ly1), Ter119 (Ter-1119), Gr1/Ly6G and Ly6C (RB6–8C5), CD19 (ID3), CD41/Itga2b (MWReg30), and CD135/Flt3 (A2F10.1) (104) (BD Biosciences Pharmingen) and NK1.1 (PK136), Sca1 (D7), CD117/c-Kit (2B8), CD16/32 (93), and CD105/Eng (MJ7/18) (eBioscience). Biotinylated antibodies were visualized with streptavidin-QD655 (Invitrogen) or streptavidin-tricolor (Invitrogen), and purified lineage antibodies were visualized with polyclonal goat anti-rat tricolor (Invitrogen) or polyclonal goat anti-rat-QD605 (Invitrogen). MACS column enrichment of c-Kit$^+$ cells was done using anti-CD117 immunomagnetic beads (Miltenyi Biotec) as previously described [20].

2.4. Flow Cytometric Analysis. Hematopoietic stem and progenitor cells were analyzed as previously described. [21–23]. Briefly, bone marrow (BM) cells were stained with a cocktail of purified rat antibodies against lineage markers B220, CD4, CD5, CD8α, CD11b, Gr1, and Ter119. Lineage$^+$ cells were visualized with a goat anti-rat-QD605 staining, followed by c-Kit enrichment for sorting analyses. Thereafter, hematopoietic stem/progenitor cells were defined as Lin$^-$Sca1$^+$c-Kit$^+$ (LSK) cells, pre-granulocyte-monocyte progenitors (pre-GMPs: Lin$^-$c$^-$Kit$^+$Sca1$^-$ [LSK$^-$] CD41$^-$CD16/32$^{low/-}$CD150$^-$CD105$^{low/-}$), granulocyte-monocyte progenitors (GMPs: LKS$^-$CD16/32^{hi}CD150$^-$), and multipotent progenitors (MPPs: Lin$^-$Sca1$^+$ c-Kit$^+$CD150$^-$CD105$^{low/-}$). Propidium iodide (Invitrogen) was used to exclude dead cells. Cell acquisition and analysis were performed on a 4-laser LSRII (BD Biosciences) using FlowJo version 8.8 software (TreeStar). Cell sorting was done on a FACSAria (BD Biosciences).

2.5. Quantitative Real-Time PCR. For analyzing gene expression in myeloid progenitors (pre-GM, GMPs) as well as in hematopoietic stem cells and multipotent progenitors (MPPs), cells from these populations were FACSAria-sorted directly into 75 μl of buffer RLT and frozen at −80°C. Total RNA extraction and DNase treatment were performed with the RNeasy Micro kit (Qiagen Inc., California) according to the manufacturer's instructions for samples containing ≤10^5 cells. Eluted RNA samples were reverse-transcribed using the SuperScript II Reverse Transcriptase Kit including random hexamers (Invitrogen) according to the protocol supplied by the manufacturer. For gene expression in LT-HSCs as well as in MPPs using the Slam marker staining (including CD150 and CD48), the CelluLyser™ protocol (TaTaa, Gothenburg, Sweden) was used according to the manufacturer's protocol. Shortly, cells were FACSAria-sorted into 5.5 ∝l lysis buffer where RNA was directly reverse-transcribed using the Transcriptor First-Strand cDNA synthesis kit (Roche). Q-PCR reactions with the diluted cDNA samples were analyzed with TaqMan gene expression assays (ABI, USA) according to the manufacturer's protocol. TaqMan Assays-on-Demand probes used are described in the Supplemental Experimental Procedures. All experiments were performed in triplicate and from at least two different sorts, and differences in cDNA input were compensated by normalizing against β-actin or

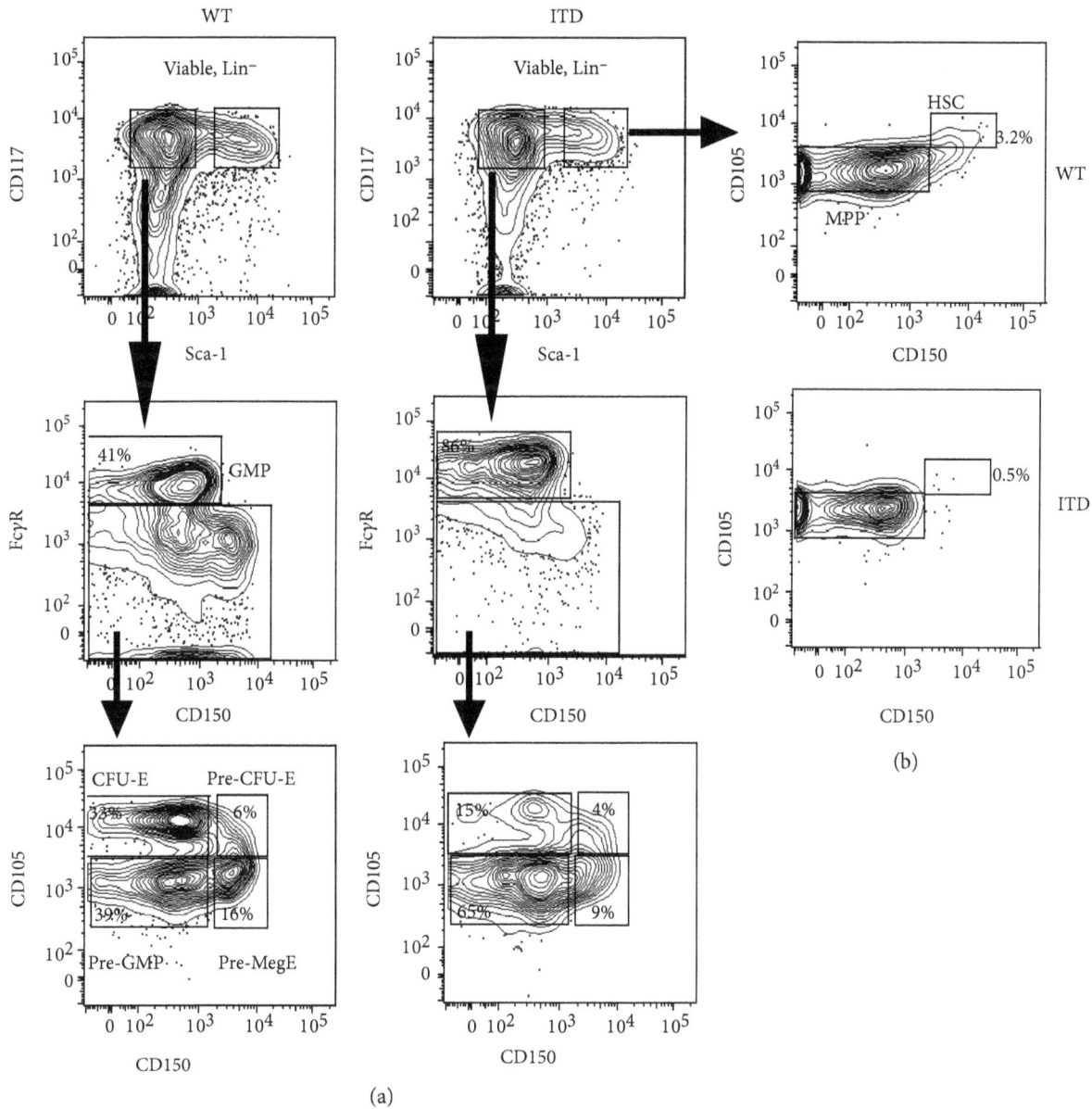

FIGURE 1: Myeloid progenitor and hematopoietic stem cell populations are changed in Flt3-ITD mice. Analysis of hematopoietic stem cell (HSC) and multipotent progenitor (MPP) subpopulations within the Lin⁻Sca-1⁺Kit⁺ (LSK) population, as well as myeloid progenitors including pre-GM and granulocytic myeloid progenitors (GMPs), in the bone marrow of Flt3-ITD and wild-type (WT) mice, was performed using a staining procedure including endoglin and the SLAM receptor CD150.

HPRT expression levels. The fold induction ratio was calculated by the Pfaffl equation:

$$\text{ratio} = \frac{(E_{\text{target}})\Delta Ct \, \text{target(control} - \text{sample})}{(E_{\text{ref}})\Delta Ct \, \text{ref(control} - \text{sample})}. \quad (1)$$

Statistical analysis was performed with two-tailed unpaired Student's t-test on log-converted values ($^*p < 0.05$, $^{**}p < 0.01$).

3. Results

3.1. Myeloid Progenitor and Hematopoietic Stem Cell Populations Are Changed in Flt3-ITD Mice. To evaluate the gene expression of the *MYC* network genes in the bone marrow of Flt3-ITD mice

compared with wild-type (WT) mice, hematopoietic stem cell and myeloid progenitor (MPP) subpopulations were identified by staining for surface markers, analyzed by fluorescence-activated cell sorting (FACS), and subsequently sorted. Initially, myeloid progenitors including pre-GM and granulocytic myeloid progenitors (GMPs), as well as Lin⁻Sca-1⁺Kit⁺ (LSK) cells, within which hematopoietic stem cells reside, were sorted using a staining procedure including endoglin and the SLAM receptor CD150, as described previously [23].

The Flt3-ITD mouse has a myeloproliferative disease with expanded myeloid populations [19]. Consistently, we observed that myeloid progenitors (MPs/LK; Lin⁻Sca-1⁻Kit⁺ cells) in Flt3-ITD mice are increased to 69.5% in comparison with 54.9% MPs in WT mice (Figure 1(a)). Moreover, we

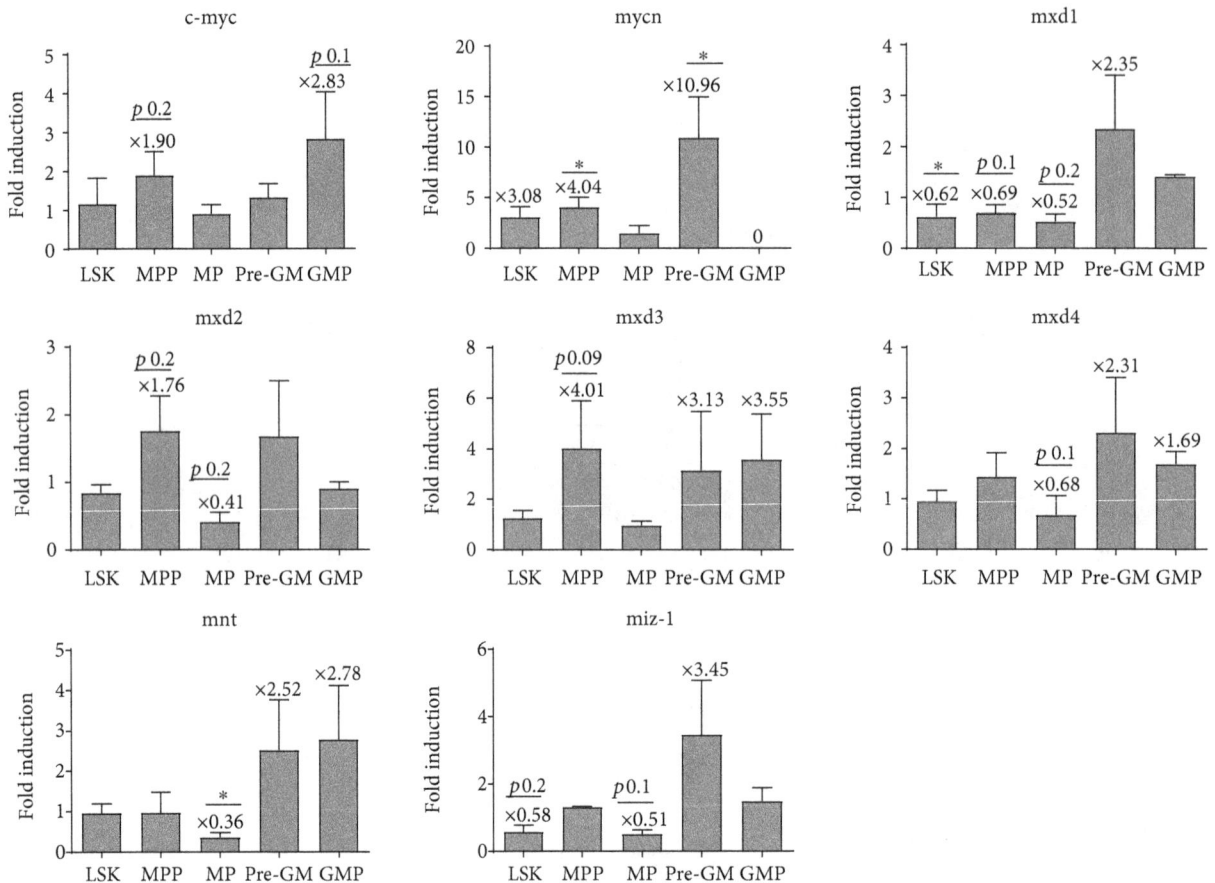

FIGURE 2: Myeloid and multipotent progenitors have altered Myc network genes in Flt3-ITD mice. The expression of Myc network genes was carried out with reverse transcription quantitative PCR (RT-Q-PCR) in sorted subpopulations of murine hematopoietic stem and progenitor cells. Fold induction was calculated as a ratio of Flt3-ITD : WT samples. Statistical analysis was performed with Student's t-test on log-converted values ($^*p < 0.05$). Significance was shown in many of the described altered expression levels; however, some changes showed low p values but did not quite reach statistically significance due to variances in the expression levels.

observed that the relative distribution of subpopulations within the MP compartment was altered as well. Importantly, progenitors of the granulocytic/monocytic pathway (pre-GM and GMPs) were increased in Flt3-ITD mice in comparison to WT mice, as we observed that pre-GMs were increased from 39% in WT to 65% in Flt3-ITD mice and GMPs were increased from 41% in WT to 86% in ITD mice (Figure 1(a)). Consistent with our previous data [24], the progenitors of the megakaryocytic and erythroid pathway were diminished (Figure 1(a)). The expression of Flt3 is altered or diminished due to the ITD mutation; therefore, staining to identify HSC subpopulations by utilizing the expression of the Flt3 receptor is not feasible. Here, we identified long-term (LT-) HSCs as CD150$^+$CD105$^+$ utilizing CD150 and endoglin (CD105), while MPPs were identified as CD150$^-$/CD105$^+$. Intriguingly, we observed a decrease in LT-HSCs in favor of MPPs in the ITD mice (Figure 1(b)). Collectively, the above data set indicates that ITD mutation in Flt3 results in the expansion of the pre-GM, GMP, and MPP compartments.

3.2. Myeloid and Multipotent Progenitors Have Altered Myc Network Genes in Flt3-ITD Mice. Next, we evaluated the expression of the Myc network genes including cMyc and

Mycn, as well as the Mxd family of Myc antagonists (Mxd1, Mxd2/Mxi1, Mxd3, and Mxd4), in stem and progenitor subpopulations in mice with the Flt3-ITD mutation and littermate WT controls by quantitative real-time PCR (Q-RT-PCR) (Figure 2). The mRNA of the cMyc gene was increased in Flt3-ITD MPPs (1.9-fold induction), as well as in Flt3-ITD GMPs (2.83-fold induction). Of note, the Mycn expression was increased in all the populations investigated in Flt3-ITD mice, except for GMPs where the expression of Mycn was turned off. Mycn was most prominently upregulated in MPPs and pre-GM cells (4.04- and 10.96-fold induction, respectively). Furthermore, analysis of the expression of the Myc antagonists, the Mad family genes, showed downregulation of Mxd1 in LSK cells (0.62-fold reduction), MPPs (0.69-fold reduction), and MPs (0.52-fold reduction). Mxd2/Mxi1 was downregulated in LSK (0.77-fold reduction) and MP (0.41-fold reduction) cells and Mxd4 in MPs (0.68-fold reduction). Additionally, Mxd2/Mxi1 and Mxd3 were upregulated in MPPs. The MNT gene, an MXD family-related gene, which is coexpressed with Myc in proliferating cells and functions as a repressor of Myc target genes [25] was downregulated (0.36-fold reduction) in myeloid progenitors (MPs) in Flt3-ITD mice. Similarly, the MIZ-1 gene, a

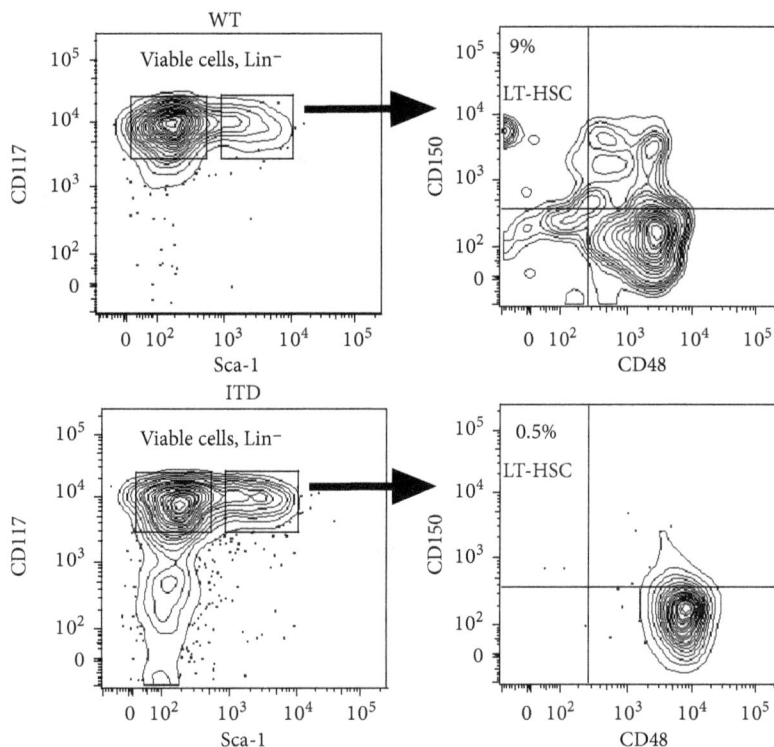

FIGURE 3: Flt3-ITD mice have altered frequencies of hematopoietic stem and progenitor cells. Next, we subdivided the hematopoietic stem cell compartment into long-term HSCs (LT-HSCs) and MPPs, utilizing the SLAM receptor staining with CD150 and CD48, and cells were sorted by flow cytometry for subsequent gene expression analysis.

transcriptional activator which is involved in upregulating growth-repressing genes such as p21, was downregulated in LSK cells (0.58-fold reduction) and MPs (0.51-fold reduction). *Max*, the Myc- and Mxd-interacting partner, was significantly increased in MPPs (1.75-fold induction) and significantly decreased in MPs (0.48-fold reduction) (data not shown). Collectively, these data indicate that the ITD mutation in Flt3 results in the alteration of Myc network genes.

3.3. Hematopoietic Stem Cells in Flt3-ITD Mice Have Altered Myc Network Expression. Next, we subdivided the hematopoietic stem cell compartment into long-term HSCs (LT-HSCs) and MPPs, utilizing the SLAM receptor staining with CD150 and CD48 [22], and cells were sorted by flow cytometry for subsequent gene expression analysis. Of note, the LT-HSCs (LSKCD150$^+$CD48$^-$) were decreased in the Flt3-ITD cells, as described previously [26], and the MPPs were increased. Intriguingly, MPPs expressed higher levels of CD48 (Figure 3).

Expression of the *Myc* network genes was evaluated in LSK, LT-HSC (CD150$^+$CD48$^-$), MPP (CD150$^-$CD48$^+$), and MP cells. Intriguingly, the expression of the *cMyc* gene did not change in LSK, LT-HSC, MPP, and MP cells as identified in the SLAM receptor-based staining in contrast to the staining including the endoglin marker (Figures 4 and 1). Conversely, the *Mycn* mRNA was increased in MPP cells (2.98-fold induction) (Figure 4), comparative with the results from the analysis in the endoglin/CD150 staining

protocol (Figure 2). However, the results in this staining did not quite reach significant values due to variations. Importantly, *Mxd1* showed a significant decrease in expression in LT-HSCs (0.63-fold reduction), as well as in MPPs (0.62-fold reduction) and the LSK compartment (0.64-fold reduction), which, however, did not reach significant levels (Figure 4). Of note, *Mxd2/Mxi1* and *Mxd4* were significantly decreased in the LSK compartment; however, their expression did not change in LT-HSCs, MPPs, and MPs. Conversely, *Mxd3* did not change significantly in any of the subpopulations (Figure 4).

3.4. Small Molecule Inhibitor, PKC412, Modulates the Expression of Myc Network Genes in Human MV4-11 Cells. PKC412 is an inhibitor of FLT3 autophosphorylation, thereby inhibiting downstream signaling [27]. It has shown to inhibit growth of primary Flt3-ITD mutant blasts [28]. To investigate whether Flt3-ITD inhibition exerts antileukemic activity via modulation of the Myc network, we treated the human Flt3-ITD mutated leukemia cell line, MV4-11, with PKC412 at two different concentrations (0.1 mM and 1 mM) and analyzed the expression of Myc network genes. Of note, PKC412 reduced *cMyc* expression to the same extent at both concentrations. Conversely, the expression of the Myc antagonists *Mxd1* and *Mxd2* was increased in a dose-dependent manner in MV4-11 cells treated with PKC412 (Figure 5), as well as the expression of *Mxd4*, but to a lesser extent. Intriguingly, MV4-11 cells do not express *Mycn* (Figure 5).

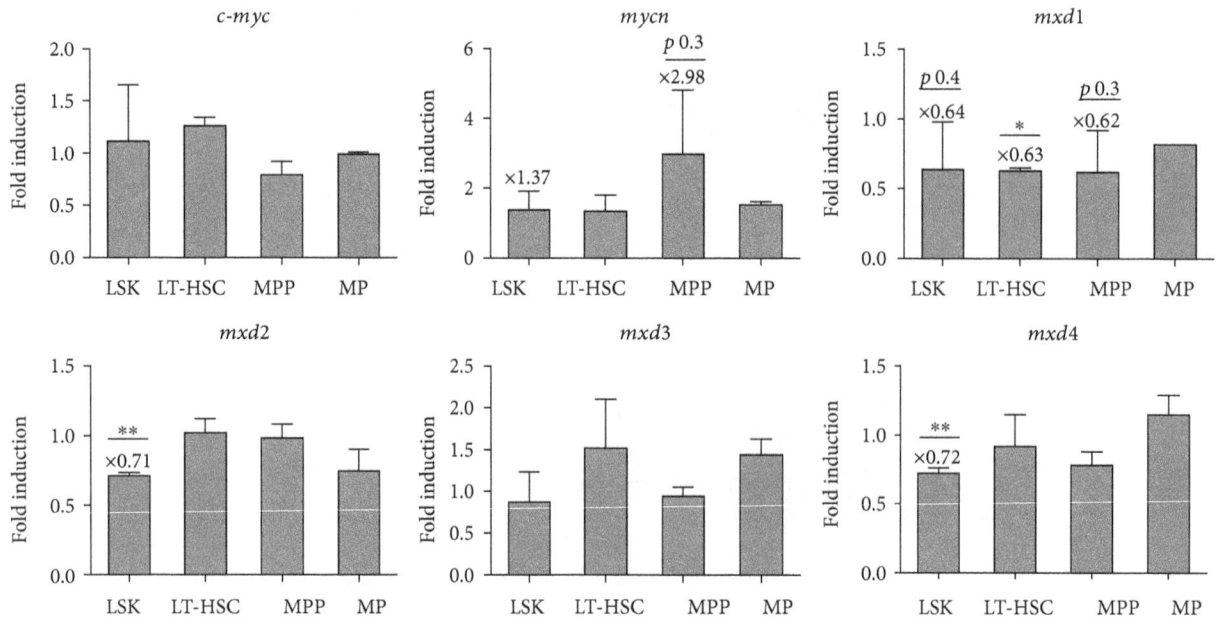

FIGURE 4: Hematopoietic stem cells in Flt3-ITD mice have altered Myc network expression. The expression of Myc network genes was carried out with reverse transcription quantitative PCR (RT-Q-PCR) in hematopoietic stem cells. Fold induction was calculated as a ratio of Flt3-ITD : WT samples. Statistical analysis was performed with Student's t-test on log-converted values ($^*p < 0.05$, $^{**}p < 0.01$).

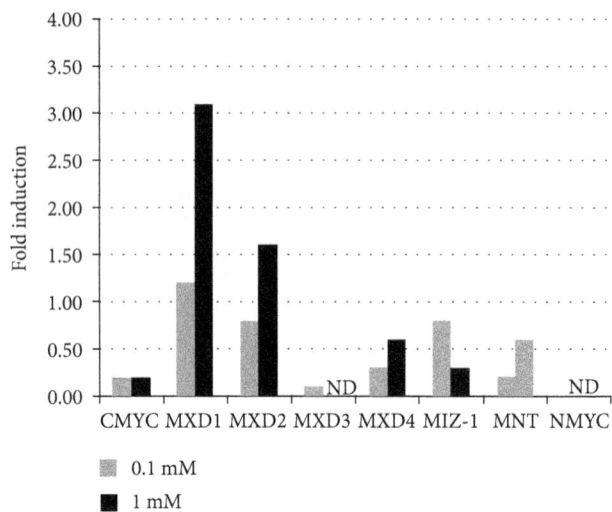

FIGURE 5: Small molecule inhibitor, PKC412, modulates the expression of *Myc* network genes in human MV4-11 cells. The human Flt3-ITD mutated leukemia cell line, MV4-11, was treated with the Flt3-inhibitor PKC412 at two different concentrations (0.1 mM and 1 mM) for 15 minutes. Expression analysis of the Myc network genes was carried out with RT-Q-PCR. ND: not detected.

4. Discussion

Currently, a rapid development of targeted therapies against specifically overexpressed or mutated molecules in AML is ongoing. Clinical trials against mutated molecules found in AML, e.g., IDH1 and IDH2, have recently been initiated [29]. Considering the risk of relapse with the current treatment, it is important to identify pathways regulated by the activated Flt3 receptor for the identification of new treatment targets. The Myc network of oncogenes and tumor suppressors is often changed in a plethora of tumors. The overexpression of the *MYC* and *MYCN* oncogenes is mostly not due to actual mutations in the genes, but their expression is deregulated due to upstream activated pathways and molecules [30]. However, there are exceptions to the rule, as *MYCN* is amplified in neuroblastomas [31]. *Myc* and *Mycn* overexpression has been shown to initiate myeloid and lymphoid neoplasms and could therefore be possible targets for inhibiting leukemic cell proliferation and viability. The Mxd network of tumor suppressors has been shown to be downregulated or deleted in different tumor types including prostate adenocarcinoma [32]. In this study, we have analyzed the possible role of the Myc network in Flt3-ITD-induced myeloproliferative disease. Flt3-ITD is one of the most common mutations in AML and is correlated with poor prognosis. Strategies of inhibiting the overactivated Flt3-ITD tyrosine kinase or pathways downstream of this receptor would therefore be of interest in treating AML patients with this mutation. Efforts with Flt3-ITD inhibitors to treat AML are ongoing. However, results have shown that the Flt3-ITD inhibitor should be used in combination with other treatments to avoid the development of drug resistance.

Herein, we report that myeloid progenitors (MPs) are increased in adult Flt-3ITD mice, which is consistent with other reports. Intriguingly, fetal Flt3-ITD mice have a normal MP compartment and are protected from leukemic transformation [33]. Similarly, LT-HSCs (LSKCD150$^+$48$^-$) were reported to be present in normal numbers in Flt3-ITD fetal livers before the onset of myeloproliferative disease. However, we here show that LT-HSCs decrease in favor of MPPs in Flt3-ITD mice which has developed a myeloproliferative disease, which has also been shown in other reports ([34, 35, 26]). Evidence has shown that the effect of Flt3-ITD on LT-HSC homeostasis is cell autonomous [26]. Changes in the expression of the *Myc* network genes downstream of Flt3-ITD could therefore be responsible for an expansion of leukemic multipotent progenitors. Of note, STAT3 is upregulated in Flt3-ITD MPPs [34]. Moreover, in adult progenitors, Flt3-ITD induces self-renewal in a STAT5-dependent manner [36]. Interestingly, lineage-specific STAT5 activation in hematopoietic progenitor cells predicts the FLT3+-mediated leukemic phenotype in mice [37], and the STAT signaling pathway has been reported to increase Myc activity. These data highlight the involvement of STAT signaling in connection with the Myc network in aberrant hematopoietic stem and progenitor cell populations in Flt3-ITD, which is thus also a potential therapeutic target in Flt3-ITD leukemia.

We found that the Myc network of oncogenes and tumor suppressors is changed in Flt3-ITD myeloproliferative mice compared with wild-type mice. Generally, the *Myc* gene expression was increased, and the expression of the Myc antagonists, mainly *Mxd1*, *Mxd2/Mxi1*, *Mxd4*, *Mnt*, and *Miz-1*, was decreased. Myc has been shown to be involved in displacing quiescent hematopoietic stem cells from their niche to more proliferative progenitor cells [38]. This can be correlated with our results showing the change in hematopoietic stem and progenitor cell subpopulation distribution, where the long-term hematopoietic stem cells are decreased in Flt3-ITD mice and the multipotent progenitors increased. Our data shows that *cMyc* was increased in Flt3-ITD multipotent progenitors (MPPs) as was *Mycn* in LSK, MPP, and pre-GM cells. Importantly, c-MYC has been reported to induce the expression of the deubiquitinase USP22, which in turn reduced ubiquitination and enhanced the stability of SIRT1 in CD34+ Flt3-ITD cells. Of note, inhibition of SIRT1 expression or activity reduced the growth of Flt3-ITD AML [39]. Additionally, c-MYC generates repair errors by regulating transcriptional activation and expression of the alternative nonhomologous end-joining pathway resulting in aberrant DNA repair in Flt3-ITD leukemia [40]. Further, N-Myc overexpression mechanistically results in the hyperproliferation of myeloid cells by decreasing transforming growth factor β signaling and increasing c-Jun-NH2-kinase signaling to cause AML [14]. Collectively, these data underscore the importance of inhibition of the Myc molecules in treating Flt3-ITD mutated AML. Furthermore, we observed the downregulation of *Mxd* family genes, i.e., *Mxd1*, *Mxd2/Mxi1*, and *Mxd4*. Interestingly, Krüppel-like factor 4 (KLF4) has been identified as an upstream transcriptional regulator of *Mxd1* and *Myc* in myeloid leukemias [41]. Intriguingly, while SIRT1 was shown to regulate c-MYC in Flt3-ITD mutated leukemia [39], it has been demonstrated to regulate *Mxd1* in malignant melanoma [42]. Similarly, we found that *Mnt* and *Miz-1* were also downregulated in Flt3-ITD MPs. Of note, *Miz-1* serves as a platform to inhibit the expression of cell cycle regulators ([43, 44]). Flt3-ITD mutated leukemic cells have enhanced activity of Cdc25, which overrides the replication checkpoint leading to arrest in the S phase [45]. These findings could point to the possibility that reduced levels of Miz-1 result in enhanced activity of Cdc25 thereby deregulating the cell

cycle in Flt3-ITD leukemia. Given that compromised DNA damage response and weakened cell cycle checkpoint promote the progression of AML, our data points to the potential role of *Myc* and *Miz-1* in regulating these pathways in Flt3-ITD leukemia.

As the phosphorylation status of FLT3 is associated with its functional activity [46], the inhibition of FLT3 phosphorylation will affect FLT3-dependent pathways such as RAS/MAPK, JAK/STAT, and Wnt pathways [9]. Given that Myc oncogenes are downstream effectors of these pathways and based on our results that *Myc* oncogenes are altered upon ITD mutation in *FLT3*, we hypothesized that modulation of FLT3 phosphorylation will result in transcriptional reprogramming of the Myc network. Our data showed that PKC412-mediated inhibition of FLT3 signaling increased *Mxd1* and *Mxd2* expression, as well as the expression of *Mxd4* and *Mnt* to a lesser degree, while it reduced *cMyc* expression in Flt3-ITD AML cells. During the course of preparation of this manuscript, Zhang et al. reported that PKC412-induced Myc downregulation results in decreased telomerase reverse transcriptase (hTERT) activity [47]. Additionally, inhibition of cMyc has several therapeutic implications in solid tumors and hematological malignancies. It has been reported that cMyc inhibition overcomes radio- and chemotherapy resistance in pediatric medulloblastoma [48]. Similarly, cMyc inhibition has been shown to negatively impact lymphoma growth [49] and overcome drug-resistant AML [33]. Furthermore, cMyc inhibition prevents leukemia initiation in mice and impairs the growth of relapsed and induction failure pediatric T-ALL cells [50]. Our data showed that selective inhibition of Flt3-ITD downstream signaling induced c-Myc inhibition, which is consistent with a recent report [47]. Furthermore, our data also shows that *Mnt* and *Miz-1* of the *Mxd* family are targets of Flt3-ITD signaling pointing to the Myc network as a whole being a target of activated Flt3-ITD. Additionally, our data showed that *nMyc* expression is increased in LSK, MPP, and pre-GM cells from Flt3-ITD mice. Reports supporting the important role of the inhibition of the Mxd family of tumor suppressors include studies showing that Mxd1 promotes cell cycle arrest and differentiation [30]; also, several studies showed deletion of the 10q24-q25 chromosome, where the *MXD2* gene is located in solid tumors [51]. Furthermore, *MXD2* is mutated in hematological malignancies [52], as well as in solid tumors. Interestingly, reintroduction of Mxd2 in glioblastoma cells deficient in Mxd2 results in reduced glioblastoma cell growth and clonogenicity [53]. Our study points to the fact that alterations in the Myc network by Flt3-ITD signaling are involved in myeloid leukemogenesis and that PKC412-mediated Flt3-ITD inhibition partly exerts its antileukemic activity by affecting the Myc/Max/Mxd network.

Authors' Contributions

F. B. and A. H. conceived the project, designed the experiments, analyzed the data, and wrote the manuscript. F. B., M. A., and A. H. performed the experiments. All authors read and approved the manuscript.

Acknowledgments

A. H. is supported by the Swedish Cancer Society, the Pediatric Cancer Society, and the Swedish Society of Physicians. The work was also supported by the Lions Foundation, Skåne, Sweden; Georg Danielsson s fund for blood disease; the Physician Society of Lund; Olof Eliasson's Foundation; the Crafoord Foundation; the Knut and Alice Wallenbergs Foundation; the Royal Physiographic Society; and the Lundberg Research Foundation. We thank the members of the Stein Eirik Jacobsen Laboratory for their helpful discussions. We thank Lilian Wittman, Zhi Ma, and Anna Fossum for their excellent technical support.

References

[1] M. R. Luskin and D. J. DeAngelo, "Midostaurin/PKC412 for the treatment of newly diagnosed FLT3 mutation-positive acute myeloid leukemia," *Expert Review of Hematology*, vol. 10, no. 12, pp. 1033–1045, 2017.

[2] C. H. Brandts, B. Sargin, M. Rode et al., "Constitutive activation of Akt by Flt3 internal tandem duplications is necessary for increased survival, proliferation, and myeloid transformation," *Cancer Research*, vol. 65, no. 21, pp. 9643–9650, 2005.

[3] F. M. Abu-Duhier, A. C. Goodeve, G. A. Wilson et al., "FLT3 internal tandem duplication mutations in adult acute myeloid leukaemia define a high-risk group," *British Journal of Haematology*, vol. 111, no. 1, pp. 190–195, 2000.

[4] C. Thiede, C. Steudel, B. Mohr et al., "Analysis of FLT3-activating mutations in 979 patients with acute myelogenous leukemia: association with FAB subtypes and identification of subgroups with poor prognosis," *Blood*, vol. 99, no. 12, pp. 4326–4335, 2002.

[5] M. A. Hospital, A. S. Green, T. T. Maciel et al., "FLT3 inhibitors: clinical potential in acute myeloid leukemia," *OncoTargets and Therapy*, vol. 10, pp. 607–615, 2017.

[6] R. Swords, C. Freeman, and F. Giles, "Targeting the FMS-like tyrosine kinase 3 in acute myeloid leukemia," *Leukemia*, vol. 26, no. 10, pp. 2176–2185, 2012.

[7] C. Choudhary, J. Schwable, C. Brandts et al., "AML-associated Flt3 kinase domain mutations show signal transduction differences compared with Flt3 ITD mutations," *Blood*, vol. 106, no. 1, pp. 265–273, 2005.

[8] L. Tickenbrock, J. Schwable, M. Wiedehage et al., "Flt3 tandem duplication mutations cooperate with Wnt signaling in leukemic signal transduction," *Blood*, vol. 105, no. 9, pp. 3699–3706, 2005.

[9] K. T. Kim, K. Baird, S. Davis et al., "Constitutive Fms-like tyrosine kinase 3 activation results in specific changes in gene expression in myeloid leukaemic cells," *British Journal of Haematology*, vol. 138, no. 5, pp. 603–615, 2007.

[10] X. Li, X. Zhang, W. Xie, X. Li, and S. Huang, "MYC-mediated synthetic lethality for treatment of hematological malignancies," *Current Cancer Drug Targets*, vol. 15, no. 1, pp. 53–70, 2015.

[11] M. Schick, S. Habringer, J. A. Nilsson, and U. Keller, "Pathogenesis and therapeutic targeting of aberrant MYC expression in haematological cancers," *British Journal of Haematology*, vol. 179, no. 5, pp. 724–738, 2017.

[12] A. Sommer, K. Bousset, E. Kremmer, M. Austen, and B. Luscher, "Identification and characterization of specific DNA-binding complexes containing members of the Myc/Max/Mad network of transcriptional regulators," *The Journal of Biological Chemistry*, vol. 273, no. 12, pp. 6632–6642, 1998.

[13] S. Herold, M. Wanzel, V. Beuger et al., "Negative regulation of the mammalian UV response by Myc through association with Miz-1," *Molecular Cell*, vol. 10, no. 3, pp. 509–521, 2002.

[14] H. Kawagoe, A. Kandilci, T. A. Kranenburg, and G. C. Grosveld, "Overexpression of N-Myc rapidly causes acute myeloid leukemia in mice," *Cancer Research*, vol. 67, no. 22, pp. 10677–10685, 2007.

[15] M. D. Delgado, M. Albajar, M. T. Gomez-Casares, A. Batlle, and J. Leon, "MYC oncogene in myeloid neoplasias," *Clinical & Translational Oncology*, vol. 15, no. 2, pp. 87–94, 2013.

[16] B. Scheijen, H. T. Ngo, H. Kang, and J. D. Griffin, "FLT3 receptors with internal tandem duplications promote cell viability and proliferation by signaling through Foxo proteins," *Oncogene*, vol. 23, no. 19, pp. 3338–3349, 2004.

[17] O. Delpuech, B. Griffiths, P. East et al., "Induction of Mxi1-SRα by FOXO3a contributes to repression of Myc-dependent gene expression," *Molecular and Cellular Biology*, vol. 27, no. 13, pp. 4917–4930, 2007.

[18] E. Laurenti, B. Varnum-Finney, A. Wilson et al., "Hematopoietic stem cell function and survival depend on c-Myc and N-Myc activity," *Cell Stem Cell*, vol. 3, no. 6, pp. 611–624, 2008.

[19] B. H. Lee, Z. Tothova, R. L. Levine et al., "FLT3 mutations confer enhanced proliferation and survival properties to multipotent progenitors in a murine model of chronic myelomonocytic leukemia," *Cancer Cell*, vol. 12, no. 4, pp. 367–380, 2007.

[20] E. Sitnicka, N. Buza-Vidas, H. Ahlenius et al., "Critical role of FLT3 ligand in IL-7 receptor independent T lymphopoiesis and regulation of lymphoid-primed multipotent progenitors," *Blood*, vol. 110, no. 8, pp. 2955–2964, 2007.

[21] J. Adolfsson, R. Månsson, N. Buza-Vidas et al., "Identification of Flt 3+ lympho-myeloid stem cells lacking erythro-megakaryocytic potential a revised road map for adult blood lineage commitment," *Cell*, vol. 121, no. 2, pp. 295–306, 2005.

[22] M. J. Kiel, O. H. Yilmaz, T. Iwashita, O. H. Yilmaz, C. Terhorst, and S. J. Morrison, "SLAM family receptors distinguish hematopoietic stem and progenitor cells and reveal endothelial niches for stem cells," *Cell*, vol. 121, no. 7, pp. 1109–1121, 2005.

[23] C. J. H. Pronk, D. J. Rossi, R. Månsson et al., "Elucidation of the phenotypic, functional, and molecular topography of a myeloerythroid progenitor cell hierarchy," *Cell Stem Cell*, vol. 1, no. 4, pp. 428–442, 2007.

[24] S. Kharazi, A. J. Mead, A. Mansour et al., "Impact of gene dosage, loss of wild-type allele, and FLT3 ligand on *Flt3-ITD*-

induced myeloproliferation," *Blood*, vol. 118, no. 13, pp. 3613–3621, 2011.

[25] G. Yang and P. J. Hurlin, "MNT and emerging concepts of MNT-MYC antagonism," *Genes (Basel)*, vol. 8, no. 2, 2017.

[26] S. H. Chu, D. Heiser, L. Li et al., "FLT3-ITD knockin impairs hematopoietic stem cell quiescence/homeostasis, leading to myeloproliferative neoplasm," *Cell Stem Cell*, vol. 11, no. 3, pp. 346–358, 2012.

[27] E. Weisberg, C. Boulton, L. M. Kelly et al., "Inhibition of mutant FLT3 receptors in leukemia cells by the small molecule tyrosine kinase inhibitor PKC412," *Cancer Cell*, vol. 1, no. 5, pp. 433–443, 2002.

[28] C. B. Williams, S. Kambhampati, W. Fiskus et al., "Preclinical and phase I results of decitabine in combination with midostaurin (PKC412) for newly diagnosed elderly or relapsed/refractory adult patients with acute myeloid leukemia," *Pharmacotherapy*, vol. 33, no. 12, pp. 1341–1352, 2013.

[29] J. P. Sasine and G. J. Schiller, "Emerging strategies for high-risk and relapsed/refractory acute myeloid leukemia: novel agents and approaches currently in clinical trials," *Blood Reviews*, vol. 29, no. 1, pp. 1–9, 2015.

[30] D. Diolaiti, L. McFerrin, P. A. Carroll, and R. N. Eisenman, "Functional interactions among members of the MAX and MLX transcriptional network during oncogenesis," *Biochimica et Biophysica Acta*, vol. 1849, no. 5, pp. 484–500, 2015.

[31] B. R. Oppedal, O. Oien, T. Jahnsen, and P. Brandtzaeg, "N-myc amplification in neuroblastomas: histopathological, DNA ploidy, and clinical variables," *Journal of Clinical Pathology*, vol. 42, no. 11, pp. 1148–1152, 1989.

[32] C. W. Hooker and P. J. Hurlin, "Of Myc and Mnt," *Journal of Cell Science*, vol. 119, no. 2, pp. 208–216, 2006.

[33] X. N. Pan, J. J. Chen, L. X. Wang et al., "Inhibition of c-Myc overcomes cytotoxic drug resistance in acute myeloid leukemia cells by promoting differentiation," *PLoS One*, vol. 9, no. 8, article e105381, 2014.

[34] A. J. Mead, S. Kharazi, D. Atkinson et al., "FLT3-ITDs instruct a myeloid differentiation and transformation bias in lympho-myeloid multipotent progenitors," *Cell Reports*, vol. 3, no. 6, pp. 1766–1776, 2013.

[35] A. J. Mead, W. H. Neo, N. Barkas et al., "Niche-mediated depletion of the normal hematopoietic stem cell reservoir by Flt3-ITD–induced myeloproliferation," *The Journal of Experimental Medicine*, vol. 214, no. 7, pp. 2005–2021, 2017.

[36] S. N. Porter, A. S. Cluster, W. Yang et al., "Fetal and neonatal hematopoietic progenitors are functionally and transcriptionally resistant to *Flt3*-ITD mutations," *eLife*, vol. 5, article e18882, 2016.

[37] T. A. Müller, R. Grundler, R. Istvanffy et al., "Lineage-specific STAT5 target gene activation in hematopoietic progenitor cells predicts the FLT3⁺-mediated leukemic phenotype," *Leukemia*, vol. 30, no. 8, pp. 1725–1733, 2016.

[38] A. Wilson, M. J. Murphy, T. Oskarsson et al., "c-Myc controls the balance between hematopoietic stem cell self-renewal and differentiation," *Genes & Development*, vol. 18, no. 22, pp. 2747–2763, 2004.

[39] L. Li, T. Osdal, Y. Ho et al., "SIRT1 activation by a c-MYC oncogenic network promotes the maintenance and drug resistance of human FLT3-ITD acute myeloid leukemia stem cells," *Cell Stem Cell*, vol. 15, no. 4, pp. 431–446, 2014.

[40] N. Muvarak, S. Kelley, C. Robert et al., "c-MYC generates repair errors via increased transcription of alternative-NHEJ

factors, LIG3 and PARP1, in tyrosine kinase-activated leukemias," *Molecular Cancer Research*, vol. 13, no. 4, pp. 699–712, 2015.

[41] V. A. Morris, C. L. Cummings, B. Korb, S. Boaglio, and V. G. Oehler, "Deregulated KLF4 expression in myeloid leukemias alters cell proliferation and differentiation through microRNA and gene targets," *Molecular and Cellular Biology*, vol. 36, no. 4, pp. 559–573, 2016.

[42] F. M. Meliso, D. Micali, C. T. Silva et al., "SIRT1 regulates Mxd 1 during malignant melanoma progression," *Oncotarget*, vol. 8, no. 70, pp. 114540–114553, 2017.

[43] R. T. Phan, M. Saito, K. Basso, H. Niu, and R. Dalla-Favera, "BCL6 interacts with the transcription factor Miz-1 to suppress the cyclin-dependent kinase inhibitor p 21 and cell cycle arrest in germinal center B cells," *Nature Immunology*, vol. 6, no. 10, pp. 1054–1060, 2005.

[44] S. Basu, Q. Liu, Y. Qiu, and F. Dong, "Gfi-1 represses *CDKN2B* encoding p15^{INK4B} through interaction with Miz-1," *Proceedings of the National Academy of Sciences of the United States of America*, vol. 106, no. 5, pp. 1433–1438, 2009.

[45] C. Seedhouse, M. Grundy, S. Shang et al., "Impaired S-phase arrest in acute myeloid leukemia cells with a FLT3 internal tandem duplication treated with clofarabine," *Clinical Cancer Research*, vol. 15, no. 23, pp. 7291–7298, 2009.

[46] S. Meshinchi and F. R. Appelbaum, "Structural and functional alterations of FLT3 in acute myeloid leukemia," *Clinical Cancer Research*, vol. 15, no. 13, pp. 4263–4269, 2009.

[47] X. Zhang, B. Li, J. Yu et al., "MYC-dependent downregulation of telomerase by FLT3 inhibitors is required for their therapeutic efficacy on acute myeloid leukemia," *Annals of Hematology*, vol. 97, no. 1, pp. 63–72, 2018.

[48] A. O. von Bueren, T. Shalaby, C. Oehler-Jänne et al., "RNA interference-mediated c-MYC inhibition prevents cell growth and decreases sensitivity to radio- and chemotherapy in childhood medulloblastoma cells," *BMC Cancer*, vol. 9, no. 1, p. 10, 2009.

[49] I. Gomez-Curet, R. S. Perkins, R. Bennett, K. L. Feidler, S. P. Dunn, and L. J. Krueger, "c-Myc inhibition negatively impacts lymphoma growth," *Journal of Pediatric Surgery*, vol. 41, no. 1, pp. 207–211, 2006.

[50] J. E. Roderick, J. Tesell, L. D. Shultz et al., "c-Myc inhibition prevents leukemia initiation in mice and impairs the growth of relapsed and induction failure pediatric T-ALL cells," *Blood*, vol. 123, no. 7, pp. 1040–1050, 2014.

[51] N. Kawamata, D. Park, S. Wilczynski, J. Yokota, and H. P. Koeffler, "Point mutations of the Mxil gene are rare in prostate cancers," *Prostate*, vol. 29, no. 3, pp. 191–193, 1996.

[52] X. L. Guo, L. Pan PhD, MD, X. J. Zhang et al., "Expression and mutation analysis of genes that encode the Myc antagonists Mad 1, Mxi 1 and Rox in acute leukaemia," *Leukemia & Lymphoma*, vol. 48, no. 6, pp. 1200–1207, 2007.

[53] D. S. Wechsler, C. A. Shelly, C. A. Petroff, and C. V. Dang, "MXI1, a putative tumor suppressor gene, suppresses growth of human glioblastoma cells," *Cancer Research*, vol. 57, no. 21, pp. 4905–4912, 1997.

12

Insights into Endothelial Progenitor Cells: Origin, Classification, Potentials, and Prospects

H. Chopra ⓘ,[1] M. K. Hung ⓘ,[2] D. L. Kwong,[3] C. F. Zhang,[4] and E. H. N. Pow ⓘ[5]

[1]B.D.S., M.D.S. (Conservative Dentistry and Endodontics), Research Postgraduate Student, Discipline of Prosthodontics, Faculty of Dentistry, The University of Hong Kong, Pok Fu Lam, Hong Kong

[2]BChinMed, Research Assistant, Department of Surgery, Queen Mary Hospital, The University of Hong Kong, Pok Fu Lam, Hong Kong

[3]MBBS, MD, FRCR, FHKCR, FHKAM, Clinical Professor, Department of Clinical Oncology, Li Ka Shing Faculty of Medicine, The University of Hong Kong, Pok Fu Lam, Hong Kong

[4]D.D.S, Ph.D. (Med), Clinical Professor, Discipline of Endodontics, Faculty of Dentistry, The University of Hong Kong, Pok Fu Lam, Hong Kong

[5]B.D.S., M.D.S. (Prosthetic Dentistry), MRACDS (Pros), FRACDS, FCDHK (Pros), FHKAM (Dental Surgery), Clinical Associate Professor, Discipline of Prosthodontics, Faculty of Dentistry, The University of Hong Kong, Pok Fu Lam, Hong Kong

Correspondence should be addressed to H. Chopra; hiteshchoprasmile@gmail.com and E. H. N. Pow; ehnpow@hku.hk

Academic Editor: Georgina Ellison

With the discovery of endothelial progenitor cells (EPCs) in the late 1990s, a paradigm shift in the concept of neoangiogenesis occurred. The identification of circulating EPCs in peripheral blood marked the beginning of a new era with enormous potential in the rapidly transforming regenerative field. Overwhelmed with the revelation, researchers across the globe focused on isolating, defining, and interpreting the role of EPCs in various physiological and pathological conditions. Consequently, controversies emerged regarding the isolation techniques and classification of EPCs. Nevertheless, the potential of using EPCs in tissue engineering as an angiogenic source has been extensively explored. Concomitantly, the impact of EPCs on various diseases, such as diabetes, cancer, and cardiovascular diseases, has been studied. Within the limitations of the current knowledge, this review attempts to delineate the concept of EPCs in a sequential manner from the speculative history to a definitive presence (origin, sources of EPCs, isolation, and identification) and significance of these EPCs. Additionally, this review is aimed at serving as a guide for investigators, identifying potential research gaps, and summarizing our current and future prospects regarding EPCs.

1. Introduction

Prevascularization is one of the critical approaches to enhance the success of tissue-engineered grafts [1]. A lack of vascular perfusion compromises the oxygen and nutrient supply as well as the disposal of wastes and toxins, leading to cell death, poor integration, and graft failure [2]. Therefore, neovascularization is currently considered the fourth pillar of the preexisting tissue engineering triad: stem cells, growth factors, and scaffold [3]. The term "haemangioblast" was proposed almost

a century ago to describe the common origin of haematopoietic/endothelial progenitor cells [4]. However, the existence of haemangioblast was substantiated only two decades ago by Asahara and his colleagues [5], whom successfully isolated "endothelial progenitor cells" (EPCs) from the human peripheral blood. This discovery resulted in a mammoth global exploration of EPCs by researchers. Concurrently, controversies regarding the origin of EPCs, ambiguity in the phenotyping of EPCs, and nonstandardized isolation techniques have emerged besides difficulties in the isolation of EPCs.

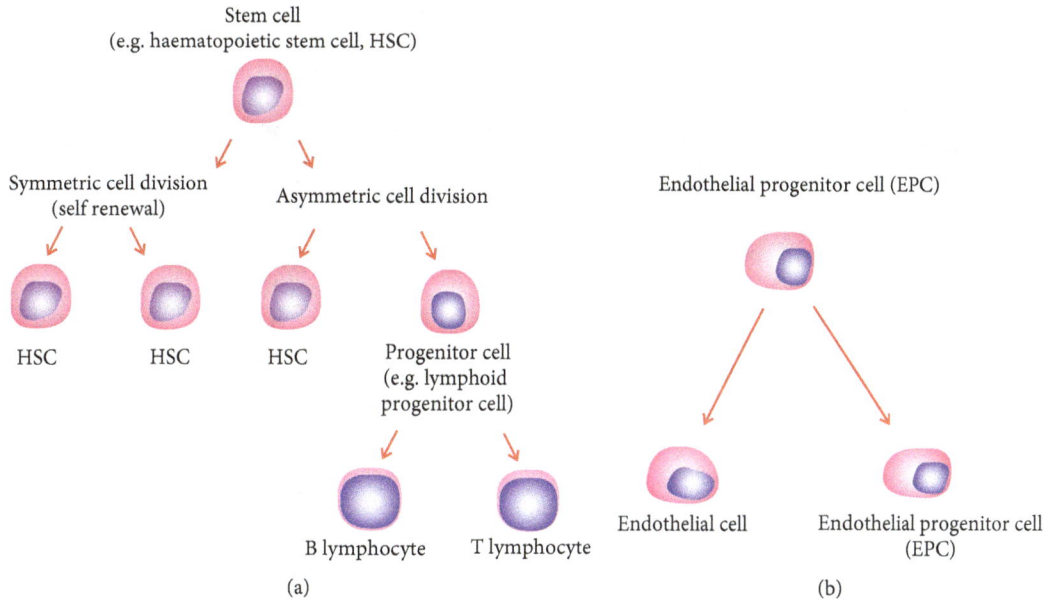

FIGURE 1: Difference between stem cells and progenitor cells.

This review is aimed at providing comprehensive insight into endothelial cells (ECs) from basic terminologies to its origin, the source of EPCs, EPC isolation techniques, the impact of EPCs on various therapies, and future prospects. Furthermore, this review will discuss the potentially unaddressed areas where research could have a substantial influence on the domain of neovascularization, and in turn, EPCs.

2. What Is Neovascularization?

Most of the tissue engineering studies and modern disease interventions are based on the augmentation or inhibition of angiogenesis. For example, in tissue-engineered grafts, amplification of angiogenesis is desired, whereas in tumours, suppression of angiogenesis is considered as an essential therapeutic application. However, the word "angiogenesis" is a misnomer, as it is a generic term that does not apply to all cases. Therefore, it is pragmatic to clarify the mechanism of blood vessel formation. Angiogenesis is defined as the formation of new capillaries from preexisting vessels [6]. De novo blood vessel formation during embryonic development is called "vasculogenesis," while "postnatal vasculogenesis" describes new blood vessel formation in adults [7]. On the other hand, "arteriogenesis" is defined as the maturation and formation of larger-diameter arteries from preexisting capillaries or collateral arteries [8]. The novel term "neovascularization" has been suggested to embody all types of vessel formation in adults [9].

3. Endothelial Progenitor Cells

Stem cells have been traditionally characterized based on three properties: self-renewability, clonogenicity, and plasticity (differentiation capacity). In sharp contrast, progenitor cells lack self-renewability. EPCs are unique, as they are distinctly different from progenitors but are similar to stem cells

with a similar triad of self-renewability, clonogenicity, and differentiation capacity (Figure 1).

Further, EPCs are mostly unipotent stem cells which can uptake acetylated low-density lipoproteins (acLDL), bind with *Ulex europaeus* agglutinin-1 (UEA-1), and take part in neovascularization through either paracrine or autocrine mechanisms. To date, two different types of EPCs have been recognized and are described according to their morphologies, time of appearance, and expression of proteins. Both types of EPCs, along with other ECs, will be discussed later in the section for better insight.

4. Origin of Endothelial Cells (ECs)

It has been contemplated that during embryogenesis, a special type of cell called "haemangioblast" is the precursor of both endothelial and haematopoietic cell lineages. The term "haemangioblast" was coined by Murray [4] and is different from "angioblast," as initially suggested by Sabin [10]. Accordingly, the term "angioblast" should be restricted to the vessels only, i.e., to the endothelium, whereas the term "haemangioblast" refers to a solid mass of cells that gives rise to both endothelium and blood cells. The hypothesis that ECs originate from haemangioblast is based on the close developmental association of the haematopoietic and endothelial lineages within blood islands [4, 10, 11]. However, these studies failed to reach a definite conclusion due to the complexities in acquiring chick embryos before the development of blood islands and the negligible number of cells present during this stage.

Nevertheless, rapid advances in medical field by the end of the twentieth century spurred the studies with embryonic stem cell differentiation models (ESCDM) [12–14], genetics, and newer animal models [15] and reported a spatiotemporal association between haematopoietic and endothelial lineages during earlier stages of life.

The earliest ESCDM was a mouse wherein an embryonic stem cell (ESC) line isolated from a mouse [16, 17] laid the foundation for studying mammalian developmental biology [18]. Differentiation of these ESCs has distinct advantages for examining the sequelae of initial cellular and molecular changes at the onset [12]. For example, mESC differentiation studies identified blast colony-forming cells (BL-CFCs), a type of progenitor cell that is the precursor of both haematopoietic cells and ECs [13]. Further, kinetic analysis has demonstrated that BL-CFCs represent the establishment of primitive erythroid and other lineage-restricted precursors [19]. Additionally, embryoid bodies (EBs), which are differentiated ESCs, have also indicated that multiple haematopoietic lineages can originate from ESCs in culture [20]. With these intriguing results and persistent efforts, hESCs were successfully isolated after almost two decades and their *in vitro* differentiation also leads to both haematopoietic and EC lineages [21, 22]. However, the first evidence that human haemangioblasts are comparable to mouse haemangioblasts was only recently reported in a study showing that human BL-CFCs, similar to mouse BL-CFCs, have both haematopoietic and vascular potential [23].

In conjunction with the cell culture studies, the study of various receptors and transcription factors and biochemical analyses of regulatory factors have provided detailed insight into the hypothesis that ECs originate from haemangioblasts. Receptor tyrosine kinases (RTKs) are considered as key regulators of developmental processes. Foetal liver kinase 1 (FLK-1) (also known as KDR) is an RTK that has been identified in primitive and more mature haematopoietic cells as well as in a wide variety of nonhaematopoietic tissues [24]. Functional analysis of FLK-1 revealed that FLK-1 is expressed in blood islands in mouse embryos and is therefore pivotal in regulating both vasculogenesis and angiogenesis [25]. In a knockdown experiment, *FLK-1* gene-deficient mouse embryos failed to generate blood islands as well as endothelial and haematopoietic cells [26]. Cell sorting further confirmed that FLK-1$^+$ cells represent the earliest precursors of embryonic haematopoiesis [27, 28], whereas FLK-1$^+$VE cadherin$^+$ cells signify a diverging point of haematopoietic and endothelial cell lineages [28]. Vascular endothelial growth factor (VEGF) is a potent angiogenic factor whose interaction with FLK-1 is responsible for the formation of BL-CFCs [13, 19]. TIE-2, an endothelial cell marker, is not expressed in the mesoderm of the primitive streak but is present in the haemangioblast [29]. Therefore, expression of TIE-2 substantiates the presence of an intermediate stage that gives rise to both haemogenic endothelium (HE) and angioblasts [30].

Another receptor that is expressed at the onset of primitive and definitive haematopoiesis (PH and DH) is CD41 [31–33]. CD41 is a platelet glycoprotein receptor that is required for normal platelet haemostatic function [34]. Although CD41 was previously thought to be lineage restricted, various studies have demonstrated differential expression of CD41, indicating a dynamic regulation of CD41 in haematopoietic development [31–33]. The phenotype of HE was found to be C-KIT$^+$TIE-2$^+$CD41$^-$ of which two-third contributes to ECs with the same gene expression while the rest of the population differentiates to hematopoietic precursors, i.e.,

haematopoietic stem cells (HSCs). This transition from HE to haematopoietic cells does not occur by asymmetric cell division but by a unique method referred to as endothelial to haematopoietic cell transition (EHT) [35, 36]. On the other hand, PH is speculated to evolve from angioblasts with a C-KIT$^+$TIE-2$^+$CD41$^+$ signature [30].

There are also myriad TFs that play a significant role in haematopoiesis. Of these, TFs from the GATA family and RUNX-1 are most commonly involved. Some TFs have distinct roles in either PH or DH, whereas some are imperative for both. For example, it has been reported that GATA-1$^-$ progenitor cells give rise to PH, whereas the GATA-1$^+$ subpopulation differentiates into VE cadherin$^+$ cells that give rise to both endothelial and haematopoietic cells [37]. On the other hand, RUNX-1 is essential for DH but does not affect PH [38–40]. However, SCL/TAL-1 (stem cell leukaemia/T cell acute lymphocytic leukaemia 1) and *LMO-2* (LIM domain TF) are necessary for both PH and DH as well as vascular remodelling [41, 42]. Functional studies have shown that forced expression of SCL mRNA in zebrafish embryos resulted in the development of both haematopoietic and endothelial precursors, suggesting a role for the *SCL* gene in haemangioblast formation [43]. Furthermore, both SCL/TAL-1 and LMO-2 act synergistically to stimulate the formation of haemangioblasts [44, 45], which in the absence of GATA-1 differentiate into ECs only [44].

Significant results from chick and mouse embryos encouraged researchers to explore other animal models. As a result, haemangioblasts were also identified in Drosophila [46] and zebrafish [47]. Zebrafish has a distinct advantage as a vertebrate which makes it a perfect model for genetic analysis and experimental embryology [48–50]. Further, as zebrafish embryos are transparent, tracing techniques emerged for mapping embryonic development until cardiac development [51–53]. In fact, by fate mapping in zebrafish, haemangioblasts and cardiomyocytes were found to work antagonistically [54].

Although the existence of haemangioblasts was proposed a century ago, it is still a matter of extensive research and debate. Despite these controversies, the above-discussed findings support the existence of haemangioblasts. In summary, HE and angioblasts are intermediate stages of haemangioblasts. Angioblasts give rise to the first wave of PH, whereas HE gives rise to the second wave of DH. A detailed model is shown in Figure 2, explaining the origin of EPCs as well as the blood cell hierarchy.

5. Types of EPCs

5.1. Based on the Source. As discussed above, EPCs shared a common precursor with other lineages. Therefore, it is plausible that these EPCs can be isolated/transdifferentiated from various sources and, hence, are sharing similar phenotypic characteristics. Therefore, we are providing a comprehensive outline of different sources of EPCs (Figure 3).

5.1.1. Haematopoietic EPCs

(1) Bone Marrow-Derived Endothelial Cells (BMECs). Bone marrow is a complex microenvironment consisting of

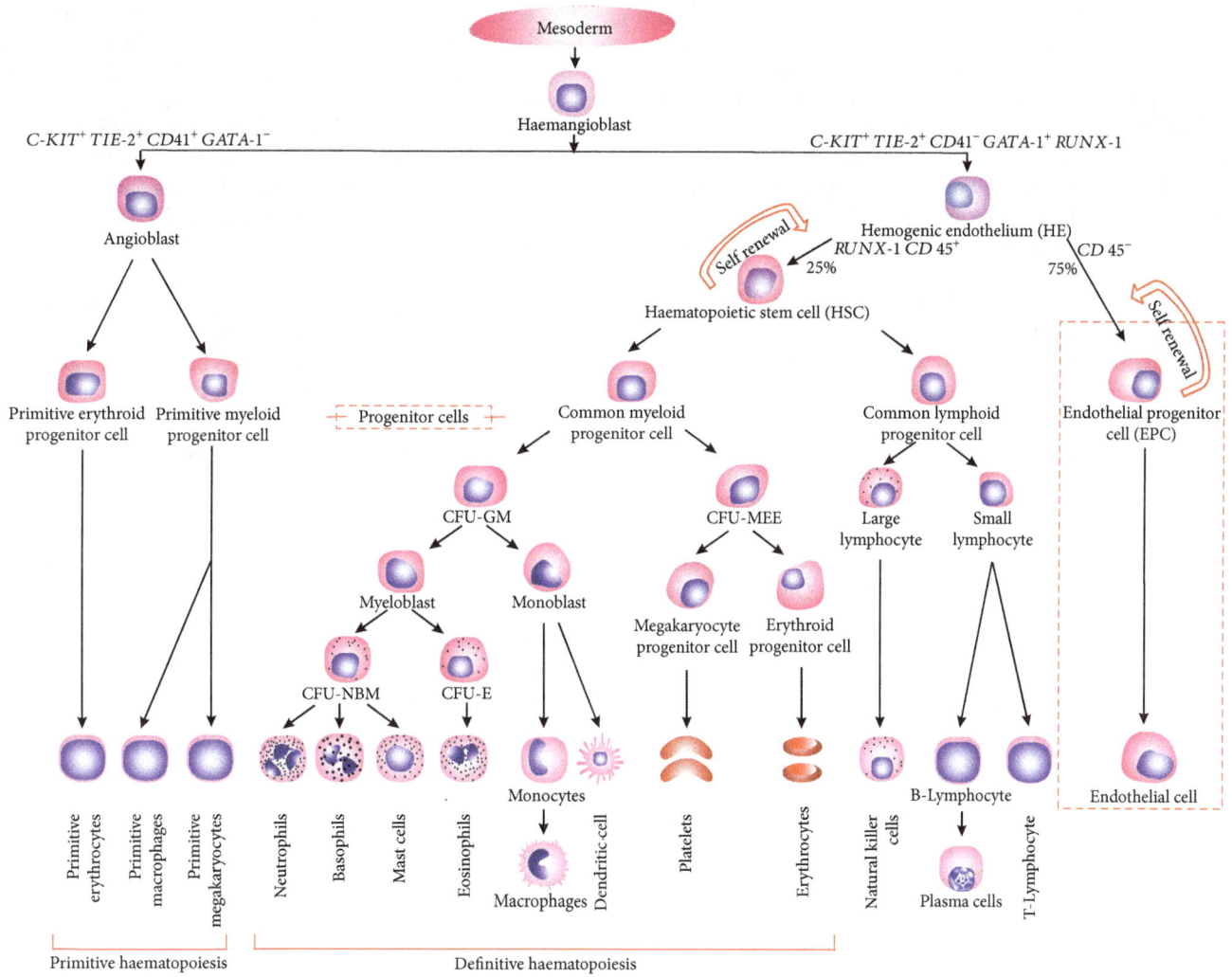

FIGURE 2: Origin of ECs from haemangioblast: haematopoiesis.

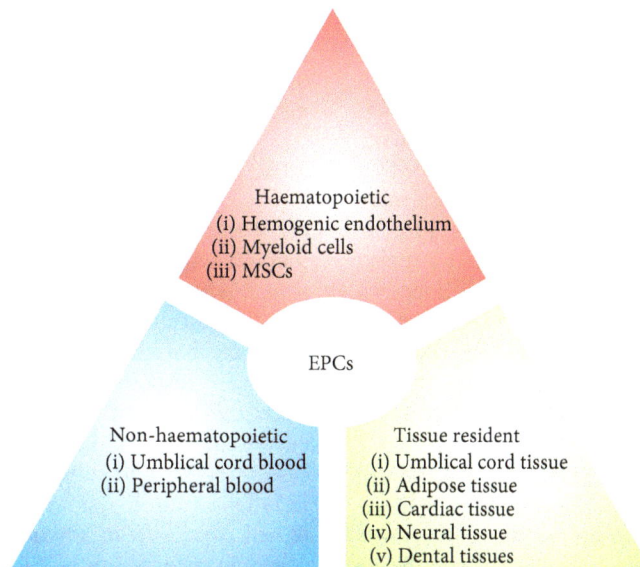

FIGURE 3: Different sources of EPCs.

different cells (Figure 2). BMECs reside in close association with various cell types, which makes the isolation of ECs very challenging. BMECs were first isolated from rat [55] or murine [56] bone marrow by the density centrifugation method or differential phagocytosis of magnetic beads, respectively. On the other hand, human BMECs were isolated either directly from bone marrow aspirate or indirectly (enzymatic digestion of spicules present in the bone marrow followed by culture of cells) using the magnetic-activated cell sorting (MACS) assay via selective binding of ECs to UEA-1 [57, 58]. Later, the isolation of human BMECs was simplified by using mononuclear cells (MNCs) obtained by density centrifugation of bone marrow aspirate and then subjecting MNCs to either MACS (using UEA-1-, CD146-, and BNH9-coated beads) or fluorescence-activated cell sorting (FACS; using CD146 or BNH9). It was found that ECs were best obtained with FACS and constituted 0.05% of MNCs [59]. The isolated ECs in variously mentioned studies were characterized by immunofluorescence staining, such as factor VIII, vWF (von Willebrand factor), CD34, CD31, E-selectin (CD62E), ICAM-1 (CD54), and VCAM-1 (CD106) [55–58]; biochemical analysis where ECs were found to be alkaline phosphatase negative but were acid phosphatase positive [56]; ultrastructural identification of Weibel-Palade bodies by electron microscopy [55, 57, 58]; positive lectin binding (UEA-1) [56]; and analysis of surface markers by flow cytometry, such as vWF, CD34, CD31, CD14, ICAM-1, and VCAM-1 [58, 59]. Further, examination of surface morphology revealed different types of cells, for example, spindle-shaped [57–59], round shaped [56, 57], or cobblestone-shaped cells [58]. However, these cell shapes and indeed ECs were not well defined until ECs were isolated from peripheral blood [5], which portrays how a momentous research leads to an escalated renaissance in haematology.

There has been a radical shift of focus from BMECs to ECs in blood because peripheral blood ECs were stated to originate from BMECs [60, 61], although it is controversial and disputed at times [62]. In addition, withdrawing blood is a relatively noninvasive procedure. The movement of cells from bone marrow to peripheral blood that contributes to circulating endothelial progenitors (CEPs) is referred to as mobilization. As a result, ECs in the peripheral blood serve as the biomarker of various pathophysiological conditions, whereas BMECs represent the hot target zone. For example, ablating bone marrow endothelial progenitors not only does impair tumour growth associated with reduced vascularization [63] but also endorses the notion that ECs originate from bone marrow. However, there are other studies which substantiate that bone marrow-derived ECs do not contribute to vascular endothelium and tumour growth [64]. Nevertheless, despite controversies, BMECs still play a major role in neovascularization.

(2) Myeloid Cells. Myeloid cells are CD14+, and EPCs are CD14−. However, when CD14+ monocytes were isolated and grown under endothelial conditions for four weeks, there was an 80% reduction in CD14 expression with a significant increase in the expression of endothelial cell markers, such as vWf, VE, and eNOS (endothelial nitric oxide synthase/endothelial protein kinase A). Furthermore, these stimulated

cells also developed cord- and tubular-like structures in vitro. Therefore, monocytes or cells with the CD14+ phenotype can also acquire an endothelial phenotype under angiogenic conditions [65]. Also, when EPCs derived from induced CD14− mononuclear cells were implanted into ischaemic hind limbs, immediate neovascularization was observed but neovascularization did not occur when uninduced CD14+ cells or macrophages and dendritic cells derived from CD14+ cells were introduced [66].

(3) Mesenchymal Stem Cells (MSCs). As discussed above, adult bone marrow is a heterogenous mixture of haematopoietic as well as mesenchymal stem cells. Friedenstein and coworkers were the first to isolate colony-forming unit fibroblasts (CFU-Fs) from bone marrow [67]. The name CFU-F has been progressively replaced by various indistinct terms, such as marrow stromal fibroblasts (MSF), marrow stromal stem cells [68], mesenchymal adult progenitor cell (MAPC) [69], or the now widely accepted term mesenchymal stem cells (MSCs). These MSCs were isolated by two techniques: either by density centrifugation [70] or by isolating CD45−/ glycophorin A−/TERR119− cells from bone marrow cells [69, 71]. Flow cytometric analysis revealed that these MSCs were positive for CD29, CD71, CD73 (SH3), CD90, CD105 (SH2), CD106, CD144, CD120a, and CD 124 [69–72], while they were negative for CD34, CD31, VEGFR2, CD62E, vWF, VE-cadherin, VCAM-1, and ICAM-1 [69–72]. CD44 was present in some studies [70, 72], whereas it was absent in others [69].

When these MSCs were grown under endothelial conditions, they acquired characteristics of ECs and were found to be positive for VEGFR2, vWF, and VE-cadherin [69, 71, 72]. It is noteworthy that CD31 was expressed late [69, 72]. Also, it was found that these differentiated ECs contributed to neovascularization in tumour models [69, 71] and wound healing models [69]. Moreover, when undifferentiated MSCs were injected, they not only contributed to increased vascularity [69, 73] but also augmented cardiac function in chronic ischaemic models suggesting that transdifferentiation of MSCs to ECs is mediated through a paracrine mechanism [74].

5.1.2. Nonhaematopoietic EPCs

(1) Peripheral Blood. Blood vessels are lined by the endothelium which was initially perceived to be a fixed structure having limited or no self-renewal ability. However, the hypothesis changed with the earliest study providing evidence that there are certain cells present in the blood which are responsible for endothelial turnover [75]. Thereafter, the levels of ECs or EC remnants were reported to be raised in the blood of patients with cardiovascular diseases [76, 77] and cancer [78]. At that time, the method of EC identification was crude using either cytologic staining of cell smears from leukocyte concentrate [76, 78] or morphologic recognition of EC-like "carcasses" in platelet-rich plasma [77]. The earliest method to quantify ECs was based on the separation of ECs from the whole blood based by density gradient sedimentation. However, this method

TABLE 1: Differences between eEPCs and lEPCs.

	Early EPCs	Late EPCs
Synonyms	CACs [82]	OECs [83, 91] or ECFCs [84]
Cell population [81, 91]	Heterogeneous	Homogenous
Cell morphology [81]	Spindle-shaped cells	Cobblestone-like cells
Appearance in culture	<1 week [5, 81]	2–4 weeks [81]
Lifespan [81]	3-4 weeks	≈12 weeks
Morphogenic potential [81]	Low	High
Angiogenic potential [81]	Good	Good
Tube formation *in vitro* [5, 92, 134]		
Tube formation by EPCs alone	*Absent*	*Present*
Tube formation by EPCs with HUVECs	*Absent*	*Present*
Tube formation *in vivo* [92]	Absent	Present
Neovascularization *in vivo* [82, 92, 93, 134]	Indirect paracrine fashion	Directly providing ECs; hence can be referred to as "true EPCs"
Surface expression		
CD34 [88, 134]	+	+
CD45 [81, 88, 134]	+	−
CD14	+ and − [91, 93]/+ [92]	−
CD133	− [88] and + [89, 136]	− [88, 89, 136]
CD31 (PECAM 1) [81, 134, 137]	−/+	++
VEGFR-2 [81, 92, 93, 134, 137]	−/+	++
VE cadherin [81, 93, 134]	−/+	++
vWf [81]	−/+	+
Phenotype [90]	Monocytic	Endothelial
AcLDL uptake [5]	+	++
Lectin binding [5]	+	++
NO production [5]	+	++

+: present; ++: strongly present; −: absent; and −/+: limited/weak/focal.

was not EC specific [79], and therefore, another method was followed which used indirect immunofluorescence with the CLB-HEC 19 antibody to specifically identify EC cells [80]. In this study, it was reported that the minimal detectable concentration of CECs was 0.06 cells/mL of whole blood [80].

However, it was not until the end of the twentieth century when Asahara et al. revolutionized haematopoiesis and neovascularization by isolating and culturing endothelial cells from the peripheral blood [5]. These ECs have "spindle-shaped" morphology and were characterized by various markers, an ability to uptake acLDL and an ability to bind UEA-1. These "spindle-shaped" ECs were later termed early EPCs (eEPCs) [81] or circulating angiogenic cells (CACs) [82]. However, if the MNCs are cultured for a longer period, such as >2 weeks, ECs with a "cobblestone" morphology appear and are referred to as outgrowth endothelial cells (OECs) [83], late EPCs (lEPCs) [81], or endothelial colony-forming cells (ECFCs) [84]. Collectively, these cells are termed as circulating endothelial progenitors (CEPs). After the experiments by Asahara and his coworkers [5], numerous studies were conducted to isolate, classify, and define these eEPCs and lEPCs. We have enumerated the differences between eEPCs and lEPCs in Table 1.

Although there is no accord between the phenotype of CECs and CEPs, emerging evidence from the plethora of studies indicate that CECs are distinctly different from CEPs. CECs are mature cells that are not culturable and might consist of two types of the population of cells: firstly, the majority of the cells that are sloughed off from the vessel wall either normally or abnormally and secondly, cells that are matured from lEPCs or in various stages of maturation from CEPs that may or may not reside in the vessel wall. In normal cases, CECs as well as CEPs are extremely low. However, their concentration is influenced by various exogenous factors, endogenous factors, and pathological conditions which are discussed elaborately in this review. For example, CECs in healthy subjects were <3 cells/mL of whole blood. However, in patients with sickle cell anaemia, their concentration increases to 5–10-fold [85]. Similarly, lEPCs were found to be in between 0.05 and 0.2 cells/mL [84]; however, their concentration increases markedly after exercise [86]. Therefore, it is quite obvious that CECs originated from the vessel wall (e.g., conditions related to endothelial dysfunction) and represent biomarkers for vascular injury (e.g., CVD), whereas CEPs originate from bone marrow with conditions that will either stimulate bone marrow (such as tissue ischaemia in exercise) or suppress bone marrow (e.g., diabetes) and may

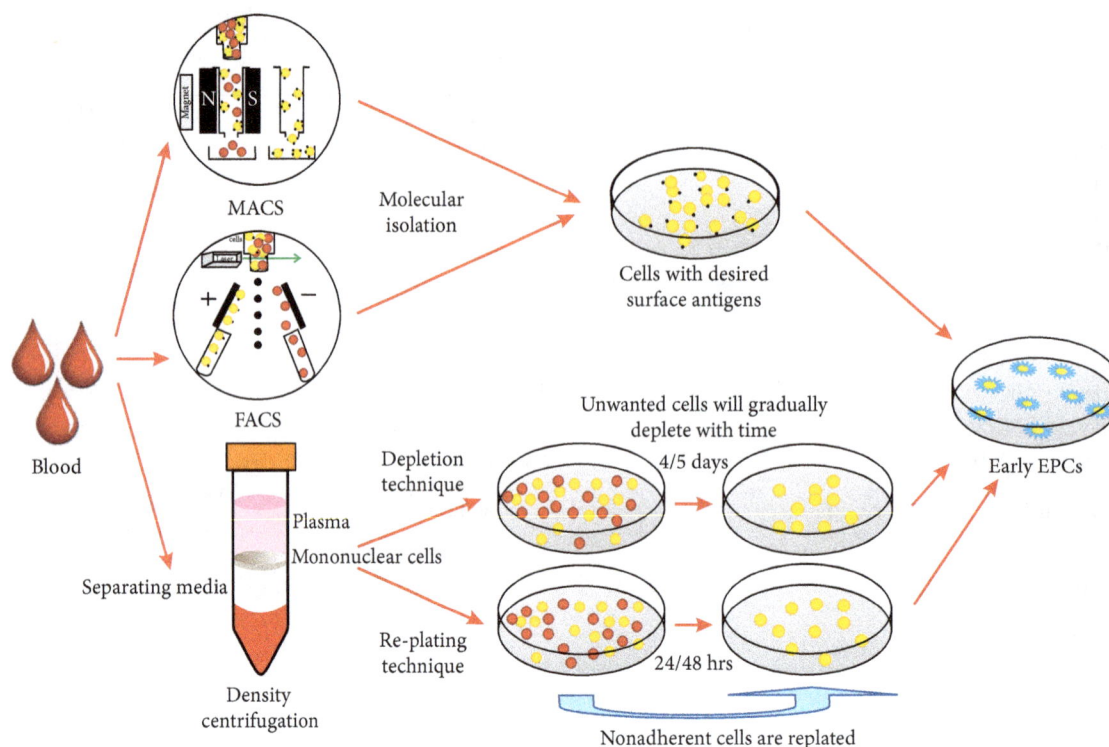

FIGURE 4: Isolation of EPCs by various techniques.

(e.g., myocardial infarction) or may not (e.g., tumour) contribute to vascular repair.

Nevertheless, the isolation of these ECs can be summarized into three basic techniques, which were later modified by various researchers (Figure 4).

(1.1) Molecular Isolation. In this technique, cells are identified based on their expression of cell surface markers. There are two methods that facilitate molecular recognition; one is MACS which employs the use of magnetic beads coated with the antibody/protein of choice, and another is FACS, which works on the principle of excitation and emission of fluorochromes bonded to the antibody/protein. Isolation of BMECs by MACS using UEA-1 was the earliest evidence in the literature of ECs [57, 58]. In fact, MACS was also used in the landmark study to isolate $CD34^+$ cells from human peripheral blood with the aim to identify putative ECs [5]. When these $CD34^+$ cells were plated on FN-coated dishes, they became spindle shaped within three days. However, when both $CD34^+$ cells and $CD34^-$ cells were cocultured, clusters of round cells appeared centrally with spindle-shaped cells at the periphery. This morphology represented reminiscent of the blood island-like groups typically found in the developing embryonic yolk sac [87]. Additionally, when these $CD34^+$ cells were injected into rabbits or ischaemic mouse hind limbs, DiI-labelled $CD34^+$ cells were localized exclusively at the neovascular zones of the ischaemic limb [5]. The assay can also now be performed using a commercially available kit (EndoCult; STEMCELL Technologies, Vancouver, BC, Canada).

On the other hand, FACS is relatively technique sensitive but with rapid advancement in technology; instead of MACS,

FACS has not only gained significant attention but is now the mainstay to isolate, classify, and analyse CEPs as well as CECs [88–90] because of its versatility and ease in obtaining a high percentage of pure populations.

(1.2) Depletion Technique. The depletion technique involves plating MNCs on FN-coated dishes for approximately four days. The nonadherent cells are then removed by washing with PBS, leaving MNCs on the dish. The four-day period is selected because the unwanted platelets, red blood cells, or monocytes are gradually depleted over this period. The number of days is, however, not fixed and has been modified by various researchers. Spindle-shaped cells, referred to as eEPCs, will appear after 6-7 days of culture [81], whereas "cobblestone" cells, referred to as lEPCs, will appear after four weeks in culture [81]. This procedure is not only used widely to isolate and characterize EPCs but has also been modified by various researchers [81, 82, 91, 92].

(1.3) Replating Technique. The fundamental principle of the replating method is to replate the nonadherent cells after plating the MNCs. The rationale for preplating the MNCs is to remove any monocytes, macrophages, or circulating mature ECs that might be present in the MNC sample [93]. The nonadherent cells were recovered either after 24 hours [94] or after 48 hours [95] and then replated and assessed. The later assay has been commercialized and is referred to as colony-forming unit Hill assay. CFU-Hill assay has demonstrated a significant inverse correlation between the circulating CFU-Hill concentration and Framingham cardiovascular risk score in human subjects [95]. However, the use of this technique for the isolation of

EPCs has not garnered significant attention as it has resulted in mixed results.

(2) Umbilical Cord Blood (UCB) EPCs. Human cord blood is a rich source of HPs [96]. EPCs have been successfully isolated from UCB [84, 97]. In fact, when the same volumes of UCB and peripheral blood were taken for isolating EPCs, not only the EC colonies appeared earlier in UCB but also these colonies were larger in size as well as 15 times more than that found in adult peripheral blood [84]. Additionally, the plasticity and telomerase activity of UCB-derived EPCs are also much higher than those of peripheral blood-derived EPCs. Moreover, when UCB-derived EPCs were transplanted in the ischaemic hind limb of immunodeficient nude rats, it promoted limb recovery by neovascularization of ischaemic hind limbs [97].

5.1.3. Tissue-Resident EPCs

(1) Umbilical Cord. In the Wharton's jelly (the connective tissue within the umbilical cord), abundant cells that exhibit MSC markers (SH2 and SH3) but not markers of haematopoietic differentiation (CD34 and CD45) were found and they were named umbilical cord stem cells (UCSCs) [98]. Furthermore, MSC-like cells were also isolated from the subendothelial layer of the umbilical cord vein [99]. When these UCSCs were subjected to endothelial conditions, they differentiated into ECs with a phenotype and function-like lEPCs. Additionally, when these EPCs were transplanted in murine ischaemic hind limbs, they promoted neovascularization [100].

(2) Adipose Tissue. Human adipose tissue also contains multipotent stem cells that can be easily harvested. Processed lipoaspirate contains cells that show multidifferentiation potential similar to MSCs but have a different phenotypic characterization [101, 102]. This unique population of cells distinct from MSCs is called adipose-derived stem cells (ADSCs) [101, 102]. The $CD34^+CD31^-$ ADSCs can differentiate into ECs and augment postnatal neovascularization [103, 104]. Interestingly, $CD34^-CD31^-$ ADSCs are also shown to differentiate into ECs and contribute to neovascularization, suggesting a common ancestor for a phenotypically different subpopulation of ADSCs [105].

(3) Cardiac Tissue. The perception that the adult heart is a postmitotic organ without regenerative capacity has changed dramatically after the isolation of $C-KIT^+Lin^-$ cells from the heart of adult rats [106]. These cells were shown to be self-renewing, clonogenic, and multipotent, exhibiting cardiogenic differentiation potential into three main cell types: cardiomyocytes (CMs), smooth muscle cells (SMCs), and ECs [106], which represent the cardiogenic lineage. When these $C-KIT^+Lin^-$ cells were injected into the ischaemic hearts of rats, functional myocardium was regenerated and more animal survived [106]. In contrast, another study demonstrated that $SCA-1^+C-KIT^-$ cells from mouse hearts could be induced by 5-azacytidine *in vitro* to differentiate towards the cardiac myogenic lineage. Furthermore, when administered intravenously, $SCA-1^+C-KIT^-$ cells ameliorated myocardial injury by differentiating into CMs [107]. Unlike C-KIT, SCA-1 is not expressed in humans. The first evidence of human cardiac stem cells (hCSCs) was found by isolating $C-KIT^+$ cells from myocardial samples and observing that these $C-KIT^+$ cells differentiated predominantly into CMs and, to a lesser extent, into SMCs and ECs. When these $C-KIT^+$ cells were injected into the infarcted myocardium of immunodeficient mice and immunosuppressed rats, they could generate a chimeric heart containing human myocardium composed of myocytes, coronary resistance arterioles, and capillaries [108]. However, in recent studies by lineage tracing analysis in murine models, it was found that $C-KIT^+$ cells generated significant numbers of ECs but insignificant numbers of CMs [109, 110]. Therefore, although research on the ideal signature of cardiac stem cells (CSCs) continues [111], it is pertinent to note that ECs are a component of the triad of the cardiogenic lineage (CMs, SMCs, and ECs). Whether the EC lineage is analogous to the haematopoietic lineage that gives rise to all blood cells or follows distinct pathways requires further research. {For ongoing research in cardiac stem cells and myocardial regeneration, which is beyond the scope of this review, readers can consider reviewing articles [111, 112].}

(4) Neural Tissue. Neuronal cells were thought to be tissue specific and unipotent until the transdifferentiation of adult neuronal stem cells (NSCs) into HSCs was demonstrated following their transplantation into the haematopoietic niche of mice [113]. However, the first evidence that neuroangiogenesis is a closely related phenomenon was uncovered by studying the fate of neuronal cells present in the subgranular zone (SGZ) of adult rats. During the first two hours after injecting BrdU- (bromodeoxyuridine-) labelled nonmitotic cells into the hippocampus of adult rats, approximately 37% of these cells exhibited endothelial markers, which gradually decreased to 9% after one month when more than 90% of the transplanted cells exhibited neural markers [114]. In fact, NSCs from the human embryo have also been shown to express several endothelial and haematopoietic markers [115]. *In vitro* studies supported that both NSCs [116, 117] and peripheral nerve-derived adult pluripotent stem cells (NEDAPS) [118] can be transdifferentiated to ECs. When NSCs were cocultured with ECs, only 6% of the NSCs differentiated into ECs. These differentiated ECs do not show any neurological markers; instead, they phenotypically express markers of the endothelial lineage [119]. Studies using an *in vivo* mouse model have shown that NSCs contribute to both neurogenesis and vasculogenesis in not only neuronal tissue but also non-neural tissue in adults [117]. All the above studies reflect two important findings: first, both NSCs and ECs share a common progenitor, and second, the local environment is crucial in governing the transdifferentiation of NSCs to ECs.

(5) Dental Tissues. Various types of stem cells have been found in the teeth and are referred to as dental stem cells [120].

(5.1) Dental Pulp Stem Cells (DPSCs). Stem cells from dental tissue were initially isolated from the dental pulp and are

termed as DPSCs. When DPSCs differentiated into osteogenic progenitors, some of the cells exhibit EC-like phenotypes and, therefore, gave rise to both osteoblasts and endotheliocytes [121]. This observation was further confirmed by another study showing that DPSCs form capillary-like structures in the presence of VEGFR and form vascular tubes on Matrigel, thereby suggesting their potential for EC differentiation [122].

Furthermore, when these DPSCs were transplanted *in vivo*, in the form of either woven bone tissue explants [121] or implanted as such in the chicken chorioallantoic membrane (CAM) assay [123], a significant increase in blood vessel density and infiltration within the host tissues was observed. In a recent study, it was also substantiated that these DPSCs can be used without any other ECs for regenerative purposes [124]. Moreover, the angiogenic potential of DPSCs was significantly increased when they were cocultured with ECs [125].

Another unique subset of stem cells referred to as side population cells (SPCs) has been identified in DPSCs. These SPCs are similar to EPCs as they express VEGFR-2 but not haematopoietic markers, such as CD45; however, unlike EPCs, SPCs do not express CD31 and CD146. SPCs also show multilineage differentiation potential and can be induced to form ECs with the expression of VEGFR-1$^+$ and VEGFR-2$^+$ and capacity to uptake acetylated-LDL and form a capillary-like network [126]. Furthermore, *in vivo* transplantation of SPCs can promote neovascularization of ischaemic mouse hind limbs [126, 127].

(5.2) Stem Cells from Human Exfoliated Deciduous Teeth (SHED). Human deciduous teeth are excellent and most readily available sources of stem cells [128]. SHED can differentiate into ECs and form functional blood vessels that anastomose with the host vasculature [129, 130]. Although there was no significant difference in the number of new blood vessels formed by SHED alone or SHED in combination with human dermal microvascular ECs (HDMECs), the microvascular organization was significantly improved when SHED were cocultured with HDMECs, thus increasing the chances of survival after transplantation [129]. The mechanism by which SHED differentiate into ECs depends on the crosstalk between STAT3 and MEK-1/ERK signalling. Unstimulated SHED express high levels of phosphorylated STAT3, which has an inverse relationship with the *MEK-1/ERK* gene. Inhibition of STAT3 activity by VEGFR induces MEK-1/ERK phosphorylation, resulting in differentiation of SHED into ECs, whereas inhibition of *MEK-1/ERK* gene results in the maintenance of STAT3 activity or the stemness of SHED [130].

(5.3) Stem Cells from Apical Papilla (SCAP). When SCAP and DPSCs were cocultured with ECs, the proangiogenic effect of SCAP was significantly weaker than that of DPSCs. In particular, although EC proliferation was not observed, significantly greater endothelial migration and tubulogenesis were noticed in DPSCs than in SCAP. Furthermore, both SCAP and DPSCs promoted angiogenesis in the CAM assay [131].

(5.4) Periodontal Ligament Stem Cells (PDLSCs). Similar to MSCs, PDLSCs have been shown to produce more VEGFR than SHED. *In vitro* Matrigel assay has shown no significant difference in the number of blood vessels formed from PDLSCs, MSCs, and SHED [132]. In coculture experiments, the angiogenic potential of PDLSCs cultured with ECs was significantly enhanced [132, 133] compared to ECs alone, which is similar to the above-discussed dental stem cells.

In summary, EPCs are either housed (e.g., in bone marrow, peripheral blood, and umbilical cord blood) or produced by transdifferentiation from various sources under the influence of microenvironments suitable for endothelial differentiation (Figure 3). The four phases of neovascularization include differentiation, proliferation, migration, and attachment of EPCs to form tubes. In general, the above studies reflected that both housed and transdifferentiated EPCs act via a paracrine mechanism; however, proliferation is significantly higher in housed EPCs than in transdifferentiated EPCs.

6. Role of the Surface Markers in ECs

Cell surface markers are proteins and carbohydrates attached to the cell membrane which play an important role in identification and investigation of cells by providing a specific target. In brief, these cell surface markers are like a fingerprint, specific to each kind of cell and capable of being identified through immunophenotyping. Various types of cell markers have been identified in ECs, such as CD34, a haematopoietic stem cell marker which is present in all types of ECs [88, 134]. CD45, a pan leukocytic marker is present only on eEPCs and not on lEPCs or CECs [81, 88, 134]. AC133/CD133 which is expressed on both haematopoietic stem and progenitor cells (HSCs) [135] is also expressed on eEPCs, while on CECs it is absent, reflecting that it is an early marker. On the other hand, conflicting reports exist on the expression of CD133 by lEPCs [88, 89, 136]. CD14 is a monocytic lineage marker. Various studies have confirmed that CD14 is present on eEPCs but not on lEPCs and CECs [93, 137]. VEGFR-2 (Flk-1 in mouse or KDR in humans) is a prominent endothelial cell marker. eEPCs show weak expression (focal expression) of VEGFR-2, but VEGFR-2 is strongly expressed in lEPCs and CECs [81, 92, 93, 134, 137]. Human endothelium constitutively expressed CD146 (also referred to as MUC18, MCAM, Mel-CAM, S-Endo-1, or P1H12 antigen) irrespectively of the anatomical localization [138–140]. Therefore, CECs can be defined by their ability to express CD146. In fact, various studies were carried out to isolate and define CECs by the expression of CD146 [83, 85, 141], and then these CD146$^+$ CEC cells were hypothesized to determine the prognosis of disease [142–144]. However, there is another caveat—CD146 can also be found on EPCs or even pericytes thereby further complicating the definitions. Additionally, various other markers, such as CD36, CD106, and vWf, have also been used infrequently in the literature. Therefore, in summary, a true definition of distinct ECs needs further investigation. Nevertheless, based upon the current evidence, we are here proposing the phenotypic definition of ECs which can apparently guide the researchers and scientific community in this field (Figure 5).

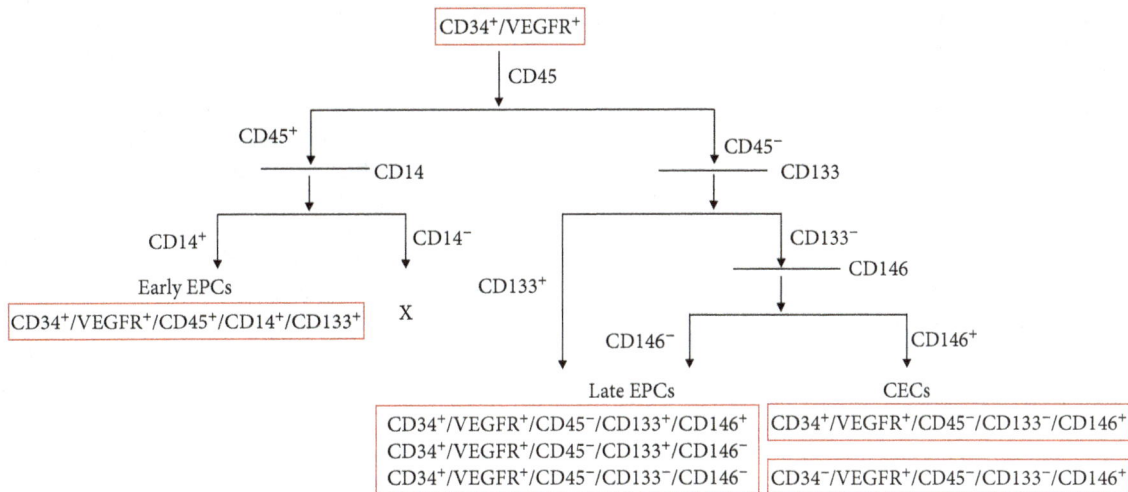

FIGURE 5: Phenotypic identity of ECs.

7. Current Prospects

The regulation of endothelial function by circulating EPCs opens a new avenue with immense potential in almost every realm of therapeutics because these circulating EPCs are affected by not only a plethora of exogenous and endogenous factors but also various pathological conditions. Therefore, EPCs are direct indicators of endothelial function.

7.1. Exogenous Factors

7.1.1. Exercise. Exercise is considered to be indispensable and vital for maintaining normal physiological functions. It has been observed that exercise for 10 minutes increases the level of EPCs in circulation by up to four times [86]. At the same time, *in vivo* studies on mice and subsequently humans with stable coronary artery diseases have also found that exercise increases the level of EPCs [145]. The increased EPC count was due to the mobilization of EPCs which has been shown to be NO dependent in a knockout mouse model (eNOS$^{-/-}$ mice) [145], wherein exercise enhances the phosphorylation of eNOS by activation of the PI3K (phosphatidylinositol 3 kinase/protein kinase B) pathway [146]. Further, it has also been demonstrated that hypoxia in tissues induced by exercise causes upregulation of hypoxia-inducible factor-1α (HIF-1α) which is responsible for the increased levels of proangiogenic cytokines, such as VEGF [147] and stromal-derived factor-1 (SDF) [148] with concomitant EPC mobilization.

Moreover, exercise also has a hormonal effect where it upregulated β2 adrenergic receptor signalling resulting in proliferation, migration, and differentiation by stimulation of proapoptosis and antiapoptosis pathways involving p38 MAPK (mitogen-activated protein kinases) and PI3K/AKT activation augmenting angiogenesis, both *in vitro* and *in vivo*, resulting in amelioration of neovascularization in animal models of hind limb ischaemia [149, 150].

It is also apparent through various observational and interventional studies that exercise helps in reducing inflammatory markers, such as C-reactive protein (CRP) and TNF-α [151]. CRP promotes apoptosis and attenuates the function and differentiation of EPCs [152], whereas TNF-α causes the diminution of proliferation and differentiation of EPCs [153]. As a result, exercise has a positive influence on EPCs by regulating inflammatory markers.

Subsequently, a positive correlation is established between exercise and EPCs in human subjects with acute myocardial infarction [154], chronic heart failure [155], peripheral arterial diseases [156], microvascular angina [157], and acute coronary syndrome [158] because all the above diseases have one common underlying pathogenesis, endothelial dysfunction, and reduced EPC number. Therefore, exercise is a major modifiable risk factor for cardiovascular disease (CVD) [159] where exercise plays a key role in attenuating the incidence and risk of CVD. Additionally, exercise is one of the components in the triad of "cardiac rehabilitation" (exercise counselling and training, education for heart-healthy living, and counselling to reduce stress) which according to American Heart Association (AHA) is a "medically supervised programme to improve cardiovascular health in case you have any experienced heart attack, heart failure, angioplasty, or heart surgery." In fact, various studies have proven a beneficial effect on endothelial function by improving the number of EPCs [158, 160].

Hence, it can be acknowledged that a sedentary lifestyle is the root cause of many problems and exercise has a holistic effect on health and on EPCs through mobilization, proliferation, differentiation, function, and survival.

7.1.2. Fasting. Fasting is an important ritual that is practised by many communities in the world. A certain degree of fasting may elicit profound and sustained beneficial metabolic, hormonal, and functional changes [161]. Recently, the effect of fasting on EPC regulation has been evaluated using a fasting stroke mouse model. In this study, focal cerebral ischaemia was induced in mice that subsequently underwent prolonged fasting (PF) or periodic PF. It was observed that PF not only significantly improved EPC-mediated angiogenesis, but also improved neurobehavioral outcomes. EPC functions, such as adhesion, migration and tube formation, as well as eNOS activity were significantly enhanced.

Moreover, the volume of the atrophied brain and the size of the cerebral infarct were reduced compared to the control group. Furthermore, transplantation of EPCs from PF mice ameliorated the cerebral ischaemic injury in the same PF mouse models [162].

However, there is a difference in the effects of fasting between rodents and humans because it was found that in rodents, fasting decreases serum insulin growth factor-1 (IGF-1) concentration by approximately 30–40%, whereas in humans, fasting did not reduce total and free IGF-1 levels unless protein intake was also reduced [163]. Therefore, it is interesting to identify the cumulative effect of fasting on human EPCs because it is known that IGF-1 causes proliferation of EPCs via the PI3K/AKT signalling pathway [164].

7.1.3. Smoking.
Smoking is hazardous to human health and is a major risk factor for many diseases. Moreover, smoking has been shown to significantly impair endothelial function and integrity [165, 166] as well as the number of circulating EPCs [165]. Subsequently, other studies have also confirmed that the number of EPCs is reduced in chronic smokers and cessation of smoking leads to restoration of the normal EPC level [167, 168].

It is intriguing to note that nicotine, a primary addictive agent in cigarettes, is considered to have a beneficial effect at low concentrations but concentrations above 10^{-6} mol/L are cytotoxic [169]. Nicotine increases EPC number and enhances EPC proliferation, migration, adhesion, and vasculogenesis *in vitro* in a dose-dependent manner with maximum activity peaking at concentrations equivalent to 10^{-8} mol/L [169]. A study investigated the impact of nicotine on EPCs in an *in vivo* murine model where it was found that EPC counts were not only significantly increased when nicotine was administered for three weeks, but when nicotine was administered in ischaemic hind limbs for four weeks, there was a significant improvement in blood perfusion compared to controls. It was hypothesized that the increased EPC activity was due to the antiapoptotic effect of nicotine on EPCs via activation of the nicotinic acetylcholine receptor (nAChR) [170]. However, in another study, it was postulated that nicotine activates telomerase activity through either the PI3K/AKT pathway (by increased phosphorylation of human telomerase reverse transcriptase (hTERT) [171, 172] or upregulation of sirtuin type 1 (SIRT1) protein expression [172]. Telomerase activity may be responsible for cellular senescence [173]. Therefore, the increased proliferative capacity of EPCs is due to the prevention of cellular senescence by nicotine. It is important to note that the above conclusions were drawn from short-term studies evaluating the effect of nicotine on EPCs after nicotine exposure of fewer than four weeks.

Recently, the effect of nicotine exposure on EPCs was evaluated for six months. It was observed that short-term nicotine exposure increased the proliferative capacity of EPCs, which is consistent with the above-described studies. However, at six months, there was a marked reversal in the number, functional impairment, and telomerase activity of EPCs [172].

Therefore, nicotine exposure causes an increase in EPC count for one month. After that, prolonged exposure results in decreased EPC number. It is noteworthy that the increase in EPCs during the first four weeks does not warrant that smoking is good because tobacco smoke has >4000 chemical constituents of which majority of them are deleterious to ECs [174]. Thus, the net effect of smoking is detrimental to ECs. Instead, the results validated the previous study conducted almost seven years back which found that nicotine patches (as a part of smoking cessation therapy) in patients had a significant reduction in exercise-induced myocardial ischaemia [175]. On the other hand, the second statement, i.e., "prolonged exposure to nicotine resulted in decreased EPC number," is an affirmation that smoking is injurious to health. As a result, the above study [172] underscores the cessation of smoking to prevent endothelial dysregulation.

7.1.4. Psychosocial Factors.
Depression is a common illness that has a negative impact on one's health and society [176]. It was observed that the number of mature and immature EPCs was reduced in patients with depression [177]. Furthermore, there was a significant inverse relationship between EPC levels and the severity of depressive symptoms [177].

In depression, the reduced EPC count is related to the increase in plasma concentrations of TNF-α and CRP [178]. CRP promotes apoptosis and attenuates the function and differentiation of EPCs [152], whereas TNF-α reduces the number of EPCs [153]. However, only TNF-α showed a statistically significant inverse correlation with EPC counts [177].

A study was conducted on healthy subjects (with no symptoms of angina or a history of CVD or diabetes mellitus) to explore the possible effect of depression on brachial artery flow-mediated dilation (FMD) and EPCs. It was found that depression was an independent predictor of decreased brachial FMD. Furthermore, impaired FMD was ultimately related to low levels of circulating EPCs [179]. Another study also reported similar results in patients with stable angina [180].

Therefore, endothelial dysregulation is also associated with depression.

7.2. Endogenous Factors

7.2.1. Serum Cholesterol.
Numerous studies have described the relationship of EPCs with lipid metabolism. Increased cholesterol level or hypercholesterolemia (HC) is one of the established risk factors for atherosclerotic vascular disease. It has been reported that HC attenuates angiogenesis and collateral vessel formation [181, 182]. Oxidized low-density lipoproteins (ox-LDL) induce dephosphorylation of the AKT kinase at Ser^{473} by activation of a serine/threonine phosphatase, resulting in deactivation of a downstream pathway or dephosphorylation of phosphorylated products of PI3K by either phosphatase and tensin homologue deleted on chromosome 10 (*PTEN*) or SH2-domain-containing inositol 5-phosphatase-2 (*SHIP-2*) [183]. PI3K is at the topmost of the endothelial regulation pathway and is composed of 2 protein subunits, p83 and p110. Both of these protein subunits must remain together for downstream activity [184]. However, ox-LDL causes nitrosylation of the P85 subunit,

thereby impairing PI3K function and inactivating downstream pathways [185]. It is also important to note that the PI3K pathway functions in close association with the p38 MAPK pathway. PI3K induces cytoprotective effects, whereas the p38 MAPK pathway has proapoptotic effects. Therefore, dysregulation of the PI3K pathway by ox-LDL causes upregulation of the MAPK pathway, resulting in EPC apoptosis [186].

ox-LDL also causes upregulation of LOX-1 receptor expression in ECs, resulting in downregulation of eNOS expression and activity followed by AKT dephosphorylation [187]. The above findings are further confirmed by using mice genetically deficient in AKT [188] or eNOS [189], in which EPC function is reduced and postischaemic angiogenesis is compromised.

However, administration of VEGFR [181] or L-arginine [182] has been shown to augment angiogenesis in hypercholesterolemia partially. L-Arginine is the substrate for eNOS which in turn is responsible for the production of nitric oxide and plays a crucial role in the proliferation, migration, and delayed senescence of EPCs [190]. On the other hand, VEGFR or statins (HMG-CoA reductase inhibitors) induce EPC differentiation by stimulating the PI3K/AKT pathway [191]. Further, VEGFR also stimulates the p38 MAPK pathway. Therefore, the level of either p38 MAPK or PI3K activation decides whether EPCs undergo apoptosis or cell proliferation, respectively [192].

In summary, HC and, in particular, ox-LDL have a marked impact on the functional characteristics of EPCs, including proliferation, migration, and apoptosis.

7.3. Pathological Diseases/Conditions

7.3.1. Hypertension.
Chronic hypertension (CH) is one of the most prevalent diseases worldwide. Studies have shown that hypertension has an adverse effect on various stages of EPC regulation. For example, functional impairment (reduced mobilization) in EPCs is the most significant independent predictor of CH [95]. Furthermore, the levels of EPCs are significantly reduced in patients with hypertension. However, functional decline in EPCs seems to occur more commonly and earlier than the reduction in EPC quantity [193, 194] and lEPCs exhibit more significant declines in proliferative activity than other types of EPCs [195]. The relationship between hypertension and EPC function is further strengthened by the effect of antihypertensive drugs on EPCs through their different mechanisms of action [196–199] {readers can read the review by Luo et al. [200] to acquire more detailed insight on matters beyond the scope of this review}.

7.3.2. Diabetes Mellitus.
Diabetes mellitus is a metabolic anomaly characterized by increased glucose intolerance. Patients with type 1 and type 2 diabetes have fewer circulating EPCs compared to matched healthy subjects because of the reduced mobilization of EPCs from bone marrow either due to insufficient release of marrow-stimulating factors, such as VEGFR and SDF-1, which resulted in downregulation of hypoxia-induced factor (HIF-1) [201] or through the PI3K-AKT-eNOS pathway [190, 191]. Moreover, EPCs

of diabetic patients exhibit reduced proliferation, adhesion, migration, and incorporation into tubular structures [202, 203]. Additionally, there is an increase in EPC apoptosis due to the upregulation of ROS (reactive oxygen species) caused by hyperglycaemia and oxidative stress [204–206]. Therefore, diabetes affects all EPC regulatory pathways.

Also, many complications of diabetes, such as diabetic vasculopathy, cardiomyopathy, neuropathy, nephropathy, and retinopathy, are closely linked to the problem of vascularization [207]. Interestingly, among all these complications, there is a marked reduction in EPCs, except for retinopathy, which follows a reverse pattern [207]. Hence, diabetes is an "angiogenic paradox" in which the same diabetic patient at the same time can present with the complications of pervasive angiogenesis (for example, diabetic retinopathy) and of diminished angiogenesis (for example, symptomatic peripheral arterial disease (PAD) in diabetic vasculopathy). It is further convoluted that the integration of different complications might result in different outcomes from the one which is expected. For example, diabetic foot syndrome (DFS) can be due to the combination of neuropathy and PAD, and therefore, presumably, there should be a reduction in EPCs. However, it was found that the number of circulating EPCs in patients with diabetes and manifesting DFS was higher than that in patients with uncomplicated diabetes [208]. A positive correlation of VEGF-A, a proinflammatory cytokine, has been found to be associated with EPCs in diabetic patients [208, 209]. It has been postulated that the ischaemic tissues are responsible for the elevated levels of VEGF-A which in turn is responsible for the increase in circulating EPCs [208, 209]. Hence, comprehending the regulatory mechanism of angiogenesis and their association with EPCs might lead to EPC-based therapies, a clinical reality in treating diabetes.

7.3.3. Cardiovascular Diseases.
Endothelial dysfunction has been shown to be closely associated with CVDs, such as coronary artery disease (CAD), myocardial infarction (MI), and ischaemia [176]. The correlation was first reported by Shintani et al., where they identified that the CD34+ cells did not differ between the MI patients and controls on day 1 but CD34+ cell levels appeared to linearly grow, reaching a peak after seven days with a statistically significant difference as compared to controls [210]. In sharp contrast, another study found that the number of CD34+ cells was significantly higher in patients with MI at admission than in controls. This study even showed a decreasing trend in the number of circulating CD34+ cells in patients with MI, with the number of CD34+ cells significantly lower on day seven than at admission but still higher than those in control patients [211]. It is noticeable that in the first study, authors presumed that EPCs originate from CD34+ cells and did not quantify EPCs and, instead, performed a cell culture assay and stated that EPCs and their putative precursor, MNC CD34+, were mobilized into PB during an acute ischaemic event in humans peaking at 7 days [210]. However, in another study, authors quantify EPCs which were at a higher level at admission than at day 7 [211]. It is also interesting to note that the level of VEGF is proportional to that of CD34+

TABLE 2: Current status of EPC clinical trials related to various disorders and diseases. The table outlines the total number of clinical trials reported on ClinicalTrials.gov till 30/1/2018.

	Completed	Recruiting	Active, but not recruiting	Not yet recruiting	Terminated	Withdrawn	Unknown status	NA	Enrolled by invitation
Single parameter of a disease or disorder	90	37	13	8	14	10	38	0	1
Different parameters in a disease or combination of diseases with single or multiple parameters in each disease	47	17	3	3	7	1	12	1	0
Total(302)	137	54	16	11	21	11	50	1	1

in both studies [210, 211], but the VEGF level in first study peaked at day 7 [210], while in another study, it was highest at day 0 [211]. Nevertheless, in both studies, release of VEGF from ischaemic tissues was implicated as the primary factor responsible for increased EPCs.

In cases of chronic ischaemic cardiomyopathy, there was no significant difference in the number of progenitor cells between chronic ischaemic cardiomyopathic patients and controls, except in *in vitro* studies, where the functional capacity of EPCs (evaluated as colony-forming activity and the migratory response) appeared to be significantly reduced in chronic ischaemia patients as compared to controls [212]. However, patients with unstable angina had a significantly greater number of circulating EPCs and EPC-CFUs than patients with stable angina [213]. In this study, the authors discovered a positive correlation between CRP levels and EPC levels. However, they did not notice any interaction between EPCs and VEGF.

To elucidate the role of EPCs in CVD, preclinical pig or rat models with ischaemic and infarct conditions were used [214, 215]. EPCs improved cardiomyocyte survival, increased myocardial contractility, and decreased the infarct size. Furthermore, thymosin $\beta4$, which is an essential paracrine factor of EPCs, also ameliorated the prognosis of myocardial infarction by reducing cardiomyocyte apoptosis, increasing myocardial contractility and decreasing the infarct size [214, 215]. Therefore, EPCs not only are considered a prognostic marker but also are of therapeutic value in CVD.

7.3.4. Cerebrovascular Diseases. There is a well-established relationship between cerebrovascular disease and EPCs. The number of circulating EPCs has been shown to increase rapidly in the acute phase of ischaemic stroke [216–219]. The increase in EPCs has been associated with positive neurological and functional outcomes, reduced infarct growth, and neurological improvement [219–221].

The most severe complication of stroke is intracerebral haemorrhage (ICH), which occurs in approximately 10–15% of all stroke cases. In a recent study on patients who had suffered from an acute ischaemic stroke, increased EPC count at day seven is associated with good functional outcome and reduced ICH residual volume [222]. With limited therapeutic options for ICH, studies on EPCs are important for the development of new treatment modalities.

Additionally, the fate of EPCs after transplantation into areas of ICH needs to be explored further.

7.3.5. Erectile Dysfunction. Erectile dysfunction is defined as the consistent inability to obtain or maintain an erection for satisfactory sexual relations. There are two types of erectile dysfunction: vasculogenic and neurogenic erectile dysfunctions. As endothelial dysfunction is considered one of the aetiologies of erectile dysfunction, the relationship between vasculogenic erectile dysfunction and EPCs is of interest. The number of circulating $CD34^+CD133^+$ EPCs is significantly reduced in patients with erectile dysfunction without known cardiovascular risk factors [223]. In patients with cardiovascular risk factors, although the number of $CD34^+/VEGFR-2^+$ cells is not affected, the number of $CD133^+$ circulating EPCs is reduced [224]. Furthermore, as erectile dysfunction is also a complication of overweight and type-1 DM, the number of $CD34^+VEGFR-2^+$ EPCs has been found to be correlated with the severity of erectile dysfunction [225, 226]. Therefore, EPCs might serve as a valuable diagnostic tool.

Regarding treatment strategies, a recent study showed that intracavernous injection of EPCs into the corpora cavernosa of rats with erectile dysfunction caused by bilateral cavernous nerve injury could restore erectile function [227]. In summary, the close correlation between erectile dysfunction and penile vascular dysfunction suggests that EPCs may have great therapeutic potential.

7.3.6. Cancer. Vascularization is a critical component of tumour growth and progression. Moreover, EPCs (including CECs) are increased in the peripheral blood of patients with various cancers, such as multiple myeloma [228], acute myeloid leukaemia [229, 230], nonsmall cell lung cancer (NSCLC) [231], hepatocellular carcinoma [232, 233], breast cancer [234–236], ovarian cancer [237], chronic lymphocytic leukaemia (CLL) [238], renal cell carcinoma (RCC) [239, 240], and endometrial cancer [241]. CECs have been implicated in tumour progression and aggressiveness [230, 231, 235, 237, 238, 240, 241]. Furthermore, in malignant breast carcinoma, EPCs are resistant to the cytokine TNF-α, which is responsible for inducing apoptosis [242].

Therefore, in cancer, EPCs may not only serve as a biomarker but also their regulation may be a critical therapeutic approach.

TABLE 3: Current status of clinical trials investigating EPCs and its relation to a single factor in disorders or diseases.

	Completed (90)	Recruiting (37)	Active, but not recruiting (13)	Not yet recruiting (8)	Terminated (14)	Withdrawn (10)	Unknown status (38)	NA (0)	Enrolled by invitation (1)
Disorder of CVS	47 — e.g., MI, angina, hypertension, peripheral vascular disease (PVD), arteriosclerosis, coronary artery ischaemia	15 — e.g., MI, cardiomyopathy, coronary artery disease (CAD), PVD, critical limb ischaemia (CLI), atherosclerosis	7 — e.g., CAD, CLI, atherosclerosis	1 — CLI	8 — e.g., angina, CAD	5 — e.g., ischaemic congestive heart failure (CHF), lower limb ischaemia	15 — e.g., aortic aneurysm, CHF, CAD, PVD	0	
Renal disease	2 — End-stage renal disease and chronic kidney disease	1 — Acute kidney injury							
GIT disorders	3 — Liver cirrhosis, nonalcoholic fatty liver disease, and severe hepatic venoocclusive disease	2 — End-stage liver disease and sinusoidal obstruction syndrome					1 — Crohn's disease		
Endocrine disorders	13 — e.g., type I and type II DM	4 — e.g., type II DM	2 — e.g., type II DM etc.	2 — e.g., type II DM etc.		2 — e.g., type II DM	5 — e.g., type I and type II DM		
Neoplastic disorders	3 — e.g., breast cancer, colorectal cancer, and nonsmall cell lung cancer	2 — e.g., BRCA1, BRCA2 gene mutation, cervical cancer			4 — e.g., renal cell carcinoma, multiple myeloma		5 — e.g., breast cancer, lung cancer		
Healthy subjects	7 — e.g., healthy subjects	1 — Obesity	1 — Healthy	1 — Quality of life			1 — Morbid obesity		
Respiratory disease	2 — Idiopathic pulmonary arterial hypertension	1 — Pulmonary emphysema		1 — Pulmonary hypertension			3 — e.g., chronic obstructive pulmonary disease (COPD), idiopathic pulmonary arterial hypertension		
Reproductive disorders	3 — e.g., polycystic ovary syndrome (PCOS)				1 — e.g., PCOS				

TABLE 3: Continued.

	Completed (90)	Recruiting (37)	Active, but not recruiting (13)	Not yet recruiting (8)	Terminated (14)	Withdrawn (10)	Unknown status (38)	NA (0)	Enrolled by invitation (1)
Musculoskeletal disorders	1 Ankylosing spondylitis		1 Bone defects						
Neurologic diseases	2 Central nervous system and acute ischaemic stroke	4 Stroke, aneurysmal subarachnoid haemorrhage, and mild cognitive impairment	1 Brain and central nervous system tumours			2 Traumatic brain injury	2 Ischaemic stroke and migraine with aura		1 Diabetic foot ulcer
Hematological disorders	4 Endotoxemia, sickle cell anaemia, dyslipidemia, and hypoxia	5 Sickle cell disease without crisis, hypercholesterolemia, microgravity-exposed endothelial cells, hemolytic uremic syndrome, and soft-tissue sarcoma		2 Dystrophic epidermolysis bullosa and septic shock	1 Graft-versus-host disease	1 Sickle cell anaemia	4 Exercise anaphylaxis, recurrent adult Hodgkin lymphoma, acute myeloid leukemia, and brachial plexus (pressure)		
Autoimmune disorders		1 Systemic scleroderma					1 Systemic lupus erythematosus		
Dental disorders				1 Tooth impacted					
Miscellaneous	3 Burn, bullous keratopathy, ischaemic ulcer	1 Sepsis	1 Delayed graft function				1 SDF-1		

8. Current Clinical Trials

As EPCs play a significant role in pathophysiological functions of the human body, EPC therapies for various cardiovascular, endocrine, haematological, renal, respiratory, neoplastic, and other diseases are underway. A summary of clinical trials is shown in Tables 2 and 3. The data were taken from ClinicalTrials.gov after inputting EPCs as a "*key word.*" A total of 302 trials were registered as of 30/1/2018. Out of these 302 trials, 45.36% are completed and the remaining studies are in different phases (Table 2). Furthermore, it was intriguing to find that more than one-fourth of the studies were terminated, were withdrawn, or had unknown status (Table 2). It was also noteworthy that most clinical trials studied the relationship between EPCs and CVDs followed by endocrinal disorders and other diseases (Table 3). However, only one study focused on isolating dental mesenchymal cells from impacted teeth to construct prevascularized tissue-engineered bone.

9. Future Prospects

EPCs will play a pivotal role in regenerative medicine and cancer therapy besides acting as surrogate markers of future health problems. However, collaborations among clinicians, biomaterial scientists, and engineers will be pertinent to resolve various issues and to enable quick clinical translation.

9.1. Novel Stem Cell Differentiation and Animal Models. Further exploration of molecular and cellular events underlying the regulation of EPCs using newer stem cell differentiation and animal models is the need of the hour.

9.2. Isolation and Consensus on the Identity of EPCs. Significant progress has been made in cytology, but a novel EPC marker still needs to be identified. Furthermore, it is difficult to form a conclusion from results acquired using different protocols and apply the information to future advancements/clinical trials. Therefore, when expanding the knowledge, standardizing the identification of EPCs by both phenotype and function is imperative.

9.3. Rarity of EPCs. The number of EPCs in either peripheral blood (0.01%) or bone marrow (0.05%) is low; therefore, it is notoriously difficult to isolate EPCs. New advances in EPC isolation methods are required to improve success and yield.

9.4. Expansion of EPCs. Irrespective of the source, after the isolation of EPCs, the number of cells must be increased before further applications. However, passaging will inadvertently shift stem cells towards maturity with diminished stemness. Currently, methods to increase EPC number without increasing the passage of cells are lacking.

9.5. EPC Homing and Incorporation. Homing of EPCs will enable the targeted delivery of EPCs to the site of interest. With recent advances in nanotechnology and tissue engineering, the local distribution of cells seems to be possible.

9.6. Modulation of the Host Environment. It is agreed that cell survival and function depend on the local or systemic environment of the host. Hypoxia, increased inflammation, and free radicals may have adverse effects on EPC survival. Therefore, modulation of the host environment is very crucial to the success of cell-based therapies.

9.7. Translation of Bench-Side Models. Emphasis should be given to the translation of bench-side EPC study models to clinical trials.

10. Summary and Conclusion

With the identification of EPCs, the domain of neovascularization has metamorphosed. The findings from various research studies have begun to coalesce like a jigsaw puzzle. With significant achievements over a century, the origin of EPCs, the role of EPCs in angiogenesis and the physiopathological process, and the potential EPC-based therapeutic approaches have begun to be uncovered, but still, a lot of work remains. Clinically, EPCs can be applied in three different ways:

(1) *Potential Biomarker.* Disease identification and severity

(2) *Target Cells.* Anti-EPC therapy for tumours/cancer

(3) *Neovascularization.* Either alone or cocultured with various stem cells

Although the complexity surrounding the biology of EPCs has increased, the comprehensive understanding of EPCs has also increased; therefore, EPC-based therapies may eventually become a clinical reality.

Acknowledgments

HC was supported through a seed grant (no. 201511159105) awarded to EHNP and CFZ by University Research Grants for "3D cell sheets cultured from endothelial progenitor cells and periodontal ligament stem cells" (2016).

References

[1] J. Rouwkema, N. C. Rivron, and C. A. van Blitterswijk, "Vascularization in tissue engineering," *Trends in Biotechnology*, vol. 26, no. 8, pp. 434–441, 2008.

[2] R. K. Jain, P. Au, J. Tam, D. G. Duda, and D. Fukumura, "Engineering vascularized tissue," *Nature Biotechnology*, vol. 23, no. 7, pp. 821–823, 2005.

[3] R. Lanza, R. Langer, and J. P. Vacanti, *Principles of Tissue Engineering*, Academic Press, 2011.

[4] P. D. F. Murray, "The development in vitro of the blood of the early chick embryo," *Proceedings of the Royal Society B: Biological Sciences*, vol. 111, no. 773, pp. 497–521, 1932.

[5] T. Asahara, T. Murohara, A. Sullivan et al., "Isolation of putative progenitor endothelial cells for angiogenesis," *Science*, vol. 275, no. 5302, pp. 964–966, 1997.

[6] J. Hunter, *The Works of John Hunter, FRS*, Cambridge University Press, 2015.

[7] D. Ribatti, A. Vacca, B. Nico, L. Roncali, and F. Dammacco, "Postnatal vasculogenesis," *Mechanisms of Development*, vol. 100, no. 2, pp. 157–163, 2001.

[8] A. Helisch and W. Schaper, "Arteriogenesis: the development and growth of collateral arteries," *Microcirculation*, vol. 10, no. 1, pp. 83–97, 2003.

[9] M. Simons, "Angiogenesis: where do we stand now?," *Circulation*, vol. 111, no. 12, pp. 1556–1566, 2005.

[10] F. R. Sabin, "Studies on the origin of blood vessels and of red corpuscles as seen in the living blastoderm of the chick during the second day of incubation," *Contributions to Embryology*, vol. 9, pp. 213–262, 1920.

[11] R. C. Wagner, "Endothelial cell embryology and growth," *Advances in Microcirculation*, vol. 9, pp. 45–75, 1980.

[12] G. M. Keller, "In vitro differentiation of embryonic stem cells," *Current Opinion in Cell Biology*, vol. 7, no. 6, pp. 862–869, 1995.

[13] K. Choi, M. Kennedy, A. Kazarov, J. C. Papadimitriou, and G. Keller, "A common precursor for hematopoietic and endothelial cells," *Development*, vol. 125, no. 4, pp. 725–732, 1998.

[14] D. Vittet, M. H. Prandini, R. Berthier et al., "Embryonic stem cells differentiate in vitro to endothelial cells through successive maturation steps," *Blood*, vol. 88, no. 9, pp. 3424–3431, 1996.

[15] T. Peterkin, A. Gibson, and R. Patient, "Common genetic control of haemangioblast and cardiac development in zebrafish," *Development*, vol. 136, no. 9, pp. 1465–1474, 2009.

[16] M. J. Evans and M. H. Kaufman, "Establishment in culture of pluripotential cells from mouse embryos," *Nature*, vol. 292, no. 5819, pp. 154–156, 1981.

[17] G. R. Martin, "Isolation of a pluripotent cell line from early mouse embryos cultured in medium conditioned by teratocarcinoma stem cells," *Proceedings of the National Academy of Sciences of the United States of America*, vol. 78, no. 12, pp. 7634–7638, 1981.

[18] T. C. Doetschman, H. Eistetter, M. Katz, W. Schmidt, and R. Kemler, "The in vitro development of blastocyst-derived embryonic stem cell lines: formation of visceral yolk sac, blood islands and myocardium," *Journal of Embryology and Experimental Morphology*, vol. 87, no. 1, pp. 27–45, 1985.

[19] M. Kennedy, M. Firpo, K. Choi et al., "A common precursor for primitive erythropoiesis and definitive haematopoiesis," *Nature*, vol. 386, no. 6624, pp. 488–493, 1997.

[20] M. V. Wiles and G. Keller, "Multiple hematopoietic lineages develop from embryonic stem (ES) cells in culture," *Development*, vol. 111, no. 2, pp. 259–267, 1991.

[21] D. S. Kaufman, E. T. Hanson, R. L. Lewis, R. Auerbach, and J. A. Thomson, "Hematopoietic colony-forming cells derived from human embryonic stem cells," *Proceedings of the National Academy of Sciences of the United States of America*, vol. 98, no. 19, pp. 10716–10721, 2001.

[22] S. Levenberg, J. S. Golub, J. Amit, J. Itskovitz-Eldor, and R. Langer, "Endothelial cells derived from human embryonic stem cells," *Proceedings of the National Academy of Sciences of the United States of America*, vol. 99, no. 7, pp. 4391–4396, 2002.

[23] M. Kennedy, S. L. D'Souza, M. Lynch-Kattman, S. Schwantz, and G. Keller, "Development of the hemangioblast defines the onset of hematopoiesis in human ES cell differentiation cultures," *Blood*, vol. 109, no. 7, pp. 2679–2687, 2007.

[24] W. Matthews, C. T. Jordan, M. Gavin, N. A. Jenkins, N. G. Copeland, and I. R. Lemischka, "A receptor tyrosine kinase cDNA isolated from a population of enriched primitive hematopoietic cells and exhibiting close genetic linkage to c-kit," *Proceedings of the National Academy of Sciences of the United States of America*, vol. 88, no. 20, pp. 9026–9030, 1991.

[25] B. Millauer, S. Wizigmann-Voos, H. Schnürch et al., "High affinity VEGF binding and developmental expression suggest Flk-1 as a major regulator of vasculogenesis and angiogenesis," *Cell*, vol. 72, no. 6, pp. 835–846, 1993.

[26] F. Shalaby, J. Rossant, T. P. Yamaguchi et al., "Failure of blood-island formation and vasculogenesis in Flk-1-deficient mice," *Nature*, vol. 376, no. 6535, pp. 62–66, 1995.

[27] N. Kabrun, H. J. Buhring, K. Choi, A. Ullrich, W. Risau, and G. Keller, "Flk-1 expression defines a population of early embryonic hematopoietic precursors," *Development*, vol. 124, no. 10, pp. 2039–2048, 1997.

[28] S. Nishikawa, S. Nishikawa, M. Hirashima, N. Matsuyoshi, and H. Kodama, "Progressive lineage analysis by cell sorting and culture identifies FLK1$^+$VE-cadherin$^+$ cells at a diverging point of endothelial and hemopoietic lineages," *Development*, vol. 125, no. 9, pp. 1747–1757, 1998.

[29] T. L. Huber, V. Kouskoff, H. Joerg Fehling, J. Palis, and G. Keller, "Haemangioblast commitment is initiated in the primitive streak of the mouse embryo," *Nature*, vol. 432, no. 7017, pp. 625–630, 2004.

[30] C. Lancrin, P. Sroczynska, C. Stephenson, T. Allen, V. Kouskoff, and G. Lacaud, "The haemangioblast generates haematopoietic cells through a haemogenic endothelium stage," *Nature*, vol. 457, no. 7231, pp. 892–895, 2009.

[31] M. J. Ferkowicz, M. Starr, X. Xie et al., "CD41 expression defines the onset of primitive and definitive hematopoiesis in the murine embryo," *Development*, vol. 130, no. 18, pp. 4393–4403, 2003.

[32] M. T. Mitjavila-Garcia, M. Cailleret, I. Godin et al., "Expression of CD41 on hematopoietic progenitors derived from embryonic hematopoietic cells," *Development*, vol. 129, no. 8, pp. 2003–2013, 2002.

[33] H. K. Mikkola, Y. Fujiwara, T. M. Schlaeger, D. Traver, and S. H. Orkin, "Expression of CD41 marks the initiation of definitive hematopoiesis in the mouse embryo," *Blood*, vol. 101, no. 2, pp. 508–516, 2003.

[34] D. R. Phillips, L. A. Fitzgerald, I. F. Chard, and L. V. Parise, "The platelet membrane glycoprotein IIb/IIIa complex. Structure, function, and relationship to adhesive protein receptors in nucleated cells," *Annals of the New York Academy of Sciences*, vol. 509, no. 1, pp. 177–187, 1987.

[35] H. M. Eilken, S. I. Nishikawa, and T. Schroeder, "Continuous single-cell imaging of blood generation from haemogenic endothelium," *Nature*, vol. 457, no. 7231, pp. 896–900, 2009.

[36] K. Kissa and P. Herbomel, "Blood stem cells emerge from aortic endothelium by a novel type of cell transition," *Nature*, vol. 464, no. 7285, pp. 112–115, 2010.

[37] T. Fujimoto, M. Ogawa, N. Minegishi et al., "Step-wise divergence of primitive and definitive haematopoietic and endothelial cell lineages during embryonic stem cell differentiation," *Genes to Cells*, vol. 6, no. 12, pp. 1113–1127, 2001.

[38] T. Okuda, J. van Deursen, S. W. Hiebert, G. Grosveld, and J. R. Downing, "AML1, the target of multiple chromosomal translocations in human leukemia, is essential for normal fetal liver hematopoiesis," *Cell*, vol. 84, no. 2, pp. 321–330, 1996.

[39] Q. Wang, T. Stacy, M. Binder, M. Marin-Padilla, A. H. Sharpe, and N. A. Speck, "Disruption of the Cbfa2 gene causes necrosis and hemorrhaging in the central nervous system and blocks definitive hematopoiesis," *Proceedings of the National Academy of Sciences of the United States of America*, vol. 93, no. 8, pp. 3444–3449, 1996.

[40] T. North, T. L. Gu, T. Stacy et al., "Cbfa2 is required for the formation of intra-aortic hematopoietic clusters," *Development*, vol. 126, no. 11, pp. 2563–2575, 1999.

[41] A. J. Warren, W. H. Colledge, M. B. L. Carlton, M. J. Evans, A. J. H. Smith, and T. H. Rabbitts, "The oncogenic cysteine-rich LIM domain protein rbtn2 is essential for erythroid development," *Cell*, vol. 78, no. 1, pp. 45–57, 1994.

[42] Y. Yamada, A. J. Warren, C. Dobson, A. Forster, R. Pannell, and T. H. Rabbitts, "The T cell leukemia LIM protein Lmo2 is necessary for adult mouse hematopoiesis," *Proceedings of the National Academy of Sciences of the United States of America*, vol. 95, no. 7, pp. 3890–3895, 1998.

[43] M. Gering, A. R. F. Rodaway, B. Göttgens, R. K. Patient, and A. R. Green, "The *SCL* gene specifies haemangioblast development from early mesoderm," *The EMBO Journal*, vol. 17, no. 14, pp. 4029–4045, 1998.

[44] M. Gering, Y. Yamada, T. H. Rabbitts, and R. K. Patient, "Lmo2 and Scl/Tal1 convert non-axial mesoderm into haemangioblasts which differentiate into endothelial cells in the absence of Gata1," *Development*, vol. 130, no. 25, pp. 6187–6199, 2003.

[45] L. J. Patterson, M. Gering, C. E. Eckfeldt et al., "The transcription factors Scl and Lmo2 act together during development of the hemangioblast in zebrafish," *Blood*, vol. 109, no. 6, pp. 2389–2398, 2007.

[46] L. Mandal, U. Banerjee, and V. Hartenstein, "Evidence for a fruit fly hemangioblast and similarities between lymph-gland hematopoiesis in fruit fly and mammal aorta-gonadal-mesonephros mesoderm," *Nature Genetics*, vol. 36, no. 9, pp. 1019–1023, 2004.

[47] K. M. Vogeli, S. W. Jin, G. R. Martin, and D. Y. R. Stainier, "A common progenitor for haematopoietic and endothelial lineages in the zebrafish gastrula," *Nature*, vol. 443, no. 7109, pp. 337–339, 2006.

[48] C. B. Kimmel, "Genetics and early development of zebrafish," *Trends in Genetics*, vol. 5, no. 8, pp. 283–288, 1989.

[49] W. Driever, D. Stemple, A. Schier, and L. Solnica-Krezel, "Zebrafish: genetic tools for studying vertebrate development," *Trends in Genetics*, vol. 10, no. 5, pp. 152–159, 1994.

[50] M. C. Fishman, "Zebrafish genetics: the enigma of arrival," *Proceedings of the National Academy of Sciences of the United States of America*, vol. 96, no. 19, pp. 10554–10556, 1999.

[51] C. B. Kimmel, R. M. Warga, and T. F. Schilling, "Origin and organization of the zebrafish fate map," *Development*, vol. 108, no. 4, pp. 581–594, 1990.

[52] R. K. Lee, D. Y. Stainier, B. M. Weinstein, and M. C. Fishman, "Cardiovascular development in the zebrafish. II. Endocardial progenitors are sequestered within the heart field," *Development*, vol. 120, no. 12, pp. 3361–3366, 1994.

[53] D. Y. R. Stainier and M. C. Fishman, "The zebrafish as a model system to study cardiovascular development," *Trends in Cardiovascular Medicine*, vol. 4, no. 5, pp. 207–212, 1994.

[54] J. J. Schoenebeck, B. R. Keegan, and D. Yelon, "Vessel and blood specification override cardiac potential in anterior mesoderm," *Developmental Cell*, vol. 13, no. 2, pp. 254–267, 2007.

[55] S. Irie and M. Tavassoli, "Purification and characterization of rat bone marrow endothelial cells," *Experimental Hematology*, vol. 14, no. 10, pp. 912–918, 1986.

[56] R. G. Fei, P. E. Penn, and N. S. Wolf, "A method to establish pure fibroblast and endothelial cell colony cultures from murine bone marrow," *Experimental Hematology*, vol. 18, no. 8, pp. 953–957, 1990.

[57] L. C. Masek and J. W. Sweetenham, "Isolation and culture of endothelial cells from human bone marrow," *British Journal of Haematology*, vol. 88, no. 4, pp. 855–865, 1994.

[58] S. Rafii, F. Shapiro, J. Rimarachin et al., "Isolation and characterization of human bone marrow microvascular endothelial cells: hematopoietic progenitor cell adhesion," *Blood*, vol. 84, no. 1, pp. 10–19, 1994.

[59] C. M. Schweitzer, C. van der Schoot, A. M. Dräger et al., "Isolation and culture of human bone marrow endothelial cells," *Experimental Hematology*, vol. 23, no. 1, pp. 41–48, 1995.

[60] Q. Shi, S. Rafii, M. H. Wu et al., "Evidence for circulating bone marrow-derived endothelial cells," *Blood*, vol. 92, no. 2, pp. 362–367, 1998.

[61] T. Asahara, H. Masuda, T. Takahashi et al., "Bone marrow origin of endothelial progenitor cells responsible for postnatal vasculogenesis in physiological and pathological neovascularization," *Circulation Research*, vol. 85, no. 3, pp. 221–228, 1999.

[62] O. Tura, E. M. Skinner, G. R. Barclay et al., "Late outgrowth endothelial cells resemble mature endothelial cells and are not derived from bone marrow," *Stem Cells*, vol. 31, no. 2, pp. 338–348, 2013.

[63] D. J. Nolan, A. Ciarrocchi, A. S. Mellick et al., "Bone marrow-derived endothelial progenitor cells are a major determinant of nascent tumor neovascularization," *Genes & Development*, vol. 21, no. 12, pp. 1546–1558, 2007.

[64] S. Purhonen, J. Palm, D. Rossi et al., "Bone marrow-derived circulating endothelial precursors do not contribute to vascular endothelium and are not needed for tumor growth," *Proceedings of the National Academy of Sciences of the United States of America*, vol. 105, no. 18, pp. 6620–6625, 2008.

[65] A. Schmeisser, C. D. Garlichs, H. Zhang et al., "Monocytes coexpress endothelial and macrophagocytic lineage markers and form cord-like structures in Matrigel® under angiogenic conditions," *Cardiovascular Research*, vol. 49, no. 3, pp. 671–680, 2001.

[66] C. Urbich, C. Heeschen, A. Aicher, E. Dernbach, A. M. Zeiher, and S. Dimmeler, "Relevance of monocytic features for neovascularization capacity of circulating endothelial progenitor cells," *Circulation*, vol. 108, no. 20, pp. 2511–2516, 2003.

[67] A. J. Friedenstein, J. F. Gorskaja, and N. N. Kulagina, "Fibroblast precursors in normal and irradiated mouse hematopoietic organs," *Experimental Hematology*, vol. 4, no. 5, pp. 267–274, 1976.

[68] M. Owen, "Marrow stromal stem cells," *Journal of Cell Science*, vol. 1988, pp. 63–76, 1988.

[69] M. Reyes, A. Dudek, B. Jahagirdar, L. Koodie, P. H. Marker, and C. M. Verfaillie, "Origin of endothelial progenitors in human postnatal bone marrow," *The Journal of Clinical Investigation*, vol. 109, no. 3, pp. 337–346, 2002.

[70] M. F. Pittenger, A. M. Mackay, S. C. Beck et al., "Multilineage potential of adult human mesenchymal stem cells," *Science*, vol. 284, no. 5411, pp. 143–147, 1999.

[71] Y. Jiang, B. N. Jahagirdar, R. L. Reinhardt et al., "Pluripotency of mesenchymal stem cells derived from adult marrow," *Nature*, vol. 418, no. 6893, pp. 41–49, 2002.

[72] J. Oswald, S. Boxberger, B. Jorgensen et al., "Mesenchymal stem cells can be differentiated into endothelial cells in vitro," *Stem Cells*, vol. 22, no. 3, pp. 377–384, 2004.

[73] G. V. Silva, S. Litovsky, J. A. Assad et al., "Mesenchymal stem cells differentiate into an endothelial phenotype, enhance vascular density, and improve heart function in a canine chronic ischemia model," *Circulation*, vol. 111, no. 2, pp. 150–156, 2005.

[74] T. Kinnaird, E. Stabile, M. S. Burnett et al., "Local delivery of marrow-derived stromal cells augments collateral perfusion through paracrine mechanisms," *Circulation*, vol. 109, no. 12, pp. 1543–1549, 2004.

[75] M. M. Stump, G. L. Jordan Jr., M. E. De Bakey, and B. Halpert, "Endothelium grown from circulating blood on isolated intravascular Dacron hub," *The American Journal of Pathology*, vol. 43, no. 3, pp. 361–367, 1963.

[76] C. A. Bouvier, "Circulating endothelium as an indication of vascular injury," *Thrombosis et Diathesis Haemorrhagica*, vol. 40, p. 163, 1970.

[77] J. Hladovec, I. Prerovsky, V. Stanek, and J. Fabian, "Circulating endothelial cells in acute myocardial infarction and angina pectoris," *Klinische Wochenschrift*, vol. 56, no. 20, pp. 1033–1036, 1978.

[78] J. Valaitis, E. McGrew, R. McGrath, and S. S. Roberts, "Capillary cell clusters in peripheral blood of postoperative cancer and noncancer patients," *Acta Cytologica*, vol. 12, no. 6, pp. 439–444, 1968.

[79] H. Takahashi and L. A. Harker, "Measurement of human endothelial cells in whole blood," *Thrombosis Research*, vol. 31, no. 1, pp. 1–12, 1983.

[80] R. Sbarbati, M. de Boer, M. Marzilli, M. Scarlattini, G. Rossi, and J. van Mourik, "Immunologic detection of endothelial cells in human whole blood," *Blood*, vol. 77, no. 4, pp. 764–769, 1991.

[81] J. Hur, C. H. Yoon, H. S. Kim et al., "Characterization of two types of endothelial progenitor cells and their different contributions to neovasculogenesis," *Arteriosclerosis, Thrombosis, and Vascular Biology*, vol. 24, no. 2, pp. 288–293, 2004.

[82] J. Rehman, J. Li, C. M. Orschell, and K. L. March, "Peripheral blood "endothelial progenitor cells" are derived from monocyte/macrophages and secrete angiogenic growth factors," *Circulation*, vol. 107, no. 8, pp. 1164–1169, 2003.

[83] Y. Lin, D. J. Weisdorf, A. Solovey, and R. P. Hebbel, "Origins of circulating endothelial cells and endothelial outgrowth from blood," *The Journal of Clinical Investigation*, vol. 105, no. 1, pp. 71–77, 2000.

[84] D. A. Ingram, L. E. Mead, H. Tanaka et al., "Identification of a novel hierarchy of endothelial progenitor cells using human peripheral and umbilical cord blood," *Blood*, vol. 104, no. 9, pp. 2752–2760, 2004.

[85] A. Solovey, Y. Lin, P. Browne, S. Choong, E. Wayner, and R. P. Hebbel, "Circulating activated endothelial cells in sickle cell anemia," *The New England Journal of Medicine*, vol. 337, no. 22, pp. 1584–1590, 1997.

[86] J. Rehman, J. Li, L. Parvathaneni et al., "Exercise acutely increases circulating endothelial progenitor cells and monocyte-/macrophage-derived angiogenic cells," *Journal of the American College of Cardiology*, vol. 43, no. 12, pp. 2314–2318, 2004.

[87] I. Flamme and W. Risau, "Induction of vasculogenesis and hematopoiesis in vitro," *Development*, vol. 116, no. 2, pp. 435–439, 1992.

[88] F. Timmermans, F. Van Hauwermeiren, M. De Smedt et al., "Endothelial outgrowth cells are not derived from CD133$^+$ cells or CD45$^+$ hematopoietic precursors," *Arteriosclerosis, Thrombosis, and Vascular Biology*, vol. 27, no. 7, pp. 1572–1579, 2007.

[89] M. Peichev, A. J. Naiyer, D. Pereira et al., "Expression of VEGFR-2 and AC133 by circulating human CD34$^+$ cells identifies a population of functional endothelial precursors," *Blood*, vol. 95, no. 3, pp. 952–958, 2000.

[90] R. J. Medina, C. L. O'Neill, M. Sweeney et al., "Molecular analysis of endothelial progenitor cell (EPC) subtypes reveals two distinct cell populations with different identities," *BMC Medical Genomics*, vol. 3, no. 1, p. 18, 2010.

[91] R. Gulati, D. Jevremovic, T. E. Peterson et al., "Diverse origin and function of cells with endothelial phenotype obtained from adult human blood," *Circulation Research*, vol. 93, no. 11, pp. 1023–1025, 2003.

[92] N. Mukai, T. Akahori, M. Komaki et al., "A comparison of the tube forming potentials of early and late endothelial progenitor cells," *Experimental Cell Research*, vol. 314, no. 3, pp. 430–440, 2008.

[93] C. H. Yoon, J. Hur, K. W. Park et al., "Synergistic neovascularization by mixed transplantation of early endothelial progenitor cells and late outgrowth endothelial cells: the role of angiogenic cytokines and matrix metalloproteinases," *Circulation*, vol. 112, no. 11, pp. 1618–1627, 2005.

[94] H. Ito, I. I. Rovira, M. L. Bloom et al., "Endothelial progenitor cells as putative targets for angiostatin," *Cancer Research*, vol. 59, no. 23, pp. 5875–5877, 1999.

[95] J. M. Hill, G. Zalos, J. P. J. Halcox et al., "Circulating endothelial progenitor cells, vascular function, and cardiovascular risk," *The New England Journal of Medicine*, vol. 348, no. 7, pp. 593–600, 2003.

[96] T. Nakahata and M. Ogawa, "Hemopoietic colony-forming cells in umbilical cord blood with extensive capability to generate mono- and multipotential hemopoietic progenitors," *The Journal of Clinical Investigation*, vol. 70, no. 6, pp. 1324–1328, 1982.

[97] T. Murohara, H. Ikeda, J. Duan et al., "Transplanted cord blood-derived endothelial precursor cells augment postnatal neovascularization," *The Journal of Clinical Investigation*, vol. 105, no. 11, pp. 1527–1536, 2000.

[98] H. S. Wang, S. C. Hung, S. T. Peng et al., "Mesenchymal stem cells in the Wharton's jelly of the human umbilical cord," *Stem Cells*, vol. 22, no. 7, pp. 1330–1337, 2004.

[99] Y. A. Romanov, V. A. Svintsitskaya, and V. N. Smirnov, "Searching for alternative sources of postnatal human mesenchymal stem cells: candidate MSC-like cells from umbilical cord," *Stem Cells*, vol. 21, no. 1, pp. 105–110, 2003.

[100] K. H. Wu, B. Zhou, S. H. Lu et al., "In vitro and in vivo differentiation of human umbilical cord derived stem cells into endothelial cells," *Journal of Cellular Biochemistry*, vol. 100, no. 3, pp. 608–616, 2007.

[101] P. A. Zuk, M. Zhu, H. Mizuno et al., "Multilineage cells from human adipose tissue: implications for cell-based therapies," *Tissue Engineering*, vol. 7, no. 2, pp. 211–228, 2001.

[102] P. A. Zuk, M. Zhu, P. Ashjian et al., "Human adipose tissue is a source of multipotent stem cells," *Molecular Biology of the Cell*, vol. 13, no. 12, pp. 4279–4295, 2002.

[103] A. Miranville, C. Heeschen, C. Sengenes, C. A. Curat, R. Busse, and A. Bouloumie, "Improvement of postnatal neovascularization by human adipose tissue-derived stem cells," *Circulation*, vol. 110, no. 3, pp. 349–355, 2004.

[104] V. Planat-Benard, J. S. Silvestre, B. Cousin et al., "Plasticity of human adipose lineage cells toward endothelial cells: physiological and therapeutic perspectives," *Circulation*, vol. 109, no. 5, pp. 656–663, 2004.

[105] Y. Cao, Z. Sun, L. Liao, Y. Meng, Q. Han, and R. C. Zhao, "Human adipose tissue-derived stem cells differentiate into endothelial cells in vitro and improve postnatal neovascularization in vivo," *Biochemical and Biophysical Research Communications*, vol. 332, no. 2, pp. 370–379, 2005.

[106] A. P. Beltrami, L. Barlucchi, D. Torella et al., "Adult cardiac stem cells are multipotent and support myocardial regeneration," *Cell*, vol. 114, no. 6, pp. 763–776, 2003.

[107] H. Oh, S. B. Bradfute, T. D. Gallardo et al., "Cardiac progenitor cells from adult myocardium: homing, differentiation, and fusion after infarction," *Proceedings of the National Academy of Sciences of the United States of America*, vol. 100, no. 21, pp. 12313–12318, 2003.

[108] C. Bearzi, M. Rota, T. Hosoda et al., "Human cardiac stem cells," *Proceedings of the National Academy of Sciences of the United States of America*, vol. 104, no. 35, pp. 14068–14073, 2007.

[109] J. H. van Berlo, O. Kanisicak, M. Maillet et al., "c-kit$^+$ cells minimally contribute cardiomyocytes to the heart," *Nature*, vol. 509, no. 7500, pp. 337–341, 2014.

[110] N. Sultana, L. Zhang, J. Yan et al., "Resident c-kit$^+$ cells in the heart are not cardiac stem cells," *Nature Communications*, vol. 6, no. 1, p. 8701, 2015.

[111] S. A. J. Chamuleau, K. R. Vrijsen, D. G. Rokosh, X. L. Tang, J. J. Piek, and R. Bolli, "Cell therapy for ischaemic heart disease: focus on the role of resident cardiac stem cells," *Netherlands Heart Journal*, vol. 17, no. 5, pp. 199–207, 2009.

[112] J. Lader, M. Stachel, and L. Bu, "Cardiac stem cells for myocardial regeneration: promising but not ready for prime time," *Current Opinion in Biotechnology*, vol. 47, pp. 30–35, 2017.

[113] C. R. Bjornson, R. L. Rietze, B. A. Reynolds, M. C. Magli, and A. L. Vescovi, "Turning brain into blood: a hematopoietic fate adopted by adult neural stem cells in vivo," *Science*, vol. 283, no. 5401, pp. 534–537, 1999.

[114] T. D. Palmer, A. R. Willhoite, and F. H. Gage, "Vascular niche for adult hippocampal neurogenesis," *The Journal of Comparative Neurology*, vol. 425, no. 4, pp. 479–494, 2000.

[115] E. A. Parati, A. Bez, D. Ponti et al., "Human neural stem cells express extra-neural markers," *Brain Research*, vol. 925, no. 2, pp. 213–221, 2002.

[116] K. Oishi, A. Kobayashi, K. Fujii, D. Kanehira, Y. Ito, and M. K. Uchida, "Angiogenesis in vitro: vascular tube formation from the differentiation of neural stem cells," *Journal of Pharmacological Sciences*, vol. 96, no. 2, pp. 208–218, 2004.

[117] M. Ii, H. Nishimura, H. Sekiguchi et al., "Concurrent vasculogenesis and neurogenesis from adult neural stem cells," *Circulation Research*, vol. 105, no. 9, pp. 860–868, 2009.

[118] S. Y. Yang, N. Strong, X. Gong, and M. H. Heggeness, "Differentiation of nerve-derived adult pluripotent stem cells into osteoblastic and endothelial cells," *The Spine Journal*, vol. 17, no. 2, pp. 277–281, 2017.

[119] A. E. Wurmser, K. Nakashima, R. G. Summers et al., "Cell fusion-independent differentiation of neural stem cells to the endothelial lineage," *Nature*, vol. 430, no. 6997, pp. 350–356, 2004.

[120] H. Chopra, M. K. Hans, and S. Shetty, "Stem cells-the hidden treasure: a strategic review," *Dental Research Journal*, vol. 10, no. 4, pp. 421–427, 2013.

[121] R. d'Aquino, A. Graziano, M. Sampaolesi et al., "Human postnatal dental pulp cells co-differentiate into osteoblasts and endotheliocytes: a pivotal synergy leading to adult bone tissue formation," *Cell Death & Differentiation*, vol. 14, no. 6, pp. 1162–1171, 2007.

[122] C. Marchionni, L. Bonsi, F. Alviano et al., "Angiogenic potential of human dental pulp stromal (STEM) cells," *International Journal of Immunopathology and Pharmacology*, vol. 22, no. 3, pp. 699–706, 2009.

[123] A. Bronckaers, P. Hilkens, Y. Fanton et al., "Angiogenic properties of human dental pulp stem cells," *PLoS One*, vol. 8, no. 8, article e71104, 2013.

[124] H. Aksel and G. T. J. Huang, "Human and swine dental pulp stem cells form a vascularlike network after angiogenic differentiation in comparison with endothelial cells: a quantitative analysis," *Journal of Endodontia*, vol. 43, no. 4, pp. 588–595, 2017.

[125] W. L. Dissanayaka, X. Zhan, C. Zhang, K. M. Hargreaves, L. Jin, and E. H. Y. Tong, "Coculture of dental pulp stem cells with endothelial cells enhances osteo-/odontogenic and angiogenic potential in vitro," *Journal of Endodontia*, vol. 38, no. 4, pp. 454–463, 2012.

[126] K. Iohara, L. Zheng, H. Wake et al., "A novel stem cell source for vasculogenesis in ischemia: subfraction of side population cells from dental pulp," *Stem Cells*, vol. 26, no. 9, pp. 2408–2418, 2008.

[127] R. Ishizaka, Y. Hayashi, K. Iohara et al., "Stimulation of angiogenesis, neurogenesis and regeneration by side population cells from dental pulp," *Biomaterials*, vol. 34, no. 8, pp. 1888–1897, 2013.

[128] M. Miura, S. Gronthos, M. Zhao et al., "SHED: stem cells from human exfoliated deciduous teeth," *Proceedings of the National Academy of Sciences of the United States of America*, vol. 100, no. 10, pp. 5807–5812, 2003.

[129] M. M. Cordeiro, Z. Dong, T. Kaneko et al., "Dental pulp tissue engineering with stem cells from exfoliated deciduous teeth," *Journal of Endodontia*, vol. 34, no. 8, pp. 962–969, 2008.

[130] V. T. Sakai, Z. Zhang, Z. Dong et al., "SHED differentiate into functional odontoblasts and endothelium," *Journal of Dental Research*, vol. 89, no. 8, pp. 791–796, 2010.

[131] P. Hilkens, Y. Fanton, W. Martens et al., "Pro-angiogenic impact of dental stem cells in vitro and in vivo," *Stem Cell Research*, vol. 12, no. 3, pp. 778–790, 2014.

[132] S. Yeasmin, J. Ceccarelli, M. Vigen et al., "Stem cells derived from tooth periodontal ligament enhance functional angiogenesis by endothelial cells," *Tissue Engineering Part A*, vol. 20, no. 7-8, pp. 1188–1196, 2014.

[133] Y. K. Bae, G. H. Kim, J. C. Lee et al., "The significance of SDF-1α-CXCR4 axis in in vivo angiogenic ability of human periodontal ligament stem cells," *Molecules and Cells*, vol. 40, no. 6, pp. 386–392, 2017.

[134] C. C. Cheng, S. J. Chang, Y. N. Chueh et al., "Distinct angiogenesis roles and surface markers of early and late endothelial progenitor cells revealed by functional group analyses," *BMC Genomics*, vol. 14, no. 1, p. 182, 2013.

[135] A. H. Yin, S. Miraglia, E. D. Zanjani et al., "AC133, a novel marker for human hematopoietic stem and progenitor cells," *Blood*, vol. 90, no. 12, pp. 5002–5012, 1997.

[136] U. M. Gehling, S. Ergun, U. Schumacher et al., "In vitro differentiation of endothelial cells from AC133-positive progenitor cells," *Blood*, vol. 95, no. 10, pp. 3106–3112, 2000.

[137] S. M. Cheng, S. J. Chang, T. N. Tsai et al., "Differential expression of distinct surface markers in early endothelial progenitor cells and monocyte-derived macrophages," *Gene Expression*, vol. 16, no. 1, pp. 15–24, 2013.

[138] J. M. Lehmann, G. Riethmuller, and J. P. Johnson, "MUC18, a marker of tumor progression in human melanoma, shows sequence similarity to the neural cell adhesion molecules of the immunoglobulin superfamily," *Proceedings of the National Academy of Sciences of the United States of America*, vol. 86, no. 24, pp. 9891–9895, 1989.

[139] N. Bardin, F. George, M. Mutin et al., "S-Endo 1, a pan-endothelial monoclonal antibody recognizing a novel human endothelial antigen," *Tissue Antigens*, vol. 48, no. 5, pp. 531–539, 1996.

[140] N. Bardin, V. Moal, F. Anfosso et al., "Soluble CD146, a novel endothelial marker, is increased in physiopathological settings linked to endothelial junctional alteration," *Thrombosis and Haemostasis*, vol. 90, no. 5, pp. 915–920, 2003.

[141] M. Danova, G. Comolli, M. Manzoni, M. Torchio, and G. Mazzini, "Flow cytometric analysis of circulating endothelial cells and endothelial progenitors for clinical purposes in oncology: a critical evaluation," *Molecular and Clinical Oncology*, vol. 4, no. 6, pp. 909–917, 2016.

[142] C. Li, Q. Wu, B. Liu et al., "Detection and validation of circulating endothelial cells, a blood-based diagnostic marker of acute myocardial infarction," *PLoS One*, vol. 8, no. 3, article e58478, 2013.

[143] D. M. Yuan, Q. Zhang, Y. L. Lv et al., "Predictive and prognostic significance of circulating endothelial cells in advanced non-small cell lung cancer patients," *Tumour Biology*, vol. 36, no. 11, pp. 9031–9037, 2015.

[144] K. Yoneda, F. Tanaka, N. Kondo et al., "Circulating endothelial cell (CEC) as a diagnostic and prognostic marker in malignant pleural mesothelioma (MPM)," *Annals of Surgical Oncology*, vol. 19, no. 13, pp. 4229–4237, 2012.

[145] U. Laufs, N. Werner, A. Link et al., "Physical training increases endothelial progenitor cells, inhibits neointima formation, and enhances angiogenesis," *Circulation*, vol. 109, no. 2, pp. 220–226, 2004.

[146] R. Hambrecht, V. Adams, S. Erbs et al., "Regular physical activity improves endothelial function in patients with coronary artery disease by increasing phosphorylation of endothelial nitric oxide synthase," *Circulation*, vol. 107, no. 25, pp. 3152–3158, 2003.

[147] J. A. Forsythe, B. H. Jiang, N. V. Iyer et al., "Activation of vascular endothelial growth factor gene transcription by hypoxia-inducible factor 1," *Molecular and Cellular Biology*, vol. 16, no. 9, pp. 4604–4613, 1996.

[148] D. J. Ceradini, A. R. Kulkarni, M. J. Callaghan et al., "Progenitor cell trafficking is regulated by hypoxic gradients through HIF-1 induction of SDF-1," *Nature Medicine*, vol. 10, no. 8, pp. 858–864, 2004.

[149] G. Iaccarino, M. Ciccarelli, D. Sorriento et al., "Ischemic neoangiogenesis enhanced by β_2-adrenergic receptor overexpression: a novel role for the endothelial adrenergic system," *Circulation Research*, vol. 97, no. 11, pp. 1182–1189, 2005.

[150] G. Galasso, R. De Rosa, M. Ciccarelli et al., "β_2-Adrenergic receptor stimulation improves endothelial progenitor cell-mediated ischemic neoangiogenesis," *Circulation Research*, vol. 112, no. 7, pp. 1026–1034, 2013.

[151] K. M. Beavers, T. E. Brinkley, and B. J. Nicklas, "Effect of exercise training on chronic inflammation," *Clinica Chimica Acta*, vol. 411, no. 11-12, pp. 785–793, 2010.

[152] S. Verma, M. A. Kuliszewski, S. H. Li et al., "C-reactive protein attenuates endothelial progenitor cell survival, differentiation, and function: further evidence of a mechanistic link between C-reactive protein and cardiovascular disease," *Circulation*, vol. 109, no. 17, pp. 2058–2067, 2004.

[153] F. H. Seeger, J. Haendeler, D. H. Walter et al., "p38 mitogen-activated protein kinase downregulates endothelial progenitor cells," *Circulation*, vol. 111, no. 9, pp. 1184–1191, 2005.

[154] M. Brehm, F. Picard, P. Ebner et al., "Effects of exercise training on mobilization and functional activity of blood-derived progenitor cells in patients with acute myocardial infarction," *European Journal of Medical Research*, vol. 14, no. 9, pp. 393–405, 2009.

[155] E. M. Craenenbroeck, V. Y. Hoymans, P. J. Beckers et al., "Exercise training improves function of circulating angiogenic cells in patients with chronic heart failure," *Basic Research in Cardiology*, vol. 105, no. 5, pp. 665–676, 2010.

[156] O. Schlager, A. Giurgea, O. Schuhfried et al., "Exercise training increases endothelial progenitor cells and decreases asymmetric dimethylarginine in peripheral arterial disease: a randomized controlled trial," *Atherosclerosis*, vol. 217, no. 1, pp. 240–248, 2011.

[157] G. Scalone, A. de Caterina, A. M. Leone et al., "Effect of exercise on circulating endothelial progenitor cells in microvascular angina," *Circulation Journal*, vol. 77, no. 7, pp. 1777–1782, 2013.

[158] F. Cesari, R. Marcucci, A. M. Gori et al., "Impact of a cardiac rehabilitation program and inflammatory state on endothelial progenitor cells in acute coronary syndrome patients," *International Journal of Cardiology*, vol. 167, no. 5, pp. 1854–1859, 2013.

[159] M. Mack and A. Gopal, "Epidemiology, traditional and novel risk factors in coronary artery disease," *Cardiology Clinics*, vol. 32, no. 3, pp. 323–332, 2014.

[160] F. Cesari, R. Marcucci, A. M. Gori et al., "Adherence to lifestyle modifications after a cardiac rehabilitation program and endothelial progenitor cells. A six-month follow-up study," *Thrombosis and Haemostasis*, vol. 112, no. 1, pp. 196–204, 2014.

[161] L. Fontana and S. Klein, "Aging, adiposity, and calorie restriction," *JAMA*, vol. 297, no. 9, pp. 986–994, 2007.

[162] B. Xin, C. L. Liu, H. Yang et al., "Prolonged fasting improves endothelial progenitor cell-mediated ischemic angiogenesis in mice," *Cellular Physiology and Biochemistry*, vol. 40, no. 3-4, pp. 693–706, 2016.

[163] L. Fontana, E. P. Weiss, D. T. Villareal, S. Klein, and J. O. Holloszy, "Long-term effects of calorie or protein restriction on serum IGF-1 and IGFBP-3 concentration in humans," *Aging Cell*, vol. 7, no. 5, pp. 681–687, 2008.

[164] J. Hou, X. Peng, J. Wang et al., "Mesenchymal stem cells promote endothelial progenitor cell proliferation by secreting insulin-like growth factor-1," *Molecular Medicine Reports*, vol. 16, no. 2, pp. 1502–1508, 2017.

[165] M. Vasa, S. Fichtlscherer, A. Aicher et al., "Number and migratory activity of circulating endothelial progenitor cells inversely correlate with risk factors for coronary artery disease," *Circulation Research*, vol. 89, no. 1, pp. E1–E7, 2001.

[166] J. T. Powell, "Vascular damage from smoking: disease mechanisms at the arterial wall," *Vascular Medicine*, vol. 3, no. 1, pp. 21–28, 1998.

[167] T. Kondo, M. Hayashi, K. Takeshita et al., "Smoking cessation rapidly increases circulating progenitor cells in peripheral blood in chronic smokers," *Arteriosclerosis, Thrombosis, and Vascular Biology*, vol. 24, no. 8, pp. 1442–1447, 2004.

[168] M. Puls, M. R. Schroeter, J. Steier et al., "Effect of smoking cessation on the number and adhesive properties of early outgrowth endothelial progenitor cells," *International Journal of Cardiology*, vol. 152, no. 1, pp. 61–69, 2011.

[169] X. Wang, J. Zhu, J. Chen, and Y. Shang, "Effects of nicotine on the number and activity of circulating endothelial progenitor cells," *Journal of Clinical Pharmacology*, vol. 44, no. 8, pp. 881–889, 2004.

[170] A. Sugimoto, H. Masuda, M. Eguchi, H. Iwaguro, T. Tanabe, and T. Asahara, "Nicotine enlivenment of blood flow recovery following endothelial progenitor cell transplantation into ischemic hindlimb," *Stem Cells and Development*, vol. 16, no. 4, pp. 649–656, 2007.

[171] Z. Junhui, H. Xiaojing, Z. Binquan, X. Xudong, C. Junzhu, and F. Guosheng, "Nicotine-reduced endothelial progenitor cell senescence through augmentation of telomerase activity via the PI3K/Akt pathway," *Cytotherapy*, vol. 11, no. 4, pp. 485–491, 2009.

[172] W. Li, D. Y. Du, Y. Liu, F. Jiang, P. Zhang, and Y. T. Li, "Long-term nicotine exposure induces dysfunction of mouse endothelial progenitor cells," *Experimental and Therapeutic Medicine*, vol. 13, no. 1, pp. 85–90, 2017.

[173] C. W. Greider, "Telomeres, telomerase and senescence," *BioEssays*, vol. 12, no. 8, pp. 363–369, 1990.

[174] R. L. Stedman, "Chemical composition of tobacco and tobacco smoke," *Chemical Reviews*, vol. 68, no. 2, pp. 153–207, 1968.

[175] J. J. Mahmarian, L. A. Moye, G. A. Nasser et al., "Nicotine patch therapy in smoking cessation reduces the extent of exercise-induced myocardial ischemia," *Journal of the American College of Cardiology*, vol. 30, no. 1, pp. 125–130, 1997.

[176] J. F. Greden, "Physical symptoms of depression: unmet needs," *The Journal of Clinical Psychiatry*, vol. 64, pp. 5–11, 2003.

[177] P. Dome, Z. Teleki, Z. Rihmer et al., "Circulating endothelial progenitor cells and depression: a possible novel link between heart and soul," *Molecular Psychiatry*, vol. 14, no. 5, pp. 523–531, 2009.

[178] C. Tuglu, S. H. Kara, O. Caliyurt, E. Vardar, and E. Abay, "Increased serum tumor necrosis factor-alpha levels and treatment response in major depressive disorder," *Psychopharmacology*, vol. 170, no. 4, pp. 429–433, 2003.

[179] H. Chen, K. H. Yiu, and H. F. Tse, "Relationships between vascular dysfunction, circulating endothelial progenitor cells, and psychological status in healthy subjects," *Depression and Anxiety*, vol. 28, no. 8, pp. 719–727, 2011.

[180] H. Chen, L. Zhang, M. Zhang et al., "Relationship of depression, stress and endothelial function in stable angina patients," *Physiology & Behavior*, vol. 118, pp. 152–158, 2013.

[181] E. Van Belle, A. Rivard, D. Chen et al., "Hypercholesterolemia attenuates angiogenesis but does not preclude augmentation by angiogenic cytokines," *Circulation*, vol. 96, no. 8, pp. 2667–2674, 1997.

[182] J. Duan, T. Murohara, H. Ikeda et al., "Hypercholesterolemia inhibits angiogenesis in response to hindlimb ischemia: nitric oxide-dependent mechanism," *Circulation*, vol. 102, no. 19, Supplement 3, pp. III370–III376, 2000.

[183] T. Imanishi, T. Hano, Y. Matsuo, and I. Nishio, "Oxidized low-density lipoprotein inhibits vascular endothelial growth factor-induced endothelial progenitor cell differentiation," *Clinical and Experimental Pharmacology & Physiology*, vol. 30, no. 9, pp. 665–670, 2003.

[184] N. R. Leslie, "The redox regulation of PI 3-kinase–dependent signaling," *Antioxidants & Redox Signaling*, vol. 8, no. 9-10, pp. 1765–1774, 2006.

[185] G. Tie, J. Yan, Y. Yang et al., "Oxidized low-density lipoprotein induces apoptosis in endothelial progenitor cells by inactivating the phosphoinositide 3-kinase/Akt pathway," *Journal of Vascular Research*, vol. 47, no. 6, pp. 519–530, 2010.

[186] Y. Wu, Q. Wang, L. Cheng, J. Wang, and G. Lu, "Effect of oxidized low-density lipoprotein on survival and function of endothelial progenitor cell mediated by p38 signal pathway," *Journal of Cardiovascular Pharmacology*, vol. 53, no. 2, pp. 151–156, 2009.

[187] F. X. Ma, B. Zhou, Z. Chen et al., "Oxidized low density lipoprotein impairs endothelial progenitor cells by regulation of endothelial nitric oxide synthase," *Journal of Lipid Research*, vol. 47, no. 6, pp. 1227–1237, 2006.

[188] E. Ackah, J. Yu, S. Zoellner et al., "Akt1/protein kinase Bα is critical for ischemic and VEGF-mediated angiogenesis," *The Journal of Clinical Investigation*, vol. 115, no. 8, pp. 2119–2127, 2005.

[189] T. Murohara, T. Asahara, M. Silver et al., "Nitric oxide synthase modulates angiogenesis in response to tissue ischemia," *The Journal of Clinical Investigation*, vol. 101, no. 11, pp. 2567–2578, 1998.

[190] A. Aicher, C. Heeschen, C. Mildner-Rihm et al., "Essential role of endothelial nitric oxide synthase for mobilization of stem and progenitor cells," *Nature Medicine*, vol. 9, no. 11, pp. 1370–1376, 2003.

[191] S. Dimmeler, A. Aicher, M. Vasa et al., "HMG-CoA reductase inhibitors (statins) increase endothelial progenitor cells via the PI 3-kinase/Akt pathway," *The Journal of Clinical Investigation*, vol. 108, no. 3, pp. 391–397, 2001.

[192] J. P. Gratton, M. Morales-Ruiz, Y. Kureishi, D. Fulton, K. Walsh, and W. C. Sessa, "Akt down-regulation of p38

signaling provides a novel mechanism of vascular endothelial growth factor-mediated cytoprotection in endothelial cells," *Journal of Biological Chemistry*, vol. 276, no. 32, pp. 30359–30365, 2001.

[193] G. Giannotti, C. Doerries, P. S. Mocharla et al., "Impaired endothelial repair capacity of early endothelial progenitor cells in prehypertension: relation to endothelial dysfunction," *Hypertension*, vol. 55, no. 6, pp. 1389–1397, 2010.

[194] O. J. MacEneaney, C. A. DeSouza, B. R. Weil et al., "Prehypertension and endothelial progenitor cell function," *Journal of Human Hypertension*, vol. 25, no. 1, pp. 57–62, 2011.

[195] E. M. V. de Cavanagh, S. A. González, F. Inserra et al., "Sympathetic predominance is associated with impaired endothelial progenitor cells and tunneling nanotubes in controlled-hypertensive patients," *American Journal of Physiology-Heart and Circulatory Physiology*, vol. 307, no. 2, pp. H207–H215, 2014.

[196] E. H. Yao, N. Fukuda, T. Matsumoto et al., "Effects of the antioxidative β-blocker celiprolol on endothelial progenitor cells in hypertensive rats," *American Journal of Hypertension*, vol. 21, no. 9, pp. 1062–1068, 2008.

[197] A. Honda, K. Matsuura, N. Fukushima, Y. Tsurumi, H. Kasanuki, and N. Hagiwara, "Telmisartan induces proliferation of human endothelial progenitor cells via PPARγ-dependent PI3K/Akt pathway," *Atherosclerosis*, vol. 205, no. 2, pp. 376–384, 2009.

[198] R. Suzuki, N. Fukuda, M. Katakawa et al., "Effects of an angiotensin II receptor blocker on the impaired function of endothelial progenitor cells in patients with essential hypertension," *American Journal of Hypertension*, vol. 27, no. 5, pp. 695–701, 2014.

[199] Y. Li, G. Alatan, Z. Ge, and D. Liu, "Effects of benazepril on functional activity of endothelial progenitor cells from hypertension patients," *Clinical and Experimental Hypertension*, vol. 36, no. 8, pp. 545–549, 2014.

[200] S. Luo, W. Xia, C. Chen, E. A. Robinson, and J. Tao, "Endothelial progenitor cells and hypertension: current concepts and future implications," *Clinical Science*, vol. 130, no. 22, pp. 2029–2042, 2016.

[201] G. P. Fadini, S. Sartore, M. Schiavon et al., "Diabetes impairs progenitor cell mobilisation after hindlimb ischaemia-reperfusion injury in rats," *Diabetologia*, vol. 49, no. 12, pp. 3075–3084, 2006.

[202] O. M. Tepper, R. D. Galiano, J. M. Capla et al., "Human endothelial progenitor cells from type II diabetics exhibit impaired proliferation, adhesion, and incorporation into vascular structures," *Circulation*, vol. 106, no. 22, pp. 2781–2786, 2002.

[203] G. P. Fadini, M. Miorin, M. Facco et al., "Circulating endothelial progenitor cells are reduced in peripheral vascular complications of type 2 diabetes mellitus," *Journal of the American College of Cardiology*, vol. 45, no. 9, pp. 1449–1457, 2005.

[204] T. Nishikawa, D. Edelstein, X. L. Du et al., "Normalizing mitochondrial superoxide production blocks three pathways of hyperglycaemic damage," *Nature*, vol. 404, no. 6779, pp. 787–790, 2000.

[205] M. Brownlee, "Biochemistry and molecular cell biology of diabetic complications," *Nature*, vol. 414, no. 6865, pp. 813–820, 2001.

[206] I. A. M. van den Oever, H. G. Raterman, M. T. Nurmohamed, and S. Simsek, "Endothelial dysfunction, inflammation, and apoptosis in diabetes mellitus," *Mediators of Inflammation*, vol. 2010, Article ID 792393, 15 pages, 2010.

[207] G. P. Fadini, S. Sartore, C. Agostini, and A. Avogaro, "Significance of endothelial progenitor cells in subjects with diabetes," *Diabetes Care*, vol. 30, no. 5, pp. 1305–1313, 2007.

[208] A. Kulwas, E. Drela, W. Jundzill, B. Goralczyk, B. Ruszkowska-Ciastek, and D. Rosc, "Circulating endothelial progenitor cells and angiogenic factors in diabetes complicated diabetic foot and without foot complications," *Journal of Diabetes and its Complications*, vol. 29, no. 5, pp. 686–690, 2015.

[209] S. Choksy, A. G. Pockley, Y. E. Wajeh, and P. Chan, "VEGF and VEGF receptor expression in human chronic critical limb ischaemia," *European Journal of Vascular and Endovascular Surgery*, vol. 28, no. 6, pp. 660–669, 2004.

[210] S. Shintani, T. Murohara, H. Ikeda et al., "Mobilization of endothelial progenitor cells in patients with acute myocardial infarction," *Circulation*, vol. 103, no. 23, pp. 2776–2779, 2001.

[211] M. Massa, V. Rosti, M. Ferrario et al., "Increased circulating hematopoietic and endothelial progenitor cells in the early phase of acute myocardial infarction," *Blood*, vol. 105, no. 1, pp. 199–206, 2005.

[212] C. Heeschen, R. Lehmann, J. Honold et al., "Profoundly reduced neovascularization capacity of bone marrow mononuclear cells derived from patients with chronic ischemic heart disease," *Circulation*, vol. 109, no. 13, pp. 1615–1622, 2004.

[213] J. George, E. Goldstein, S. Abashidze et al., "Circulating endothelial progenitor cells in patients with unstable angina: association with systemic inflammation," *European Heart Journal*, vol. 25, no. 12, pp. 1003–1008, 2004.

[214] R. Hinkel, C. el-Aouni, T. Olson et al., "Thymosin β4 is an essential paracrine factor of embryonic endothelial progenitor cell–mediated cardioprotection," *Circulation*, vol. 117, no. 17, pp. 2232–2240, 2008.

[215] Z. T. Chang, L. Hong, H. Wang, H. L. Lai, L. F. Li, and Q. L. Yin, "Application of peripheral-blood-derived endothelial progenitor cell for treating ischemia-reperfusion injury and infarction: a preclinical study in rat models," *Journal of Cardiothoracic Surgery*, vol. 8, no. 1, p. 33, 2013.

[216] K. Chu, K. H. Jung, S. T. Lee et al., "Circulating endothelial progenitor cells as a new marker of endothelial dysfunction or repair in acute stroke," *Stroke*, vol. 39, no. 5, pp. 1441–1447, 2008.

[217] E. Paczkowska, M. Golab-Janowska, A. Bajer-Czajkowska et al., "Increased circulating endothelial progenitor cells in patients with haemorrhagic and ischaemic stroke: the role of endothelin-1," *Journal of the Neurological Sciences*, vol. 325, no. 1-2, pp. 90–99, 2013.

[218] A. Taguchi, T. Matsuyama, H. Moriwaki et al., "Circulating CD34-positive cells provide an index of cerebrovascular function," *Circulation*, vol. 109, no. 24, pp. 2972–2975, 2004.

[219] H. K. Yip, L. T. Chang, W. N. Chang et al., "Level and value of circulating endothelial progenitor cells in patients after acute ischemic stroke," *Stroke*, vol. 39, no. 1, pp. 69–74, 2008.

[220] T. Sobrino, O. Hurtado, M. A. Moro et al., "The increase of circulating endothelial progenitor cells after acute ischemic stroke is associated with good outcome," *Stroke*, vol. 38, no. 10, pp. 2759–2764, 2007.

[221] F. Cesari, P. Nencini, M. Nesi et al., "Bone marrow-derived progenitor cells in the early phase of ischemic stroke: relation with stroke severity and discharge outcome," *Journal of Cerebral Blood Flow & Metabolism*, vol. 29, no. 12, pp. 1983–1990, 2009.

[222] J. Pias-Peleteiro, M. Perez-Mato, E. Lopez-Arias et al., "Increased endothelial progenitor cell levels are associated with good outcome in intracerebral hemorrhage," *Scientific Reports*, vol. 6, no. 1, article 28724, 2016.

[223] C. Foresta, N. Caretta, A. Lana, A. Cabrelle, G. Palu, and A. Ferlin, "Circulating endothelial progenitor cells in subjects with erectile dysfunction," *International Journal of Impotence Research*, vol. 17, no. 3, pp. 288–290, 2005.

[224] M. Baumhakel, N. Werner, M. Bohm, and G. Nickenig, "Circulating endothelial progenitor cells correlate with erectile function in patients with coronary heart disease," *European Heart Journal*, vol. 27, no. 18, pp. 2184–2188, 2006.

[225] K. Esposito, M. Ciotola, M. I. Maiorino et al., "Circulating CD34$^+$KDR$^+$ endothelial progenitor cells correlate with erectile function and endothelial function in overweight men," *The Journal of Sexual Medicine*, vol. 6, no. 1, pp. 107–114, 2009.

[226] M. I. Maiorino, G. Bellastella, M. Petrizzo et al., "Circulating endothelial progenitor cells in type 1 diabetic patients with erectile dysfunction," *Endocrine*, vol. 49, no. 2, pp. 415–421, 2015.

[227] C. H. Liao, Y. N. Wu, Y. H. Lin, R. F. Syu Huang, S. P. Liu, and H. S. Chiang, "Restoration of erectile function with intracavernous injections of endothelial progenitor cells after bilateral cavernous nerve injury in rats," *Andrology*, vol. 3, no. 5, pp. 924–932, 2015.

[228] H. Zhang, V. Vakil, M. Braunstein et al., "Circulating endothelial progenitor cells in multiple myeloma: implications and significance," *Blood*, vol. 105, no. 8, pp. 3286–3294, 2005.

[229] A. Wierzbowska, T. Robak, A. Krawczynska et al., "Circulating endothelial cells in patients with acute myeloid leukemia," *European Journal of Haematology*, vol. 75, no. 6, pp. 492–497, 2005.

[230] A. M. Zahran, S. S. Aly, H. A. Altayeb, and A. M. Ali, "Circulating endothelial cells and their progenitors in acute myeloid leukemia," *Oncology Letters*, vol. 12, no. 3, pp. 1965–1970, 2016.

[231] B. Dome, J. Timar, J. Dobos et al., "Identification and clinical significance of circulating endothelial progenitor cells in human non-small cell lung cancer," *Cancer Research*, vol. 66, no. 14, pp. 7341–7347, 2006.

[232] J. W. Y. Ho, R. W. C. Pang, C. Lau et al., "Significance of circulating endothelial progenitor cells in hepatocellular carcinoma," *Hepatology*, vol. 44, no. 4, pp. 836–843, 2006.

[233] D. Yu, X. Sun, Y. Qiu et al., "Identification and clinical significance of mobilized endothelial progenitor cells in tumor vasculogenesis of hepatocellular carcinoma," *Clinical Cancer Research*, vol. 13, no. 13, pp. 3814–3824, 2007.

[234] C. Richter-Ehrenstein, J. Rentzsch, S. Runkel, A. Schneider, and G. Schonfelder, "Endothelial progenitor cells in breast cancer patients," *Breast Cancer Research and Treatment*, vol. 106, no. 3, pp. 343–349, 2007.

[235] R. P. Naik, D. Jin, E. Chuang et al., "Circulating endothelial progenitor cells correlate to stage in patients with invasive breast cancer," *Breast Cancer Research and Treatment*, vol. 107, no. 1, pp. 133–138, 2008.

[236] P. Rhone, B. Ruszkowska-Ciastek, M. Celmer et al., "Increased number of endothelial progenitors in peripheral blood as a possible early marker of tumour growth in postmenopausal breast cancer patients," *Journal of Physiology and Pharmacology*, vol. 68, no. 1, pp. 139–148, 2017.

[237] Y. Su, L. Zheng, Q. Wang et al., "Quantity and clinical relevance of circulating endothelial progenitor cells in human ovarian cancer," *Journal of Experimental & Clinical Cancer Research*, vol. 29, no. 1, p. 27, 2010.

[238] G. M. Rigolin, R. Maffei, L. Rizzotto et al., "Circulating endothelial cells in patients with chronic lymphocytic leukemia: clinical-prognostic and biologic significance," *Cancer*, vol. 116, no. 8, pp. 1926–1937, 2010.

[239] R. S. Bhatt, A. J. Zurita, A. O'Neill et al., "Increased mobilisation of circulating endothelial progenitors in von Hippel-Lindau disease and renal cell carcinoma," *British Journal of Cancer*, vol. 105, no. 1, pp. 112–117, 2011.

[240] P. Yu, Y. Z. Ge, Y. Zhao et al., "Identification and significance of mobilized endothelial progenitor cells in tumor neovascularization of renal cell carcinoma," *Tumour Biology*, vol. 35, no. 9, pp. 9331–9341, 2014.

[241] M. Paprocka, C. Kieda, A. Kantor et al., "Increased endothelial progenitor cell number in early stage of endometrial cancer," *International Journal of Gynecological Cancer*, vol. 27, no. 5, pp. 947–952, 2017.

[242] C. P. Chou, S. S. Jiang, H. B. Pan et al., "Endothelial cell colony forming units derived from malignant breast diseases are resistant to tumor necrosis factor-α-induced apoptosis," *Scientific Reports*, vol. 6, no. 1, article 37450, 2016.

13

Safety of Autologous Cord Blood Cells for Preterms: A Descriptive Study

Jie Yang[ID],[1] Zhuxiao Ren,[1] Chunyi Zhang,[1] Yunbei Rao,[1] Junjuan Zhong,[1] Zhu Wang,[1] Zhipeng Liu,[2] Wei Wei,[2] Lijuang Lu,[3] Jiying Wen,[3] Guocheng Liu,[3] Kaiyan Liu[ID],[4] and Qi Wang[ID][1,2]

[1]Department of Neonatology, Guangdong Women and Children Hospital, Guangzhou, China
[2]Guangdong Cord Blood and Stem Cell Bank, Guangzhou, China
[3]Department of Obstetrics, Guangdong Women and Children Hospital, Guangzhou, China
[4]Institute of Hematology, People's Hospital, Peking University, Beijing, China

Correspondence should be addressed to Kaiyan Liu; liukaiyan@medmail.com.cn and Qi Wang; wangqigz@21cn.com

Academic Editor: Leonora Buzanska

Background. Preterm birth complications are one of the leading causes of death among children under 5 years of age. Despite advances in medical care, many survivors face a lifetime of disability, including mental and physical retardation, and chronic lung disease. More recently, both allogenic and autogenic cord blood cells have been applied in the treatment of neonatal conditions such as hypoxic-ischemic encephalopathy (HIE) and bronchopulmonary dysplasia (BPD). *Objective.* To assess the safety of autologous, volume- and red blood cell- (RBC-) reduced, noncryopreserved umbilical cord blood (UCB) cell infusion to preterm infants. *Method.* This study was a phase I, open-label, single-arm, single-center trial to evaluate the safety of autologous, volume- and RBC-reduced, noncryopreserved UCB cell (5×10^7cells/kg) infusion for preterm infants <37 weeks gestational age. UCB cell characteristics, pre- and postinfusion vital signs, and laboratory investigations were recorded. Clinical data including mortality rates and preterm complications were recorded. *Results.* After processing, (22.67 ± 4.05) ml UCB cells in volume, $(2.67 \pm 2.00) \times 10^8$ cells in number, with $(22.67 \pm 4.05) \times 10^6$ CD34+, $(3.72 \pm 3.25) \times 10^5$ colony forming cells (CFU-GM), and $(99.7 \pm 0.17\%)$ vitality were infused to 15 preterm infants within 8 hours after birth. No adverse effects were noticed during treatment. All fifteen patients who received UCB infusion survived. The duration of hospitalization ranged from 4 to 65 (30 ± 23.6) days. Regarding preterm complications, no BPD, necrotizing enterocolitis (NEC), retinopathy of prematurity (ROP) was observed. There were 1/15 (7%) infant with intraventricular hemorrhage (IVH), 5/15 (33.3%) infants with ventilation-associated pneumonia, and 10/15 (66.67%) with anemia, respectively. *Conclusions.* Collection, preparation, and infusion of fresh autologous UCB cells to preterm infants is feasible and safe. Adequately powered randomized controlled studies are needed.

1. Introduction

Preterm delivery is a global health problem. The rate of preterm birth ranges from 5% to 18% of babies born across 184 countries. An estimated 15 million babies are born preterm every year [1]. Preterm birth complications are the leading cause of death among children under 5 years of age, which are responsible for nearly 1 million deaths in 2015. The morbidity associated with preterm birth often extends to later life, resulting in enormous physical, psychological, and economic costs [2]. Inflammation, ischemia, and free radical toxicity

lead to multiorgan damage in preterm infants, characterized by reduced numbers of tissue cells, blood vessels, and progenitor cell [3–6]. Current management has been shown to reduce preterm complications and overall morbidity. However, many survivors still face a lifetime of disability, including mental and physical retardation, and chronic lung disease [1]. It has been reported that among infants born with gestational ages of 22 to 28 weeks, 16% are complicated with severe intraventricular hemorrhage (IVH), 36% with late-onset sepsis (LOS), and 68% with bronchopulmonary dysplasia (BPD) [7]. The current treatments such as pulmonary surfactant administration, noninvasive respiratory support, and antibiotic administration are single-organ or symptom-targeted. Neonatologists are in urgent need for new systemic multiorgan-targeted treatments.

Human umbilical cord blood cells (UCBC) are abundant in stem cells. These primitive cells can home into damaged tissues, produce anti-inflammatory and immune-modulatory factors by paracrine effects, and differentiate into tissue cells [8]. Potential effects on respiratory distress syndrome (RDS), sepsis, and hypoxic-ischemic brain damage have been suggested in animal models [9–11]. Recently, these potential effects have been proved to be safe and feasible in clinical applications. Allogenic umbilical cord blood-derived mesenchymal stem cells (MSCs) have been applied in adults with acute RDS [12] and preterm infants with BPD [13], and autologous UCBC has been applied to neonates with HIE [14].

Recently, delayed cord clamping in premature neonates have been reported to improve neonatal mortality and morbidity. The American College of Obstetricians and Gynecologists now recommends a delay in umbilical cord clamping in preterm infants for at least 30–60 seconds after birth [15]. The potential mechanism was that delayed cord clamping was accompanied by an increased supply of RBCs and valuable progenitor cells [16].

Based on these evidence, we hypothesized that autologous cord blood infusion was safe for preterm infants. We report the outcomes of the infusion of autologous, volume- and RBC-reduced, noncryopreserved cord blood cell to 15 premature neonates.

2. Methods

This study was a phase I, open-label, single-arm, single-center trial to evaluate the safety of autologous, volume- and red blood cell- (RBC-) reduced, noncryopreserved umbilical cord blood cells (UCBC) (5×10^7 cells/kg) infusion for preterm infants <37 weeks gestational age.

2.1. Patients. We initiated this pilot study in December 2009. Inborn infants admitted to the Neonatal Intensive Care Unit (NICU) of Guangdong Women and Children's Hospital were eligible if they were (1) preterm: <37 weeks gestation, (2) without congenital abnormalities, (3) without maternal chorioamnionitis, (4) had available UCB, and (5) the mother was negative for hepatitis B (HBsAg and/or HBeAg) and C virus (anti-HCV), syphilis, HIV (anti-HIV-1 and -2) and IgM against Cytomegalovirus, rubella, toxoplasma, and herpes simplex virus. The study protocol was approved by the ethics committee of Guangdong Women and Children's Hospital. All patients in the study were given an intensive care therapy in accordance with the departmental guidelines which included therapies including positive pressure mechanical ventilation, noninvasive respiratory support, oxygen therapy, and exogenous surfactant (Curosurf, Chiesi, Parma, Italy) replacement. Chest radiographs were performed at admission and 8 hours after CBT on the first day of life in all surviving patients. Blood gas was monitored every 24 hours until weaning from ventilation. All clinical

diagnoses were defined according to a standard reference [17]. Soon after the preterm infant was delivered, written consent was signed by the parents, and autologous cord blood infusion was applied to the baby in addition to routine pulmonary surfactant replacement and mechanical ventilation support as indicated.

2.2. Cord Blood Process. Guangdong Cord Blood and Stem Cell Bank is a public provincial blood bank affiliated to the Guangdong Women and Children's Hospital, which collects cord blood of every delivery in this hospital. Therefore, the cord blood of all the subjects had been routinely collected during the delivery. The procedure of cord blood collection and transfusion was performed in accordance with the cord blood bank guidance [18]. The umbilical cord was clamped for the collection using a blood-collection bag (WEGO, China) containing 28 ml of citrate-phosphate-dextrose anticoagulant right after the baby was born and before the placenta was delivered. The umbilical vein was sterilized and punctured with a 17-gauge needle. UCB collections were made by trained obstetricians or cord blood bank collection staff who were present at the hospital during weekdays for 8–12 hours per day. When collection was completed, the blood bag tubing was closed and sealed. Cord blood labeled with the full name of the donor, group type, and volume of the blood product was stored in 4 degree and sent to the Cord Blood and Stem Cell Bank for processing immediately. Before processing, 2 ml samples were taken from all collected CB units to test for the presence of virus (human immunodeficiency virus, hepatitis B virus, hepatitis C virus, and Cytomegalovirus) and bacterial infections (including Treponema Pallidum). A sample of peripheral blood was collected from the mother and tested for the presence of maternal transmissible diseases. And the results were obtained soon before the transfusion started. After the sample was taken, it was volume- and RBC-reduced after 30 minute incubation with 6% Hespan (Bethlehem, USA) following established CBB procedures using the SEPAX S-100 automated processing system (Biosafe, Geneva, Switzerland) if the unit contained >30 ml of UCB or manually if the unit was <30 ml. The mononuclear layer was isolated by density gradient centrifugation ($1000g$, 30 min, RT, Beckman, American), then was transferred to cryobags. Excessive nucleated cell-poor plasma was expelled. Meanwhile, MNC count, CD34 cell, CFU-GM, and sterility detection (Sheldon Manufacturing Inc., Cornelius, OR, USA) were performed. Cell viability was measured via 7-aminoactinomycin D (7-AAD) detection kit through flow cytometry analysis (BD Bioscience, USA). All infusions were administered in Guangdong Women and Children Hospital. Infusate and subject identities were double-checked by the research and clinical nursing staff. Infusions were also monitored by the research and clinical staff. Cells were infused over 15 minutes, followed by a 2 ml saline flush to clear the intravascular line.

2.2.1. Assessment of Safety. Shortly, before, during, and until 24 hours after transfusion, heart rate, systolic, diastolic, and mean arterial blood pressure and arterial blood oxygen saturation level were monitored in peripheral blood continually and documented. Moreover, laboratory investigations in peripheral blood were monitored and kept stable during the whole treatment period, detailed in Table 1. Infusion reactions and signs of circulatory overload were checked.

2.2.2. Results. From January 1, 2009, till June 5, 2016, fifteen infants were enrolled for the treatment, gestational age ranged from 28 2/7 to 34 1/7 (31.2 ± 1.62) weeks and birth weight ranged from 1200 to 2220 (1582.7 ± 252.8) grams; 12/15 (80%) were delivered by cesarean section. All 15 patients who received the cord blood infusion survived. The duration of hospitalization ranged from 4 to 65 (30 ± 23.6) days. Details were shown in Table 2.

2.3. Characteristics of Cord Blood Processing. Cord blood volume collected ranged from 27 to 76 ml, mean (47.13 ± 19.10) ml; volume postprocessing ranged from 16 to 30 ml, mean (22.67 ± 4.05) ml; cells collected ranged from 0.97 to 8.11 ($\times 10^8$), mean ($3.10 \pm 2.17 \times 10^8$); cells postprocessing ranged from 0.86 to 7.83 ($\times 10^8$), mean ($2.67 \pm 2.00 \times 10^8$); cells concentration postprocessing ranged from 5.85 to 40.8×10^6/ml, mean ($13.10 \pm 10.35 \times 10^6$/ml); CFU-GM ranged from 0.72 to 11.27 ($\times 10^5$), mean ($3.72 \pm 3.25 \times 10^5$); amount of CD34+ cells in units varied widely, ranged from 0.1 to 16.22×10^6, mean (22.67 ± 4.05) ml; and viability of postprocessing units was high, ranged from 99.5 to 100%, mean (99.7 ± 0.17%). Details are shown in Table 3.

2.4. Infusion. Infused NC ranged from 4.48 to 5.0×10^7/kg, mean ($4.97 \pm 0.13 \times 10^6$/ml); time between collection (birth) and initiation of infusion ranged from 4.5 to 9 hours after birth, mean (6.77 ± 1.52 h); infused volume ranged from 2 to 28 ml, mean (10.27 ± 6.18 ml); pathogen detection (including bacteria culture, fungus culture, human immunodeficiency virus, hepatitis B virus, hepatitis C virus, Cytomegalovirus, and Treponema Pallidum) results were all negative.

2.5. Cord Blood Safety. The patient's vital signs and laboratory investigations were monitored during the whole treatment period, details were shown in Table 1. No significant infusion reactions were noted. No signs of circulatory overload and graft-versus-host disease (GVHD) were detected. Heart rate, mean arterial pressure, and oxygen saturation did not vary significantly before and after infusions.

2.6. Clinical Presentation and Complications

2.6.1. Mortality. The fifteen patients who received infusions all survived.

2.6.2. Nervous System. Three patients had birth asphyxia, among them one suffered from IVH. None of the patients developed abnormal clinical features of central nervous system disorders such as convulsions, apnea, or dysphagia.

2.6.3. Respiratory System. 12/15 (80%) presented with tachypnea and grunting soon after birth. The infants were diagnosed with RDS, 2/15 (13.3%) cases were grade I, 5/15 (33.3%) cases were grade II, 6/15 (40%) cases were grade III, and 2/15 (13.3%) cases were grade IV; and 12/15 (80%) received one dose PS replacement and 8/15 (53.3%) received

intubation-surfactant replacement extubation–nasal continuous positive airway pressure (INSURE) therapy; however, one patient needed reintubation. 4/15 (26.7%) received mechanical ventilation; the median duration was 3.2 ± 1.8 days. The duration of oxygen therapy was (5.3 ± 3.0) days. No patient suffered from BPD, and chest radiographs showed improvement.

2.6.4. Infection. 5/15 suffered from ventilation-associated pneumonia (VAP), of which two were cases of Klebsiella pneumonia, one was a case of *Pseudomonas aeruginosa* pneumonia, one was a case of *Acinetobacter baumannii* pneumonia, and 1 suffered from late onset sepsis, infected with Klebsiella pneumonia proved by blood culture.

2.6.5. ROP. No patients suffered from ROP.

2.6.6. NEC. No patients suffered from NEC.

2.6.7. Anemia. 10/15 (66.67%) suffered from anemia (≤140 g/l); 2/15 (13.33%) needed RBC transfusion.

3. Discussion

In our study, we treated 15 preterm infants with autologous, volume and RBC-reduced cord blood cells. The treatment was started within 8 hours after birth. No adverse effect of cell therapy was noticed. No patient died during treatment. No preterm complications such as BPD, NEC, or ROP were observed. Our study presents preliminary data on the safety of autologous cord blood cell therapy in preterm infants. We postulated that several factors contributed to the safety issue, among them, the most important one was the autologous cell source. Based on the autologous cell source, no GVHD-related complication was observed. Moreover, autologous cell source avoided ethical issues. A second factor that contributed to the safety issue was cord blood minimal-processing procedure. In our study, only density gradient centrifugation was employed to separate nucleated cells. Since our cell infusions were started within 8 hours after birth, no cryopreservation was needed; thus, no chemicals were added into the cord blood cells for cryopreservation. This minimal-processing procedure and immediate transfusion after processing helped to avoid contamination and possible chemical toxicity. It also alleviated decrease of viability which may happen during storage.

In our study, mean (47.13 ± 19.10) ml cord blood with a total TNC of $(3.10 \pm 2.17) \times 10^8$ mononuclear cells was collected before processing. After processing, cord blood volume and TNC were reduced to (22.67 ± 4.05) ml and $(2.67 \pm 2.00) \times 10^8$, respectively, including $(22.67 \pm 4.05) \times 10^6$ CD34+ and $(3.72 \pm 3.25) \times 10^5$ colony forming cells (CFU-GM) in a vitality (99.7 ± 0.17%).

Recently, delayed umbilical cord clamping 30–60 seconds after birth in preterms had been recommended by the American College of Obstetricians and Gynecologists and had been reported to reduce preterm-related complications. It is possible that delayed cord clamping increases supply of RBC and valuable stem and progenitor cells (SPC), thus may improve mortality and morbidity in premature neonates

TABLE 1: Clinical findings previous and post infusion.

Serial number	Blood routine								pH			Blood gas								
	HB		HCT		WBC		PLT					PO2			PCO2			Fio2		
	Pre	Post	Pre	Post	Pre	Post	Pre	Post	Pre	Post-12h	Post-24h	Pre	Post-12h	Post-24h	Pre	Post-12h	Post-24h	Pre	Post-12h	Post-24h
1	177	144	50	37.3	10.8	9.2	304	335	7.34	7.27	7.45	9.3	8.9	8.9	4.8	7	3.2	0.3	0.21	0.21
2	167	137	49	37.4	10.9	10.2	284	243	7.26	7.4	7.37	6.7	12.7	6.4	6.8	3.7	4.6	0.4	0.25	0.21
3	135	132	37	15.3	14.9	13.2	252	248	7.25	7.2	7.33	4.64	5.07	9.9	7.25	8.02	4.26	0.35	0.25	0.21
4	145	144	39	39.9	8.8	10.1	405	336	7.25	7.28	7.39	6.5	9.1	6.1	7.6	6.6	4.4	0.35	0.21	0.21
5	171	180	50	50.6	9.6	17.9	265	161	7.42	7.39	7.34	3.9	4.5	6.4	3.7	3.9	5.1	0.55	0.3	0.23
6	120	116	35	34	14	13.5	320	256	7.34	7.36	7.49	8.3	6.6	5.6	5.9	4.8	3.2	0.45	0.21	0.21
7	148	139	44	39.1	35	14.2	274	446	7.3	7.34	7.37	11.6	11.3	6.95	5.1	4.28	4.34	0.35	0.21	0.21
8	212	203	60.5	54.3	13.7	14	413	420	7.42	7.28	7.45	10.48	10.25	8.31	4.78	4.82	3.62	0.25	0.21	0.21
9	149	136	43.7	42.1	9.62	10.3	338	340	7.28	7.42	7.43	9.77	8.23	7.14	7.82	4.5	4.23	0.25	0.21	0.21
10	166	158	47.6	46.7	12.3	16.3	271	189	7.32	7.3	7.3	9.84	10.2	8.13	6.66	5.45	6.03	0.5	0.4	0.35
11	164	109	49	31.8	14.4	9.4	229	154	7.34	7.35	7.36	6.4	5.3	5	5.2	4.9	4.5	0.5	0.3	0.21
12	169	136	49	41.9	7.1	17	296	318	7.32	7.5	7.37	9	14	7.6	4.7	2.5	3.4	0.25	0.21	0.21
13	159	105	46	31.2	12.9	10.6	329	465	7.28	7.5	7.48	8.3	6.2	8	7.6	3	4.1	0.3	0.21	0.21
14	142	136	46	42	11.8	9.6	235	245	7.39	7.4	7.58	10.06	9.82	6.17	5.3	4.82	2.92	0.25	0.21	0.21
15	136	122	48	46.3	11.3	9.3	236	240	7.32	7.36	7.4	11.1	10.95	10.32	6.47	5.37	4.83	0.45	0.25	0.21
Mean	157	139	46.3	39.3	13.1	12.3	296.7	293.1	7.32	7.36	7.40	8.39	8.87	7.39	5.98	4.91	4.18	0.37	0.24	0.22
SD	22.04	25.5	6.18	9.30	6.4	3.03	56.70	97.88	0.06	0.08	0.07	2.31	2.86	1.54	1.28	1.5	0.82	0.10	0.05	0.034

TABLE 2

	Sex	GA (weeks)	BW (g)	Delivery mode	APGAR		RDS grade	PS		Respiratory support			Time return to BW (D)	Complications						Duration of hospitalization (D)	Prognosis
					1 minute	5 minute			Times	Duration of mechanical ventilation (D)	Duration of oxygen therapy (D)	Reintubation		BPD	VAP	IVH	ROP	LOS	NEC		
1	M	30+5	1630	CS	9	9	3	Y	1	5	5	N	20	Nil	Nil	Nil	Nil	Nil	Nil	18	Cured
2	M	30+5	1510	CS	5	9	4	Y	1	3	9	N	21	Nil	Nil	Nil	Nil	Nil	Nil	53	Cured
3	M	33	1630	VD	8	6	3	Y	1	4	11	N	36	Nil	Y	Nil	Nil	Y	Nil	46	Cured
4	M	31+2	1510	VD	9	10	2	Y	1	2.5	3	N	20	Nil	Y	Nil	Nil	Nil	Nil	65	Cured
5	F	28+2	1400	CS	9	10	3	Y	1	4	9	Y	32	Nil	Y	Nil	Nil	Nil	Nil	30	Cured
6	M	30+1	1600	CS	8	10	4	Y	1	2.5	4	N	26	Nil	Y	Nil	Nil	Nil	Nil	4	Cured
7	M	29+1	1450	CS	9	10	2	Y	1	7	8	N	28	Nil	Nil	Nil	Nil	Nil	Nil	10	Cured
8	M	31+5	1700	CS	8	9	1	Y	1	2	2	N	14	Nil	Nil	Nil	Nil	Nil	Nil	47	Cured
9	M	32+5	1940	CS	9	10	2	Y	1	3	3	N	13	Nil	Nil	Nil	Nil	Nil	Nil	24	Cured
10	M	29+6	1400	CS	10	10	1	N	0	0	3	N	14	Nil	Y	Nil	Nil	Nil	Nil	82	Cured
11	M	32+5	1660	CS	9	10	3	Y	1	5.5	9	N	12	Nil	Nil	Nil	Nil	Nil	Nil	23	Cured
12	M	31	1240	VD	9	9	2	Y	1	4	5	N	14	Nil	Y	Y	Nil	Nil	Nil	20	Cured
13	M	30	1600	CS	9	10	3	Y	1	3	4.5	N	12	Nil	Nil	Nil	Nil	Nil	Nil	19	Cured
14	F	32+2	1450	CS	9	10	2	N	0	1.5	2.5	N	16	Nil	Nil	Nil	Nil	Nil	Nil	5	Cured
15	F	34+1	2220	VD	9	10	3	N	0	1	2	N	14	Nil	Nil	Nil	Nil	Nil	Nil	4	Cured
MEAN±SD										3.2±1.8	5.3±3.0									30±23.6	

TABLE 3

No	Volume collected	Volume postprocessing	Cells collected (108)	Cells postprocessing (108)	Cell concentration postprocessing*106/ml	CFU-GM/105	CD34+/106	Viability	Infused NC*107/kg	Infused age (H)	Infused volume	Pathogen detection
1	34	22	1.82	1.46	6.65	1.84	1.1	100	4.48	5	11	Negative
2	35	20	1.6	1.32	5.82	1.98	0.7	99.5	5	6	13	Negative
3	61	24	2.44	1.67	6.95	2.3	1.14	99.8	5	7	12	Negative
4	33	16	0.97	0.86	5.4	0.72	0.31	99.8	5	4	14	Negative
5	36	22	1.43	1.21	5.5	1.57	0.59	99.8	5	9	13	Negative
6	28	16	1.43	1.23	7.7	1.53	0.9	99.5	5	4.5	11	Negative
7	55	28	5.81	5.43	26.3	11.27	5.69	99.8	5	6	3	Negative
8	65	20	2.99	2.37	11.85	1.66	1.66	99.9	5	7	8	Negative
9	81	20	6.14	4.33	21.65	9.96	3.9	99.9	5	8	5	Negative
10	27	28	2.21	1.97	7.05	3.35	0.55	99.8	5	8	28	Negative
11	46	24	2.96	2.65	13.6	3.32	1.01	99.5	5	7	6	Negative
12	37	24	1.51	1.4	5.85	1.04	0.08	99.9	5	9	12	Negative
13	24	22	1.72	1.58	8.53	2.82	1.1	99.8	5	6	9	Negative
14	69	24	8.11	7.83	40.8	6.08	16.22	99.8	5	7	2	Negative
15	76	30	5.3	4.7	22.8	6.39	1	99.5	5	8	7	Negative
Mean	47.13	22.67	3.10	2.67	13.10	3.72	2.40	99.7	4.97	6.77	10.27	
SD	19.10	4.05	2.17	2.00	10.35	3.25	4.10	0.17	0.13	1.52	6.18	

[15, 16]. However, delayed umbilical cord clamping mainly supply RBC instead of MNC to the infants. Therefore, we used noncryopreserved autologous cord blood cells infusion soon after preterm birth which contains mainly MNC with a lower volume. As is known that SPC mainly exits in MNC layer. It is considered as the most effective component in cord blood and strongly associated with a lower risk of developing preterm complications [19, 20]. Further, in view of the vulnerable heart function of preterm infants, they could only accept limited volume of infusion. Therefore, to achieve more MNC in a lower volume, we used volume- and RBC-reduced cord blood cells in our study to decrease the burden to the heart.

BPD is the main complication that contributes to morbidity and mortality in extremely premature newborns. It has been reported that among infants born with gestational ages of 22 to 28 weeks, 68% suffered from BPD [7]. The pathophysiologic features of BPD include abnormal lung growth characterized by reduced numbers of alveoli, blood vessels, prominent fibrosis, and secondary pulmonary hypertension [21]. Cord blood angiogenic progenitor cells and endothelial progenitor cells were reported to be decreased in preterm infants with BPD [5, 6]. Current therapy for BPD included noninvasive ventilation strategies, inhaled nitric oxide, antioxidants, vitamin A, caffeine, and corticosteroids. However, so far there are no specific therapies that have been widely adopted. It has been reported that MSCs may release anti-inflammatory paracrine factors. These factors have effect on both lung injury and sepsis [22, 23]. Periventricular leukomalacia (PVL) is another severe preterm complication, affecting 16% infants born with gestational age of 22 to 28 weeks [7]. PVL reflected perinatal damage from inflammation and oxidation to the developing brain, which was one of main reasons responsible for cerebral palsy [24]. Current therapy for hypoxic-ischemic damage was hypothermia. However, hypothermia therapy is contraindicated in preterm infants because of their immature thermoregulation [25, 26]. HUCBC has been shown to be effective in newborn models of hypoxic injury [4]; furthermore, autologous intravenous UCB infusion is safe and feasible in neonates with HIE and young children with acquired neurological disorders [7, 27]. In our study, there was one case complicated with IVH; however, no clinical presentation related to the central nervous system was observed. The underlying mechanism might be that the UCBC migrate to damaged sites, form anti-inflammatory or immunomodulatory factors, then proliferate into neurons [28, 29]. Sepsis is a common and major cause of death in preterm infants [30, 31]. Among very low birth weight infants (VLBW; < 1500 g), rates of sepsis range between 11% and 46% [32]. Neonatal sepsis and systemic inflammatory response syndrome (SIRS) are associated with brain damage [31, 33]. Current therapy for neonatal sepsis is the antibiotic administration. However, antibiotic resistance is a therapeutic problem in preterms. Substantial evidence from models of both lung injury and sepsis suggested that MSCs have an anti-inflammatory effect on host tissue, partly through the release of paracrine factors, reprogramming host macrophages [22, 23, 34]. In addition, MSCs reduced alveolar bacterial counts and improved alveolar macrophage

phagocytosis after direct bacterial injury mediated by FGF7, LL-37 [35, 36]. All these investigations have laid down the foundation for cord blood cell therapy for preterms with pulmonary disorders complicated with sepsis and brain damage. NEC and ROP are two main complications of preterm infants; however, there were no cases observed in our study; the underlying reason might be the limited enrolled number and relatively large gestational age of infants enrolled in our study. To achieve more evidence regarding NEC and ROP, a large cohort study will be needed in our future study.

Studies on safety and feasibility of whole autologous cord blood transplant in preterm were also reported [19, 20]. Rudnicki and colleagues compared whole autologous cord blood infusion with allogeneic red blood cells in the treatment of preterm with anemia and showed autologous CB infusion was as effective and safe as allogeneic RBC transfusion [19]. In our study, 10/15 (66.67%) infants suffered from anemia (≤140 g/l); 2/15 (13.33%) needed RBC transfusion. Allogeneic RBCs transfusion is the main therapy for severe anemia [17]. In this study, we explore the safety of volume- and RBC-reduced cord blood cells to treat preterm infants. Both autologous cord blood infusion possess its advantage. However, further multiple center randomized controlled studies are needed regarding short-term and long-term outcomes.

Regarding the administration route, there were reports on the advantage of damaged site administration when compared to intravenous infusion. However, on the one hand, the potential preterm complications were due to multiorgan damage. To achieve the multiorgan-targeted effect, we used intravenous infusion as the administration route, which may result in cells being trapped in organs such as lung and brain. On the other hand, in the report supported site administration, allogenic-MSC was used in intratracheal administration to treat hyperoxia-induced lung damage; it seemed to attenuate the side effects of rejection.

In our study, we chose the infusion timing to be very soon after birth which is within the first 8 postnatal hours. Although some infants were delivered at midnight, we tried to process as early as within 8 hours after their birth. As it had been reported that it would take more than 1 week for progenitor cells to differentiate into damaged tissue cells, we administered CBC during the first hours after birth, so that it might provide enough time for these cells for differentiation.

In conclusion, we demonstrated autologous, volume- and RBC-reduced, noncryopreserved cord blood cells transfusion soon after birth was safe and feasible in preterm infants. Autologous cord blood infusion avoid GVHD; meanwhile, the reduced volume would protect the fragile cardio-function of the preterm infants. This autologous, volume- and RBC-reduced, method guaranteed the safety of application. In addition, this was an autologous transfusion instead of "cell transplantation therapy", and therefore it was not regulated by the FDA regulation licensing public cord blood banks distributing unrelated banked cord blood units for allogeneic transplantation in 2012. However, our study was the single-center descriptive study with limited number of preterm infants, further multicenter randomized controlled trials are needed to prove the effectiveness.

Authors' Contributions

Jie Yang and Zhuxiao Ren has equivalent contribution to the study.

Acknowledgments

This work was supported by Guangzhou Technology Program (grant numbers 201707010398, 201804010380).

References

[1] H. Blencowe, S. Cousens, M. Z. Oestergaard et al., "National, regional, and worldwide estimates of preterm birth rates in the year 2010 with time trends since 1990 for selected countries: a systematic analysis and implications," *The Lancet*, vol. 379, no. 9832, pp. 2162–2172, 2012.

[2] S. Petrou, Z. Mehta, C. Hockley, P. Cook-Mozaffari, J. Henderson, and M. Goldacre, "The impact of preterm birth on hospital inpatient admissions and costs during the first 5 years of life," *Pediatrics*, vol. 112, no. 6, pp. 1290–1297, 2003.

[3] O. Khwaja and J. J. Volpe, "Pathogenesis of cerebral white matter injury of prematurity," *Archives of Disease in Childhood - Fetal and Neonatal Edition*, vol. 93, no. 2, pp. F153–F161, 2008.

[4] S. A. Mitsialis and S. Kourembanas, "Stem cell-based therapies for the newborn lung and brain: possibilities and challenges," *Seminars in Perinatology*, vol. 40, no. 3, pp. 138–151, 2016.

[5] C. D. Baker, V. Balasubramaniam, P. M. Mourani et al., "Cord blood angiogenic progenitor cells are decreased in bronchopulmonary dysplasia," *The European Respiratory Journal*, vol. 40, no. 6, pp. 1516–1522, 2012.

[6] A. Borghesi, M. Massa, R. Campanelli et al., "Circulating endothelial progenitor cells in preterm infants with bronchopulmonary dysplasia," *American Journal of Respiratory and Critical Care Medicine*, vol. 180, no. 6, pp. 540–546, 2009.

[7] B. J. Stoll, N. I. Hansen, E. F. Bell et al., "Neonatal outcomes of extremely preterm infants from the NICHD neonatal research network," *Pediatrics*, vol. 126, no. 3, pp. 443–456, 2010.

[8] T. C. Lund, A. E. Boitano, C. S. Delaney, E. J. Shpall, and J. E. Wagner, "Advances in umbilical cord blood manipulation-from niche to bedside," *Nature Reviews. Clinical Oncology*, vol. 12, no. 3, pp. 163–174, 2015.

[9] J. Walter, L. B. Ware, and M. A. Matthay, "Mesenchymal stem cells: mechanisms of potential therapeutic benefit in ARDS and sepsis," *The Lancet Respiratory Medicine*, vol. 2, no. 12, pp. 1016–1026, 2014.

[10] R. S. Alphonse, S. Rajabali, and B. Thebaud, "Lung injury in preterm neonates: the role and therapeutic potential of stem cells," *Antioxidants & Redox Signaling*, vol. 17, no. 7, pp. 1013–1040, 2012.

[11] A. Drobyshevsky, C. M. Cotten, Z. Shi et al., "Human umbilical cord blood cells ameliorate motor deficits in rabbits in a cerebral palsy model," *Developmental Neuroscience*, vol. 37, no. 4-5, pp. 349–362, 2015.

[12] Y. Chang, S. H. Park, J. W. Huh, C. M. Lim, Y. Koh, and S. B. Hong, "Intratracheal administration of umbilical cord blood-derived mesenchymal stem cells in a patient with acute respiratory distress syndrome," *Journal of Korean Medical Science*, vol. 29, no. 3, pp. 438–440, 2014.

[13] Y. S. Chang, S. Y. Ahn, H. S. Yoo et al., "Mesenchymal stem cells for bronchopulmonary dysplasia: phase 1 dose-escalation clinical trial," *The Journal of Pediatrics*, vol. 164, no. 5, pp. 966–972.e6, 2014.

[14] C. M. Cotten, A. P. Murtha, R. N. Goldberg et al., "Feasibility of autologous cord blood cells for infants with hypoxic-ischemic encephalopathy," *The Journal of Pediatrics*, vol. 164, no. 5, pp. 973–979.e1, 2014.

[15] "Committee opinion no. 684 summary: delayed umbilical cord clamping after birth," *Obstetrics & Gynecology*, vol. 129, no. 1, pp. 232-233, 2017.

[16] C. Lawton, S. Acosta, N. Watson et al., "Enhancing endogenous stem cells in the newborn via delayed umbilical cord clamping," *Neural Regeneration Research*, vol. 10, no. 9, pp. 1359–1362, 2015.

[17] T. Gomella, M. Cummingham, and E. Fabien, *Neonatology*, Lange, New York, 6th edition, 2009.

[18] National Health and Family Planning Commission of the People's Republic of China, "Umbilical cord blood and stem cell bank management regulation," http://www.Moh.Gov.cn/zhuzhan/wsbmgz/201308/9da745d55fe749a2b82b95ee65294b55.shtml (Chinese).

[19] M. Kotowski, Z. Litwinska, P. Klos et al., "Autologus cord blood transfusion in preterm infants-could its humoral effect be the key to control prematurity-related complications? A preliminary study," *Journal of Physiology and Pharmacology*, vol. 68, no. 6, pp. 921–927, 2017.

[20] J. Rudnicki, M. P. Kawa, M. Kotowski et al., "Clinical evaluation of the safety and feasibility of whole autologous cord blood transplant as a source of stem and progenitor cells for extremely premature neonates: preliminary report," *Experimental and Clinical Transplantation*, vol. 13, no. 6, pp. 563–572, 2015.

[21] W. H. Northway Jr, R. C. Rosan, and D. Y. Porter, "Pulmonary disease following respirator therapy of hyaline-membrane disease — bronchopulmonary dysplasia," *The New England Journal of Medicine*, vol. 276, no. 7, pp. 357–368, 1967.

[22] L. A. Ortiz, M. DuTreil, C. Fattman et al., "Interleukin 1 receptor antagonist mediates the antiinflammatory and antifibrotic effect of mesenchymal stem cells during lung injury," *Proceedings of the National Academy of Sciences of the United States of America*, vol. 104, no. 26, pp. 11002–11007, 2007.

[23] S. Danchuk, J. H. Ylostalo, F. Hossain et al., "Human multipotent stromal cells attenuate lipopolysaccharide-induced acute lung injury in mice via secretion of tumor necrosis factor-α-induced protein 6," *Stem Cell Research & Therapy*, vol. 2, no. 3, p. 27, 2011.

[24] A. H. MacLennan, S. C. Thompson, and J. Gecz, "Cerebral palsy: causes, pathways, and the role of genetic variants," *American Journal of Obstetrics and Gynecology*, vol. 213, no. 6, pp. 779–788, 2015.

[25] S. Shankaran, A. R. Laptook, R. A. Ehrenkranz et al., "Whole-body hypothermia for neonates with hypoxic-ischemic encephalopathy," *The New England Journal of Medicine*, vol. 353, no. 15, pp. 1574–1584, 2005.

[26] R. P. Sutsko, K. C. Young, A. Ribeiro et al., "Long-term reparative effects of mesenchymal stem cell therapy following neonatal hyperoxia-induced lung injury," *Pediatric Research*, vol. 73, no. 1, pp. 46–53, 2013.

[27] W. Sun, L. Buzanska, K. Domanska-Janik, R. J. Salvi, and
      M. K. Stachowiak, "Voltage-sensitive and ligand-gated chan-
      nels in differentiating neural stem-like cells derived from the
      nonhematopoietic fraction of human umbilical cord blood,"
      Stem Cells, vol. 23, no. 7, pp. 931–945, 2005.

[28] A. Saha, S. Buntz, P. Scotland et al., "A cord blood monocyte-
      derived cell therapy product accelerates brain remyelination,"
      JCI Insight, vol. 1, no. 13, article e86667, 2016.

[29] Z. A. Englander, J. Sun, Laura Case, M. A. Mikati, J. Kurtzberg,
      and A. W. Song, "Brain structural connectivity increases con-
      current with functional improvement: evidence from diffusion
      tensor MRI in children with cerebral palsy during therapy,"
      NeuroImage: Clinical, vol. 7, pp. 315–324, 2015.

[30] J. E. Lawn, S. Cousens, J. Zupan, and Lancet Neonatal Survival
      Steering Team, "4 million neonatal deaths: when? Where?
      Why?," *The Lancet*, vol. 365, no. 9462, pp. 891–900, 2005.

[31] S. Vergnano, E. Menson, N. Kennea et al., "Neonatal infections
      in England: the NeonIN surveillance network," *Archives of
      Disease in Childhood - Fetal and Neonatal Edition*, vol. 96,
      no. 1, pp. F9–14, 2011.

[32] B. Alshaikh, K. Yusuf, and R. Sauve, "Neurodevelopmental
      outcomes of very low birth weight infants with neonatal sepsis:
      systematic review and meta-analysis," *Journal of Perinatology*,
      vol. 33, no. 7, pp. 558–564, 2013.

[33] B. J. Stoll, N. I. Hansen, I. Adams-Chapman et al., "Neurode-
      velopmental and growth impairment among extremely low-
      birth-weight infants with neonatal infection," *Journal of the
      American Medical Association*, vol. 292, no. 19, pp. 2357–
      2365, 2004.

[34] K. Németh, A. Leelahavanichkul, P. S. T. Yuen et al., "Bone
      marrow stromal cells attenuate sepsis via prostaglandin E_2-
      dependent reprogramming of host macrophages to increase
      their interleukin-10 production," *Nature Medicine*, vol. 15,
      no. 1, pp. 42–49, 2009.

[35] J. W. Lee, A. Krasnodembskaya, D. H. McKenna, Y. Song,
      J. Abbott, and M. A. Matthay, "Therapeutic effects of human
      mesenchymal stem cells in *ex vivo* human lungs injured with
      live bacteria," *American Journal of Respiratory and Critical
      Care Medicine*, vol. 187, no. 7, pp. 751–760, 2013.

[36] A. Krasnodembskaya, Y. Song, X. Fang et al., "Antibacterial
      effect of human mesenchymal stem cells is mediated in part
      from secretion of the antimicrobial peptide LL-37," *Stem Cells*,
      vol. 28, no. 12, pp. 2229–2238, 2010.

14

The Effect of Chronic Inflammation and Oxidative and Endoplasmic Reticulum Stress in the Course of Metabolic Syndrome and its Therapy

Michalina Alicka ⓘD[1] **and Krzysztof Marycz** ⓘD[1,2]

[1]*Department of Experimental Biology, The Faculty of Biology and Animal Science, University of Environmental and Life Sciences Wroclaw, Wroclaw, Poland*
[2]*Faculty of Veterinary Medicine, Equine Clinic-Equine Surgery, Justus-Liebig-University, 35392 Gießen, Germany*

Correspondence should be addressed to Krzysztof Marycz; krzysztof.marycz@upwr.edu.pl

Academic Editor: Stan Gronthos

Metabolic syndrome (MetS) is highly associated with a modern lifestyle. The prevalence of MetS has reached epidemic proportion and is still rising. The main cause of MetS and finally type 2 diabetes occurrence is excessive nutrient intake, lack of physical activity, and inflammatory cytokines secretion. These factors lead to redistribution of body fat and oxidative and endoplasmic reticulum (ER) stress occurrence, resulting in insulin resistance, increase adipocyte differentiation, and much elevated levels of proinflammatory cytokines. Cellular therapies, especially mesenchymal stem cell (MSC) transplantation, seem to be promising in the MetS and type 2 diabetes treatments, due to their immunomodulatory effect and multipotent capacity; adipose-derived stem cells (ASCs) play a crucial role in MSC-based cellular therapies. In this review, we focused on etiopathology of MetS, especially on the crosstalk between chronic inflammation, oxidative stress, and ER stress and their effect on MetS-related disease occurrence, as well as future perspectives of cellular therapies. We also provide an overview of therapeutic approaches that target endoplasmic reticulum and oxidative stress.

1. Introduction

Metabolic syndrome—also called insulin resistance syndrome or syndrome X—was described for the first time in 1988 [1]. The term describes all of the metabolic disorders that are associated with visceral adiposity. The metabolic syndrome frequency depends on sociodemographic and 132#geographic factors. The conditions that have been described as metabolic risk factors of MetS development involve insulin resistance, hypertension, dyslipidemia (hypertriglyceridemia, low high-density lipoprotein cholesterol), abdominal obesity, elevated glucose levels, high blood pressure, and proinflammatory and prothrombotic state [2]. Characteristics of insulin-resistant phenotype include impaired glucose metabolism or tolerance, elevated fasting glucose levels and/or hyperglycemia, and decreased insulin-mediated glucose reductions in the suppression of glucose production inside the body [3]. Genetics, postmenopausal status [4], excessive alcohol consumption [5], prolonged chronic stress [6], and physical inactivity [7] may have a causal effect, but these depend on the ethnic group [8].

Nutrition Examination Survey and National Health data estimate that the highest MetS prevalence has Mexican-American women. The data estimates that 34% of adults in the United States had a diagnosis of MetS [9]. International Diabetes Federation extrapolates that MetS prevalence in European population is 41% in men and 38% in women [10]. MetS is associated with a high risk of developing several lifestyle diseases including type 2 diabetes and cerebrovascular disease. Moreover, individuals with the MetS carry an approximately twofold increase in the risk of cardiovascular disease [2]. Globally, 8.3% of adults (382 mln) live with type 2 diabetes but the number is still rising. It is estimated that the number of diabetes patients will increase to 592 mln in

20 years (IDF). Furthermore, it is well known that type 2 diabetes is currently the leading cause of death among people under 60 years of age. The emerging problem has become the reason for new drug development, such as dipeptidyl-peptidase-4 (DPP-4) inhibitors, sodium glucose transporter-2 (SGLT2) inhibitors, glucagon-like peptide (GLP-1) mimesis, and cellular therapy (MSC) application [11]. Although it is obvious that the accumulation of visceral and ectopic fat is an important contributing factor to metabolic and cardiovascular risk implementation of fat distribution, assessment into clinical practice is still a challenge. Moreover, the prevalence of obesity has increased over the last 20 years [12]. The main recommendation for metabolic syndrome prevention and treatment is changes in the lifestyle. The changes include regular physical activity [13, 14] and calorie restriction [15]. Herein, we demonstrated the effect of chronic inflammation, oxidative stress, and prolonged endoplasmic reticulum stress on MetS development, as well as the potential of cellular therapy on MetS-associated diseases, especially type 2 diabetes treatment.

2. Adipose Tissue and Metabolic Syndrome: Chronic Inflammation

Adipose tissue is an active metabolic and endocrine organ responsible for the cross-talk between various systems, including the immune and the cardiovascular systems [16]. Adipocytes play an important role in the control of energy balance and lipid/glucose homeostasis. Adipose tissue excess or obesity has an effect of pathology in caloric balance in susceptible individuals that contribute to metabolic syndrome [17]. The adipocyte is the only cell whose size evolves drastically. Studies have reported that the degree of inflammation in the adipose tissue depends on the size of the adipocytes [18]. Prolonged obesity causes cell hypertrophy (cell size increase), which might lead to MetS occurrence. Because of the alternations, new adipocytes are required to work against the hypertrophic adipocytes [19, 20]. Probably, the adipose tissue depots of overweight individuals have already committed the resource of their stem cells to the adipocyte lineage and, consequently, have no capacity to create new adipose cells [21]. Adipocyte hypertrophy leads to local adipose tissue hypoxia, caused by relative deficiency of vasculature [22, 23]. Furthermore, hypoxia can induce cell necrosis with the production of adipokines [24].

Adipose tissue is a type of connective tissue which consists predominantly of mature adipocytes and stromal vascular fraction (SVF) cells, such as preadipocytes, fibroblasts, blood cells, macrophages, and endothelial cells [25]. Furthermore, the adipocyte tissue is a source of multipotent adipose tissue-derived mesenchymal stem cells (ASCs). ASCs were first described by Zuk and colleagues at the beginning of the 21st century [26] as multipotent, self-renewing, and undifferentiated progenitor cells that are phenotypically and morphologically similar to bone marrow-derived mesenchymal stem cells (BMSCs). Moreover, the cells have an ability to form single colonies (CFU-Fs) and adhere to the plastic surface. The Internal Fat Applied Technology Society has

suggested that both ASCs and BMSCs display the stem cell-specific types of surface markers, including CD90, CD105, CD73, CD44, and CD166, and lack of the typical hematopoietic markers CD45 and CD34. Moreover, ASCs have an ability to differentiate into cells of mesoderm, including adipocytes, osteocytes, chondrocytes, and myocytes, that exhibit their potential for cell-based therapies [27, 28]. Both populations of MSCs, because of their immunomodulatory activity and the potential to differentiate into insulin-producing cells, might become a potential therapy strategy in the course of type 2 diabetes and MetS [29–31]. Bone marrow-derived MSCs are suboptimal for clinical use in regenerative medicine because of a highly invasive aspiration procedure [32]. ASC isolation from subcutaneous adipose tissue is a minimally invasive method [33, 34]. The group [26] has demonstrated that the adipose tissue is an alternative source of MSC.

Abdominal obesity is associated with an increase in both adipocyte size and adipocyte number; furthermore, MSCs are able to differentiate into adipocytes. Thus, new adipocytes arise from ASC pools regardless of age [34]. Furthermore, Liechty and colleagues have demonstrated that xenotransplantation of MSCs from human into fetal sheep marrow was successfully performed. Moreover, the cells were able to differentiate into adipocytes in adipose tissue, confirming that MSCs are an important cell source for adipogenesis [35, 36]. As mentioned above, proliferations and differentiation capacity decrease with the age because of both an accumulation of multiple oxidative stress factors and decrease antioxidative protection. The events lead to the decrease of proliferation activity, decreased differentiation capacity, and higher sensitivity to apoptosis. The alternations very limit their therapeutic potential [11, 37–39].

MetS progression is associated with decreased CD34, as well as endothelial progenitor cell level. Furthermore, some factors, like elevated proinflammatory cytokine, including IL-6 and IFNα induce MSC proliferation, although normally they are in an undifferentiated and inactive state [40]. Thus, both increased caloric uptake and inflammation can cause a constant providing of alarm factors and MSC activity. Furthermore, reduction of MSC pool can lead to irreparable impairment of body regeneration [41]. A equine model has shown that MSCs isolated from EMS (equine metabolic syndrome) horses exhibited decreased clonogenic potential, increased population doubling time (PDT), and depletion of MSC-specific surface markers, such as CD90, CD105, and CD73 [42–45]. Moreover, murine studies have demonstrated decreased CD105 expression consistent with decreased potential for chondrogenic differentiation in obese mice [46]. It is interesting that MetS cells were characterized by overexpression of immune cell receptor CD44, a cell surface marker which plays an important role in inflammatory cell activation. Interestingly, other independent studies have confirmed the theory of overexpression CD44 in an obese mouse. Moreover, knockout CD44 mouse did not develop neither obesity nor type 2 diabetes despite high-fat diet feeding [47–49]. Another research has revealed that overexpression of CD44 is significantly correlated with local inflammation and systemic insulin resistance in human adipose tissue [49] (Table 1).

TABLE 1: Characterization of specific MSC surface biomarkers in non-MetS and MetS individuals.

	Specific surface markers	Characterization/effects	References
Non-MetS	(−) CD34, CD45	(−) hematopoetic stem cell-specific markers	[27, 28]
	(+) CD105, CD90, CD73, CD44, CD166	(+) mesenchymal stem cell-specific markers	
MetS	↓ CD90, CD105, CD73	↓ decreased clonogenic potential, increased PDT, decreased potential for chondrogenesis	[42–46]
	↑ CD44	↑ inflammatory response	[47–49]

MetS: metabolic syndrome; (+): presence; (−): lack; ↑: increase; ↓: decrease.

Multiple scientists described the function of the immune system in metabolic syndrome. It is not still clear what causes MetS, but it is known that a chronic inflammatory state is associated with metabolic syndrome occurrences. The report is based on evidence of increased various proinflammatory cytokines (e.g., interleukin 1β (IL-1β), IL-8, monocyte chemoattractant protein-1 (MCP-1), tumor necrosis factor α (TNFα), and prothrombotic mediator plasminogen activator inhibitor-1 (PAI-1)), as well as biomarkers of inflammation (e.g. C-reactive protein (CRP)) concentration in MetS individuals [50, 51]. There are three major sites that have been involved in initiating of chronic inflammation in MetS: liver, intestine, and adipose tissue [52–55]. Moreover, the secretion of inflammatory mediators from one tissue promotes inflammation in other sites, thereby increasing the chronic inflammation in the body causing tissue dysfunction/injury [54].

Recently, many studies reported that adipocyte hypertrophy and hyperplasia in response to nutritional excess result in abnormal adipose cell function and cause insulin resistance [25, 56, 57]. Hypertrophic adipocytes secrete proinflammatory cytokines, such as TNFα, IL-6, IL-8, and MCP-1. High levels of proinflammatory cytokines cause serine phosphorylation of insulin receptor substrate-1 via nuclear factor κB and Jun N-terminal kinase signaling. The reaction leads to the development of insulin resistance [58, 59] (Table 2). Hypoxia can contribute to the induction of cell necrosis with the production of TNFα, IL-6, PAI-6, and macrophage infiltration [22].

TNFα acts as a paracrine mediator to enhance insulin resistance in adipose cells. Furthermore, it is an important mediator of several cardiovascular events, such as heart failure and atherosclerosis [60]. TNFα is also key in the pathophysiology of inflammatory dermatoses associated with MetS, including hidradenitis suppurativa and psoriasis [61].

IL-6 is a potent cytokine that plays a significant role in the pathogenesis of insulin resistance and type 2 diabetes. An excess of IL-6 has been measured in adipose tissue in patients with obesity and type 2 diabetes, as well as in patients with MetS [62]. Moreover, a murine model has shown that elevated IL-6 level is associated with several diseases which include cardiovascular events, atherosclerosis, and hypertension and chronic IL-6 exposure causes hyperglycemia associated with insulin resistance [63, 64].

PAI-1 is a serine protease inhibitor that exhibits inhibitory activity toward the plasminogen activator urokinase. Elevated circulating PAI-1 has been reported in both obese MetS patients and patients with type 2 diabetes. Additionally,

TABLE 2: Functions of adipokines and biomarkers in metabolic syndrome.

Adipokines/ biomarkers	Function in metabolic syndrome	References
TNFα	↑ systemic insulin resistance via NFκB/JNK signaling	[56, 58, 59]
	↓ insulin signal transduction	[68]
IL-6	↑ production of hepatic CRP	[69]
	↑ hyperglycemia, atherosclerosis	[63, 64]
	↓ insulin signal transduction	[70]
	↑ insulin resistance via NFκB/JNK signaling	[58, 59]
PAI-1	↑ adipose tissue development	[65]
	↓ insulin signal transduction	[65]
MCP1	↑ insulin resistance via NFκB/JNK signaling	[58, 59]
CRP	↑ atherosclerosis	[60]

TNFα: tumor necrosis factor-α; IL: interleukin; MCP-1: monocyte chemoattractant protein 1; PAI-1: plasminogen-activator inhibitor 1; CRP: C-reactive protein; ↑: increase; ↓: decrease.

there is a positive correlation between intension of the plasma concentration of PAI-1 and MetS. The mechanism of the inhibitor overexpression in MetS involves several mediators, but the exact way is still unknown. Recent studies have suggested that PAI-1 is committed in control of insulin signaling and adipose tissue development [65].

MCP-1 is chemokine that allures macrophages into the adipose tissue in obesity. A murine model has exhibited that both MCP-1-deficient and MCP-1 receptor CCR2-deficient mice are protected against inflammation and macrophage accumulation in adipose tissue and display resistance to DIO-caused insulin resistance [66, 67]. MCP-1 secretion depends on the size of adipocytes; large adipocytes exhibit elevated secretion, which means that MCP-1 expression and secretion are upregulated in obesity and reduction after weight loss [18].

3. Impact of Oxidative Stress in the Course of MetS

The detailed mechanism of adipocyte dysregulation occurrences is not clear, but scientists postulated that both inflammatory mediators and obesity-induced oxidative stress affect MetS development. Oxidative stress (OS) is defined as an imbalance between antioxidant and prooxidant factors. The imbalance can lead to oxidative damage to proteins, nucleic acids, and lipids in different biological systems, therefore causing structural and functional impairment of many molecules [71, 72]. OS plays an important role in MetS and MetS-related diseases. Elevated oxidative damage, such depressed α-tocopherol and vitamin C concentration, decreased antioxidant protection and superoxide dismutase (SOD) activity, and increased malondialdehyde levels, lipid peroxidation, protein carbonyls, and xanthine oxidase activity are strongly correlated with MetS occurrence [73, 74].

Several animal and human studies have shown a positive correlation between adipose tissue accumulations an oxidative stress which has resulted in increased production of reactive oxygen species (ROS) and overexpression of NADPH oxidase with simultaneous decreased expression of antioxidant enzymes. Moreover, *in vitro* research has revealed that the application of higher concentration of fatty acids in adipocytes culture leads to the increase in oxidative stress via the NADPH pathway. An animal model has shown that feeding mice with a high-glucose diet which suffered from hyperglycemia resulted in free radicals production and, consequently, oxidative stress occurrence [75]. Furthermore, overweight mice treated with NADPH oxidase inhibitor have decreased ROS production with a reduction of diabetes symptoms [76, 77]. There is a close correlation between oxidative stress in the metabolic syndrome patients and the progress of complications, like vascular endothelial activation that can cause atherosclerosis [78]. Moreover, type 2 diabetes mellitus patients have elevated lipid peroxidation in comparison to age-matched control subject and reduced plasma glutathione (GSH) level, as well as GSH-metabolizing enzymes [79, 80]. Furthermore, several studies have shown that mitochondrial dysfunction is highly associated with obesity, strictly linked to increased ROS production and the progression of insulin resistance [81]. Similar to the murine model, a number of studies have provided that treatment reducing reactive oxygen species production increases insulin sensitivity and decreases hyperlipidemia and hepatic steatosis [76, 82, 83]. Oxidative stress is also highly associated with endoplasmic reticulum stress occurrence.

4. Endoplasmatic Reticulum Stress in the Course of MetS

The endoplasmic reticulum (ER) is an intracellular organelle responsible for lipid and protein biosynthesis, protein folding, maturation, and quality control. Moreover, it is a critical site for calcium cation (Ca^{2+}) homeostasis. The Ca^{2+} are maintained at relatively high concentrations inside the lumen and can be released out of the ER during cell signaling responses [84]. There are two conceptual types of ER membranes: smooth and rough. The smooth ER is a key site for the biosynthesis of lipids, while the rough ER is studded with ribosomes which are responsible for protein synthesis. In addition, the protein folds and matures in the ER lumen with the assistance of ER luminal chaperone proteins [85]. The accumulation of unfolded and incompletely folded proteins changes to redox status and luminal Ca^{2+} concentration

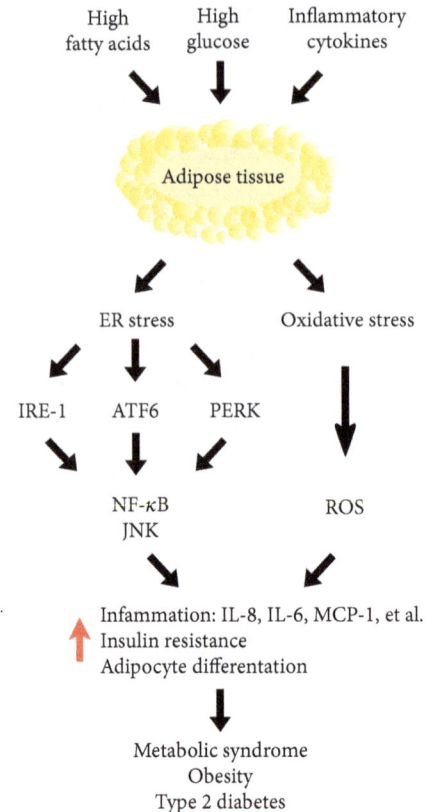

FIGURE 1: Schema of the correlation between excessive intake of fatty acids and glucose and inflammatory cytokine secretion on metabolic syndrome occurrence. Overconsumption of fat and sugar and proinflammatory cytokine production play a crucial role in ER and oxidative stress occurrence. Elevated NF-κB, JNK, and ROS concentration leads to increase inflammation, insulin resistance, and adipocyte differentiation, which cause MetS and finally obesity and type 2 diabetes.

(ER stress) and activates intracellular signaling pathways to restore homeostasis. In the ER, the unfolded protein response (UPR) acts to increase the capacity of ER protein folding and posttranslational modification [86, 87]. The UPR has three signaling arms: the inositol-requiring enzyme 1α (IRE1α), the protein kinase RNA-like endoplasmic reticulum kinase (PERK), and the activating transcription factor 6 (ATF6). Studies in the last decade indicate that impairment of sensing and signaling pathway downstream of ER stress has a significant impact on the pathogenesis of numerous human metabolic disorders, including insulin resistance (IR), obesity, and diabetes [87, 88] (Figure 1).

4.1. IRE1α Signaling Pathway. IRE1α is the most evolutionarily conserved UPR branch and exhibits endoribonuclease activity. There are two *IRE1* genes (*IRE1α* and *IRE1β*), but only *IRE1α* is expressed ubiquitously. Under physiologic conditions, it remains in an inactive form, because of an interaction with immunoglobulin heavy chain-binding protein (BiP). Upon activation (accumulation of unfolded and misfolded proteins), BiP dissociates from IRE1α, leading to dimerization, transautophosphorylation of the luminal domain of IRE1α, and activation of the RNase and kinase activities. The protein kinase and RNase domains are localized within their cytosolic region and splice X-box binding protein 1 (XBP-1) transcripts. Thus, IRE1α leads to the generation of the transcription factor XBP-1 and indirectly causes overexpression of ER luminal chaperones, as well as ER-associated degradation (ERAD) machinery elements [89]. Moreover, XBP-1 increases biogenesis capacity of ER and Golgi apparatus, thereby increasing the pace of protein secretion [90]. Recent studies indicate that *IRE1* is able to microRNA (miR) degradation causing activation of inflammatory and apoptotic pathways [91]. Interestingly, as a protein kinase, *IRE1* contributes the ER protein folding, thereby leading to inflammation through interaction with TNFα receptor-associated factor 2 (TRAF2). The process activates the nuclear factor κB (NFκB) and c-Jun N-terminal kinase (JNK) pathways through apoptosis signal-regulating kinase-1 (ASK1) [92–94].

4.2. PERK Branch of the ER Stress Response. PERK is a serine threonine kinase that phosphorylates downstream targets such as IRE1. Interestingly, PERK signaling pathway activation occurs with a slower kinetic than IRE1α and ATF6 [95, 96]. It has a luminal ER stress-sensing domain activated through transautophosphorylation and, upon activation, phosphorylates eukaryotic translation initiation factor 2 alpha (eIF2α). The process causes reduction of global protein biosynthesis and ER protein folding load [97]. Activated eIF2α enhances the translation of activating transcription factor-4 (ATF4) which leads to induction of the UPR effector C/EBPα-homologous protein (CHOP). Interestingly, in pathological states, prolonged CHOP expression causes apoptosis occurrence through several mechanisms, such as decreased expression of the antiapoptotic factor B cell lymphoma-2 (Bcl-2) [88].

4.3. ATF6 Signaling Arm. Unlike both the IRE1α and PERK, ATF6 is released from BiP/Grp78 binding and translocates to Golgi complex after ER stress. In the Golgi apparatus, ATF6 is cleaved by site 1 and site 2 proteases (S1P and S2P) at the transmembrane site to generate a transcriptionally active polypeptide. The released ATF6 cytosolic fragment p50 can translocate to the nucleus to increase the expression of numerous ER chaperone genes, such as *BiP*, ERAD components, and *XBP-1* mRNA [86, 92, 97].

ER stress is highly correlated with metabolic disorders including type 2 diabetes and obesity. Recent studies have revealed that ER stress-mediated activation of JNK has been associated with insulin resistance through phosphorylation of insulin receptor substrate-1 (IRS1) on Ser307, which leads to the reduction of tyrosine phosphorylation and IRS1 activation. In addition, ER stress factors, such as XBP-1s, phosphor-JNK, and phosphor-eIF2α, exhibit upregulation in the adipose tissue and liver of obese insulin-resistant nondiabetic individuals. Moreover, the factor levels significantly decreased after weight loss [98, 99]. In addition, ER stress-induced insulin resistance in the muscle requires the induction of the mTORC1 pathway [100].

The number of evidence that ER stress is associated with the pathogenesis of metabolic syndrome has been increased in the last few years, and several drugs, especially UPR regulators, have been tested [101]. BiP is a major regulator of the UPR, and the regulation of BiP expression plays an important role in ER stress modulation [102]. For example, valproate, a small molecule BiP activator, protects beta cells from palmitate-induced ER stress apoptosis. BiP is highly expressed in the ER and can be used as the endoplasmic reticulum marker [102]. Moreover, small molecule inhibitors of PERK and eIF2α, such as GSK2606414 and GSK2656157 (preclinical candidate), have been developed. Both of them have been commonly used to reduce ER stress by inhibition of receptor-interacting serine/threonine-protein kinase 1 (RIPK1) and thereby apoptosis [102, 103]. Guanabenz has been discovered as a molecule that targets eIF2α phosphorylation and leads to the reduction of protein production and thus reduces ER stress. Furthermore, salubrinal protects cells from ER stress-induced apoptosis by inhibition of dephosphorylation of eIF2α [104]. Integrated stress response inhibitor (ISRIB) has been described as an eIF2B activator and UPR inhibitor in the PERK branch [105]. Moreover, specific inhibitors of CHOP have also been developed. CHOP is activated through phosphorylation mediated by p38 mitogen-activated protein kinase (MAPK) and its inhibition may be beneficial to diabetes patients because of reduction of ER stress-mediated apoptosis [106, 107]. Two chemical compounds with similar structures named STF-083010 and 4μ8C selectively inhibit IRE1's RNase capacity and thus inhibits UPR [108]. Furthermore, both drugs are safe for human that make them promising candidates for clinical treatment. Other studies have shown that both compounds have been used in cells to protect them from apoptosis and ER stress [109]. Each ER stress signaling pathway carries out specialized function in metabolic diseases, and new drugs specific to the ER stress branches have been described as promising candidates in ER stress therapy and are currently being developed [101].

ER stress can lead to mitochondrial damage and oxidative stress induction. IRE1α interacts with Bak and Bax (proapoptotic Bcl-2 family members) and enhances mitochondrial-dependent cellular death. In addition, during ER stress, calcium cations released from the ER lumen can be taken up by the nearby mitochondria, which causes mitochondrial damage and thereby increases the production of ROS and proapoptotic signaling. Moreover, both mitochondria and ER are physically and functionally linked by mitochondria-associated ER membranes (MAMs) [110]. Recent studies have pointed out that ER protein folding process is highly associated to ROS production. Redox homeostasis is essential in the protein folding pathway as well as disulfide bone formation [111–113]. Some alternations in that process lead to ROS imbalance and increase ROS production. Disulfide bone formation, crucial for the production of mature and functional proteins, is a reversible process catalyzed by several ER oxidoreductases (e.g., ER protein (ERP) 57 and ERP72) [114]. The redox state is modulated by numerous redox mechanisms. The GSH/GSSG cycle is one of the redox mechanisms that plays a crucial role in the protein folding process. GSH can undergo oxidation to GSSG maintaining redox homeostasis. The balance between GSH and GSSG (1:1 in the RE lumen and 1:50 in the cytoplasm, respectively) is essential in maintaining ER redox homeostasis [113]. If production of misfolded proteins occurs, GSH can reduce nonnative bonds allowing them to refold again. The protein refolding process is very slow and needs electron acceptors. When large numbers of misfolded proteins are accumulated in the ER, GSH mechanism is compromised; ROS production and ER stress occur [112, 115]. Beyond the GSH/GSSG mechanism, protein disulfide-isomerase (PDI) can cause ER stress and OS occurrence. PDI catalyzes the formation of disulfide bone as a multifunctional oxidoreductase chaperone protein. During the oxidative protein folding process, two electrons are transferred to the oxygen molecules, thereby producing hydrogen peroxide (a type of ROS) that leads to OS [116]. The process leads to redox balance alternation and thus ER stress [112, 117]. Both of the two mechanisms can provide an important indicator of the oxidative stress in ER.

Interestingly, the interdependence of ER stress and oxidative stress often causes the activation of inflammation [118]. Inflammation can activate UPR by all three branches (PERK, IRE1α, and AT6 signaling). In turn, UPR can modulate crucial proinflammatory pathways, such as the JNK/activator protein 1 (AP1) and NFκB [119]. The NFκB pathway can be triggered through PERK, IRE1α, and AT6, whereas the JNK/AP1 is mainly induced by IRE1 [101]. Recent studies have pointed out that a high-fat diet can induce inflammatory response in obese rats and mice by ER stress and downstream of the Toll-like receptor 4 (TLR4) signaling pathway [120, 121]. Levels of some interleukins, like IL-23, IL-24, and IL-33, are increased in diabetic beta cells and can lead to activation of ER stress and therefore induction of autophagy [101, 122]. Adipose-secreted hormone leptin enhances IL-1β secretion in beta cells, inhibits the secretion of IL-1Rα (its natural antagonist), and therefore triggers the innate immune system in type 2 diabetes individuals [123, 124]. Moreover, IL-1β increases inflammation in beta cells by the IRE1α signaling pathway [125]. Elevated expression of TNFα and interferon gamma (IFN-γ) activates ER stress in human, rat, and mouse beta cells and nitric oxide (NO) production in rat [126]. Recent studies have demonstrated that salubrinal (a selective inhibitor of the PERK-eIF2α pathway) blocks TNFα, but not IL-1β, and thereby inhibits the NFκB signaling [127]. Manganese (III) meso-tetrakis (N-ethylpyridinium-2-yl) porphyrin (MnP) (manganese metalloporphyrin SOD mimetic) decreases iNOS, TNFα, and MCP-1 levels by blockade of NFκB in type 2 diabetes individuals [128]. Moreover, no pharmaceutical treatment but aerobic training decreased serum levels of IL-6, IFN-γ, TNFα, advanced oxidation protein products (AOPP), and thiobarbituric acid-reactive substances (TBARS) and in addition elevated levels of IL-10 and total thiol content (T-SH) in obese patients [129]. A better understanding of the ER stress response molecular mechanisms carries potential strategies to various metabolic disease treatments [130].

5. Future Perspective for Cellular Therapies

Stem cell transplantation is an excellent platform to metabolic syndrome-associated disease therapy, including obesity and type 2 diabetes [131, 132]. Recent preclinical and clinical studies have revealed that stem cell therapy had been applied successfully in diabetes mellitus individuals. Preclinical studies on an animal model have shown that MSC treatment exhibited a promising therapeutic effect on glycemic control through recovering islet function and improving insulin resistance. Approximately 100 registered phase I/II clinical trials among type 2 diabetes mellitus documented patients have been found with the clinical study registry [132, 133].

Because of their multipotential capacity, MSC is the most popular stem cell type used in diabetes treatment. A small amount of diabetic MSCs (6%) expresses both proinsulin and C-peptide; thus, MSCs possess the potential to differentiate into physiologically functional insulin-producing cells (IPCs) [30, 134, 135]. Moreover, MSCs promote the regeneration of endogenous pancreatic islet cells by secreting numerous cytokines and growth factors. The MSCs migrate to impaired islet cells and secrete paracrine factor, including insulin-like growth factor 1 (IGF-1), vascular endothelial growth factor (VEGF), angiopoietin-1, and platelet-derived growth factor BB (PDGF-BB) [136, 137]. MSCs have also immunoregulatory capacity because of the low intracellular expression of MHC class II [138]. Moreover, they suppress the proliferation of T lymphocytes and promote T-cell tolerance [139]. Additionally, MSCs inhibit the proliferation of B lymphocytes, thereby decreasing cytokine secretion, cytotoxicity of natural killer (NK) cell, and lymphocytes T, as well as B cell maturation and antibody production [140]. Additionally, MSCs promote autophagosome and autolysosome formation and thereby protect the islet cells [141].

MSCs have enzymatic and nonenzymatic mechanisms to inactivate ROS and to improve damages of genome and proteasome caused by reactive species that guarantee an efficiently managed OS [142, 143]. Studies have shown that rat MSCs, human BMSCs, and the immortalized cell line human MSC-telomerase reverse transcriptase (TERT) cultivated in the presence of ascorbate revealed expression of active thioredoxin reductases, catalase (CAT), glutathione peroxidases (GPXs), SOD1, and SOD2 [144, 145]. Calió et al. have reported that BMSC-based therapy reduces apoptosis rate and reactive oxygen species in the cell of rats with high blood pressure [146]. Furthermore, MSCs promote pancreatic islet against oxidative stress and hypoxia that cause cell destruction. Chandravanshi and colleagues have demonstrated that after 48 h of coculture with Wharton's jelly-derived MSCs, pancreatic islet cells exhibited increased viability, reduced apoptosis rate, and decreased levels of ROS, NO, and superoxide ions in comparison to the control group (without MSCs). In contrast to pharmaceutical antioxidant therapy, MSC can not only reduce oxidative stress (elimination of reactive oxygen species, free radicals) but also promote regeneration of previously damaged tissue [147, 148]. MSC transplantation was proven to be a very useful tool in the therapy of pathologies in which cell damage is linked to OS occurrence.

Unique properties of mesenchymal stem cells make them a suitable candidate for a number of metabolic disease therapies. However, some reports have demonstrated that MSC allogenic transplantation can lead to increased tumor transformation due to their immunosuppressive and multipotent features [132, 149]. Interestingly, most studies revealed that allogenic application is much more efficient in diabetes treatment than autologous transplantation [29, 150]. Moreover, aspects like the survival time of engrafted MSC *in vivo*, optimal dosing regimen, and the long-time effect of repeated dosing need further investigation [132]. In the future, mesenchymal stem cell therapy is expected to become a new level of therapeutic option for MetS-related diseases, but more controlled and advanced clinical trials are needed to optimize the application process.

6. Conclusions

Nowadays, metabolic syndrome and type 2 diabetes have become the leading causes of death among adults under the age of 60 and are highly associated with lifestyle. Excessive intake of sugar and fatty acids causes increased inflammation, ROS accumulation, and ER stress occurrence. A better understanding of the relationship between UPR, oxidative stress, insulin resistance, and inflammation will give new approach of the course of MetS. Application of ASC, as a promising tool for MetS and type 2 diabetes therapeutic intervention, is still hindered by technical and biological barriers.

Abbreviations

MetS: Metabolic syndrome
ER: Endoplasmic reticulum
MSC: Mesenchymal stem cell
DPP-4:   Dipeptyl-peptidase-4
SGLT2:   Sodium glucose transporter-2
GLP-1:   Glucagon-like peptide
SVF: Stromal vascular fraction
ASC: Adipose tissue-derived mesenchymal stem cell
BMSC: Bone marrow-derived mesenchymal stem cell
CFU-Fs: Fibroblast colony-forming units
PDT: Population doubling time
IL-1β: Interleukin 1β
MCP-1:   Monocyte chemoattractant protein-1
TNFα: Tumor necrosis factor α
PAI-1:   Plasminogen activator inhibitor-1
CRP: C-reactive protein
OS: Oxidative stress
SOD: Superoxide dismutase
ROS: Reactive oxygen species
GSH: Glutathione
Ca^{2+}:   Calcium cation
UPR: Unfolded protein response
IRE1α: Inositol-requiring enzyme 1α
PERK: Protein kinase RNA-like endoplasmic reticulum kinase
ATF6:   Activating transcription factor 6
IR: Insulin resistance
BiP: Chain-binding protein
XBP-1:   X-box binding protein 1
ERAD: ER-associated degradation
TRAF2:   TNFα receptor-associated factor 2
JNK: Jun N-terminal kinase
ASK1:   Apoptosis signal-regulating kinase-1
eIF2α: Eukaryotic translation initiation factor 2 alpha
ATF4:   Activating transcription factor-4
CHOP: C/EBPα-homologous protein
Bcl-2:   B cell lymphoma-2
S1P: Site 1 proteases
S2P: Site 2 proteases
IRS: Insulin receptor substrate-1
Bix: BIP inducer X
MAPK: P38 mitogen-activated protein kinase
RIPK1:   Receptor-interacting serine/threonine-protein kinase 1
ISRIB: Integrated stress response inhibitor
MAMs: Mitochondria-associated ER membranes
PDI: Protein disulfide isomerase
AP1:   Activator protein 1
NFκB: Nuclear factor κB
TLR4:   Toll-like receptors 4
IFN-γ: Interferon gamma
NO: Nitric oxide
MnP: Manganese metalloporphyrin SOD mimetic
AOPP: Advanced oxidation protein products
TBARS: Thiobarbituric acid-reactive substances
T-SH: Total thiol
IPCs: Insulin-producing cells
IGF-1:   Insulin-like growth factor 1
VEGF: Vascular endothelial growth factor
PDGF-BB: Platelet-derived growth factor BB
NK: Natural killer
TERT: Telomerase reverse transcriptase
CAT: Catalase
GPX: Glutathione peroxidase
EMS: Equine metabolic syndrome.

Acknowledgments

This research was supported by the National Science Centre, Poland, Grant no. 2016/21/B/NZ7/01111, "Modulation mitochondrial metabolism and dynamics and targeting DNA methylation of adipose derived mesenchymal stromal stem cell (ASC) using resveratrol and 5-azacytydine as a therapeutic strategy in the course of equine metabolic syndrome (EMS)." Publication was supported by the Wroclaw Centre of Biotechnology programme the Leading National Research Centre (KNOW) for years 2014–2018.

References

[1] G. M. Reaven, "Banting lecture 1988. Role of insulin resistance in human disease," *Diabetes*, vol. 37, no. 12, pp. 1595–1607, 1988.

[2] K. G. M. M. Alberti, R. H. Eckel, S. M. Grundy et al., "Harmonizing the metabolic syndrome: a joint interim statement of the International Diabetes Federation Task Force on Epidemiology and Prevention; National Heart, Lung, and Blood Institute; American Heart Association; World Heart Federation; International Atherosclerosis Society; and International Association for the Study of Obesity," *Circulation*, vol. 120, no. 16, pp. 1640–1645, 2009.

[3] J. Kaur, "A comprehensive review on metabolic syndrome," *Cardiology Research and Practice*, vol. 2014, Article ID 943162, 21 pages, 2014.

[4] Y.-W. Park, S. Zhu, L. Palaniappan, S. Heshka, M. R. Carnethon, and S. B. Heymsfield, "The metabolic syndrome," *Archives of Internal Medicine*, vol. 163, no. 4, pp. 427–436, 2003.

[5] A. Z. Fan, M. Russell, T. Naimi et al., "Patterns of alcohol consumption and the metabolic syndrome," *The Journal of Clinical Endocrinology & Metabolism*, vol. 93, no. 10, pp. 3833–3838, 2008.

[6] B. C. Gohil, L. A. Rosenblum, J. D. Coplan, and J. G. Kral, "Hypothalamic-pituitary-adrenal axis function and the metabolic syndrome X of obesity," *CNS Spectrums*, vol. 6, no. 7, pp. 581–589, 2001.

[7] K. P. Gennuso, R. E. Gangnon, K. M. Thraen-Borowski, and L. H. Colbert, "Dose-response relationships between sedentary behaviour and the metabolic syndrome and its components," *Diabetologia*, vol. 58, no. 3, pp. 485–492, 2015.

[8] P. Zimmet, K. G. Alberti, and J. Shaw, "Global and societal implications of the diabetes epidemic," *Nature*, vol. 414, no. 6865, pp. 782–787, 2001.

[9] A. Mozumdar and G. Liguori, "Persistent increase of prevalence of metabolic syndrome among U.S. adults: NHANES III to NHANES 1999–2006," *Diabetes Care*, vol. 34, no. 1, pp. 216–219, 2011.

[10] W. Gao and DECODE Study Group, "Does the constellation of risk factors with and without abdominal adiposity associate with different cardiovascular mortality risk?," *International Journal of Obesity*, vol. 32, no. 5, pp. 757–762, 2008.

[11] K. Kornicka, J. Houston, and K. Marycz, "Dysfunction of mesenchymal stem cells isolated from metabolic syndrome and type 2 diabetic patients as result of oxidative stress and autophagy may limit their potential therapeutic use," *Stem Cell Reviews*, vol. 14, no. 3, pp. 337–345, 2018.

[12] I. J. Neeland, P. Poirier, and J.-P. Després, "Cardiovascular and metabolic heterogeneity of obesity: clinical challenges and implications for management," *Circulation*, vol. 137, no. 13, pp. 1391–1406, 2018.

[13] M. Marędziak, A. Śmieszek, K. Chrząstek, K. Basinska, and K. Marycz, "Physical activity increases the total number of bone-marrow-derived mesenchymal stem cells, enhances their osteogenic potential, and inhibits their adipogenic properties," *Stem Cells International*, vol. 2015, Article ID 379093, 11 pages, 2015.

[14] K. Marycz, K. Mierzejewska, A. Śmieszek et al., "Endurance exercise mobilizes developmentally early stem cells into peripheral blood and increases their number in bone marrow:

implications for tissue regeneration," *Stem Cells International*, vol. 2016, Article ID 5756901, 10 pages, 2016.

[15] E. S. Ford, W. H. Giles, and W. H. Dietz, "Prevalence of the metabolic syndrome among US adults: findings from the third National Health and Nutrition Examination Survey," *Journal of the American Medical Association*, vol. 287, no. 3, pp. 356–359, 2002.

[16] M. E. F. Vázquez-Vela, N. Torres, and A. R. Tovar, "White adipose tissue as endocrine organ and its role in obesity," *Archives of Medical Research*, vol. 39, no. 8, pp. 715–728, 2008.

[17] O. A. MacDougald and S. Mandrup, "Adipogenesis: forces that tip the scales," *Trends in Endocrinology & Metabolism*, vol. 13, no. 1, pp. 5–11, 2002.

[18] T. Skurk, C. Alberti-Huber, C. Herder, and H. Hauner, "Relationship between adipocyte size and adipokine expression and secretion," *The Journal of Clinical Endocrinology & Metabolism*, vol. 92, no. 3, pp. 1023–1033, 2007.

[19] K. L. Spalding, E. Arner, P. O. Westermark et al., "Dynamics of fat cell turnover in humans," *Nature*, vol. 453, no. 7196, pp. 783–787, 2008.

[20] B. M. Spiegelman and J. S. Flier, "Obesity and the regulation of energy balance," *Cell*, vol. 104, no. 4, pp. 531–543, 2001.

[21] A. Cederberg and S. Enerbäck, "Insulin resistance and type 2 diabetes - an adipocentric view," *Current Molecular Medicine*, vol. 3, no. 2, pp. 107–125, 2003.

[22] N. Halberg, I. Wernstedt-Asterholm, and P. E. Scherer, "The adipocyte as an endocrine cell," *Endocrinology and Metabolism Clinics of North America*, vol. 37, no. 3, pp. 753–768, 2008.

[23] P. Trayhurn, "Hypoxia and adipose tissue function and dysfunction in obesity," *Physiological Reviews*, vol. 93, no. 1, pp. 1–21, 2013.

[24] N. Halberg, T. Khan, M. E. Trujillo et al., "Hypoxia-inducible factor 1alpha induces fibrosis and insulin resistance in white adipose tissue," *Molecular and Cellular Biology*, vol. 29, no. 16, pp. 4467–4483, 2009.

[25] H. Xu, G. T. Barnes, Q. Yang et al., "Chronic inflammation in fat plays a crucial role in the development of obesity-related insulin resistance," *The Journal of Clinical Investigation*, vol. 112, no. 12, pp. 1821–1830, 2003.

[26] P. A. Zuk, M. Zhu, P. Ashjian et al., "Human adipose tissue is a source of multipotent stem cells," *Molecular Biology of the Cell*, vol. 13, no. 12, pp. 4279–4295, 2002.

[27] M. Z. Ratajczak, K. Marycz, A. Poniewierska-Baran, K. Fiedorowicz, M. Zbucka-Kretowska, and M. Moniuszko, "Very small embryonic-like stem cells as a novel developmental concept and the hierarchy of the stem cell compartment," *Advances in Medical Sciences*, vol. 59, no. 2, pp. 273–280, 2014.

[28] D.-H. Woo, H. S. Hwang, and J. H. Shim, "Comparison of adult stem cells derived from multiple stem cell niches," *Biotechnology Letters*, vol. 38, no. 5, pp. 751–759, 2016.

[29] R. Abdi, P. Fiorina, C. N. Adra, M. Atkinson, and M. H. Sayegh, "Immunomodulation by mesenchymal stem cells: a potential therapeutic strategy for type 1 diabetes," *Diabetes*, vol. 57, no. 7, pp. 1759–1767, 2008.

[30] S. M. Phadnis, S. M. Ghaskadbi, A. A. Hardikar, and R. R. Bhonde, "Mesenchymal stem cells derived from bone marrow of diabetic patients portrait unique markers influenced by the diabetic microenvironment," *The Review of Diabetic Studies*, vol. 6, no. 4, pp. 260–270, 2009.

[31] Y. Sun, L. Chen, X. Hou et al., "Differentiation of bone marrow-derived mesenchymal stem cells from diabetic patients into insulin-producing cells *in vitro*," *Chinese Medical Journal*, vol. 120, no. 9, pp. 771–776, 2007.

[32] M. T. Koobatian, M.-S. Liang, D. D. Swartz, and S. T. Andreadis, "Differential effects of culture senescence and mechanical stimulation on the proliferation and leiomyogenic differentiation of MSC from different sources: implications for engineering vascular grafts," *Tissue Engineering Part A*, vol. 21, no. 7-8, pp. 1364–1375, 2015.

[33] O. S. Beane, V. C. Fonseca, L. L. Cooper, G. Koren, and E. M. Darling, "Impact of aging on the regenerative properties of bone marrow-, muscle-, and adipose-derived mesenchymal stem/stromal cells," *PLoS One*, vol. 9, no. 12, article e115963, 2014.

[34] P. A. Zuk, M. Zhu, H. Mizuno et al., "Multilineage cells from human adipose tissue: implications for cell-based therapies," *Tissue Engineering*, vol. 7, no. 2, pp. 211–228, 2001.

[35] K. W. Liechty, T. C. MacKenzie, A. F. Shaaban et al., "Human mesenchymal stem cells engraft and demonstrate site-specific differentiation after *in utero* transplantation in sheep," *Nature Medicine*, vol. 6, no. 11, pp. 1282–1286, 2000.

[36] L. M. Scavo, M. Karas, M. Murray, and D. Leroith, "Insulin-like growth factor-I stimulates both cell growth and lipogenesis during differentiation of human mesenchymal stem cells into adipocytes," *The Journal of Clinical Endocrinology & Metabolism*, vol. 89, no. 7, pp. 3543–3553, 2004.

[37] K. Kornicka, B. Babiarczuk, J. Krzak, and K. Marycz, "The effect of a sol–gel derived silica coating doped with vitamin E on oxidative stress and senescence of human adipose-derived mesenchymal stem cells (AMSCs)," *RSC Advances*, vol. 6, no. 35, pp. 29524–29537, 2016.

[38] K. Kornicka, K. Marycz, K. A. Tomaszewski, M. Marędziak, and A. Śmieszek, "The effect of age on osteogenic and adipogenic differentiation potential of human adipose derived stromal stem cells (hASCs) and the impact of stress factors in the course of the differentiation process," *Oxidative Medicine and Cellular Longevity*, vol. 2015, Article ID 309169, 20 pages, 2015.

[39] M. Marędziak, K. Marycz, K. A. Tomaszewski, K. Kornicka, and B. M. Henry, "The influence of aging on the regenerative potential of human adipose derived mesenchymal stem cells," *Stem Cells International*, vol. 2016, Article ID 2152435, 15 pages, 2016.

[40] H. Hemeda, M. Jakob, A.-K. Ludwig, B. Giebel, S. Lang, and S. Brandau, "Interferon-gamma and tumor necrosis factor-alpha differentially affect cytokine expression and migration properties of mesenchymal stem cells," *Stem Cells and Development*, vol. 19, no. 5, pp. 693–706, 2010.

[41] A. A. Rizvi, "Hypertension, obesity, and inflammation: the complex designs of a deadly trio," *Metabolic Syndrome and Related Disorders*, vol. 8, no. 4, pp. 287–294, 2010.

[42] K. Marycz, K. Kornicka, K. Basinska, and A. Czyrek, "Equine metabolic syndrome affects viability, senescence, and stress factors of equine adipose-derived mesenchymal stromal stem cells: new insight into EqASCs isolated from EMS horses in the context of their aging," *Oxidative Medicine and Cellular Longevity*, vol. 2016, Article ID 4710326, 17 pages, 2016.

[43] K. Marycz, K. Kornicka, M. Marędziak, P. Golonka, and J. Nicpoń, "Equine metabolic syndrome impairs adipose stem cells osteogenic differentiation by predominance of autophagy over selective mitophagy," *Journal of Cellular and Molecular Medicine*, vol. 20, no. 12, pp. 2384–2404, 2016.

[44] K. Marycz, K. Kornicka, J. Grzesiak, A. Śmieszek, and J. Szłapka, "Macroautophagy and selective mitophagy ameliorate chondrogenic differentiation potential in adipose stem cells of equine metabolic syndrome: new findings in the field of progenitor cells differentiation," *Oxidative Medicine and Cellular Longevity*, vol. 2016, Article ID 3718468, 18 pages, 2016.

[45] K. Marycz, K. Kornicka, J. Szlapka-Kosarzewska, and C. Weiss, "Excessive endoplasmic reticulum stress correlates with impaired mitochondrial dynamics, mitophagy and apoptosis, in liver and adipose tissue, but not in muscles in EMS horses," *International Journal of Molecular Sciences*, vol. 19, no. 1, 2018.

[46] C.-L. Wu, B. O. Diekman, D. Jain, and F. Guilak, "Diet-induced obesity alters the differentiation potential of stem cells isolated from bone marrow, adipose tissue, and infrapatellar fad pad: the effects of free fatty acids," *International Journal of Obesity*, vol. 37, pp. 1079–1087, 2013.

[47] K. Kodama, M. Horikoshi, K. Toda et al., "Expression-based genome-wide association study links the receptor CD44 in adipose tissue with type 2 diabetes," *Proceedings of the National Academy of Sciences of the United States of America*, vol. 109, no. 18, pp. 7049–7054, 2012.

[48] K. Kodama, K. Toda, S. Morinaga, S. Yamada, and A. J. Butte, "Anti-CD44 antibody treatment lowers hyperglycemia and improves insulin resistance, adipose inflammation, and hepatic steatosis in diet-induced obese mice," *Diabetes*, vol. 64, no. 3, pp. 867–875, 2015.

[49] L. F. Liu, K. Kodama, K. Wei et al., "The receptor CD44 is associated with systemic insulin resistance and proinflammatory macrophages in human adipose tissue," *Diabetologia*, vol. 58, no. 7, pp. 1579–1586, 2015.

[50] C. N. Lumeng, "Innate immune activation in obesity," *Molecular Aspects of Medicine*, vol. 34, pp. 12–29, 2013.

[51] L. Tornatore, A. K. Thotakura, J. Bennett, M. Moretti, and G. Franzoso, "The nuclear factor kappa B signaling pathway: integrating metabolism with inflammation," *Trends in Cell Biology*, vol. 22, no. 11, pp. 557–566, 2012.

[52] J. Henao-Mejia, E. Elinav, C. Jin et al., "Inflammasome-mediated dysbiosis regulates progression of NAFLD and obesity," *Nature*, vol. 482, no. 7384, pp. 179–185, 2012.

[53] M. M. Malagón, A. Díaz-Ruiz, R. Guzmán-Ruiz et al., "Adipobiology for novel therapeutic approaches in metabolic syndrome," *Current Vascular Pharmacology*, vol. 11, no. 6, pp. 954–967, 2013.

[54] H. Tilg and A. Kaser, "Gut microbiome, obesity, and metabolic dysfunction," *The Journal of Clinical Investigation*, vol. 121, no. 6, pp. 2126–2132, 2011.

[55] K. Basinska, K. Marycz, A. Śieszek, and J. Nicpoń, "The production and distribution of IL-6 and TNF-α in subcutaneous adipose tissue and their correlation with serum concentrations in Welsh ponies with equine metabolic syndrome," *Journal of Veterinary Science*, vol. 16, no. 1, pp. 113–120, 2015.

[56] G. S. Hotamisligil, "The role of TNFalpha and TNF receptors in obesity and insulin resistance," *Journal of Internal Medicine*, vol. 245, no. 6, pp. 621–625, 1999.

[57] V. Rotter, I. Nagaev, and U. Smith, "Interleukin-6 (IL-6) induces insulin resistance in 3T3-L1 adipocytes and is, like IL-8 and tumor necrosis factor-α, overexpressed in human fat cells from insulin-resistant subjects," *Journal*

of Biological Chemistry, vol. 278, no. 46, pp. 45777–45784, 2003.

[58] J. Hirosumi, G. Tuncman, L. Chang et al., "A central role for JNK in obesity and insulin resistance," *Nature*, vol. 420, no. 6913, pp. 333–336, 2002.

[59] M. Jernås, J. Palming, K. Sjöholm et al., "Separation of human adipocytes by size: hypertrophic fat cells display distinct gene expression," *The FASEB Journal*, vol. 20, no. 9, pp. 1540–1542, 2006.

[60] D. C. W. Lau, B. Dhillon, H. Yan, P. E. Szmitko, and S. Verma, "Adipokines: molecular links between obesity and atheroslcerosis," *American Journal of Physiology. Heart and Circulatory Physiology*, vol. 288, no. 5, pp. H2031–H2041, 2005.

[61] M. Azzawi and P. Hasleton, "Tumour necrosis factor alpha and the cardiovascular system: its role in cardiac allograft rejection and heart disease," *Cardiovascular Research*, vol. 43, no. 4, pp. 850–859, 1999.

[62] R. Testa, F. Olivieri, A. R. Bonfigli et al., "Interleukin-6-174 G > C polymorphism affects the association between IL-6 plasma levels and insulin resistance in type 2 diabetic patients," *Diabetes Research and Clinical Practice*, vol. 71, no. 3, pp. 299–305, 2006.

[63] E. Bernberg, M. A. Ulleryd, M. E. Johansson, and G. M. L. Bergström, "Social disruption stress increases IL-6 levels and accelerates atherosclerosis in ApoE$^{-/-}$ mice," *Atherosclerosis*, vol. 221, no. 2, pp. 359–365, 2012.

[64] Y. D. Kim, Y. H. Kim, Y. M. Cho et al., "Metformin ameliorates IL-6-induced hepatic insulin resistance via induction of orphan nuclear receptor small heterodimer partner (SHP) in mouse models," *Diabetologia*, vol. 55, no. 5, pp. 1482–1494, 2012.

[65] K. Srikanthan, A. Feyh, H. Visweshwar, J. I. Shapiro, and K. Sodhi, "Systematic review of metabolic syndrome biomarkers: a panel for early detection, management, and risk stratification in the West Virginian population," *International Journal of Medical Sciences*, vol. 13, no. 1, pp. 25–38, 2016.

[66] H. Kanda, S. Tateya, Y. Tamori et al., "MCP-1 contributes to macrophage infiltration into adipose tissue, insulin resistance, and hepatic steatosis in obesity," *The Journal of Clinical Investigation*, vol. 116, no. 6, pp. 1494–1505, 2006.

[67] S. P. Weisberg, D. Hunter, R. Huber et al., "CCR2 modulates inflammatory and metabolic effects of high-fat feeding," *The Journal of Clinical Investigation*, vol. 116, no. 1, pp. 115–124, 2006.

[68] F. B. Hu, M. J. Stampfer, S. M. Haffner, C. G. Solomon, W. C. Willett, and J. E. Manson, "Elevated risk of cardiovascular disease prior to clinical diagnosis of type 2 diabetes," *Diabetes Care*, vol. 25, no. 7, pp. 1129–1134, 2002.

[69] V. Mohamed-Ali, S. Goodrick, A. Rawesh et al., "Subcutaneous adipose tissue releases interleukin-6, but not tumor necrosis factor-alpha, in vivo," *The Journal of Clinical Endocrinology and Metabolism*, vol. 82, no. 12, pp. 4196–4200, 1997.

[70] J. J. Senn, P. J. Klover, I. A. Nowak et al., "Suppressor of cytokine signaling-3 (SOCS-3), a potential mediator of interleukin-6-dependent insulin resistance in hepatocytes," *The Journal of Biological Chemistry*, vol. 278, no. 16, pp. 13740–13746, 2003.

[71] A. Mancini, G. E. Martorana, M. Magini et al., "Oxidative stress and metabolic syndrome: effects of a natural antioxidants enriched diet on insulin resistance," *Clinical Nutrition ESPEN*, vol. 10, no. 2, pp. e52–e60, 2015.

[72] H. Sies, "Oxidative stress: oxidants and antioxidants," *Experimental Physiology*, vol. 82, no. 2, pp. 291–295, 1997.

[73] F. Armutcu, M. Ataymen, H. Atmaca, and A. Gurel, "Oxidative stress markers, C-reactive protein and heat shock protein 70 levels in subjects with metabolic syndrome," *Clinical Chemistry and Laboratory Medicine*, vol. 46, no. 6, pp. 785–790, 2008.

[74] V. O. Palmieri, I. Grattagliano, P. Portincasa, and G. Palasciano, "Systemic oxidative alterations are associated with visceral adiposity and liver steatosis in patients with metabolic syndrome," *The Journal of Nutrition*, vol. 136, no. 12, pp. 3022–3026, 2006.

[75] V. Folmer, J. C. M. Soares, and J. B. T. Rocha, "Oxidative stress in mice is dependent on the free glucose content of the diet," *The International Journal of Biochemistry & Cell Biology*, vol. 34, no. 10, pp. 1279–1285, 2002.

[76] S. Furukawa, T. Fujita, M. Shimabukuro et al., "Increased oxidative stress in obesity and its impact on metabolic syndrome," *The Journal of Clinical Investigation*, vol. 114, no. 12, pp. 1752–1761, 2004.

[77] E. McCracken, M. Monaghan, and S. Sreenivasan, "Pathophysiology of the metabolic syndrome," *Clinics in Dermatology*, vol. 36, no. 1, pp. 14–20, 2018.

[78] T. A. Elhadd, G. Kennedy, A. Hill et al., "Abnormal markers of endothelial cell activation and oxidative stress in children, adolescents and young adults with type 1 diabetes with no clinical vascular disease," *Diabetes/Metabolism Research and Reviews*, vol. 15, no. 6, pp. 405–411, 1999.

[79] E. Altomare, G. Vendemiale, D. Chicco, V. Procacci, and F. Cirelli, "Increased lipid peroxidation in type 2 poorly controlled diabetic patients," *Diabète & Métabolisme*, vol. 18, no. 4, pp. 264–271, 1992.

[80] R. K. Sundaram, A. Bhaskar, S. Vijayalingam, M. Viswanathan, R. Mohan, and K. R. Shanmugasundaram, "Antioxidant status and lipid peroxidation in type II diabetes mellitus with and without complications," *Clinical Science*, vol. 90, no. 4, pp. 255–260, 1996.

[81] A. De Pauw, S. Tejerina, M. Raes, J. Keijer, and T. Arnould, "Mitochondrial (dys)function in adipocyte (de)differentiation and systemic metabolic alterations," *The American Journal of Pathology*, vol. 175, no. 3, pp. 927–939, 2009.

[82] N. Houstis, E. D. Rosen, and E. S. Lander, "Reactive oxygen species have a causal role in multiple forms of insulin resistance," *Nature*, vol. 440, no. 7086, pp. 944–948, 2006.

[83] T. Konrad, P. Vicini, K. Kusterer et al., "Alpha-lipoic acid treatment decreases serum lactate and pyruvate concentrations and improves glucose effectiveness in lean and obese patients with type 2 diabetes," *Diabetes Care*, vol. 22, no. 2, pp. 280–287, 1999.

[84] M. J. Berridge, "Neuronal calcium signaling," *Neuron*, vol. 21, no. 1, pp. 13–26, 1998.

[85] J. L. Brodsky and W. R. Skach, "Protein folding and quality control in the endoplasmic reticulum: recent lessons from yeast and mammalian cell systems," *Current Opinion in Cell Biology*, vol. 23, no. 4, pp. 464–475, 2011.

[86] S. S. Cao and R. J. Kaufman, "Targeting endoplasmic reticulum stress in metabolic disease," *Expert Opinion on Therapeutic Targets*, vol. 17, no. 4, pp. 437–448, 2013.

[87] D. Lindholm, L. Korhonen, O. Eriksson, and S. Kõks, "Recent insights into the role of unfolded protein response in ER stress in health and disease," *Frontiers in Cell and Development Biology*, vol. 5, p. 48, 2017.

[88] I. Tabas and D. Ron, "Integrating the mechanisms of apoptosis induced by endoplasmic reticulum stress," *Nature Cell Biology*, vol. 13, no. 3, pp. 184–190, 2011.

[89] A.-H. Lee, N. N. Iwakoshi, and L. H. Glimcher, "XBP-1 regulates a subset of endoplasmic reticulum resident chaperone genes in the unfolded protein response," *Molecular and Cellular Biology*, vol. 23, no. 21, pp. 7448–7459, 2003.

[90] C. Hetz, E. Chevet, and S. A. Oakes, "Proteostasis control by the unfolded protein response," *Nature Cell Biology*, vol. 17, no. 7, pp. 829–838, 2015.

[91] J.-P. Upton, L. Wang, D. Han et al., "IRE1α cleaves select microRNAs during ER stress to derepress translation of proapoptotic caspase-2," *Science*, vol. 338, no. 6108, pp. 818–822, 2012.

[92] S. S. Cao and R. J. Kaufman, "Unfolded protein response," *Current Biology*, vol. 22, no. 16, pp. R622–R626, 2012.

[93] C. Hetz, "The unfolded protein response: controlling cell fate decisions under ER stress and beyond," *Nature Reviews Molecular Cell Biology*, vol. 13, no. 2, pp. 89–102, 2012.

[94] F. Urano, X. Wang, A. Bertolotti et al., "Coupling of stress in the ER to activation of JNK protein kinases by transmembrane protein kinase IRE1," *Science*, vol. 287, no. 5453, pp. 664–666, 2000.

[95] J. H. Lin, H. Li, D. Yasumura et al., "IRE1 signaling affects cell fate during the unfolded protein response," *Science*, vol. 318, no. 5852, pp. 944–949, 2007.

[96] D. T. Rutkowski, S. M. Arnold, C. N. Miller et al., "Adaptation to ER stress is mediated by differential stabilities of pro-survival and pro-apoptotic mRNAs and proteins," *PLoS Biology*, vol. 4, no. 11, article e374, 2006.

[97] D. Ron and P. Walter, "Signal integration in the endoplasmic reticulum unfolded protein response," *Nature Reviews Molecular Cell Biology*, vol. 8, no. 7, pp. 519–529, 2007.

[98] G. Boden, X. Duan, C. Homko et al., "Increase in endoplasmic reticulum stress-related proteins and genes in adipose tissue of obese, insulin-resistant individuals," *Diabetes*, vol. 57, no. 9, pp. 2438–2444, 2008.

[99] M. F. Gregor, L. Yang, E. Fabbrini et al., "Endoplasmic reticulum stress is reduced in tissues of obese subjects after weight loss," *Diabetes*, vol. 58, no. 3, pp. 693–700, 2009.

[100] M. Flamment, E. Hajduch, P. Ferré, and F. Foufelle, "New insights into ER stress-induced insulin resistance," *Trends in Endocrinology & Metabolism*, vol. 23, no. 8, pp. 381–390, 2012.

[101] R. Ghemrawi, S.-F. Battaglia-Hsu, and C. Arnold, "Endoplasmic reticulum stress in metabolic disorders," *Cell*, vol. 7, no. 6, 2018.

[102] C. M. Oslowski and F. Urano, "Chapter four - measuring ER stress and the unfolded protein response using mammalian tissue culture system," *Methods in Enzymology*, vol. 490, pp. 71–92, 2011.

[103] D. Rojas-Rivera, T. Delvaeye, R. Roelandt et al., "When PERK inhibitors turn out to be new potent RIPK1 inhibitors: critical issues on the specificity and use of GSK2606414 and GSK2656157," *Cell Death and Differentiation*, vol. 24, no. 6, pp. 1100–1110, 2017.

[104] P. Tsaytler, H. P. Harding, D. Ron, and A. Bertolotti, "Selective inhibition of a regulatory subunit of protein phosphatase 1 restores proteostasis," *Science*, vol. 332, no. 6025, pp. 91–94, 2011.

[105] L. N. Guthrie, K. Abiraman, E. S. Plyler et al., "Attenuation of PKR-like ER kinase (PERK) signaling selectively controls endoplasmic reticulum stress-induced inflammation without compromising immunological responses," *Journal of Biological Chemistry*, vol. 291, no. 30, pp. 15830–15840, 2016.

[106] S. Oyadomari, A. Koizumi, K. Takeda et al., "Targeted disruption of the *Chop* gene delays endoplasmic reticulum stress-mediated diabetes," *The Journal of Clinical Investigation*, vol. 109, no. 4, pp. 525–532, 2002.

[107] X. Z. Wang and D. Ron, "Stress-induced phosphorylation and activation of the transcription factor CHOP (GADD153) by p38 MAP kinase," *Science*, vol. 272, no. 5266, pp. 1347–1349, 1996.

[108] D. Han, A. G. Lerner, L. Vande Walle et al., "IRE1α kinase activation modes control alternate endoribonuclease outputs to determine divergent cell fates," *Cell*, vol. 138, no. 3, pp. 562–575, 2009.

[109] M. Bouchecareilh, A. Higa, S. Fribourg, M. Moenner, and E. Chevet, "Peptides derived from the bifunctional kinase/RNase enzyme IRE1α modulate IRE1α activity and protect cells from endoplasmic reticulum stress," *The FASEB Journal*, vol. 25, no. 9, pp. 3115–3129, 2011.

[110] R. Bravo, T. Gutierrez, F. Paredes et al., "Endoplasmic reticulum: ER stress regulates mitochondrial bioenergetics," *The International Journal of Biochemistry & Cell Biology*, vol. 44, no. 1, pp. 16–20, 2012.

[111] V. Plaisance, S. Brajkovic, M. Tenenbaum et al., "Endoplasmic reticulum stress links oxidative stress to impaired pancreatic beta-cell function caused by human oxidized LDL," *PLoS One*, vol. 11, no. 9, article e0163046, 2016.

[112] W. C. Chong, M. D. Shastri, and R. Eri, "Endoplasmic reticulum stress and oxidative stress: a vicious nexus implicated in bowel disease pathophysiology," *International Journal of Molecular Sciences*, vol. 18, no. 4, 2017.

[113] D. van der Vlies, M. Makkinje, A. Jansens et al., "Oxidation of ER resident proteins upon oxidative stress: effects of altering cellular redox/antioxidant status and implications for protein maturation," *Antioxidants & Redox Signaling*, vol. 5, no. 4, pp. 381–387, 2003.

[114] T. E. Creighton, D. A. Hillson, and R. B. Freedman, "Catalysis by protein-disulphide isomerase of the unfolding and refolding of proteins with disulphide bonds," *Journal of Molecular Biology*, vol. 142, no. 1, pp. 43–62, 1980.

[115] S. Chakravarthi and N. J. Bulleid, "Glutathione is required to regulate the formation of native disulfide bonds within proteins entering the secretory pathway," *Journal of Biological Chemistry*, vol. 279, no. 38, pp. 39872–39879, 2004.

[116] D. M. Ferrari and H. D. Söling, "The protein disulphide-isomerase family: unravelling a string of folds," *Biochemical Journal*, vol. 339, no. 1, pp. 1–10, 1999.

[117] M. Hagiwara and K. Nagata, "Redox-dependent protein quality control in the endoplasmic reticulum: folding to degradation," *Antioxidants & Redox Signaling*, vol. 16, no. 10, pp. 1119–1128, 2012.

[118] N. Chaudhari, P. Talwar, A. Parimisetty, C. Lefebvre d'Hellencourt, and P. Ravanan, "A molecular web: endoplasmic reticulum stress, inflammation, and oxidative stress," *Frontiers in Cellular Neuroscience*, vol. 8, p. 213, 2014.

[119] S. S. Cao, K. L. Luo, and L. Shi, "Endoplasmic reticulum stress interacts with inflammation in human diseases," *Journal of Cellular Physiology*, vol. 231, no. 2, pp. 288–294, 2016.

[120] X. Li, "Endoplasmic reticulum stress regulates inflammation in adipocyte of obese rats via toll-like receptors 4 signaling," *Iranian Journal of Basic Medical Sciences*, vol. 21, no. 5, pp. 502–507, 2018.

[121] N. Kawasaki, R. Asada, A. Saito, S. Kanemoto, and K. Imaizumi, "Obesity-induced endoplasmic reticulum stress causes chronic inflammation in adipose tissue," *Scientific Reports*, vol. 2, no. 1, article 799, 2012.

[122] S. Z. Hasnain, D. J. Borg, B. E. Harcourt et al., "Glycemic control in diabetes is restored by therapeutic manipulation of cytokines that regulate beta cell stress," *Nature Medicine*, vol. 20, no. 12, pp. 1417–1426, 2014.

[123] K. Maedler, P. Sergeev, J. A. Ehses et al., "Leptin modulates β cell expression of IL-1 receptor antagonist and release of IL-1β in human islets," *Proceedings of the National Academy of Sciences of the United States of America*, vol. 101, no. 21, pp. 8138–8143, 2004.

[124] M. Y. Donath, M. Böni-Schnetzler, H. Ellingsgaard, and J. A. Ehses, "Islet inflammation impairs the pancreatic β-cell in type 2 diabetes," *Physiology*, vol. 24, no. 6, pp. 325–331, 2009.

[125] M. Miani, J. Barthson, M. L. Colli, F. Brozzi, M. Cnop, and D. L. Eizirik, "Endoplasmic reticulum stress sensitizes pancreatic beta cells to interleukin-1β-induced apoptosis via Bim/A1 imbalance," *Cell Death & Disease*, vol. 4, no. 7, article e701, 2013.

[126] F. Brozzi, T. R. Nardelli, M. Lopes et al., "Cytokines induce endoplasmic reticulum stress in human, rat and mouse beta cells via different mechanisms," *Diabetologia*, vol. 58, no. 10, pp. 2307–2316, 2015.

[127] S. Nakajima, Y. Chi, K. Gao, K. Kono, and J. Yao, "eIF2α-independent inhibition of TNF-α-triggered NF-κB activation by Salubrinal," *Biological and Pharmaceutical Bulletin*, vol. 38, no. 9, pp. 1368–1374, 2015.

[128] G. Coudriet, M. Delmastro-Greenwood, D. Previte et al., "Treatment with a catalytic superoxide dismutase (SOD) mimetic improves liver steatosis, insulin sensitivity, and inflammation in obesity-induced type 2 diabetes," *Antioxidants*, vol. 6, no. 4, p. 85, 2017.

[129] J. B. Farinha, F. M. Steckling, S. T. Stefanello et al., "Response of oxidative stress and inflammatory biomarkers to a 12-week aerobic exercise training in women with metabolic syndrome," *Sports Medicine-Open*, vol. 1, no. 1, p. 19, 2015.

[130] L. Ozcan and I. Tabas, "Role of endoplasmic reticulum stress in metabolic disease and other disorders," *Annual Review of Medicine*, vol. 63, no. 1, pp. 317–328, 2012.

[131] K. Matsushita and V. J. Dzau, "Mesenchymal stem cells in obesity: insights for translational applications," *Laboratory Investigation*, vol. 97, no. 10, pp. 1158–1166, 2017.

[132] L. Zang, H. Hao, J. Liu, Y. Li, W. Han, and Y. Mu, "Mesenchymal stem cell therapy in type 2 diabetes mellitus," *Diabetology and Metabolic Syndrome*, vol. 9, no. 1, p. 36, 2017.

[133] "Home-ClinicalTrials.gov," April 2018, https://clinicaltrials.gov/.

[134] S. Kadam, S. Muthyala, P. Nair, and R. Bhonde, "Human placenta-derived mesenchymal stem cells and islet-like cell clusters generated from these cells as a novel source for stem cell therapy in diabetes," *Review of Diabetic Studies*, vol. 7, no. 2, pp. 168–182, 2010.

[135] S. S. Kadam, M. Sudhakar, P. D. Nair, and R. R. Bhonde, "Reversal of experimental diabetes in mice by transplantation of neo-islets generated from human amnion-derived mesenchymal stromal cells using immuno-isolatory macrocapsules," *Cytotherapy*, vol. 12, no. 8, pp. 982–991, 2010.

[136] A. I. Caplan and J. E. Dennis, "Mesenchymal stem cells as trophic mediators," *Journal of Cellular Biochemistry*, vol. 98, no. 5, pp. 1076–1084, 2006.

[137] L. Chen, E. E. Tredget, P. Y. G. Wu, and Y. Wu, "Paracrine factors of mesenchymal stem cells recruit macrophages and endothelial lineage cells and enhance wound healing," *PLoS One*, vol. 3, no. 4, article e1886, 2008.

[138] K. Le Blanc, C. Tammik, K. Rosendahl, E. Zetterberg, and O. Ringdén, "HLA expression and immunologic properties of differentiated and undifferentiated mesenchymal stem cells," *Experimental Hematology*, vol. 31, no. 10, pp. 890–896, 2003.

[139] P. Hematti, J. Kim, A. P. Stein, and D. Kaufman, "Potential role of mesenchymal stromal cells in pancreatic islet transplantation," *Transplantation Reviews*, vol. 27, no. 1, pp. 21–29, 2013.

[140] Y. Wang, X. Chen, W. Cao, and Y. Shi, "Plasticity of mesenchymal stem cells in immunomodulation: pathological and therapeutic implications," *Nature Immunology*, vol. 15, no. 11, pp. 1009–1016, 2014.

[141] K. Zhao, H. Hao, J. Liu et al., "Bone marrow-derived mesenchymal stem cells ameliorate chronic high glucose-induced β-cell injury through modulation of autophagy," *Cell Death & Disease*, vol. 6, no. 9, article e1885, 2015.

[142] A. Valle-Prieto and P. A. Conget, "Human mesenchymal stem cells efficiently manage oxidative stress," *Stem Cells and Development*, vol. 19, no. 12, pp. 1885–1893, 2010.

[143] W. A. Silva, D. T. Covas, R. A. Panepucci et al., "The profile of gene expression of human marrow mesenchymal stem cells," *Stem Cells*, vol. 21, no. 6, pp. 661–669, 2003.

[144] A. Stolzing and A. Scutt, "Effect of reduced culture temperature on antioxidant defences of mesenchymal stem cells," *Free Radical Biology & Medicine*, vol. 41, no. 2, pp. 326–338, 2006.

[145] R. Ebert, M. Ulmer, S. Zeck et al., "Selenium supplementation restores the antioxidative capacity and prevents cell damage in bone marrow stromal cells in vitro," *Stem Cells*, vol. 24, no. 5, pp. 1226–1235, 2006.

[146] M. L. Calió, D. S. Marinho, G. M. Ko et al., "Transplantation of bone marrow mesenchymal stem cells decreases oxidative stress, apoptosis, and hippocampal damage in brain of a spontaneous stroke model," *Free Radical Biology & Medicine*, vol. 70, pp. 141–154, 2014.

[147] B. Chandravanshi and R. R. Bhonde, "Shielding engineered islets with mesenchymal stem cells enhance survival under hypoxia," *Journal of Cellular Biochemistry*, vol. 118, no. 9, pp. 2672–2683, 2017.

[148] E. Wojtas, A. Zachwieja, A. Zwyrzykowska, R. KupczyńSki, and K. Marycz, "The application of mesenchymal progenitor stem cells for the reduction of oxidative stress in animals," *Turkish Journal of Biology*, vol. 41, pp. 12–19, 2017.

15

Mesenchymal Stromal/Stem Cells in Regenerative Medicine and Tissue Engineering

Ross E. B. Fitzsimmons ⓘ,[1,2] **Matthew S. Mazurek** ⓘ,[3] **Agnes Soos** ⓘ,[1,2] **and Craig A. Simmons** ⓘ[1,2,4]

[1]*Institute of Biomaterials and Biomedical Engineering, University of Toronto, 164 College Street, Toronto, ON, Canada M5S 3G9*
[2]*Translational Biology and Engineering Program, Ted Rogers Centre for Heart Research, 661 University Ave, Toronto, ON, Canada M5G 1M1*
[3]*Division of Gastroenterology and Hepatology, Department of Medicine, University of Calgary, Calgary, AB, Canada T2N 4Z6*
[4]*Department of Mechanical and Industrial Engineering, University of Toronto, 5 King's College Road, Toronto, ON, Canada M5S 3G8*

Correspondence should be addressed to Ross E. B. Fitzsimmons; ross.fitzsimmons@mail.utoronto.ca and Craig A. Simmons; c.simmons@utoronto.ca

Academic Editor: Jane Ru Choi

As a result of over five decades of investigation, mesenchymal stromal/stem cells (MSCs) have emerged as a versatile and frequently utilized cell source in the fields of regenerative medicine and tissue engineering. In this review, we summarize the history of MSC research from the initial discovery of their multipotency to the more recent recognition of their perivascular identity *in vivo* and their extraordinary capacity for immunomodulation and angiogenic signaling. As well, we discuss long-standing questions regarding their developmental origins and their capacity for differentiation toward a range of cell lineages. We also highlight important considerations and potential risks involved with their isolation, ex vivo expansion, and clinical use. Overall, this review aims to serve as an overview of the breadth of research that has demonstrated the utility of MSCs in a wide range of clinical contexts and continues to unravel the mechanisms by which these cells exert their therapeutic effects.

1. Introduction

By merit of their regenerative secretome and their capacity for differentiation toward multiple mesenchymal lineages, the fibroblastic cell type termed mesenchymal stromal/stem cells (MSCs) shows promise for a wide range of tissue engineering and regenerative medicine applications (Figure 1). As a result of their therapeutic versatility and the multitude of promising clinical results thus far, MSCs are poised to become an increasingly significant cell source for regenerative therapies as medicine evolves to focus on personalized and cell-based therapeutics. Given their emerging importance, this review aims to provide an overview of historical and ongoing work aimed at understanding and better utilizing these cells for therapeutic purposes.

2. Initial Discoveries and the Evolving Definition of "MSC"

The initial discovery of MSCs is attributed to Friedenstein et al. who discovered a fibroblastic cell type derived from mouse and guinea pig bone marrow that could produce clonal colonies capable of generating bone and reticular tissue when heterotopically transplanted [1, 2]. The subsequent discovery that colonies of this cell type can generate cartilage and adipose tissue, in addition to bone, gave rise to the descriptor *mesenchymal stem cells*, as originally coined by Arnold Caplan [3]. Finally, Pittenger et al. established that human bone marrow also contains a subpopulation of stromal cells that are genuinely multipotent stem cells by demonstrating single colonies have trilineage mesenchymal potential [4].

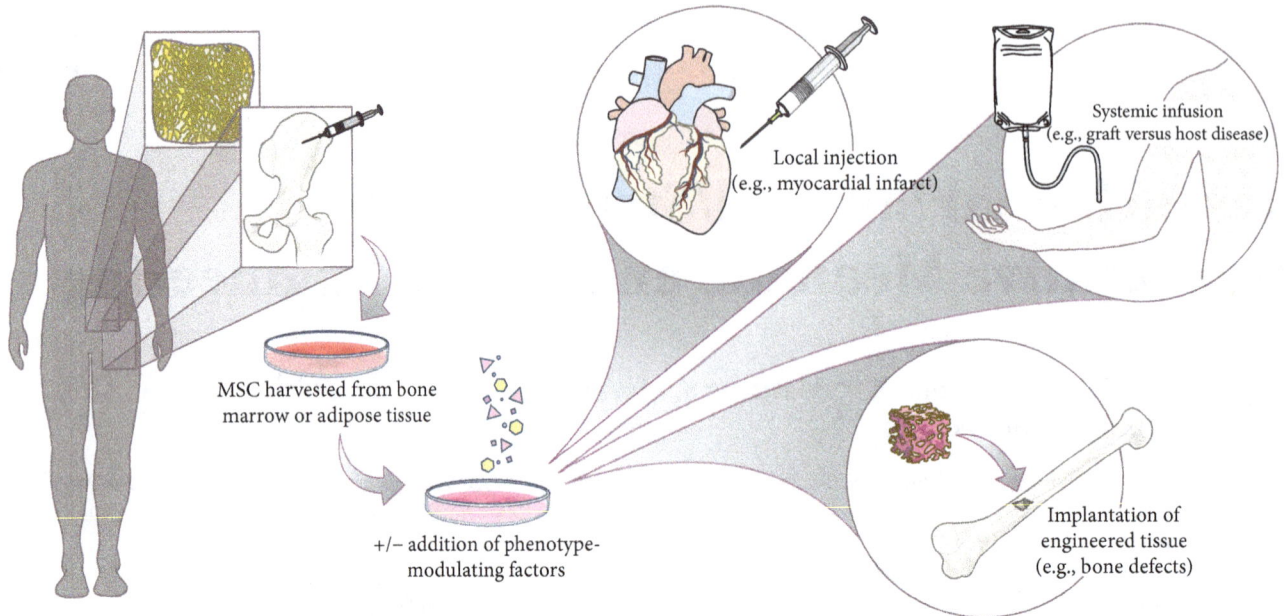

FIGURE 1: Strategies for mesenchymal stromal/stem cell- (MSC-) based therapies. MSCs may be isolated from a number of tissues (e.g., bone marrow, adipose tissue, and umbilical cord) and optionally cultured prior to clinical use. Depending on the specific application, MSC suspensions may then be introduced intravenously or by local injection to achieve the desired therapeutic effects, such as treating autoimmune diseases or stimulating local tissue repair and vascularization, respectively. MSCs may also be utilized for engineering tissues by first promoting their differentiation toward a desired cell type (e.g., osteoblasts, chondrocytes, and adipocytes) prior to being surgically implanted, often along with scaffold material.

Over time, the acronym MSC has come to take on multiple meanings including, mesenchymal stem cell, mesenchymal stromal cell, and multipotent stromal cell. To help clarify this, the International Society for Cellular Therapy (ISCT) has officially defined MSCs as *multipotent mesenchymal stromal cells* and suggests this to mean the plastic-adherent fraction from stromal tissues, while reserving the term *mesenchymal stem cells* to mean the subpopulation that actually has the two cardinal stem cell properties (*i.e.*, self-renewal and the capacity to differentiate down multiple lineages) [5]. Furthermore, ISCT has also defined MSCs as meeting several criteria including (i) being plastic adherent, (ii) having osteogenic, adipogenic, and chondrogenic trilineage differentiation potential, (iii) and being positive (>95%) and negative (<2%) for a panel of cell surface antigens. Positive markers for human MSCs include CD73 (also present on lymphocytes, endothelial cells, smooth muscle cells, and fibroblasts), CD90 (also present on hematopoietic stem cells, lymphocytes, endothelial cells, neurons, and fibroblasts), and CD105 (also found on endothelial cells, monocytes, hematopoietic progenitors, and fibroblasts) [6]. Negative markers include CD34 (present on hematopoietic progenitors and endothelial cells), CD45 (a pan-leukocyte marker), CD14 or CD11b (present on monocytes and macrophages), CD79-α or CD19 (present on B cells), and HLA-DR unless stimulated with IFN-γ (present on macrophages, B cells, and dendritic cells) [5]. It should be noted, however, that the validity of CD34 as a negative marker has recently been called into question and may require reexamination [6, 7].

As these elaborate inclusionary and exclusionary criteria highlight, no single MSC-specific epitope has been discovered, unlike for some other stem cell populations (e.g., LGR5, which labels resident stem cells in hair follicles and intestinal crypts) [8, 9]. However, some markers may be used to enrich for the stem cell population, including Stro-1, CD146, CD106, CD271, MSCA-1, and others (Table 1) [6, 10–13]. This unfortunate lack of a single definitive marker continues to confound the interpretation of a broad range of studies given that sorting out the canonical MSC population from the adherent fraction is rarely done, leading to the perennial question of which subpopulation in the adherent stromal fraction is actually eliciting the observed effects. This lack of a definitive MSC marker has also contributed to the challenge of delineating the exact *in vivo* location, function, and developmental origin of MSCs.

3. MSC Adult Anatomical Location

In the bone marrow, where MSCs were first discovered, MSCs have been reported to typically localize near the sinusoidal endothelium in close association with the resident hematopoietic stem cells (HSCs) [14, 15]. In addition to serving as osteogenic progenitors, such MSCs have been shown to play an important role in regulating HSC function by maintaining the HSC niche and by secreting trophic factors such as angiopoietin 1 (Ang1), stem cell factor (SCF), and CXC ligand 12 (CXCL12) [10]. Beyond the bone marrow, MSC/MSC-like populations have also

TABLE 1: Potential markers for MSC identification and enrichment.

Selection type (and comments)	CD No.	Name	Acronym	Reference
Negative	**CD11b**	**Integrin subunit alpha M**	**ITGAM**	[5]
Negative	**CD14**	**CD14 molecule**	**CD14**	[5]
Negative	**CD19**	**CD19 molecule**	**CD19**	[5]
Negative (not in all MSC populations)	**CD34**	**CD34 molecule**	**CD34**	[5]
Negative	**CD45**	**Protein tyrosine phosphatase, receptor type C**	**PTPRC**	[5]
Negative	**CD79a**	**CD79a molecule**	**CD79A**	[5]
Negative (unless stimulated with IFN-γ)	—	**Human leukocyte antigen, antigen D Related**	**HLA-DR**	[5]
Positive	CD9	CD9 molecule	CD9	[172]
Positive	CD10	Membrane metalloendopeptidase	MME	[173]
Positive	CD13	Alanyl aminopeptidase, membrane	ANPEP	[174]
Positive	CD29	Integrin subunit beta 1	ITGB1	[175]
Positive	CD44	CD44 molecule (Indian blood group)	CD44	[176]
Positive	CD49f	Integrin subunit alpha 6	ITGA6	[177]
Positive	CD54	Intercellular adhesion molecule 1	ICAM1	[178]
Positive	CD71	Transferrin receptor	TFRC	[179]
Positive	**CD73**	**5′-nucleotidase ecto**	**NT5E**	[5]
Positive	**CD90**	**Thy-1 cell surface antigen**	**THY1**	[5]
Positive	**CD105**	**Endoglin**	**ENG**	[5]
Positive	CD106	Vascular cell adhesion molecule 1	VCAM1	[11]
Positive	CD146	Melanoma cell adhesion molecule	MCAM	[10]
Positive	CD166	Activated leukocyte cell adhesion molecule	ALCAM	[180]
Positive	CD200	CD200 molecule	CD200	[181]
Positive	CD271	Nerve growth factor receptor	NGFR	[12]
Positive	CD349	Frizzled class receptor 9	FZD9	[173]
Positive	CD362	Syndecan 2	SDC2	[182]
Positive (a disialoganglioside, nonpeptide)	—	Ganglioside GD2	G2	[183]
Positive (also known as nucleostemin)	—	G protein nucleolar 3	GNL3	[184]
Positive (target of anti-STRO1 antibodies)	—	Heat shock protein family A (Hsp70) member 8	HSPA8	[185]
Positive	—	Heat shock protein 90 beta family member 1	HSP90B1	[186]
Positive (a glycosphingolipid, nonpeptide)	—	Stage-specific embryonic antigen-4	SSEA-4	[187]
Positive	—	Sushi domain containing 2	SUSD2	[188]
Positive	—	Alkaline phosphatase, liver/bone/kidney	ALPL	[13]

Bolded text indicates markers recommended by the International Society for Cellular Therapy (ISCT) for minimally defining human multipotent mesenchymal stromal cells by positive and negative selection.

been found in many adult tissues (*e.g.*, skin, pancreas, heart, brain, lung, kidney, adipose tissue, cartilage, and tendon) [16–19]. Such a broad anatomical distribution would suggest a common and ubiquitous MSC niche exists throughout the body. Indeed, evidence suggests that many MSC populations are specifically located near blood vessels and are in fact a subpopulation of pericytes that reside on capillaries and venules [20]. Supporting observations include the fact that pericytes and MSCs express similar surface antigens, and that cells in perivascular positions were found to express MSC markers in human bone marrow and dental pulp [16, 21]. Perhaps most definitively, Crisan et al. found that cells positive for NG2, CD146, and PDGFR-β specifically stained pericytes in multiple human tissues, and when cells with these markers were isolated, they were shown to have trilineage potential *in vitro* and were osteogenic once transplanted

in vivo [22]. The converse, that all pericytes are MSCs, is not thought to be the case [20].

In addition to being abluminal to microvessels, it should be noted that a Gli1$^+$ MSC-like population has also been found to reside within the adventitia of larger vessels in mice. The Gli1$^+$ population exhibits trilineage differentiation *in vitro* and is thought to play a role in arterial calcification *in vivo* [23–25]. Similarly, a MSC population with a CD34$^+$ CD31$^-$ CD146$^-$ CD45$^-$ phenotype has been discovered to reside within the adventitia of human arteries and veins suggesting that not all perivascular MSCs are pericyte-like cells in humans [7]. Furthermore, a MSC population has also been isolated from the perivascular tissue of umbilical cords (human umbilical cord perivascular cells (HUCPVCs)) which shows promise for tissue engineering applications given the cells' noninvasive extraction and their relatively high abundance and proliferative capacity, compared to bone marrow-derived MSCs [26–28].

Finally, despite the prevalent view that MSCs reside in perivascular niches, some MSC populations may reside in avascular regions as well. For example, a lineage tracing study focused on murine tooth repair demonstrated that while some odontoblasts descend from cells expressing the pericyte marker, NG2, the majority of odontoblasts did not, suggestive of a nonpericyte origin (or at least not from NG2-positive pericytes) [29]. Additionally, MSCs have been isolated from tissues that are typically avascular, including human synovial tissue [30–32] and porcine aortic valve [33]. However, there are fenestrated capillaries localized near the synovial surface [34], and diseased sclerotic and stenotic valves can be partially vascularized [35, 36], raising the possibility of MSCs trafficking from one anatomical location to another (*e.g.*, synovium-associated vasculature to avascular cartilage) and innate differences in the local presence or absence of perivascular MSCs. Future work focused on these questions will have important implications for understanding disease progression and potential regenerative avenues.

4. MSC Developmental Origins

Presently, there are considered to be multiple developmental origins of MSCs. Unsurprisingly, given their mesenchymal differentiation potential, certain subsets of MSCs are derived from mesodermal precursors, such as lateral plate mesoderm- (LPM-) derived mesoangioblast cells from the embryonic dorsal aorta [37, 38]. Support for this comes from the observation that mesoangioblast cells isolated from the mouse dorsal aorta and then grafted into chick embryos incorporated into several mesodermal tissues (bone, cartilage, muscle, and blood) [39].

Other reports suggest MSCs partly descend from a subpopulation of neural crest cells, with the remaining MSCs descending from unknown origins. Support for this comes from the observation that a population of murine Sox1$^+$ trunk neuroepithelial cells could undergo clonogenic expansion and maintain adipogenic, chondrogenic, and osteogenic differentiation *in vitro* [40]. This neural crest origin may help explain why MSCs have neural differentiation potential and why human bone marrow-derived MSCs can be enriched for using antibodies against nerve growth factor receptor [12, 38]. Given their lineage tracing results, the authors claimed that neural crest-derived MSCs are the earliest MSCs to arise in the embryo, but they did note that other MSCs must also arise later on in development as not all MSCs detected were found to be of a neural crest origin. Corroborating this, a lineage tracing study using the promoter from Protein-0, a neural crest-associated marker, found that only a portion of bone marrow-derived MSCs were labeled in adult mice, suggestive of both a neural crest and nonneural crest origin [41].

It is possible that the indefinite nonneural crest source of MSCs observed in these studies may be mesoangioblasts or another mesoderm-derived cell type. It has also been suggested that data indicative of a mesoangioblast origin may alternatively be explained by simply "contamination" of neural crest cells as the neural tube is close to dorsal aorta at day 9.5 [38]. With regard to human MSC origins, similar dual mesoderm and neural crest origins may also exist given that human iPSCs differentiated toward these two lineages can both give rise to MSC-like cells [42, 43]. Further study will be required to resolve these issues and to elucidate if any lasting functional dissimilarities exist between MSC subpopulations that arise from differing time periods and locations during development.

5. MSC Expansion in Culture

Once isolated from their respective *in vivo* locations, human MSC populations can be expanded up to several hundredfold while maintaining their multipotency and capacity to form fibroblastic colony-forming units (CFU-F) provided the cells are seeded at a satisfactorily low seeding density (~10–100 cell/cm^2) [44]. When cultured at low clonal density, MSCs take on a highly proliferative phenotype and maintain their trilineage potential; such cells have become commonly referred to as RS-MSCs (rapidly self-renewing MSCs). This proliferative phase is thought to be dependent on Dickkopf-related protein 1 (Dkk-1) autocrine signaling which inhibits Wnt signaling that would otherwise promote differentiation [45]. Favorable for minimizing risk to patients, *in vitro* proliferation of human MSCs exhibits a relatively low frequency of oncogenic transformation ($<10^{-9}$) [46–48]. This is in stark contrast with murine MSCs which frequently gain chromosomal defects *in vitro* and often produce fibrosarcomas when injected back into mice [49].

With time, sparsely plated human MSCs create colonies with distinct *in vitro* niches with the inner cells expressing differentiation markers and the outer cells exhibiting a more RS-MSC phenotype with high motility and proliferation [50, 51]. Yet, when replated, both inner and outer regions create colonies similar to the original, implying differentiation of the inner colony is reversible to some extent [51]. If MSCs are seeded at a higher density (~1000 cell/cm^2) and/or are cultured to confluence, RS-MSCs will decrease and SR-MSCs (slowly replicating MSCs) will increase over time, while both the CFU-F and proportion of multipotent cells will gradually decline [44, 51]. This dynamic nature during culture underlines the importance of properly maintaining MSC cultures to ensure maximum self-renewal and the maintenance of differentiation potential for downstream applications.

6. MSC Differentiation Potential

As mentioned earlier, by definition, MSCs have trilineage potential with the capacity to undergo osteogenesis, adipogenesis, and chondrogenesis contingent on their exposure to the particular soluble factors in their microenvironment. Differentiation protocols for driving differentiation toward these lineages have been routinely utilized and extensively optimized [52, 53]. For example, osteogenesis typically involves the use of dexamethasone, β-glycerolphosphate, and ascorbic acid. Adipogenesis protocols also utilize dexamethasone, in addition to isobutylmethylxanthine and indomethacin. Chondrogenesis protocols, on the other hand, typically utilize dexamethasone, ascorbic acid, sodium pyruvate, TGF-β1, and a combination of insulin-transferrin-selenium (ITS). However, variations of the components and their concentrations exist and the optimal formulations may depend on the subpopulation of MSC used and the ultimate therapeutic goal. MSCs predifferentiated toward these three lineages have been investigated extensively in the context of tissue engineering wherein cells are implanted at the site of desired repair or replacement, often along with a scaffold (Figure 1) [54–58].

Beyond the standard trilineage potential of MSCs, differentiation has also been observed toward other cell types, such as tenocytes, skeletal myocytes, cardiomyocytes, smooth muscle cells, and even neurons [59–61]. However, some of these claims have courted a degree of skepticism in regard to the frequency of differentiation and the functionality of the terminal cells produced, especially for nonmesenchymal and nonmesodermal cell types. For example, while MSCs have been shown to differentiate into neuron-like cells, the functionality of rat MSC-derived neurons has been called into question in terms of their capacity to generate normal action potentials [62, 63]. Similarly, human MSCs have also been reported to differentiate into endothelial-like cells; however, such cells have lower expression of endothelial markers compared to mature endothelial cells [64]. Further study into the differentiation frequency and normal functioning of MSC-derived terminally differentiated cells will be necessary, in addition to determining if different MSC populations are better suited to differentiate into some cell types than others. With regard to the latter, a recent study comparing human CD146$^+$/CD34$^-$/CD45$^-$ MSCs isolated from different anatomical locations (bone marrow, periosteum, and skeletal muscle) revealed that each subpopulation differed considerably in their transcriptomic signature and *in vivo* differentiation potential, hence suggesting that MSCs are not a uniform population throughout the body [65]. Moreover, MSC heterogeneity may not only exist between tissue types but also within individual tissues. For example, locationally and transcriptionally distinct subpopulations of CD34$^+$/CD146$^-$ "adventitial MSCs" and CD34$^-$/CD146$^+$ "pericyte-like MSCs" have been found to reside in human adipose tissue, a commonly used cell source for regenerative medicine [66]. Similar findings have also been noted in horses and canines, suggesting these dual perivascular subpopulations are conserved in mammals [67, 68]. Interestingly, both equine and human adipose-derived CD34$^-$/CD146$^+$ MSCs display greater angiogenicity compared to CD34$^+$/CD146$^-$ MSCs indicative of a relatively conserved functional phenotype as well, possibly due to their pericyte-like differentiation state [67, 69]. Heterogeneity among MSCs may also have important implications for treating disease resulting from inappropriate differentiation and proliferation. Of note, subsets of PDGFRβ^+ and/or PDGFRα^+ MSC-like progenitor cells with fibro-adipogenic potential have been found to be present in multiple tissues (*e.g.*, tendon, myocardium, and skeletal muscle) and may prove to be useful targets for reducing fibrotic damage after injury [70, 71].

Further investigation into MSC heterogeneity will be required to resolve if such differences are solely a result of innate differences arising from different developmental origins or if differing local microenvironments also play a role.

Unlike some other stem cell populations (e.g., hematopoietic stem cells), which have a well-established and relatively straight-forward unidirectional differentiation hierarchy, the hierarchy of MSC differentiation is currently poorly defined. To date, one of the MSC-like populations that have been most vigorously investigated in terms of hierarchy are human umbilical cord-perivascular cells (HUCPVCs). Such cells have been found to differentiate from quintipotential stem cells (with osteogenic, adipogenic, chondrogenic, myogenic, and fibrogenic potential) to a restricted fibroblast-state in a deterministic manner with a predictable order of loss in potency [72]. Whether this is true for all or some MSC populations remains to be examined, but this study should serve as a useful template for future investigation. As well, computational approaches that cluster cells according to differentially expressed genes may also help clarify the hierarchy of MSC subpopulations and their progeny cells [66] and may serve as a guide for future lineage tracing studies. That said, transdifferentiation toward nonmesodermal lineages and bidirectional phenotype switching between different mesenchymal cell types (e.g., transitions between fibroblasts and myofibroblasts or between synthetic and contractile smooth muscle cells) may further complicate any MSC hierarchical differentiation model established [73]. Regardless of any specific hierarchy and the potential for phenotypic plasticity, it should be emphasized that ultimately, the microenvironment dictates MSC behaviour, in terms of both their differentiation and their interaction with other cell types.

7. MSC Immunomodulatory Paracrine Signaling

Recently, a paradigm shift has occurred in the understanding of the therapeutic effects of MSCs. Despite the differentiation potential these cells exhibit and contrary to initial assumptions, in many therapeutic contexts, MSCs exert their healing effects not through engraftment and differentiation but rather through paracrine signaling and communication through cell-cell contacts [51, 74]. The significance of this paradigm change is reflected in the recent recommendation to rebrand MSCs as *medicinal signaling cells* by Arnold Caplan, who had originally coined the term mesenchymal stem cells [75]. Notable examples of MSC paracrine/juxtacrine-mediated treatments currently in preclinical and clinical development include injections into the myocardium after infarction, treatments for graft versus host disease (GvHD), and therapies for autoimmunity disorders (such as Crohn's disease and type I diabetes) [76–79]. Given these successes, it is becoming increasing clear that the MSC secretome has broadly beneficial effects that can be exploited for a wide range of therapeutic applications.

The MSC secretome contains a large range of molecules that are beneficial for tissue repair, including ligands that promote the proliferation and differentiation of other stem/

progenitor cells, chemoattraction, antifibrosis, antiapoptosis, angiogenesis, and immunomodulation [80]. Currently, perhaps the most impactful of these properties from a clinical perspective is their capacity for immunomodulation, which has motivated the development of intravenous injections of MSCs, such as Osiris Therapeutics' Prochymal®, which is approved for GvHD in Canada and currently in clinical trials for several autoimmune disorders in Canada and the USA. This immunomodulatory capacity has been partly attributed to the ability of MSCs to inhibit effector T-cell activation and proliferation, both directly through various cytokines and indirectly through modulating the activity of regulatory T-cells [81, 82]. MSCs have also been described as modulating the behaviors of natural killer cells, dendritic cells, B-cells, neutrophils, and monocytes/macrophages through the actions of a number of molecules, including prostaglandin E2 (PGE2), indoleamine 2,3-dioxygenase (IDO), nitric oxide (NO), interleukin-10 (IL-10), and many others [8, 80]. Notably in the context of localized tissue repair, MSCs have been implicated in promoting alternative activation of macrophages toward a regenerative and proangiogenic M2 phenotype, as opposed to a classical proinflammatory M1 phenotype [83–86]. Consequently, given the many roles MSCs play in therapeutic immunomodulation and regeneration, it is becoming increasingly acknowledged that one of the main roles of adult MSCs *in vivo* may be to coordinate healing responses and to help prevent autoimmunity after injury [8, 74, 80].

Lastly, it should be noted that MSCs are not solely anti-inflammatory. Under certain conditions, MSCs can elicit an inflammatory response by presenting antigens to induce CD8$^+$ T-cell responses, and increasing expression of MHCDII and presenting antigens to CD4$^+$ T-cells [87–89]. The "switch" between eliciting an inflammatory or anti-inflammatory response generally seems to be whether the activating signals are associated with infections or tissue injury, respectively [90].

8. MSC Angiogenic Paracrine Signaling

In addition to being proangiogenic by promoting a regenerative microenvironment via immunomodulation, MSCs also directly secrete angiogenic factors that affect endothelial cell survival, proliferation, and migration. Such factors include key growth factors critical for initial vessel formation and subsequent stabilization, such as VEGF, FGF2, SDF1, ANG1, MCP-1, HGF, and many others [91, 92]. Beyond these classical angiogenic growth factors, MSCs also secrete microvesicles (>200 μm) and exosomes (~50–200 μm) that can carry both growth factors and miRNAs and have been demonstrated to have proangiogenic activities both *in vitro* and *in vivo* [93]. Such extracellular vesicles have been shown to enhance angiogenesis and healing in a number of contexts, including murine and rat models of burn injury, cutaneous wounds, myocardial infarction, and limb ischemia [94–99]. Recent proteomic analysis has found human MSC-derived exosomes contain a number of proteins associated with angiogenesis that were upregulated when MSCs were

exposed to ischemic-like conditions, including PDGF, EGF, FGF, and NF-κB pathway-affiliated proteins [100].

Similarly, recent qPCR screening of exosomes derived from murine MSC-like cells revealed they contain a number of known proangiogenic microRNAs, several of which were found to be preferentially internalized by endothelial cells, including miR-424, miR-30c, miR-30b, and let-7f [101]. Relatedly, miR-210 has also been implicated in the therapeutic effect of MSC-derived extracellular vesicles in a mouse model of cardiac infarction, as siRNA knockdown reduced the angiogenic effect of the vesicles [102]. Delineating which specific MSC-derived exosomal miRNAs are responsible for particular aspects of angiogenesis is an ongoing area of research. Recently, for example, exosomal miRNA-125a from human adipose-derived MSCs has been implicated in enhancing angiogenesis specifically by promoting tip cell formation through the inhibition of delta-like 4 (DLL4) [103]. Ultimately, however, as is the case with angiogenic growth factors, multiple miRNAs may have to work in concert to achieve maximal effects and interrogating which subsets are critical for different stages of angiogenesis will require further inquiry.

9. Direct Cellular Involvement of MSCs in Angiogenesis

In addition to their interaction via various paracrine routes, MSCs also participate in direct cell-cell contact with endothelial cells. When cocultured on or embedded within hydrogels (e.g., fibrin or Matrigel), endothelial cells form capillary-like structures on which MSCs may adhere and assume an abluminal position akin to their perivascular position *in vivo* [104]. This maintained mural cell behavior after culture may be exploited for microvascular tissue engineering as it has beneficial effects for the nascent endothelial tubules. For example, the permeability of these *in vitro* structures is decreased in the presence of MSCs relative to simply coculturing endothelial cells with fibroblasts potentially due to tighter cell-cell junctions and VE-cadherin expression [105]. This effect may also be attributed to increased basement membrane formation, as extensive studies of pericyte-endothelial cell cocultures have demonstrated that both the expression and deposition of basement membrane proteins is upregulated through cell-cell contact *in vitro* [106, 107]. However, any specific effects of MSCs on basement membrane formation and its composition, compared to non-multipotent pericytes, has yet to be elucidated.

Under *in vivo* contexts, MSCs can also assume a perivascular cell phenotype and have beneficial effects on vessel stability and permeability. For example, when collagen-fibronectin gels containing EGFP-labeled human MSCs and HUVEC (human umbilical vein endothelial cells) were implanted in cranial windows of SCID mice, implants with MSCs resulted in a higher vessel density compared to HUVEC-only implants, and EGFP colocalized with staining for the smooth muscle cell- (SMC-) related markers, αSMA and SM22α [108]. Similarly, when embedded within submillimeter collagen rods coated with endothelial cells and then implanted in an omental pouch within rats, GFP-labeled rat MSCs were found to migrate out of the modules and began to associate with blood vessels and express αSMA at day 7 postimplantation, while at day 21, all GFP$^+$ MSCs were found to be in a perivascular position [109]. Strikingly, when examined by microCT after Microfil® injection, including MSCs within the implant created vasculature with reduced leakiness compared to endothelial cell-only controls which exhibited a leaky core.

Similarly, after subcutaneous injection of HUVEC and fibrin hydrogel into SCID mice, HUVEC-derived vessels formed after 7 and 14 days showed decreased permeability to 70 kDa dextran in conditions including human adipose and bone marrow-derived MSCs, compared to lung fibro-blasts or endothelial cells alone [110]. Correspondingly, with this improved barrier function, only implants with ASCs and BMSCs contained vessels with abluminal calponin staining, suggestive of SMC differentiation of the implanted stromal cells. Collectively, it is clear that not only is the presence of a mesenchymal cell type advantageous for vessel formation and stabilization, but the identity of the mesenchymal cell type and its propensity to take on an abluminal position and perivascular cell phenotype has an impact on the functionality of the resulting vessels.

10. Clinical Considerations for Using Bone or Adipose MSC Sources

As noted previously, MSCs can be isolated from many different human tissues; however, the most common adult sources for clinical use are bone marrow and adipose tissue. This is due to a number of reasons, including the total cell numbers that can be harvested, the frequency of the cells of interest, and the relatively small procedural risk associated with obtaining cells from these locations compared to other anatomical locations. As well, in the case of adipose tissue removal, if the procedure is being carried out for other purposes (*e.g.*, elective cosmetic surgery), there is no additional risk associated with the harvesting of progenitor cells which would otherwise be discarded.

In the case of bone marrow aspirate, the procedure is generally carried out at the bedside using a local anesthetic (*e.g.*, lidocaine) with the posterior superior iliac spine being the preferred collection site owing to its relative ease of access [111]. After sterilization of the overlying skin, a fine gauge trocar is used to gain access to the marrow space, which then permits the subsequent aspiration of marrow by syringe [111]. For the purposes of stem cell harvesting, it is possible to harvest as much as 20 mL of marrow from a single aspirate site [112].

Bone marrow sampling is generally considered to be safe but can frequently result in pain during and after the procedure [113]. Preventative measures, such as first ensuring that the periosteum is adequately anesthetized, can be used to reduce the pain to acceptable levels [113]. Other adverse events during bone marrow sampling are rare, with an estimated event rate of 5/10,000 and a fatality rate of 1-2/100,000 [114]. In a 2013 survey conducted by the British Society of Haematology, out of a total of 19,259 bone marrow

aspirates with or without trephine biopsies, clinically significant hemorrhage occurred in only 11 patients, while infections were seen in just two [114]. The risk of bleeding can be mitigated through careful patient selection and correction of underlying coagulopathies if necessary. When bleeding does occur, it is usually mild and can often be controlled by the manual application of pressure to the site [111]. In the event of more significant bleeding, arterial embolization has been demonstrated to be an effective hemostatic therapy [115]. The risk of infection can be mitigated by first ensuring an absence of any overlying skin or soft tissue infection or presence of osteomyelitis. In suspected occurrences of infectious complications, topical antimicrobials are generally considered to be adequate in most cases.

In contrast to bone marrow aspirate, adipose tissue—in the form of liquid fat from liposuction or solid fat from abdominoplasty—is obtained under general anesthetic with a greater risk of procedural morbidity and mortality [116]. In the case of liposuction, the targeted fat is removed via aspiration after injection of a sterile saline solution containing epinephrine and a topical anesthetic [116]. The process may be facilitated by the liquefaction of fat using ultrasound- or laser-assisted liposuction [116]. Conversely, abdominoplasty involves the surgical excision of excess solid adipose tissue and dermis.

Common adverse events for liposuction include post-operative nausea and vomiting, local nerve damage and paresthesias, intra- and postprocedural bleeding and hematomas, persistent edema, surgical wound infection, skin necrosis, and unplanned hospitalization or increased length of stay [117]. The risk of fatality of liposuction is conservatively estimated to be 1/5000 with deaths being attributable to pulmonary embolism, visceral perforation, cardiorespiratory complications associated with anesthesia, and hemorrhage (in order of decreasing frequency) [118]. Abdominoplasty is a more invasive procedure with higher rates of surgical complications, including wound dehiscence and necrosis, infection, and a fatality rate approaching 1/600 [119].

Given the relatively unfavorable risk profile associated with surgical collection of adipose tissue, the harvesting of adipose-derived MSCs is ideal for patients who are already planning on undergoing such a procedure. Otherwise, bone marrow aspirate remains a preferred option as it can permit the ad hoc collection of MSCs at a lower risk of morbidity and mortality. However, such clinical risks must be weighed against certain practical requirements as well.

In addition to considering the risks associated with the different anatomical sites and any contraindications specific to a certain patient, the preference for one tissue source over the other may also be affected by the number of desired cells that can be collected from a certain source and the quantity of cells requisite for a particular application. As summarized by Murphy et al., in the case of a bone marrow aspirate, approximately 109–664 CFU-F/mL can be obtained at a frequency of 10–83 CFU-F/10^6 nucleated cells [120]. In contrast, lipoaspirate typically yields far more cells of interest per milliliter of tissue, with 2058–9650 CFU-F/mL at a frequency of 205–51,000 CFU-F/10^6 nucleated cells

[120]. Hence, if the quantity of cells that can be obtained via bone marrow aspirate are insufficient for a particular autologous application, relying on an adipose cell source instead may be a sensible option. This is especially true in situations where *ex vivo* culture must be limited to preserve a desired cellular phenotype or when culture is not utilized at all (*i.e.*, immediate autologous use of the stromal vascular fraction (SVF) after harvesting).

Beyond differences in the quantity of cells obtainable from either bone or adipose tissues, innate differences in differentiation ability between cell types may also affect the preference of one MSC population over the other for a particular application. Unsurprisingly, given their developmental and anatomical origins, adipose-derived MSCs have been demonstrated to have an increased capacity for *in vitro* adipogenic differentiation by Oil Red O staining, possibly due to their relatively higher expression of the adipogenesis-regulating transcription factor, PPAR-γ, after exposure to adipogenic stimuli [121, 122]. Similarly, bone marrow-derived MSCs have been demonstrated to have an increased capacity for osteogenic differentiation over MSCs derived from adipose tissue via alizarin red staining [121, 122]. This may be partly attributable to their higher expression of the key osteogenic transcription factor, Runx2, during osteogenic differentiation [122]. Moreover, bone marrow-derived MSCs have also been shown to have a higher capacity for chondrogenic differentiation (by alcian blue staining and collagen II expression), as may be expected considering the close relationship between chondrogenesis and osteogenesis in the generation of osseous tissues [121–123]. It should be noted, however, that some conflicting reports to these general findings also exist and suggest that whether adipose or bone-derived MSCs have the higher capacity to differentiate toward a particular lineage may depend on the characteristics of the patient (*e.g.*, sex, age, and disease state), the isolation protocol, and the differentiation conditions [90].

Other notable functional differences between the two cell types have been documented. For example, in a comparison of the immunomodulatory capacity of adipose and bone marrow-derived MSCs isolated from the same donor, Valencia et al. found that MSCs from bone marrow had a higher capacity to inhibit natural killer cytotoxic activity, whereas adipose-derived MSCs had a higher capacity to inhibit dendritic cell differentiation [124]. Corroborating this, other reports have also described similar findings regarding these differential effects on natural killer cells and dendritic cell differentiation [125, 126]. Similarly, differences in growth factor expression between the two cell types have also been noted and may influence which cell type to use in clinical applications where MSCs are intended to provide trophic support. For example, bone marrow-derived MSCs have been shown to produce significantly more HGF compared to adipose-derived MSCs, which may be an important consideration for regenerative therapies involving the liver [122]. Overall, the choice of bone or adipose sources is complex and is influenced by factors specific to the application and the patient. As the use of MSCs becomes increasingly common, the optimal choice of cell source for specific clinical circumstances will likely become clearer.

11. iPSC Sources and Epigenetic Reprogramming of MSCs

Despite the clinical promise of MSCs in allogeneic applications (or the use of HLA-matched donor cells), some therapies may necessitate an autologous approach, such as long-term implantation of MSC-derived engineered tissues. However, this presents a significant challenge in cases where the desired cell type cannot be obtained in sufficient numbers to be clinically useful. This may occur in the case of needing to engineer particularly large replacement tissues, as MSCs have limited expansion capability in culture, partly due to their low to absent expression of telomerase [127, 128]. As well, this may occur when patients have insufficient MSCs of adequate quality due to age or disease. With regard to aging, CFU-F frequency within the bone marrow generally declines with age, and the capacity of the remaining MSCs to withstand oxidative stress appears to also decline along with their function and therapeutic efficacy [129–131]. Such functional changes may be the result of progressively shortening telomeres, accumulated molecular damage, and stochastic genetic and epigenetic changes over time [132–136]. Such age-associated epigenetic dysregulation may also contribute to alterations in the differentiation potential and heterogeneity of MSCs [137, 138]. In addition to age-induced functional decline, conditions such as type 2 diabetes and metabolic syndrome may similarly limit the therapeutic potential of MSCs for autologous use due to increased oxidative stress, mitochondrial dysfunction, and increased senescence [139].

One potential solution to address this issue is iPSC (induced pluripotent stem cell) technology in which somatic cells from a patient are first reprogrammed to a pluripotent state, usually by the overexpression of transcription factors (*e.g.*, KLF4, c-MYC, OCT4, and SOX2) [140, 141]. Favorably, such cells can then be expanded *in vitro* extensively prior to differentiation, partly due to their expression of telomerase. Also favorably, especially for cells harvested from aged patients, once harvested cells are differentiated into the desired cell type after having been in a transient pluripotent state results in longer telomeres compared to the starting donor cell along with a "rejuvenated" epigenetic landscape with reduced aging-associated epigenetic marks and increased resistance to oxidative stress [142, 143].

Multiple studies have explored methods for differentiating MSC-like cells from iPSCs [143–149]. These reports have described iPSC-MSCs as being largely comparable to mature MSCs in terms of trilineage potential, immunomodulation, and trophic support. However, some minor differences have also been noted, such as differences in adipose differentiation, T-cell regulation, sensitivity to NK cells, and their expression levels of certain genes (*e.g.*, interleukin-1 and TGFβ receptors) [143, 150–153]. Interestingly, a recent study by Chin et al. reported that differentiation of human pluripotent stem cells into MSCs results in two distinct subpopulations with different trophic phenotypes [149].

One subpopulation with higher expression of CD146 and CD73 could maintain HSCs (hematopoietic stem cells) *ex vivo* and expressed HSC niche-related genes, while a second subpopulation with lower expression of CD146 and CD73 displayed poor maintenance of HSCs. Such *in vitro* findings using iPSCs are intriguingly reminiscent of *in vivo* MSC heterogeneity and may not only help provide a source of MSCs for clinical use but may also help elucidate the developmental origins of different MSC subpopulations.

While iPSCs are a promising source of MSCs, they do carry the risk of malignant transformation during culture and teratoma formation after transplantation due to residual pluripotent cells [154]. Alternative means for returning aged or diseased MSCs to a more therapeutically effective state without relying on a transient pluripotent stage may also exist. One option may consist of using the pluripotency genes used for creating iPSCs but for a shorter duration in order to elicit partial reprogramming and reverse age-associated epigenetic marks but not loss of cellular identity. Such an approach yielded impressive results in mice in terms of improving recovery from metabolic disease and increasing muscle regeneration after transient *in vivo* overexpression [155]. It remains to be seen, however, if this approach has a beneficial effect on MSCs as well. Future work will need to focus on determining the optimal dosing regimen for human cells and examining if this method is useful for the *ex vivo* rejuvenation of human MSCs.

Alternatives for rejuvenating cells that do not rely on pluripotency genes at all also exist, which may be preferable for further mitigating tumorigenic risks. One option may be to alter the levels of beneficial or detrimental miRNAs within cultured MSCs prior to transplantation. For example, Okada et al. unveiled that miR-195 plays a key role in inducing senescence in murine bone marrow-derived MSCs by inhibiting the expression of telomerase [156]. When the authors inhibited miR-195, telomere lengths and cellular proliferation were increased compared to control cells. Most importantly though, using a mouse model of acute myocardial infarction, the authors demonstrated that when transplanted the rejuvenated cells resulted in reduced infarct size and improved left-ventricle function.

Conversely, upregulation of certain molecules, such as miR-543 and miR-590-3p may also be useful in preventing senescence given their inhibitory roles in senescence onset in MSCs [157]. Upregulation of SIRT1, a NAD^+-dependent deacetylase, has also been shown to prevent MSC senescence possibly through increasing telomerase activity and reducing DNA damage [158]. Strikingly, overexpression of telomerase and myocardin in aged murine MSCs resulted in improved therapeutic efficacy when used in a model of hindlimb ischemia, in terms of stimulating arteriogenesis and increasing blood flow [159]. Regardless of whether particular factors are upregulated or downregulated, it should be stressed that any approach that alters regulators of senescence, telomere length, and/or pluripotency will require extensive investigation in order to ensure that rejuvenation of MSCs does not come at the cost of increasing tumorigenesis.

12. Clinical Risks and Challenges

As of May 2018, there are currently 82 active and recruiting trials involving "mesenchymal stem cells" listed by ClinicalTrials.gov in the United States alone, in addition to 44 already completed studies; moreover, there are also 27 active/recruiting trials involving "mesenchymal stromal cells" with 9 already completed. Of these ongoing studies, the majority are currently in phase 1 followed by phase 2 trials. Given these appreciable number of trials and their early stages, it will be crucial to discern if any patterns of adverse effects can be detected among MSC clinical trials in order to develop effective solutions to these issues. The risks involved in these trials are partly dependent on the route of administration of MSCs (Figure 1).

In terms of risks involving the systemic infusion of MSCs, Lalu et al. conducted a meta-analysis of clinical trials with both autologous and allogeneic MSCs and concluded that this route of administration appears generally safe as their analysis did not find any significant association between MSC infusion and acute toxicity, infection, organ system complications, malignancy, or death [160]. There was, however, a significant association with transient fever in some patients. Other studies have also identified chill, infection, and liver damage as potential adverse effects of systemic administration [161, 162]. Lalu et al. also commented on the frequent absence of reporting follow-up duration for long-term adverse events in the studies they examined and noted that it is critical that future studies investigate both short-term and long-term adverse events given that experimental cell-based therapies may have serious long-term consequences (*e.g.*, immunological complications, causing/enhancing neoplastic growth). Favorably for risk mitigation, however, there is evidence to suggest that MSCs that are infused systemically generally do not persist over the long-term [163]. Also favorably, of the 13 studies examined by Lalu et al. that used unmatched allogeneic MSCs, none reported acute infusional toxicity. Such findings bode well for systemically administered therapies requiring large quantities of cells that cannot be acquired from a single patient and for cases in which a patient's own MSCs may be functionally inadequate and/or inaccessible due to underlying disease.

Regardless, while MSCs themselves appear generally safe for systemic infusion, biological and chemical components associated with the *ex vivo* culture and storage of MSCs, such as fetal bovine serum (FBS) and dimethylsulfoxide (DMSO) may introduce risks in the clinical use of MSCs. Such components warrant caution due to the possibility of infectious contamination, immunogenicity, and/or infusional toxicity [164, 165]. With regard to zoonotic concerns regarding FBS, such risks may be addressed through the use of human platelet lysate in place of FBS for supporting the *ex vivo* growth of MSCs [164, 166].

Risks and their associated challenges regarding more experimental interventions involving the local injection of MSCs and implantation of engineered tissues are currently less well defined compared to the more commonly used systemic administration route. Currently, challenges associated with these approaches often relate to first establishing clinically significant efficacy in order to justify these more invasive procedures. Some key challenges for local injections include maintaining cell viability, increasing MSC permanence after injection, and optimizing delivery to a specific location [161, 167, 168]. In regard to this, rapidly gelling injectable hydrogels have shown promise in targeting MSCs to specific anatomical locations and in maintaining their viability after injection to prolong therapeutic function [169]. Currently, investigations into generating engineered tissues are primarily focused on ensuring comparable function to native tissues (or at least, similar enough to be therapeutically useful). Key challenges include optimizing the differentiation process, developing effective scaffold materials, and ensuring sufficient maturation of the nascent tissues through chemical and mechanical cues [73, 170, 171]. As well, depending on the tissue type and its dimensions, the issue of vascularization either pre- or postimplantation must also be addressed in order to preserve function and to avoid ischemia-induced inflammation. As discussed previously in this review, MSCs themselves may be of use in this regard given their proangiogenic signaling and native perivascular phenotype. Ostensibly, some engineered tissues may be optimally composed of MSC-derived terminally differentiated cells along with angiogenic undifferentiated MSCs, in order to fully take advantage of both their differentiation and angiogenic capabilities.

13. Concluding Remarks

Efforts into understanding and exploiting MSCs for therapeutic use have garnered a multifaceted view into the capabilities of these cells, albeit sometimes in a nonlinear and even serendipitous manner. Contrary to many other clinical successes for drugs and cell therapies alike, where a comprehensive understanding of the therapeutic mechanism(s) is first established before being employed clinically, MSCs have had remarkable successes despite a limited understanding of their *in vivo* function under normal physiological conditions. To further improve and build on these early successes, future work will need to be directed toward understanding the more nuanced aspects of these cells. As alluded to earlier, this will partly involve developing an improved understanding of the differences between MSCs found in different anatomical locations and the heterogeneity that exists within these subpopulations, in addition to performing rigorous investigation into the functional differences between cells differentiated from MSCs and native terminal cells. By building on the body of MSC research that has been produced thus far, potential risks in downstream clinical applications can be mitigated and the therapeutic potential of MSCs may be further expanded upon to benefit patients in a wide range of clinical settings.

Acknowledgments

This work was financially supported by Canadian Institutes of Health Research (CIHR) operating grants MOP-102721, RMF-111624, and MOP-130481. Ross E.B. Fitzsimmons was financially supported by a CIHR Banting and Best Doctoral Scholarship.

References

[1] A. J. Friedenstein, I. I. Piatetzky-Shapiro, and K. V. Petrakova, "Osteogenesis in transplants of bone marrow cells," *Development*, vol. 16, no. 3, pp. 381–390, 1966.

[2] A. J. Friedenstein, R. K. Chailakhjan, and K. S. Lalykina, "The development of fibroblast colonies in monolayer cultures of guinea-pig bone marrow and spleen cells," *Cell Proliferation*, vol. 3, no. 4, pp. 393–403, 1970.

[3] A. I. Caplan, "Mesenchymal stem cells," *Journal of Orthopaedic Research*, vol. 9, no. 5, pp. 641–650, 1991.

[4] M. F. Pittenger, A. M. Mackay, S. C. Beck et al., "Multilineage potential of adult human mesenchymal stem cells," *Science*, vol. 284, no. 5411, pp. 143–147, 1999.

[5] M. Dominici, K. le Blanc, I. Mueller et al., "Minimal criteria for defining multipotent mesenchymal stromal cells. The International Society for Cellular Therapy position statement," *Cytotherapy*, vol. 8, no. 4, pp. 315–317, 2006.

[6] C.-S. Lin, Z.-C. Xin, J. Dai, and T. F. Lue, "Commonly used mesenchymal stem cell markers and tracking labels: limitations and challenges," *Histology and Histopathology*, vol. 28, no. 9, pp. 1109–1116, 2013.

[7] M. Corselli, C.-W. Chen, B. Sun, S. Yap, J. P. Rubin, and B. Peault, "The tunica adventitia of human arteries and veins as a source of mesenchymal stem cells," *Stem Cells and Development*, vol. 21, no. 8, pp. 1299–1308, 2012.

[8] A. J. Nauta and W. E. Fibbe, "Immunomodulatory properties of mesenchymal stromal cells," *Blood*, vol. 110, no. 10, pp. 3499–3506, 2007.

[9] N. Barker and H. Clevers, "Leucine-rich repeat-containing G-protein-coupled receptors as markers of adult stem cells," *Gastroenterology*, vol. 138, no. 5, pp. 1681–1696, 2010.

[10] B. Sacchetti, A. Funari, S. Michienzi et al., "Self-renewing osteoprogenitors in bone marrow sinusoids can organize a hematopoietic microenvironment," *Cell*, vol. 131, no. 2, pp. 324–336, 2007.

[11] S. Gronthos, A. C. W. Zannettino, S. J. Hay et al., "Molecular and cellular characterisation of highly purified stromal stem cells derived from human bone marrow," *Journal of Cell Science*, vol. 116, no. 9, pp. 1827–1835, 2003.

[12] N. Quirici, D. Soligo, P. Bossolasco, F. Servida, C. Lumini, and G. L. Deliliers, "Isolation of bone marrow mesenchymal stem cells by anti-nerve growth factor receptor antibodies," *Experimental Hematology*, vol. 30, no. 7, pp. 783–791, 2002.

[13] M. Sobiesiak, K. Sivasubramaniyan, C. Hermann et al., "The mesenchymal stem cell antigen MSCA-1 is identical to tissue non-specific alkaline phosphatase," *Stem Cells and Development*, vol. 19, no. 5, pp. 669–677, 2010.

[14] S. J. Morrison and D. T. Scadden, "The bone marrow niche for haematopoietic stem cells," *Nature*, vol. 505, no. 7483, pp. 327–334, 2014.

[15] B. A. Anthony and D. C. Link, "Regulation of hematopoietic stem cells by bone marrow stromal cells," *Trends in Immunology*, vol. 35, no. 1, pp. 32–37, 2014.

[16] C. Nombela-Arrieta, J. Ritz, and L. E. Silberstein, "The elusive nature and function of mesenchymal stem cells," *Nature Reviews Molecular Cell Biology*, vol. 12, no. 2, pp. 126–131, 2011.

[17] N. Beyer Nardi and L. da Silva Meirelles, "Mesenchymal stem cells: isolation, in vitro expansion and characterization," in *Stem Cells. Handbook of Experimental Pharmacology, vol 174*, A. M. Wobus and K. R. Boheler, Eds., pp. 249–282, Springer, Berlin, Heidelberg, 2006.

[18] W. C. W. Chen, J. E. Baily, M. Corselli et al., "Human myocardial pericytes: multipotent mesodermal precursors exhibiting cardiac specificity," *Stem Cells*, vol. 33, no. 2, pp. 557–573, 2015.

[19] A. Stefanska, C. Kenyon, H. C. Christian et al., "Human kidney pericytes produce renin," *Kidney International*, vol. 90, no. 6, pp. 1251–1261, 2016.

[20] A. I. Caplan, "All MSCs are pericytes?," *Cell Stem Cell*, vol. 3, no. 3, pp. 229–230, 2008.

[21] S. Shi and S. Gronthos, "Perivascular niche of postnatal mesenchymal stem cells in human bone marrow and dental pulp," *Journal of Bone and Mineral Research*, vol. 18, no. 4, pp. 696–704, 2003.

[22] M. Crisan, S. Yap, L. Casteilla et al., "A perivascular origin for mesenchymal stem cells in multiple human organs," *Cell Stem Cell*, vol. 3, no. 3, pp. 301–313, 2008.

[23] R. Kramann, R. K. Schneider, D. P. DiRocco et al., "Perivascular Gli1$^+$ progenitors are key contributors to injury-induced organ fibrosis," *Cell Stem Cell*, vol. 16, no. 1, pp. 51–66, 2015.

[24] R. Kramann, C. Goettsch, J. Wongboonsin et al., "Adventitial MSC-like cells are progenitors of vascular smooth muscle cells and drive vascular calcification in chronic kidney disease," *Cell Stem Cell*, vol. 19, no. 5, pp. 628–642, 2016.

[25] A. H. Baker and B. Peault, "A Gli(1) ttering role for perivascular stem cells in blood vessel remodeling," *Cell Stem Cell*, vol. 19, no. 5, pp. 563–565, 2016.

[26] R. Sarugaser, D. Lickorish, D. Baksh, M. M. Hosseini, and J. E. Davies, "Human umbilical cord perivascular (HUCPV) cells: a source of mesenchymal progenitors," *Stem Cells*, vol. 23, no. 2, pp. 220–229, 2005.

[27] J. Ennis, C. Götherström, K. Le Blanc, and J. E. Davies, "*In vitro* immunologic properties of human umbilical cord perivascular cells," *Cytotherapy*, vol. 10, no. 2, pp. 174–181, 2008.

[28] N. Zebardast, D. Lickorish, and J. E. Davies, "Human umbilical cord perivascular cells (HUCPVC): a mesenchymal cell source for dermal wound healing," *Organogenesis*, vol. 6, no. 4, pp. 197–203, 2010.

[29] J. Feng, A. Mantesso, C. De Bari, A. Nishiyama, and P. T. Sharpe, "Dual origin of mesenchymal stem cells contributing to organ growth and repair," *Proceedings of the National Academy of Sciences*, vol. 108, no. 16, pp. 6503–6508, 2011.

[30] Y. Sakaguchi, I. Sekiya, K. Yagishita, and T. Muneta, "Comparison of human stem cells derived from various mesenchymal tissues: superiority of synovium as a cell source," *Arthritis & Rheumatology*, vol. 52, no. 8, pp. 2521–2529, 2005.

[31] A. Nimura, T. Muneta, H. Koga et al., "Increased proliferation of human synovial mesenchymal stem cells with autologous human serum: comparisons with bone marrow mesenchymal stem cells and with fetal bovine serum," *Arthritis & Rheumatology*, vol. 58, no. 2, pp. 501–510, 2008.

[32] Y. Ogata, Y. Mabuchi, M. Yoshida et al., "Purified human synovium mesenchymal stem cells as a good resource for cartilage regeneration," *PLoS One*, vol. 10, no. 6, article e0129096, 2015.

[33] J.-H. Chen, C. Y. Y. Yip, E. D. Sone, and C. A. Simmons, "Identification and characterization of aortic valve mesenchymal progenitor cells with robust osteogenic calcification potential," *The American Journal of Pathology*, vol. 174, no. 3, pp. 1109–1119, 2009.

[34] J. R. Levick, "Microvascular architecture and exchange in synovial joints," *Microcirculation*, vol. 2, no. 3, pp. 217–233, 1995.

[35] K. L. Weind, C. G. Ellis, and D. R. Boughner, "The aortic valve blood supply," *The Journal of Heart Valve Disease*, vol. 9, pp. 1–7, 2000.

[36] Y. Soini, T. Salo, and J. Satta, "Angiogenesis is involved in the pathogenesis of nonrheumatic aortic valve stenosis," *Human Pathology*, vol. 34, no. 8, pp. 756–763, 2003.

[37] G. Sheng, "The developmental basis of mesenchymal stem/stromal cells (MSCs)," *BMC Developmental Biology*, vol. 15, no. 1, pp. 44–48, 2015.

[38] L. da Silva Meirelles, A. I. Caplan, and N. B. Nardi, "In search of the in vivo identity of mesenchymal stem cells," *Stem Cells*, vol. 26, no. 9, pp. 2287–2299, 2008.

[39] M. G. Minasi, M. Riminucci, L. de Angelis et al., "The mesoangioblast: a multipotent, self-renewing cell that originates from the dorsal aorta and differentiates into most mesodermal tissues," *Development*, vol. 129, no. 11, pp. 2773–2783, 2002.

[40] Y. Takashima, T. Era, K. Nakao et al., "Neuroepithelial cells supply an initial transient wave of MSC differentiation," *Cell*, vol. 129, no. 7, pp. 1377–1388, 2007.

[41] S. Morikawa, Y. Mabuchi, K. Niibe et al., "Development of mesenchymal stem cells partially originate from the neural crest," *Biochemical and Biophysical Research Communications*, vol. 379, no. 4, pp. 1114–1119, 2009.

[42] M. A. Vodyanik, J. Yu, X. Zhang et al., "A mesoderm-derived precursor for mesenchymal stem and endothelial cells," *Cell Stem Cell*, vol. 7, no. 6, pp. 718–729, 2010.

[43] R. Chijimatsu, M. Ikeya, Y. Yasui et al., "Characterization of mesenchymal stem cell-like cells derived from human iPSCs via neural crest development and their application for osteochondral repair," *Stem Cells International*, vol. 2017, Article ID 1960965, 18 pages, 2017.

[44] I. Sekiya, B. L. Larson, J. R. Smith, R. Pochampally, J.-G. Cui, and D. J. Prockop, "Expansion of human adult stem cells from bone marrow stroma: conditions that maximize the yields of early progenitors and evaluate their quality," *Stem Cells*, vol. 20, no. 6, pp. 530–541, 2002.

[45] C. A. Gregory, H. Singh, A. S. Perry, and D. J. Prockop, "The Wnt signaling inhibitor dickkopf-1 is required for reentry into the cell cycle of human adult stem cells from bone marrow," *Journal of Biological Chemistry*, vol. 278, no. 30, pp. 28067–28078, 2003.

[46] M. E. Bernardo, N. Zaffaroni, F. Novara et al., "Human bone marrow derived mesenchymal stem cells do not undergo

transformation after long-term *in vitro* culture and do not exhibit telomere maintenance mechanisms," *Cancer Research*, vol. 67, no. 19, pp. 9142–9149, 2007.

[47] D. J. Prockop, M. Brenner, W. E. Fibbe et al., "Defining the risks of mesenchymal stromal cell therapy," *Cytotherapy*, vol. 12, no. 5, pp. 576–578, 2010.

[48] A. Conforti, N. Starc, S. Biagini et al., "Resistance to neoplastic transformation of *ex-vivo* expanded human mesenchymal stromal cells after exposure to supramaximal physical and chemical stress," *Oncotarget*, vol. 7, no. 47, pp. 77416–77429, 2016.

[49] M. Miura, Y. Miura, H. M. Padilla-Nash et al., "Accumulated chromosomal instability in murine bone marrow mesenchymal stem cells leads to malignant transformation," *Stem Cells*, vol. 24, no. 4, pp. 1095–1103, 2006.

[50] C. A. Gregory, J. Ylostalo, and D. J. Prockop, "Adult bone marrow stem/progenitor cells (MSCs) are preconditioned by microenvironmental "niches" in culture: a two-stage hypothesis for regulation of MSC fate," *Science's STKE*, vol. 2005, no. 294, article pe37, 2005.

[51] D. J. Prockop, "Repair of tissues by adult stem/progenitor cells (MSCs): controversies, myths, and changing paradigms," *Molecular Therapy*, vol. 17, no. 6, pp. 939–946, 2009.

[52] M. C. Ciuffreda, G. Malpasso, P. Musarò, V. Turco, and M. Gnecchi, "Protocols for *in vitro* differentiation of human mesenchymal stem cells into osteogenic, chondrogenic and adipogenic lineages," in *Mesenchymal Stem Cells. Methods in Molecular Biology, vol 1416*, M. Gnecchi, Ed., pp. 149–158, Humana Press, New York, NY, USA, 2016.

[53] C. Vater, P. Kasten, and M. Stiehler, "Culture media for the differentiation of mesenchymal stromal cells," *Acta Biomaterialia*, vol. 7, no. 2, pp. 463–477, 2011.

[54] S. Bose, M. Roy, and A. Bandyopadhyay, "Recent advances in bone tissue engineering scaffolds," *Trends in Biotechnology*, vol. 30, no. 10, pp. 546–554, 2012.

[55] A. R. Amini, C. T. Laurencin, and S. P. Nukavarapu, "Bone tissue engineering: recent advances and challenges," *Critical Reviews™ in Biomedical Engineering*, vol. 40, no. 5, pp. 363–408, 2012.

[56] E. A. Makris, A. H. Gomoll, K. N. Malizos, J. C. Hu, and K. A. Athanasiou, "Repair and tissue engineering techniques for articular cartilage," *Nature Reviews Rheumatology*, vol. 11, no. 1, pp. 21–34, 2015.

[57] L. Zhang, J. Hu, and K. A. Athanasiou, "The role of tissue engineering in articular cartilage repair and regeneration," *Critical Reviews™ in Biomedical Engineering*, vol. 37, no. 1-2, pp. 1–57, 2009.

[58] J. H. Choi, J. M. Gimble, K. Lee et al., "Adipose tissue engineering for soft tissue regeneration," *Tissue Engineering Part B: Reviews*, vol. 16, no. 4, pp. 413–426, 2010.

[59] D. W. Youngstrom, J. E. LaDow, and J. G. Barrett, "Tenogenesis of bone marrow-, adipose-, and tendon-derived stem cells in a dynamic bioreactor," *Connective Tissue Research*, vol. 57, no. 6, pp. 454–465, 2016.

[60] D. Galli, M. Vitale, and M. Vaccarezza, "Bone marrow-derived mesenchymal cell differentiation toward myogenic lineages: facts and perspectives," *BioMed Research International*, vol. 2014, Article ID 762695, 6 pages, 2014.

[61] V. M. Tatard, G. D'Ippolito, S. Diabira et al., "Neurotrophin-directed differentiation of human adult marrow stromal cells to dopaminergic-like neurons," *Bone*, vol. 40, no. 2, pp. 360–373, 2007.

[62] S. Wislet-Gendebien, G. Hans, P. Leprince, J.-M. Rigo, G. Moonen, and B. Rogister, "Plasticity of cultured mesenchymal stem cells: switch from nestin-positive to excitable neuron-like phenotype," *Stem Cells*, vol. 23, no. 3, pp. 392–402, 2005.

[63] D. G. Phinney and D. J. Prockop, "Concise review: mesenchymal stem/multipotent stromal cells: the state of transdifferentiation and modes of tissue repair-current views," *Stem Cells*, vol. 25, no. 11, pp. 2896–2902, 2007.

[64] A.-C. Volz, B. Huber, and P. J. Kluger, "Adipose-derived stem cell differentiation as a basic tool for vascularized adipose tissue engineering," *Differentiation*, vol. 92, no. 1-2, pp. 52–64, 2016.

[65] B. Sacchetti, A. Funari, C. Remoli et al., "No identical "mesenchymal stem cells" at different times and sites: human committed progenitors of distinct origin and differentiation potential are incorporated as adventitial cells in microvessels," *Stem Cell Reports*, vol. 6, no. 6, pp. 897–913, 2016.

[66] W. R. Hardy, N. I. Moldovan, L. Moldovan et al., "Transcriptional networks in single perivascular cells sorted from human adipose tissue reveal a hierarchy of mesenchymal stem cells," *Stem Cells*, vol. 35, no. 5, pp. 1273–1289, 2017.

[67] C. L. Esteves, T. A. Sheldrake, S. P. Mesquita et al., "Isolation and characterization of equine native MSC populations," *Stem Cell Research and Therapy*, vol. 8, no. 1, p. 80, 2017.

[68] A. W. James, X. Zhang, M. Crisan et al., "Isolation and characterization of canine perivascular stem/stromal cells for bone tissue engineering," *PLoS One*, vol. 12, no. 5, pp. e0177308–e0177316, 2017.

[69] N. E. Lee, S. J. Kim, S.-J. Yang et al., "Comparative characterization of mesenchymal stromal cells from multiple abdominal adipose tissues and enrichment of angiogenic ability via CD146 molecule," *Cytotherapy*, vol. 19, no. 2, pp. 170–180, 2017.

[70] A. R. Jensen, B. V. Kelley, G. M. Mosich et al., "Neer Award 2018: platelet-derived growth factor receptor α co-expression typifies a subset of platelet-derived growth factor receptor β–positive progenitor cells that contribute to fatty degeneration and fibrosis of the murine rotator cuff," *Journal of Shoulder and Elbow Surgery*, vol. 27, no. 7, pp. 1149–1161, 2018.

[71] I. R. Murray, Z. N. Gonzalez, J. Baily et al., "αv integrins on mesenchymal cells regulate skeletal and cardiac muscle fibrosis," *Nature Communications*, vol. 8, no. 1, p. 1118, 2017.

[72] R. Sarugaser, L. Hanoun, A. Keating, W. L. Stanford, and J. E. Davies, "Human mesenchymal stem cells self-renew and differentiate according to a deterministic hierarchy," *PLoS One*, vol. 4, no. 8, article e6498, 2009.

[73] A. I. Caplan, "Adult mesenchymal stem cells for tissue engineering versus regenerative medicine," *Journal of Cellular Physiology*, vol. 213, no. 2, pp. 341–347, 2007.

[74] A. I. Caplan and D. Correa, "The MSC: an injury drugstore," *Cell Stem Cell*, vol. 9, no. 1, pp. 11–15, 2011.

[75] A. I. Caplan, "Mesenchymal stem cells: time to change the name!," *Stem Cells Translational Medicine*, vol. 6, no. 6, pp. 1445–1451, 2017.

[76] M. Cai, R. Shen, L. Song et al., "Bone marrow mesenchymal stem cells (BM-MSCs) improve heart function in swine

myocardial infarction model through paracrine effects," *Scientific Reports*, vol. 6, no. 1, pp. 1–12, 2016.

[77] B. Amorin, A. P. Alegretti, V. Valim et al., "Mesenchymal stem cell therapy and acute graft-versus-host disease: a review," *Human Cell*, vol. 27, no. 4, pp. 137–150, 2014.

[78] J. Dalal, K. Gandy, and J. Domen, "Role of mesenchymal stem cell therapy in Crohn's disease," *Pediatric Research*, vol. 71, no. 4–2, pp. 445–451, 2012.

[79] J. Katuchova, D. Harvanova, T. Spakova et al., "Mesenchymal stem cells in the treatment of type 1 diabetes mellitus," *Endocrine Pathology*, vol. 26, no. 2, pp. 95–103, 2015.

[80] N. G. Singer and A. I. Caplan, "Mesenchymal stem cells: mechanisms of inflammation," *Annual Review of Pathology: Mechanisms of Disease*, vol. 6, no. 1, pp. 457–478, 2011.

[81] M. M. Duffy, T. Ritter, R. Ceredig, and M. D. Griffin, "Mesenchymal stem cell effects on T-cell effector pathways," *Stem Cell Research & Therapy*, vol. 2, no. 4, p. 34, 2011.

[82] R. Haddad and F. Saldanha-Araujo, "Mechanisms of T-cell immunosuppression by mesenchymal stromal cells: what do we know so far?," *BioMed Research International*, vol. 2014, Article ID 216806, 14 pages, 2014.

[83] E. Eggenhofer and M. J. Hoogduijn, "Mesenchymal stem cell-educated macrophages," *Transplantation Research*, vol. 1, no. 1, p. 12, 2012.

[84] A. Mantovani, S. K. Biswas, M. R. Galdiero, A. Sica, and M. Locati, "Macrophage plasticity and polarization in tissue repair and remodelling," *The Journal of Pathology*, vol. 229, no. 2, pp. 176–185, 2013.

[85] M. E. Bernardo and W. E. Fibbe, "Mesenchymal stromal cells: sensors and switchers of inflammation," *Cell Stem Cell*, vol. 13, no. 4, pp. 392–402, 2013.

[86] E. Chung and Y. Son, "Crosstalk between mesenchymal stem cells and macrophages in tissue repair," *Tissue Engineering and Regenerative Medicine*, vol. 11, no. 6, pp. 431–438, 2014.

[87] W. K. Chan, A. S.-Y. Lau, J. C.-B. Li, H. K.-W. Law, Y. L. Lau, and G. C.-F. Chan, "MHC expression kinetics and immunogenicity of mesenchymal stromal cells after short-term IFN-γ challenge," *Experimental Hematology*, vol. 36, no. 11, pp. 1545–1555, 2008.

[88] M. François, R. Romieu-Mourez, S. Stock-Martineau, M.-N. Boivin, J. L. Bramson, and J. Galipeau, "Mesenchymal stromal cells cross-present soluble exogenous antigens as part of their antigen-presenting cell properties," *Blood*, vol. 114, no. 13, pp. 2632–2638, 2009.

[89] J. L. Chan, K. C. Tang, A. P. Patel et al., "Antigen-presenting property of mesenchymal stem cells occurs during a narrow window at low levels of interferon-γ," *Blood*, vol. 107, no. 12, pp. 4817–4824, 2006.

[90] M. Strioga, S. Viswanathan, A. Darinskas, O. Slaby, and J. Michalek, "Same or not the same? Comparison of adipose tissue-derived versus bone marrow-derived mesenchymal stem and stromal cells," *Stem Cells and Development*, vol. 21, no. 14, pp. 2724–2752, 2012.

[91] S. M. Nassiri and R. Rahbarghazi, "Interactions of mesenchymal stem cells with endothelial cells," *Stem Cells and Development*, vol. 23, no. 4, pp. 319–332, 2014.

[92] H. Tao, Z. Han, Z. C. Han, and Z. Li, "Proangiogenic features of mesenchymal stem cells and their therapeutic applications," *Stem Cells International*, vol. 2016, Article ID 1314709, 11 pages, 2016.

[93] D. G. Phinney and M. F. Pittenger, "Concise review: MSC-derived exosomes for cell-free therapy," *Stem Cells*, vol. 35, no. 4, pp. 851–858, 2017.

[94] A. Shabbir, A. Cox, L. Rodriguez-Menocal, M. Salgado, and E. V. Badiavas, "Mesenchymal stem cell exosomes induce proliferation and migration of normal and chronic wound fibroblasts, and enhance angiogenesis in vitro," *Stem Cells and Development*, vol. 24, no. 14, pp. 1635–1647, 2015.

[95] B. Zhang, X. Wu, X. Zhang et al., "Human umbilical cord mesenchymal stem cell exosomes enhance angiogenesis through the Wnt4/β-catenin pathway," *Stem Cells Translational Medicine*, vol. 4, no. 5, pp. 513–522, 2015.

[96] S. Bian, L. Zhang, L. Duan, X. Wang, Y. Min, and H. Yu, "Extracellular vesicles derived from human bone marrow mesenchymal stem cells promote angiogenesis in a rat myocardial infarction model," *Journal of Molecular Medicine*, vol. 92, no. 4, pp. 387–397, 2014.

[97] X. Teng, L. Chen, W. Chen, J. Yang, Z. Yang, and Z. Shen, "Mesenchymal stem cell-derived exosomes improve the microenvironment of infarcted myocardium contributing to angiogenesis and anti-inflammation," *Cellular Physiology and Biochemistry*, vol. 37, no. 6, pp. 2415–2424, 2015.

[98] J. Zhang, J. Guan, X. Niu et al., "Exosomes released from human induced pluripotent stem cells-derived MSCs facilitate cutaneous wound healing by promoting collagen synthesis and angiogenesis," *Journal of Translational Medicine*, vol. 13, no. 1, p. 49, 2015.

[99] G.-W. Hu, Q. Li, X. Niu et al., "Exosomes secreted by human-induced pluripotent stem cell-derived mesenchymal stem cells attenuate limb ischemia by promoting angiogenesis in mice," *Stem Cell Research & Therapy*, vol. 6, no. 1, p. 10, 2015.

[100] J. D. Anderson, H. J. Johansson, C. S. Graham et al., "Comprehensive proteomic analysis of mesenchymal stem cell exosomes reveals modulation of angiogenesis via nuclear factor-kappaB signaling," *Stem Cells*, vol. 34, no. 3, pp. 601–613, 2016.

[101] M. Gong, B. Yu, J. Wang et al., "Mesenchymal stem cells release exosomes that transfer miRNAs to endothelial cells and promote angiogenesis," *Oncotarget*, vol. 8, no. 28, pp. 45200–45212, 2017.

[102] N. Wang, C. Chen, D. Yang et al., "Mesenchymal stem cells-derived extracellular vesicles, via miR-210, improve infarcted cardiac function by promotion of angiogenesis," *Biochimica et Biophysica Acta (BBA) - Molecular Basis of Disease*, vol. 1863, no. 8, pp. 2085–2092, 2017.

[103] X. Liang, L. Zhang, S. Wang, Q. Han, and R. C. Zhao, "Exosomes secreted by mesenchymal stem cells promote endothelial cell angiogenesis by transferring miR-125a," *Journal of Cell Science*, vol. 129, no. 11, pp. 2182–2189, 2016.

[104] R. R. Rao, A. W. Peterson, J. Ceccarelli, A. J. Putnam, and J. P. Stegemann, "Matrix composition regulates three-dimensional network formation by endothelial cells and mesenchymal stem cells in collagen/fibrin materials," *Angiogenesis*, vol. 15, no. 2, pp. 253–264, 2012.

[105] S. J. Grainger and A. J. Putnam, "Assessing the permeability of engineered capillary networks in a 3D culture," *PLoS One*, vol. 6, no. 7, article e22086, 2011.

[106] A. N. Stratman, W. B. Saunders, A. Sacharidou et al., "Endothelial cell lumen and vascular guidance tunnel formation requires MT1-MMP-dependent proteolysis in 3-dimensional collagen matrices," *Blood*, vol. 114, no. 2, pp. 237–247, 2009.

[107] A. N. Stratman and G. E. Davis, "Endothelial cell-pericyte interactions stimulate basement membrane matrix assembly: influence on vascular tube remodeling, maturation, and stabilization," *Microscopy and Microanalysis*, vol. 18, no. 01, pp. 68–80, 2012.

[108] P. Au, J. Tam, D. Fukumura, and R. K. Jain, "Bone marrow-derived mesenchymal stem cells facilitate engineering of long-lasting functional vasculature," *Blood*, vol. 111, no. 9, pp. 4551–4558, 2008.

[109] M. D. Chamberlain, R. Gupta, and M. V. Sefton, "Bone marrow-derived mesenchymal stromal cells enhance chimeric vessel development driven by endothelial cell-coated microtissues," *Tissue Engineering Part A*, vol. 18, no. 3-4, pp. 285–294, 2012.

[110] S. J. Grainger, B. Carrion, J. Ceccarelli, and A. J. Putnam, "Stromal cell identity influences the *in vivo* functionality of engineered capillary networks formed by co-delivery of endothelial cells and stromal cells," *Tissue Engineering Part A*, vol. 19, no. 9-10, pp. 1209–1222, 2013.

[111] S. Malempati, S. Joshi, S. Lai, D. A. V. Braner, and K. Tegtmeyer, "Videos in clinical medicine. Bone marrow aspiration and biopsy," *The New England Journal of Medicine*, vol. 361, no. 15, article e28, 2009.

[112] E. M. Fennema, A. J. S. Renard, A. Leusink, C. A. van Blitterswijk, and J. de Boer, "The effect of bone marrow aspiration strategy on the yield and quality of human mesenchymal stem cells," *Acta Orthopaedica*, vol. 80, no. 5, pp. 618–621, 2009.

[113] N. Hjortholm, E. Jaddini, K. Hałaburda, and E. Snarski, "Strategies of pain reduction during the bone marrow biopsy," *Annals of Hematology*, vol. 92, no. 2, pp. 145–149, 2013.

[114] B. J. Bain, "Bone marrow biopsy morbidity and mortality," *British Journal of Haematology*, vol. 121, no. 6, pp. 949–951, 2003.

[115] B. J. Bain, "Morbidity associated with bone marrow aspiration and trephine biopsy - a review of UK data for 2004," *Haematologica*, vol. 91, no. 9, pp. 1293-1294, 2006.

[116] J. P. Hunstad and M. E. Aitken, "Liposuction: techniques and guidelines," *Clinics in Plastic Surgery*, vol. 33, no. 1, pp. 13–25, 2006.

[117] R. A. Yoho, J. J. Romaine, and D. O'Neil, "Review of the liposuction, abdominoplasty, and face-lift mortality and morbidity risk literature," *Dermatologic Surgery.*, vol. 31, no. 7, pp. 733–743, 2005.

[118] F. M. Grazer and R. H. de Jong, "Fatal outcomes from liposuction: census survey of cosmetic surgeons," *Plastic and Reconstructive Surgery*, vol. 105, no. 1, pp. 436–446, 2000.

[119] M. Chaouat, P. Levan, B. Lalanne, T. Buisson, P. Nicolau, and M. Mimoun, "Abdominal dermolipectomies: early postoperative complications and long-term unfavorable results," *Plastic and Reconstructive Surgery*, vol. 106, no. 7, pp. 1614–1618, 2000.

[120] M. B. Murphy, K. Moncivais, and A. I. Caplan, "Mesenchymal stem cells: environmentally responsive therapeutics for regenerative medicine," *Experimental & Molecular Medicine*, vol. 45, no. 11, article e54, 2013.

[121] T. M. Liu, M. Martina, D. W. Hutmacher, J. H. P. Hui, E. H. Lee, and B. Lim, "Identification of common pathways mediating differentiation of bone marrow- and adipose tissue-derived human mesenchymal stem cells into three mesenchymal lineages," *Stem Cells*, vol. 25, no. 3, pp. 750–760, 2007.

[122] C.-Y. Li, X.-Y. Wu, J.-B. Tong et al., "Comparative analysis of human mesenchymal stem cells from bone marrow and adipose tissue under xeno-free conditions for cell therapy," *Stem Cell Research & Therapy*, vol. 6, no. 1, p. 55, 2015.

[123] Y. Jing, J. Jing, L. Ye et al., "Chondrogenesis and osteogenesis are one continuous developmental and lineage defined biological process," *Scientific Reports*, vol. 7, no. 1, p. 10020, 2017.

[124] J. Valencia, B. Blanco, R. Yáñez et al., "Comparative analysis of the immunomodulatory capacities of human bone marrow- and adipose tissue-derived mesenchymal stromal cells from the same donor," *Cytotherapy*, vol. 18, no. 10, pp. 1297–1311, 2016.

[125] B. Blanco, M. C. Herrero-Sánchez, C. Rodríguez-Serrano et al., "Immunomodulatory effects of bone marrow versus adipose tissue-derived mesenchymal stromal cells on NK cells: implications in the transplantation setting," *European Journal of Haematology*, vol. 97, no. 6, pp. 528–537, 2016.

[126] E. Ivanova-Todorova, I. Bochev, M. Mourdjeva et al., "Adipose tissue-derived mesenchymal stem cells are more potent suppressors of dendritic cells differentiation compared to bone marrow-derived mesenchymal stem cells," *Immunology Letters*, vol. 126, no. 1-2, pp. 37–42, 2009.

[127] S. Zimmermann, M. Voss, S. Kaiser, U. Kapp, C. F. Waller, and U. M. Martens, "Lack of telomerase activity in human mesenchymal stem cells," *Leukemia*, vol. 17, no. 6, pp. 1146–1149, 2003.

[128] N. Serakinci, J. Graakjaer, and S. Kolvraa, "Telomere stability and telomerase in mesenchymal stem cells," *Biochimie*, vol. 90, no. 1, pp. 33–40, 2008.

[129] A. Stolzing, E. Jones, D. McGonagle, and A. Scutt, "Age-related changes in human bone marrow-derived mesenchymal stem cells: consequences for cell therapies," *Mechanisms of Ageing and Development*, vol. 129, no. 3, pp. 163–173, 2008.

[130] G. Kasper, L. Mao, S. Geissler et al., "Insights into mesenchymal stem cell aging: involvement of antioxidant defense and actin cytoskeleton," *Stem Cells*, vol. 27, no. 6, pp. 1288–1297, 2009.

[131] P. Ganguly, J. J. El-Jawhari, P. V. Giannoudis, A. N. Burska, F. Ponchel, and E. A. Jones, "Age-related changes in bone marrow mesenchymal stromal cells: a potential impact on osteoporosis and osteoarthritis development," *Cell Transplantation*, vol. 26, no. 9, pp. 1520–1529, 2017.

[132] Y. Li, Q. Wu, Y. Wang, L. Li, H. Bu, and J. Bao, "Senescence of mesenchymal stem cells (review)," *International Journal of Molecular Medicine*, vol. 39, no. 4, pp. 775–782, 2017.

[133] B. R. Stab, L. Martinez, A. Grismaldo et al., "Mitochondrial functional changes characterization in young and senescent human adipose derived MSCs," *Frontiers in Aging Neuroscience*, vol. 8, p. 299, 2016.

[134] M. J. Peffers, J. Collins, Y. Fang et al., "Age-related changes in mesenchymal stem cells identified using a multi-omics approach," *European Cell and Materials*, vol. 31, pp. 136–159, 2016.

[135] E. G. Toraño, G. F. Bayón, Á. del Real et al., "Age-associated hydroxymethylation in human bone-marrow mesenchymal stem cells," *Journal of Translational Medicine*, vol. 14, no. 1, p. 207, 2016.

[136] J. Franzen, W. Wagner, and E. Fernandez-Rebollo, "Epigenetic modifications upon senescence of mesenchymal stem cells," *Current Stem Cell Reports*, vol. 2, no. 3, pp. 248–254, 2016.

[137] Z. Li, C. Liu, Z. Xie et al., "Epigenetic dysregulation in mesenchymal stem cell aging and spontaneous differentiation," *PLoS One*, vol. 6, no. 6, article e20526, 2011.

[138] Z. Hamidouche, K. Rother, J. Przybilla et al., "Bistable epigenetic states explain age-dependent decline in mesenchymal stem cell heterogeneity," *Stem Cells*, vol. 35, no. 3, pp. 694–704, 2017.

[139] K. Kornicka, J. Houston, and K. Marycz, "Dysfunction of mesenchymal stem cells isolated from metabolic syndrome and type 2 diabetic patients as result of oxidative stress and autophagy may limit their potential therapeutic use," *Stem Cell Reviews and Reports*, vol. 14, no. 3, pp. 337–345, 2018.

[140] K. Takahashi and S. Yamanaka, "Induction of pluripotent stem cells from mouse embryonic and adult fibroblast cultures by defined factors," *Cell*, vol. 126, no. 4, pp. 663–676, 2006.

[141] K. Takahashi, K. Tanabe, M. Ohnuki et al., "Induction of pluripotent stem cells from adult human fibroblasts by defined factors," *Cell*, vol. 131, no. 5, pp. 861–872, 2007.

[142] L. Lapasset, O. Milhavet, A. Prieur et al., "Rejuvenating senescent and centenarian human cells by reprogramming through the pluripotent state," *Genes & Development*, vol. 25, no. 21, pp. 2248–2253, 2011.

[143] J. Frobel, H. Hemeda, M. Lenz et al., "Epigenetic rejuvenation of mesenchymal stromal cells derived from induced pluripotent stem cells," *Stem Cell Reports*, vol. 3, no. 3, pp. 414–422, 2014.

[144] L. G. Villa-Diaz, S. E. Brown, Y. Liu et al., "Derivation of mesenchymal stem cells from human induced pluripotent stem cells cultured on synthetic substrates," *Stem Cells*, vol. 30, no. 6, pp. 1174–1181, 2012.

[145] L. Zou, Y. Luo, M. Chen et al., "A simple method for deriving functional MSCs and applied for osteogenesis in 3D scaffolds," *Scientific Reports*, vol. 3, no. 1, article 2243, 2013.

[146] K. Hynes, D. Menicanin, K. Mrozik, S. Gronthos, and P. M. Bartold, "Generation of functional mesenchymal stem cells from different induced pluripotent stem cell lines," *Stem Cells and Development*, vol. 23, no. 10, pp. 1084–1096, 2014.

[147] M. Moslem, I. Eberle, I. Weber, R. Henschler, and T. Cantz, "Mesenchymal stem/stromal cells derived from induced pluripotent stem cells support CD34^pos hematopoietic stem cell propagation and suppress inflammatory reaction," *Stem Cells International*, vol. 2015, Article ID 843058, 14 pages, 2015.

[148] K. Hynes, D. Menicanin, S. Gronthos, and M. P. Bartold, "Differentiation of iPSC to mesenchymal stem-like cells and their characterization," in *Induced Pluripotent Stem (iPS) Cells. Methods in Molecular Biology, vol 1357* Humana Press, New York, NY, USA.

[149] C. J. Chin, S. Li, M. Corselli et al., "Transcriptionally and functionally distinct mesenchymal subpopulations are generated from human pluripotent stem cells," *Stem Cell Reports*, vol. 10, no. 2, pp. 436–446, 2018.

[150] R. Kang, Y. Zhou, S. Tan et al., "Mesenchymal stem cells derived from human induced pluripotent stem cells retain adequate osteogenicity and chondrogenicity but less adipogenicity," *Stem Cell Research & Therapy*, vol. 6, no. 1, p. 144, 2015.

[151] S. Diederichs and R. S. Tuan, "Functional comparison of human-induced pluripotent stem cell-derived mesenchymal cells and bone marrow-derived mesenchymal stromal cells from the same donor," *Stem Cells and Development*, vol. 23, no. 14, pp. 1594–1610, 2014.

[152] M. Giuliani, N. Oudrhiri, Z. M. Noman et al., "Human mesenchymal stem cells derived from induced pluripotent stem cells down-regulate NK-cell cytolytic machinery," *Blood*, vol. 118, no. 12, pp. 3254–3262, 2011.

[153] Q. Zhao, C. A. Gregory, R. H. Lee et al., "MSCs derived from iPSCs with a modified protocol are tumor-tropic but have much less potential to promote tumors than bone marrow MSCs," *Proceedings of the National Academy of Sciences of the United States of America*, vol. 112, no. 2, pp. 530–535, 2015.

[154] A. S. Lee, C. Tang, M. S. Rao, I. L. Weissman, and J. C. Wu, "Tumorigenicity as a clinical hurdle for pluripotent stem cell therapies," *Nature Medicine*, vol. 19, no. 8, pp. 998–1004, 2013.

[155] A. Ocampo, P. Reddy, P. Martinez-Redondo et al., "In vivo amelioration of age-associated hallmarks by partial reprogramming," *Cell*, vol. 167, no. 7, pp. 1719–1733.e12, 2016.

[156] M. Okada, H. W. Kim, K. Matsu-ura, Y.-G. Wang, M. Xu, and M. Ashraf, "Abrogation of age-induced microRNA-195 rejuvenates the senescent mesenchymal stem cells by reactivating telomerase," *Stem Cells*, vol. 34, no. 1, pp. 148–159, 2016.

[157] S. Lee, K.-R. Yu, Y.-S. Ryu et al., "miR-543 and miR-590-3p regulate human mesenchymal stem cell aging via direct targeting of AIMP3/p18," *Age*, vol. 36, no. 6, article 9724, 2014.

[158] H. Chen, X. Liu, W. Zhu et al., "SIRT1 ameliorates age-related senescence of mesenchymal stem cells via modulating telomere shelterin," *Frontiers in Aging Neuroscience*, vol. 6, p. 103, 2014.

[159] R. Madonna, D. A. Taylor, Y. J. Geng et al., "Transplantation of mesenchymal cells rejuvenated by the overexpression of telomerase and myocardin promotes revascularization and tissue repair in a murine model of hindlimb ischemia," *Circulation Research*, vol. 113, no. 7, pp. 902–914, 2013.

[160] M. M. Lalu, L. McIntyre, C. Pugliese et al., "Safety of cell therapy with mesenchymal stromal cells (SafeCell): a systematic review and meta-analysis of clinical trials," *PLoS One*, vol. 7, no. 10, pp. e47559–e47521, 2012.

[161] G. Ren, X. Chen, F. Dong et al., "Concise review: mesenchymal stem cells and translational medicine: emerging issues," *Stem Cells Translational Medicine*, vol. 1, no. 1, pp. 51–58, 2012.

[162] L. von Bahr, B. Sundberg, L. Lönnies et al., "Long-term complications, immunologic effects, and role of passage for outcome in mesenchymal stromal cell therapy," *Biology of Blood and Marrow Transplantation*, vol. 18, no. 4, pp. 557–564, 2012.

[163] E. Eggenhofer, V. Benseler, A. Kroemer et al., "Mesenchymal stem cells are short-lived and do not migrate beyond the lungs after intravenous infusion," *Frontiers in Immunology*, vol. 3, p. 297, 2012.

[164] H. Hemeda, B. Giebel, and W. Wagner, "Evaluation of human platelet lysate versus fetal bovine serum for culture of mesenchymal stromal cells," *Cytotherapy*, vol. 16, no. 2, pp. 170–180, 2014.

[165] M. Duijvestein, A. C. W. Vos, H. Roelofs et al., "Autologous bone marrow-derived mesenchymal stromal cell treatment for refractory luminal Crohn's disease: results of a phase I study," *Gut*, vol. 59, no. 12, pp. 1662–1669, 2010.

[166] E. Fernandez-Rebollo, B. Mentrup, R. Ebert et al., "Human platelet lysate versus fetal calf serum: these supplements do not select for different mesenchymal stromal cells," *Scientific Reports*, vol. 7, no. 1, p. 5132, 2017.

[167] T. J. Kean, P. Lin, A. I. Caplan, and J. E. Dennis, "MSCs: delivery routes and engraftment, cell-targeting strategies, and immune modulation," *Stem Cells International*, vol. 2013, Article ID 732742, 13 pages, 2013.

[168] S. T. Ji, H. Kim, J. Yun, J. S. Chung, and S.-M. Kwon, "Promising therapeutic strategies for mesenchymal stem cell-based cardiovascular regeneration: from cell priming to tissue engineering," *Stem Cells International*, vol. 2017, Article ID 3945403, 13 pages, 2017.

[169] L. M. Marquardt and S. C. Heilshorn, "Design of injectable materials to improve stem cell transplantation," *Current Stem Cell Reports*, vol. 2, no. 3, pp. 207–220, 2016.

[170] S. Hanson, R. N. D'Souza, and P. Hematti, "Biomaterial-mesenchymal stem cell constructs for immunomodulation in composite tissue engineering," *Tissue Engineering Part A*, vol. 20, no. 15-16, pp. 2162–2168, 2014.

[171] A. B. Castillo and C. R. Jacobs, "Mesenchymal stem cell mechanobiology," *Current Osteoporosis Reports*, vol. 8, no. 2, pp. 98–104, 2010.

[172] A. Schäffler and C. Büchler, "Concise review: adipose tissue-derived stromal cells—basic and clinical implications for novel cell-based therapies," *Stem Cells*, vol. 25, no. 4, pp. 818–827, 2007.

[173] H.-J. Bühring, V. L. Battula, S. Treml, B. Schewe, L. Kanz, and W. Vogel, "Novel markers for the prospective isolation of human MSC," *Annals of the New York Academy of Sciences*, vol. 1106, no. 1, pp. 262–271, 2007.

[174] C. Muñiz, C. Teodosio, A. Mayado et al., "Ex vivo identification and characterization of a population of CD13^{high} CD105$^+$ CD45$^-$ mesenchymal stem cells in human bone marrow," *Stem Cell Research & Therapy*, vol. 6, no. 1, p. 169, 2015.

[175] O. G. Davies, P. R. Cooper, R. M. Shelton, A. J. Smith, and B. A. Scheven, "Isolation of adipose and bone marrow mesenchymal stem cells using CD29 and CD90 modifies their capacity for osteogenic and adipogenic differentiation," *Journal of Tissue Engineering*, vol. 6, 10 pages, 2015.

[176] H. Zhu, N. Mitsuhashi, A. Klein et al., "The role of the hyaluronan receptor CD44 in mesenchymal stem cell migration in the extracellular matrix," *Stem Cells*, vol. 24, no. 4, pp. 928–935, 2006.

[177] K.-R. Yu, S.-R. Yang, J.-W. Jung et al., "CD49f enhances multipotency and maintains stemness through the direct regulation of OCT4 and SOX2," *Stem Cells*, vol. 30, no. 5, pp. 876–887, 2012.

[178] E. G. Suto, Y. Mabuchi, N. Suzuki et al., "Prospectively isolated mesenchymal stem/stromal cells are enriched in the CD73$^+$ population and exhibit efficacy after transplantation," *Scientific Reports*, vol. 7, no. 1, p. 4838, 2017.

[179] P. A. Zuk, M. Zhu, P. Ashjian et al., "Human adipose tissue is a source of multipotent stem cells," *Molecular Biology of the Cell*, vol. 13, no. 12, pp. 4279–4295, 2002.

[180] S. Halfon, N. Abramov, B. Grinblat, and I. Ginis, "Markers distinguishing mesenchymal stem cells from fibroblasts are downregulated with passaging," *Stem Cells and Development*, vol. 20, no. 1, pp. 53–66, 2011.

[181] B. Delorme, J. Ringe, N. Gallay et al., "Specific plasma membrane protein phenotype of culture-amplified and native human bone marrow mesenchymal stem cells," *Blood*, vol. 111, no. 5, pp. 2631–2635, 2008.

[182] S. F. H. de Witte, M. Franquesa, C. C. Baan, and M. J. Hoogduijn, "Toward development of iMesenchymal stem cells for immunomodulatory therapy," *Frontiers in Immunology*, vol. 6, p. 648, 2016.

[183] C. Martinez, T. J. Hofmann, R. Marino, M. Dominici, and E. M. Horwitz, "Human bone marrow mesenchymal stromal cells express the neural ganglioside GD2: a novel surface marker for the identification of MSCs," *Blood*, vol. 109, no. 10, pp. 4245–4248, 2007.

[184] P. A. Oktar, S. Yildirim, D. Balci, and A. Can, "Continual expression throughout the cell cycle and downregulation upon adipogenic differentiation makes nucleostemin a vital human MSC proliferation marker," *Stem Cell Reviews and Reports*, vol. 7, no. 2, pp. 413–424, 2011.

[185] S. Fitter, S. Gronthos, S. S. Ooi, and A. C. W. Zannettino, "The mesenchymal precursor cell marker antibody STRO-1 binds to cell surface heat shock cognate 70," *Stem Cells*, vol. 35, no. 4, pp. 940–951, 2017.

[186] S. Gronthos, R. McCarty, K. Mrozik et al., "Heat shock protein-90 beta is expressed at the surface of multipotential mesenchymal precursor cells: generation of a novel monoclonal antibody, STRO-4, with specificity for mesenchymal precursor cells from human and ovine tissues," *Stem Cells and Development*, vol. 18, no. 9, pp. 1253–1262, 2009.

[187] E. J. Gang, D. Bosnakovski, C. A. Figueiredo, J. W. Visser, and R. C. R. Perlingeiro, "SSEA-4 identifies mesenchymal stem cells from bone marrow," *Blood*, vol. 109, no. 4, pp. 1743–1751, 2007.

[188] K. Sivasubramaniyan, A. Harichandan, S. Schumann et al., "Prospective isolation of mesenchymal stem cells from human bone marrow using novel antibodies directed against sushi domain containing 2," *Stem Cells and Development*, vol. 22, no. 13, pp. 1944–1954, 2013.

16

Intraspinal Transplantation of the Adipose Tissue-Derived Regenerative Cells in Amyotrophic Lateral Sclerosis in Accordance with the Current Experts' Recommendations: Choosing Optimal Monitoring Tools

Magdalena Kuzma-Kozakiewicz,[1,2] **Andrzej Marchel,**[3] **Anna Kaminska,**[1]
Malgorzata Gawel,[1,2] **Jan Sznajder,**[4] **Anna Figiel-Dabrowska,**[5] **Arkadiusz Nowak,**[3]
Edyta Maj,[6] **Natalia Ewa Krzesniak,**[7] **Bartlomiej H. Noszczyk,**[7] **Krystyna Domanska-Janik** ⓘ,[5]
and Anna Sarnowska ⓘ[5]

[1]*Department of Neurology, Medical University of Warsaw, Zwirki i Wigury 61 Str, 02-091 Warsaw, Poland*
[2]*Neurodegenerative Diseases Research Group, Medical University of Warsaw, Zwirki i Wigury 61 Str, 02-091 Warsaw, Poland*
[3]*Department of Neurosurgery, Medical University of Warsaw, Zwirki i Wigury 61 Str, 02-091 Warsaw, Poland*
[4]*Department of Rehabilitation, Józef Piłsudski University of Physical Education in Warsaw, Marymoncka Str. 34,*
  00-968 Warsaw, Poland
[5]*Mossakowski Medical Research Centre, Polish Academy of Sciences, 5 Pawinskiego Str, 02-106 Warsaw, Poland*
[6]*2nd Department of Clinical Radiology, Medical University of Warsaw, Zwirki i Wigury 61 Str, 02-091 Warsaw, Poland*
[7]*Department of Plastic and Reconstructive Surgery, Centre of Postgraduate Medical Education, Prof. W. Orlowski Memorial Hospital,*
  Czerniakowska 231, 00-416 Warsaw, Poland

Correspondence should be addressed to Anna Sarnowska; a_sarnowska@tlen.pl

Academic Editor: Sangho Roh

Stem cells (SCs) may constitute a perspective alternative to pharmacological treatment in neurodegenerative diseases. Although the safety of SC transplantation has been widely shown, their clinical efficiency in amyotrophic lateral sclerosis (ALS) is still to be proved. It is not only due to a limited number of studies, small treatment groups, and fast but nonlinear disease progression but also due to lack of objective methods able to show subtle clinical changes. Preliminary guidelines for cell therapy have recently been proposed by a group of ALS experts. They combine clinical, neurophysiological, and functional assessment together with monitoring of the cytokine level. Here, we describe a pilot study on transplantation of autologous adipose-derived regenerative cells (ADRC) into the spinal cord of the patients with ALS and monitoring of the results in accordance with the current recommendations. To show early and/or subtle changes within the muscles of interest, a wide range of clinical and functional tests were used and compared in order to choose the most sensitive and optimal set. Additionally, an analysis of transplanted ADRC was provided to develop standards ensuring the derivation and verification of adequate quality of transplanted cells and to correlate ADRC properties with clinical outcome.

1. Introduction

Amyotrophic lateral sclerosis is a fatal neurodegenerative disease characterized by a progressive loss of motor neurons in the central and peripheral nervous system. Starting insidiously with an impairment of fine hand movements, foot drop, or slurred speech, in 2 to 5 years it leads to quadriplegia, anarthria, aphagia, and respiratory insufficiency [1]. There is no causative treatment. The first available drug, riluzole, prolongs survival by the average of 3 months, while edaravone, recently registered in Japan and US, relents disease progression in a subgroup of patients without respiratory involvement [2, 3]. Patients with mutations in the *SOD1* gene might in future profit from oligonucleotide strategy, but the clinical trials are still ongoing [4, 5]. Stem cells (SCs) may therefore constitute a perspective alternative to pharmacological treatment in ALS. Although the safety of SC transplantation has been widely shown [6–8], their efficiency in ALS is still unproven. It is not only due to a limited number of studies, high variability of transplanted cell types, small treatment groups, and fast but nonlinear disease progression but also the lack of objective methods able to prove subtle clinical changes.

The usual monitoring strategies used in clinical trials involve the combination of muscle strength assessment: MRC (Medical Research Council), grip test, functional status: ALSFRS R (amyotrophic lateral sclerosis functional rating scale-revised), Norris scale, and respiratory functions: FVC and SNIP. In a recent statement, the representatives of International Workshop on Progress in Stem Cells Research for ALS/MND recommend the use of ALSFRS R, FVC, electrophysiological quantitative motor unit assessment, and cytokine level [9].

Here, we describe a pilot study on transplantation of autologous adipose-derived regenerative cells into the spinal cord of the patients with ALS and monitoring of the results in accordance with the current recommendations. In a limited number of patients, we aimed to use a wide range of clinical and functional tests in order to identify measures able to show early and/or subtle changes within the muscles of interest.

Our choice of the material for transplantation was dictated by a relative safety, nontumorigenic history, and availability of mesenchymal cells [10]. Embryonic stem cells, despite their high ability to differentiate toward neuronal cells, can give rise to tumors. In turn, a very good and quite safe material, such as fetal cells, is still ethically controversial and difficult to obtain for wider therapy. Recent papers present promising findings of preclinical experiments with adipose-derived regenerative cell (ADRC) transplantation. The ADRCs constitute a freshly isolated, heterogeneous population, characterized and described also by our group [10], not cultivated in vitro (in contrast to ADSC) to enhance or keep their high immunomodulatory properties [11]. These cells may be isolated under a moderate level of invasiveness and with comparatively high efficiency per number of cells. Authors demonstrate their remarkably strong adjuvant properties that are thought to be responsible for the positive results in regenerative medicine [12]. Scientific data suggest that ADRCs improve blood flow, modulate the inflammatory response, and protect tissues from dying. Furthermore, compared with the bone marrow stromal cells, ADRCs show greater plasticity, longer survival times, and higher vasculogenetic potential. An ADRC can be induced to differentiate, not only into adipocytes, bone, and chondrocytes in line with basic MSC properties but also under defined conditions into neuroectodermal cell lineages [13]. However, the protective properties of ADRCs depend strictly on their stage-related differentiation. Our data gathered in preclinical and clinical experimentation indicate that freshly isolated, undifferentiated, and highly proliferating MSC have the highest adjuvant properties [11]. With time of culture, cells differentiate and their protective effect declines in parallel with changes in their paracrine/adjuvant capabilities [14].

To correlate properties of freshly isolated ADRC with clinical outcome, each ADRC fraction obtained and ready for transplantation was divided into portions assigned to transplantation and basic research.

2. Material and Methods

2.1. Study Design. The study was registered at http://ClinicalTrials.gov (NCT03296501). It was designed as a nonrandomized, prospective, single-center, open-label study, with no placebo control, to assess safety and efficacy of ADRC transplantation into the individuals with ALS. After a minimum of 3 months of clinical, functional, and electrophysiological monitoring, the patients underwent ADRC injection followed by 2 subsequent intrathecal infusions. Safety, adverse events, and efficacy were confirmed by clinical, electrophysiological, neuroimaging, and pulmonary function assessment together with functional and objective motor assessment. The quality of life (QoL) and depression were monitored throughout the study.

Both the study protocol and the informed consent procedure were approved by the Bioethics Committee of the Medical University of Warsaw. Prior to enrollment to the study, each participant was given detailed "Information for the study participant" and signed an informed consent in 2 copies, one for each party. The procedure was repeated before each surgical intervention.

2.2. Patients. Patients with ALS were diagnosed and followed at the Department of Neurology, Medical University of Warsaw. The qualification procedure included three steps. The first step was a register-based-approach. The patients' clinical data was taken from the Warsaw ALS/MND registry, which collects demographic and clinical information of all ALS/MND patients diagnosed and followed at the Department of Neurology, Medical University of Warsaw, since 2003 ($n = 780$). By using inclusion and exclusion criteria as search filters (Table 1), a group of potentially eligible patients was identified. The second step involved updated clinical assessment. In case of positive verification, the patients signed an informed consent (third step) and were included into the study.

2.3. Surgical Procedures

2.3.1. Liposuction. The fat tissue was harvested from the abdomen or inner thighs after infiltration with Klein solution (based on lactated Ringers solution with lidocaine and epinephrine) under local anesthesia. In order to preserve regenerative properties of cells, fat collection was performed in low pressure (250 kPa), using syringe liposuction. We obtained approximately 250 ml of lipoaspirate during each procedure using 3 mm harvesting cannulas [15–17].

TABLE 1: Inclusion and exclusion criteria for the intraspinal and intrathecal ADRC transplantation.

Inclusion criteria	Exclusion criteria
(i) Clinically definite or probable ALS	(i) PEG or indications for PEG insertion
(ii) Age 18–65 years	(ii) Respiratory insufficiency, NIPPV, IV, or indications
(iii) ALS – FRS > 25	(iii) *SOD1* and *C9orf72* mutation
(iv) FVC > 70%	(iv) Concomitant disorders with contraindications for neurosurgery
(v) Stable dose of riluzole for the past 30 days	(v) Pregnancy or lactation
(vi) Disease duration 6–24 months	(vi) Unable to provide informed consent
(vii) Pretreatment observation period of >3 months (neurological and physiotherapist assessment, ALSFRS R, and MUNIX)	
(viii) In females with childbearing potential at least two efficient contraceptive methods	
(ix) Able to provide informed consent	

2.3.2. Lumbar Laminectomy. The patient was placed in the prone position, and the operative field was aseptically prepared. Fluoroscopy was used to obtain positive confirmation of the appropriate levels for thoracolumbar (T10/11) exposure. A standard midline posterior approach was used with completion of a Th10–Th11 laminectomy. A Surgicel® was used as a hemostatic aid when necessary. A 4–5 cm incision was made through the dura, exposing the spinal cord. Following the dura opening, a microinjection platform was fixed to the operating table. The platform itself consists of 2 rigid bars spaced to provide easy visualization of the dura and the spinal cord. Originally designed gondola was positioned along these rods. It was equipped with universal joints that allowed for correction of the sagittal and coronal angles. The device also allowed for adjustment in the mediolateral and rostrocaudal direction. The dura was reflected away from the pial layer and secured to the operative drape. The dorsal root entry zone was identified, and the pial surface was opened with a microscalpel under operating microscope magnification. The spinal cord was penetrated on an orthogonal trajectory to the cord surface at a point 1 mm medial to the dorsal root entry zone. Patients received four bilateral (8 total) injections performed at 4 mm intervals along the rostrocaudal axis at Th10–Th11. For intraspinal transplantation, the patient received $8 \times 10 \mu l$ at the concentration of 2000,000/10 μl which resulted in the total cell number of 16,000 cells/80 μl. The injection rate was programmed to 10 μl/min, using a precalibrated microinjector pump. Doses were administered through the pump connected to a syringe and needle assembly. The cell suspension was infused at an average depth of 4 mm from contact at the pial surface after an initial needle introduction to an average depth of 5 mm. Depth coordinates were individualized based on preoperative MRI results and ranged from 3 to 5 mm. By passing to a depth of 5 mm and then pulling back 1 mm, a small reservoir was created to reduce reflux. During the injection process, the mechanical ventilation of the patient was kept shallow in order to reduce ventilation-associated cord excursion. Following infusion, the needle was left in place for 1 extra minute to minimize the potential for cell suspension reflux along the needle track. Following watertight dural closure,

muscular and fascial layers were closed. Finally, skin closure was completed. Somatosensory evoked potentials (SSEPs) were monitored throughout the procedure.

2.3.3. Intrathecal Stem Cell Injection. Intrathecal stem cell injections were performed with the use of a lumbar drainage system. Lumbar drain was placed at the level of the L3 or L4 vertebrae, so that the introducing needle entered below the level at which the spinal cord ended. An average of 15 cm of drain was introduced into the subarachnoid space of the vertebral canal thus positioning its end at the level of the Th12 vertebrae. The tubing was then secured onto the skin with a stitch and covered with a clear sterile dressing. A total cell suspension volume of 4 ml (approx. 14,000,000 cells/ml, 56,000,000 cells/4 ml in total) was injected over 2 minutes followed by saline injection (1 ml over 30 sec). The drain was left in place for 24 hours to reduce suspension reflux through the punctured dura.

2.4. Patients' Evaluation. The patients' evaluation was divided into three sections: clinical assessment, psychological evaluation, and laboratory tests (Figure 1). The functional assessment was performed by the same physical therapist specialized in neuromuscular diseases. The timetable of the assessments is presented in Table 2. The assessments performed at the visits that involved intervention (either intraspinal or intrathecal ADRC transplantation) were performed 3–7 days prior to a respective intervention.

2.5. Muscle Strength

2.5.1. Manual Muscle Test. The manual muscle test was performed according to the Medical Research Council (MRC) [18]. Every assessed muscle group was rated from 0 (no visible contraction) to 5 (normal).

2.5.2. Handheld Dynamometer. (HHD)—MicroFET 2 was used to assess arm flexors, elbow flexors, wrist extensors, finger extensors, abductors of digitus secundus and hip flexors, knee extensors, and ankle dorsiflexors. The result was an average score of three attempts in each muscle group [19].

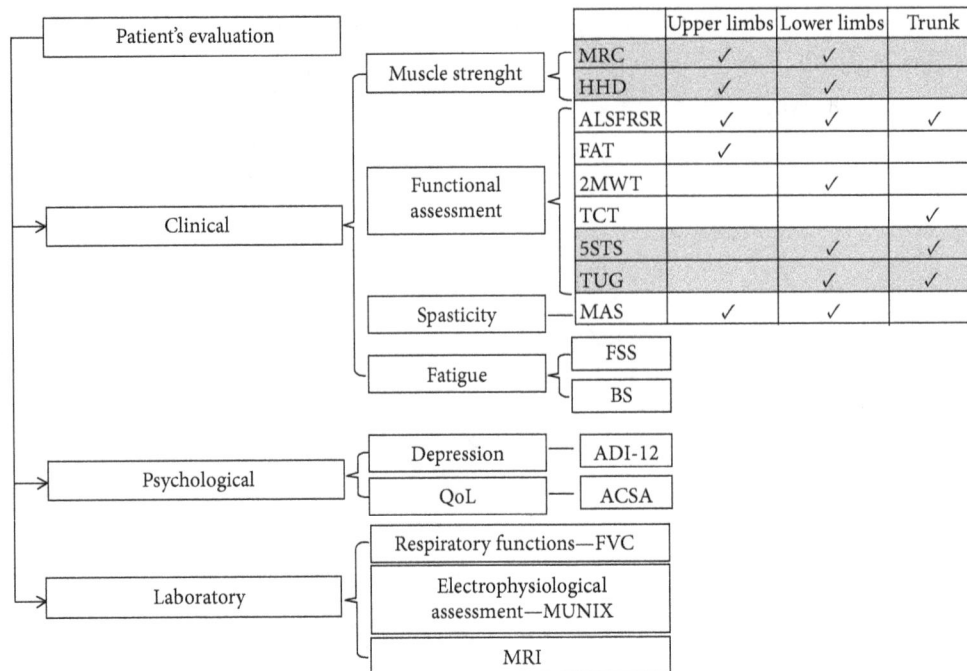

	Upper limbs	Lower limbs	Trunk
MRC	✓	✓	
HHD	✓	✓	
ALSFRSR	✓	✓	✓
FAT	✓		
2MWT		✓	
TCT			✓
5STS		✓	✓
TUG		✓	✓
MAS	✓	✓	

FIGURE 1: Patient's assessment paradigm. The diagram presents the applied electrophysiological methods, psychological assessment, and functional tests, along with their assignment to specific functions.

2.6. Functional Assessment

2.6.1. Amyotrophic Lateral Sclerosis Functional Rating Scale-Revised (ALSFRS R).
ALSFRS R contains 12 functional items concerning bulbar function, upper limb, lower limb, trunk, and respiratory functions. Each item is scored from 0 (unable to) to 4 (normal) [20]. The scale was independently applied by a neurologist specializing in ALS and a physiotherapist—interrater differences were discussed prior to final scoring.

2.6.2. Frenchay Arm Test (FAT).
The Frenchay Arm Test was used to assess the function of the upper limbs. It consists of five simple tasks: drawing a line with a ruler, picking up a pin, picking up a glass of water and drinking some, fixing a clothespin to the stick and removing it, and combing hair with scores 0 (unable to) to 1 (able to perform) [21]. It was performed in both upper limbs, and the average score was used in further analysis. In the original version, the affected hand was assessed.

2.6.3. Trunk Control Test (TCT).
The trunk control test was administrated to evaluate functions of the muscles of the trunk [22]. It involves completion of four tasks: rolling to a weak side, rolling to a strong side, balancing in a sitting position, and sitting up from lying down. Each task is scored from 0 (unable to) to 12 (able with help or in abnormal style) to 25 (fully able). The result was expressed in a sum of item scores.

2.6.4. Two-Minute Walk Test (2MWT).
The two-minute walk test was used to evaluate the function of lower limbs and trunk muscles. The results were expressed in distance (meters); the patient was able to cover in 2 minutes [23]. The level of fatigue was additionally estimated before and after the test by rate of perceived exertion (Borg scale (BS)) [24].

2.6.5. Five Times Sit to Stand Test (5STS).
5STS was also used to measure functional muscle strength of lower extremities and trunk [25]. A patient's task was to rise from a chair five times as fast as possible with arms crossed on the chest. The results were expressed in seconds as a mean of 3 independent attempts.

2.6.6. Timed Up and Go (TUG).
TUG similarly assessed the functional use of the lower extremity and trunk when a patient was asked to rise from an armchair, walk 3 meters, turn, walk back, and sit down again [26, 27]. The results were expressed in seconds as a mean of 3 independent attempts.

2.7. Spasticity

2.7.1. Modified Ashworth Scale (MAS).
MAS assesses muscle tone in the upper and lower limbs [28, 29]. It is scored from 0 (normal muscle tone) to 4 (affected part rigid in flexion or extension of extremity). The results were expressed as a mean of the results obtained in all limbs.

2.8. Fatigue

2.8.1. Fatigue Severity Scale (FSS).
FSS consists of 9 points scored from 1 (definitely disagree) to 7 (definitely agree). A result of >36 is considered positive [30].

2.9. Depression

2.9.1. ALS Depression Inventory (ADI-12).
ADI-12 is a self-reported questionnaire developed specifically to screen for depression in ALS [31], describing mood, anhedonia,

TABLE 2: Timetable of the adipose-derived regenerative cell (ADRC) isolation and transplantation study.

Action visit	V1 screening	V2	V3	V4	V5	V6	V7
Week	−24	−12	0	12	24	36	48
Permitted delta in weeks to V1		+2		+2	+2	+/−2	+/−2
Interventions							
Intraspinal transplantation			X				
Intrathecal transplantation				X	X		
Screening assessment							
Patient information, informed consent	X		X	X	X		
Inclusion/exclusion criteria	X						
Medical history	X		X	X	X	X	X
Diagnosis according to EEC	X		X	X	X	X	X
Physical and neurological examination	X	X	X	X	X	X	X
EMG	X						
MUNIX	X	X	X	X	X	X	X
Spinal MRI C with contrast			X				
Spinal MRI Th with contrast			X	X	X		X
Spinal MRI S with contrast			X	X	X		X
Spinal MRI Th			X*	X*	X*		
Spinal MRI LS			X*	X*	X*		
Spirometry	X	X	X	X	X	X	X
Chest X-ray			X				
Laboratory studies	X		X	X	X		
Muscle strength assessment							
MRC	X	X	X	X	X	X	X
HHD	X	X	X	X	X	X	X
Functional assessment							
ALSFRS R	X	X	X	X	X	X	X
2MWT (with concomitant BS)	X	X	X	X	X	X	X
5STS	X	X	X	X	X	X	X
TUG	X	X	X	X	X	X	X
TCT	X	X	X	X	X	X	X
FAT	X	X	X	X	X	X	X
Other examinations							
FSS	X	X	X	X	X	X	X
MAS	X	X	X	X	X	X	X
Psychological assessment							
ADI-12	X		X		X		X
ACSA	X		X		X		X

MUNIX: motor unit number index (MUNIX). *Examination performer 48 h after the ARDC transplantation. MRC: Manual Muscle Test Medical Research Council; HHD: handheld dynamometer (HHD); ALSFRS R: amyotrophic lateral sclerosis functional rating scale-revised; 2MWT: two-minute walk test; BS: Borg scale; 5STS: Five Times Sit to Stand test; TUG: Timed Up and Go; FAT: Frenchay Arm Test; TCT: Trunk Control Test; MAS: Modified Ashworth Scale; FSS: Fatigue Severity Scale; ADI-12: ALS Depression Inventory; ACSA: Anamnestic Comparative Self-Assessment.

and energy, without referring to motor-related symptoms. It consists of 12 statements concerning the past two weeks, scoring from 12 (best possible) to 48 (worst possible). Scores between 23 and 29 indicate mild depression and 30 as severe depression.

2.10. Quality of Life 2.11. Anamnestic Comparative Self-Assessment (ACSA). ACSA assesses global QoL compared

to the worse and the best time of a lifetime scoring from −5 (as bad as possible) to +5 (as good as possible) [32].

2.12. Electrophysiological Evaluation

2.12.1. Motor Unit Number Index (MUNIX). The MUNIX was performed according to the protocol developed by Neuwirth and Weber [33]. Six muscles were examined on both

sides: abductor pollicis brevis, abductor digiti minimi, biceps brachii, tibialis anterior, extensor digitorum brevis, and abductor hallucis muscles after supramaximal distal stimulation of the median, ulnar, musculocutaneous, peroneal, and tibial nerves, respectively. The results (CMAP amplitude in mV) and motor unit number index were analyzed by a certified neurophysiologist. The results were expressed as the sum of results from all extremities (total MUNIX), upper and lower limbs (MUNIX upper limbs and MUNIX lower limbs).

2.13. Cell Isolation and Analysis

2.13.1. Adipose-Derived Regenerative Cell (ADRC) Isolation. Preclinical characterisation of ADRC cellular composition, rate of proliferation (PDT), genetic stability under 5% oxygen, and maintenance of stemness properties together with commitment to cell differentiation toward mesodermal direction were described in our previous publication [10].

Under operating room conditions, immediately after collection, the lipoaspirate was processed in the CellCelution 800 System (Cytori Therapeutics Inc., San Diego, CA). It was washed to remove free blood and lipids and digested with Celase 800 (Cytori Therapeutics Inc.) enzyme to release the stromal vascular fraction. After a series of centrifugation steps and passing through a system of sieves with various pores, the stromal fraction was concentrated, and 5 ml of ADRC suspended in Ringer solution was prepared for transplantation: 4 ml was intended for patient's treatment, while 1 ml of remnant stromal vascular fraction was used for *in vitro* analysis.

2.13.2. CFU-F Assay. The ADRC at 0 passage was seeded on 6-well plates at a density 100 cells/well. The seeded cells were cultured in standard culture condition for 10 days. Then, the cells were fixed with 4% PFA for 15 minutes and stained with 0.5% toluidine blue for 20 minutes. The 1% stock solution of dye was prepared in 70% ethanol, and distilled water was added in proportion 1 : 1 to obtain the final 0.5%-mixture concentration. After incubation, the stain was directly washed with distilled water. The ADRC-stained colonies containing 50 or more cells were counted, and CFU-F frequency (number of colonies per number seeded cells) was calculated.

2.13.3. Determination of Chemokine and Cytokine Profile. The analysis of 102 chemokines or cytokines was performed on CSF samples using the Proteome Profiler Human XL Cytokine Array Kit (R&D Systems) following manufacturers' protocol (Table 3). The kit consists of 4 membranes, which were incubated overnight with 300 μl of every sample and a binding buffer. The membranes were washed and incubated with the detection cocktail, with streptavidin-conjugated horseradish peroxidase (R&D Systems) for 30 min and finally incubation with the chemiluminescence reagent. The spots were visualized by Fusion FX6 (Vilber Lourmat) with EvolutionCapt FX6. The signal readings were proportional to the amount of the bound analyte. The results were analyzed by Zen Software (Zeiss) based on densitometric analysis (Figure 2). The graph bars

TABLE 3: Cytokine array assay.

Adiponectin/Acrp30	INF-gamma	Lipocalin-2/NGAL
Aggrecan	IGFBP-2	CCL2/MCP-1
Angiogenin	IGFBP-3	CCL7/MCP-3
Angiopoietin-1	IL-1 alpha/IL-1F1	M-CSF
Angiopoietin-2	IL-1 beta/IL-1F2	MIF
BAFF/BLyS/TNFSF13B	IL-1ra/IL-1F3	CXCL9/MIG
BDNF	IL-2	CCL3/CCL4 MIP-1 alpha/beta
CD14	IL-3	CCL20/MIP-3 alpha
CD30	IL-4	CCL19/MIP-3 beta
CD40 ligand/TNFSF5	IL-5	MMP-9
Chitinase 3-like	IL-6	Myeloperoxidase
Complement component C5/C5a	IL-8	Osteopontin (OPN)
Complement factor D	IL-10	PDGF-AA
C-reactive protein (CRP)	IL-11	PDGF-AB/BB
Cripto-1	IL-12 p70	Pentraxin 3/TSF-14
Cystatin C	IL-13	CXCL4/PF4
Dkk-1	IL-15	RAGE
DPPIV/CD26	IL-16	CCL5/RANTES
EGF	IL-17A	RBP4
CXCL5/ENA-78	IL-18 BPa	Relaxin-2
Endoglin/CD105	IL-19	Resistin
EMMPRIN	IL-22	CXCL12/SDF-1 alpha
Fas ligand	IL-23	Serpin E1/PAI-1
FGF basic	IL-24	SHBG
KGF/FGF-7	IL-27	ST2/IL1 R4
FGF-19	IL-31	CCL17/TARC
Flt-3 ligand	IL-32alpha/beta/gamma	TFF3
G-CSF	IL-33	TfR
GDF-15	IL-34	TGF-alpha
GM-CSF	CXCL10/IP-10	Thrombospondin-1
CXCL1/GRO alpha	CXCL11/I-TAC	TNF-alpha
Growth hormone (GH)	Kallikrein 3/PSA	uPAR
HGF	Leptin	VEGF
ICAM-1/CD54	LIF	Vitamin D BP

present means from two spots captured with analyzed antibody according to the following formula: mean density of analyzed spots/mean density of control spots × 100%−mean density of background.

2.14. Statistical Analysis.
Statistical analysis of the raw data was conducted using the GraphPad Prism version 5 software (La Jolla, CA, USA). The mean ± SEM was calculated for all samples, and significance was determined using one-way ANOVA followed by adequate post hoc test. For data of MUNIX and HHD evaluation, the Pearson coefficient was calculated. The values were considered as significant

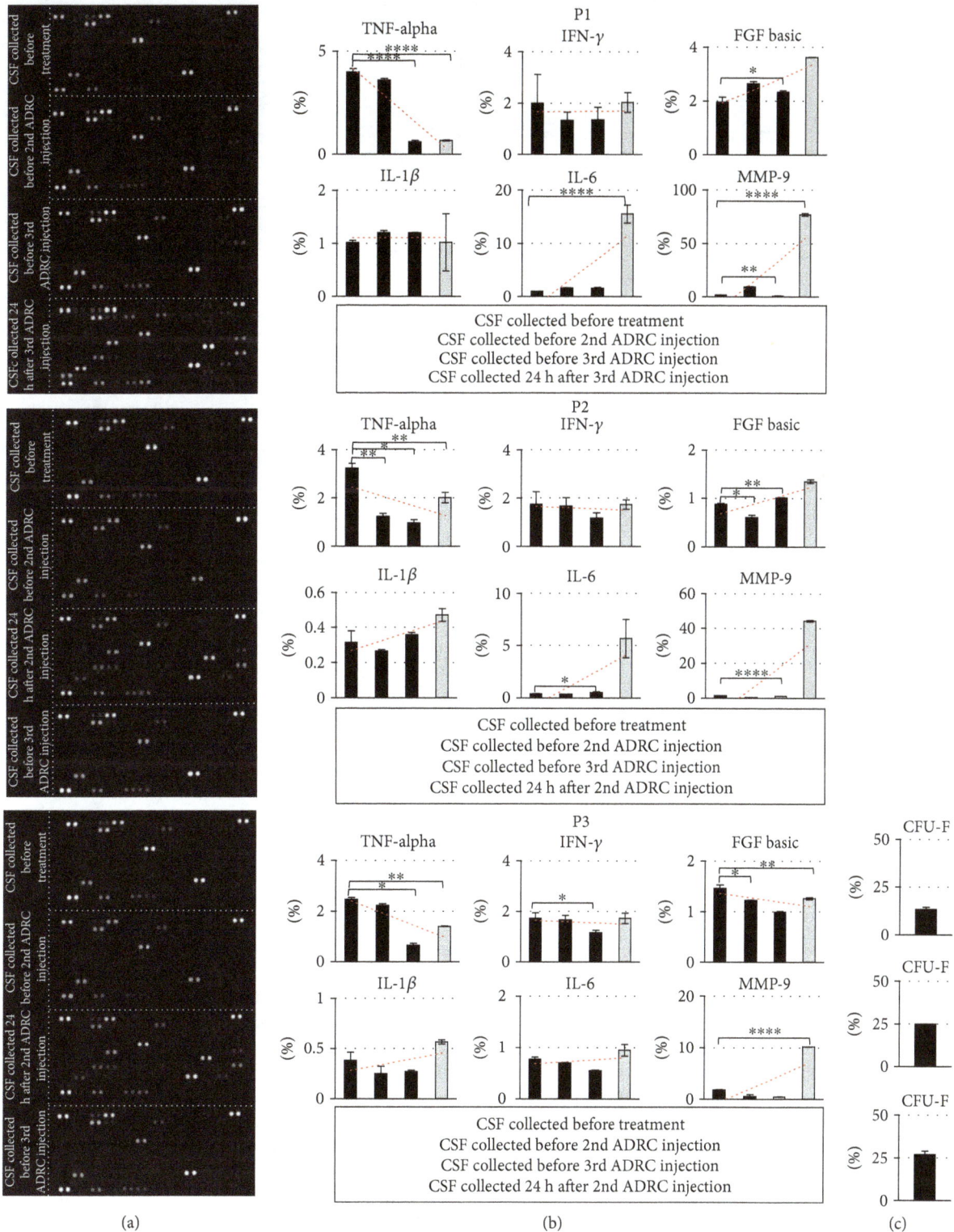

FIGURE 2: Cytokine and chemokine level in CSF after ADRC application. (a) Membrane-based antibody arrays for the parallel determination of the relative levels of human cytokines and chemokines from CSF of ALS patients (resp. P1, P2, and P3). (b) Comparison of TNFα, IFN-γ, IL-1β, IL-6, bFGF, and MMP-9 level after MSC transplantation (black graph bars—3 months after ADRC application, grey bars—24 hours after cell application). (c) Quantification of CFU frequency. ADRCs obtained after enzymatic isolation were analyzed to evaluate the stem cell/clonogenic population among a heterogeneous stromal cell population.

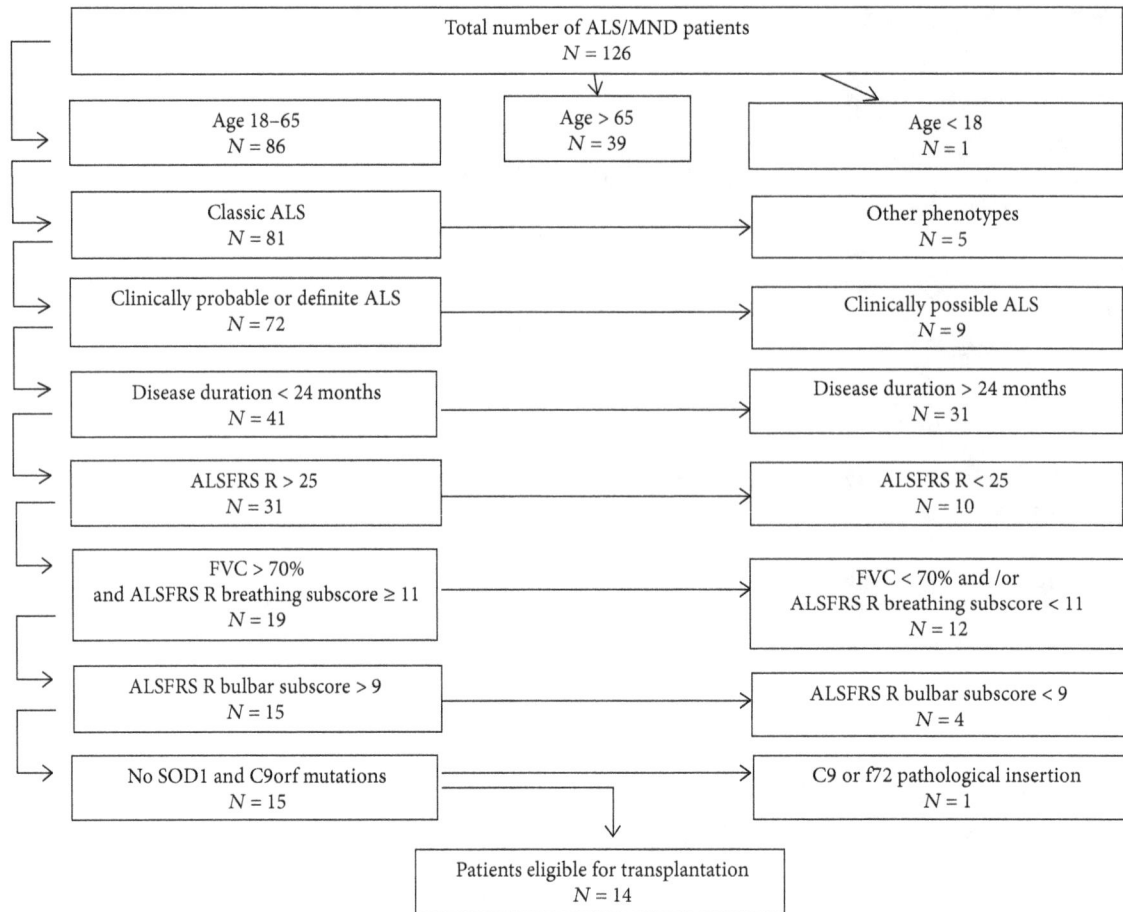

FIGURE 3: The qualification scheme of patients according to the proposal during the International Workshop on Progress in Stem Cells Research for ALS/MND in 2016.

with a value of $p < 0.05$ ($^*p < 0.05$, $^{**}p < 0.01$, $^*p < 0.001$, and $^{****}p < 0.0001$).

3. Results

3.1. Clinical Outcome. One hundred and twenty six patients were diagnosed with MND between January 2015 and November 2017 at the Department of Neurology and/or at the University MND outpatient clinic. Of these, 86 patients were at the age 18–65 (Figure 3). From the remaining group, 5 patients had clinical phenotypes other than classic ALS: progressive muscle atrophy ($n = 2$), flail arm or flail leg syndrome ($n = 2$), or primary lateral sclerosis ($n = 1$). Nine patients presented clinically possible ALS according to the El Escorial criteria [34], 31 had a disease duration longer than 24 months, and 10 patients were at the advanced disease stage (ALSFRS R < 25). From the remaining group of 31 patients, 12 had respiratory insufficiency and 4 a marked bulbar involvement. One patient was excluded from the study due to a mutation in the C9orf72 gene. All in all, only 11% of patients ($n = 14$) fulfilled the inclusion criteria. The updated clinical assessment disqualified 9 patients as no longer eligible for the study due to either gastrostomy, respiratory insufficiency, or loss of walking capacity. One patient decided to rebuff the transplantation.

The transplantation of ADRC into the spinal cord at the level of Th10–11 was performed in four patients (3.2%, 3 males/1 female, mean age 37.2, site of onset—upper limbs (4/4), mean diagnosis delay 14.7 months, and mean disease duration 19.0 months). One patient underwent additionally intraspinal transplantation into the cervical part. The results of this application will be published separately. In all cases, intraspinal injection was followed by two intrathecal cell infusions performed in subsequent 3-month intervals. The patients were followed every 3 months.

There was no death related to the transplantation procedure. One patient died 29 months after the first transplantation, two days after gastrostomy insertion. The autopsy was not performed. The adverse events (AEs) included abdominal pain (2/4 patients, severity 1–3/10) in the area of liposuction, which resolved within 24–36 hours after the intervention, and a persistent superficial sensation impairment in the close surrounding of the site of cannula insertion. In case of the intraspinal transplantation, all patients experienced pain at the site of laminectomy (severity 5–6/10), which required analgesic therapy for 7–10 days. One patient reported intubation-induced speech difficulties, which resolved within 10 days without treatment. Following intrathecal infusion, one patient experienced headache without signs of meningeal irritation.

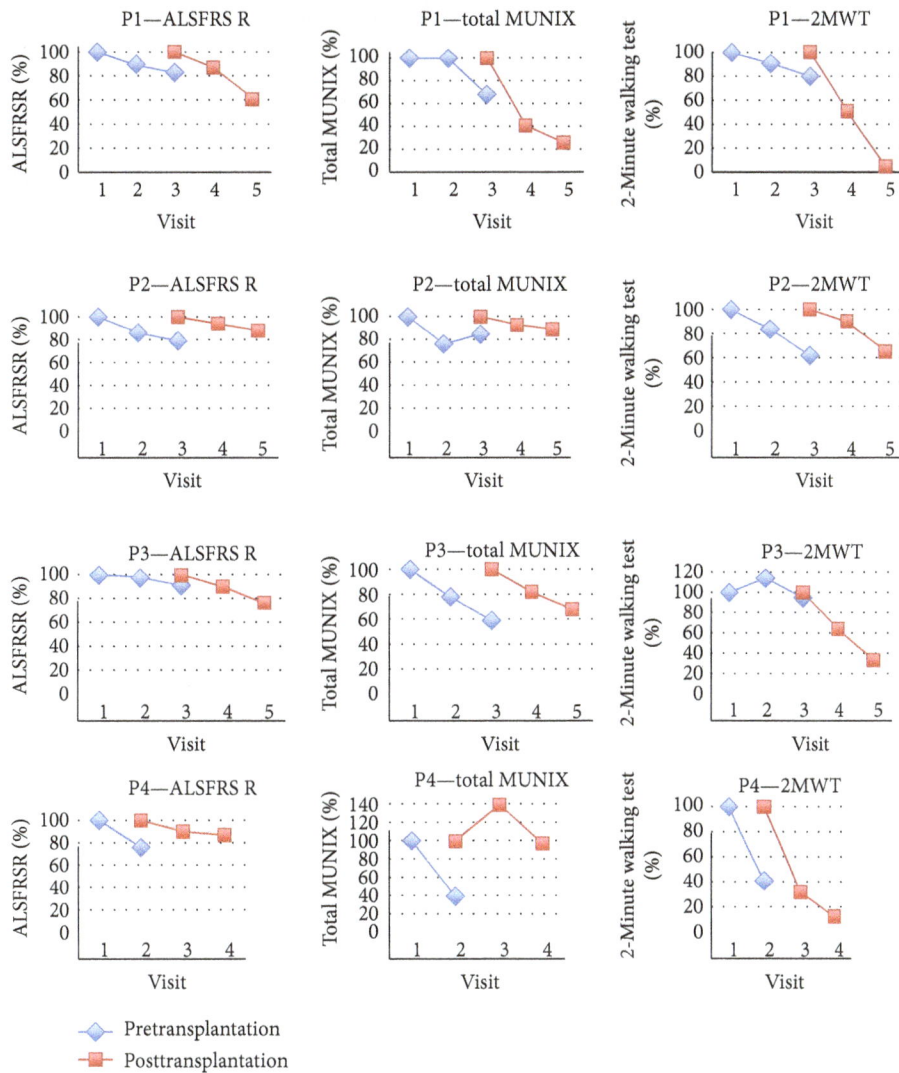

FIGURE 4: Functional tests. According to Figure 1, functional tests evaluating muscle efficiency in the upper (FAT) and lower limbs (2MWT, TUG, and 5STS) and trunk (TCT) were performed in several time points before, in the course of, and after ADRC therapy. The stability or decrease in these functions was compared with the trajectory of the ALSFRS scale. Impairment in all functional tests was observed faster than decrease in ALSFRS. Although 5STS and TUG showed good correlation with other functional parameters, their longitudinal use was limited in patients who were no longer able to stand up without the help of their arms/hands (on average 6–9 months after the first transplantation; P3 and P4).

Two patients reported reduction of previously increased muscle tone immediately after intraspinal ADRC infusion. Although the study timetable did not include 2MWT and BS evaluation directly after the intervention, in case of patient P2, the tests were additionally carried following the patient-reported walking improvement. The outcome of the 2WMT improved from 100.5 m (fatigability of 8 at BS) prior to transplantation to 128.0 m (with markedly reduced fatigability—BS of 5) seven days after the procedure. There was a slight reduction in the progression of walking impairment: from a 30% reduction of the 2MWT in the 3 months before the operation to a 10% drop in the following observation period (Figure 4). Patient P4 reported improved walking, arm movement, and speech from the second week after transplantation. An objectification in the direct postoperative period was not possible due to the pain in the lumbar region.

At three months after transplantation, there was no apparent reduction of a walking capacity slope. According to both patients, the effects persisted for 4 weeks and did not occur after any of the intrathecal infusions.

Both pre- and posttransplantation monitoring showed a physical, functional, and respiratory decline in all studied patients (Figure 4, Table 4).

ALSFRS R and MRC shared a similar deterioration pattern reaching down to 50 and 40% (resp.) of their initial value within 21 months of observation. The slope of decline was much steeper in the case of both MUNIX and muscle strength as examined by HHD (Figure 5). So was the range of decrease exceeding 90% in the observation period. There was a positive correlation between MUNIX and HHD throughout the study in merged results of all our patients ($r = 0.8856$, $p < 0.0001$). The MUNIX and HHD showed a

TABLE 4: Longitudinal forced vital capacity assessment in ALS patients prior to and after ADRC administration.

	Patient/visit	V1	V2	V3 (prior to intraspinal tx)	V4 (prior to 1st intrathecal tx)	V5 (prior to 2nd intrathecal tx)	V6	V7
FVC (%)	P1	110	105	100	100	90	85	80
	P2	89	89	84	88	85	75	65 (NIV)
	P3	128	128	106	106	100	90	83
	P4		90	71	65	44		

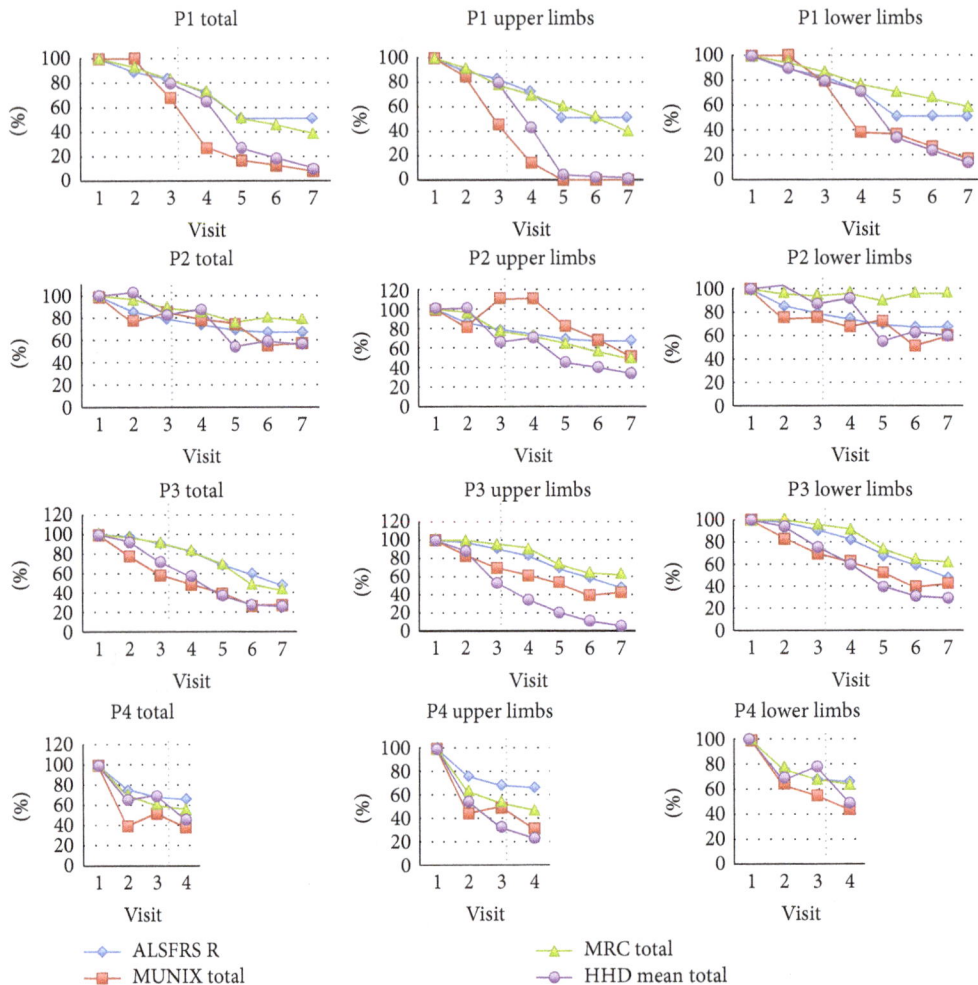

FIGURE 5: Muscle strength and electrophysiological assessment. The detailed clinical evaluation performed within one week of the neurosurgery procedure and repeated every 3 months throughout the project was complemented with ALS-FRS-R, MRC, MUNIX, and HHD evaluation. ALSFRS R and MRC shared a similar deterioration pattern. The slope of decline was much steeper in the case of both MUNIX and muscle strength as examined by HHD. The MUNIX and HHD showed a marked decline even when the values of ALSFRS R and MRC were still stable (P1, P2, and P3—resp. patient 1, patient 2, and patient 3).

marked decline even when the values of ALSFRS R and MRC were still stable. At the time of transplantation (from 3 to 6 months after the inclusion to the study), the ALSFRS R was 83%, 79%, 91%, and 68% of the value obtained at visit 1 (V1), whereas total MUNIX was as low as 68%, 85%, 59%, and 52% in patients P1, P2, P3, and P4, respectively (Figure 5). The above pattern was also present when upper and lower limbs were analyzed separately.

The values of three functional tests, which separately assessed the upper limbs, lower limbs, and the trunk,

decreased faster and earlier than ALSFRS R. In patient P1, they all reached 50% of their initial value prior to V4, in patient P2 and P3 at V5 (except for TCT in P3), whereas ALSFRS R reached the same level at V5 (P1) and V7 (P3), or did not reach it yet (P2). Patient P4 only had 3 visits to date; his results could not be analyzed in this aspect.

The results of 2MWT matched those of MUNIX and HHD, but not MRC in the same extremities (Figures 4–6). The reduction of MUNIX values was an earlier event; however, the magnitude of 2MWT drop was higher. To

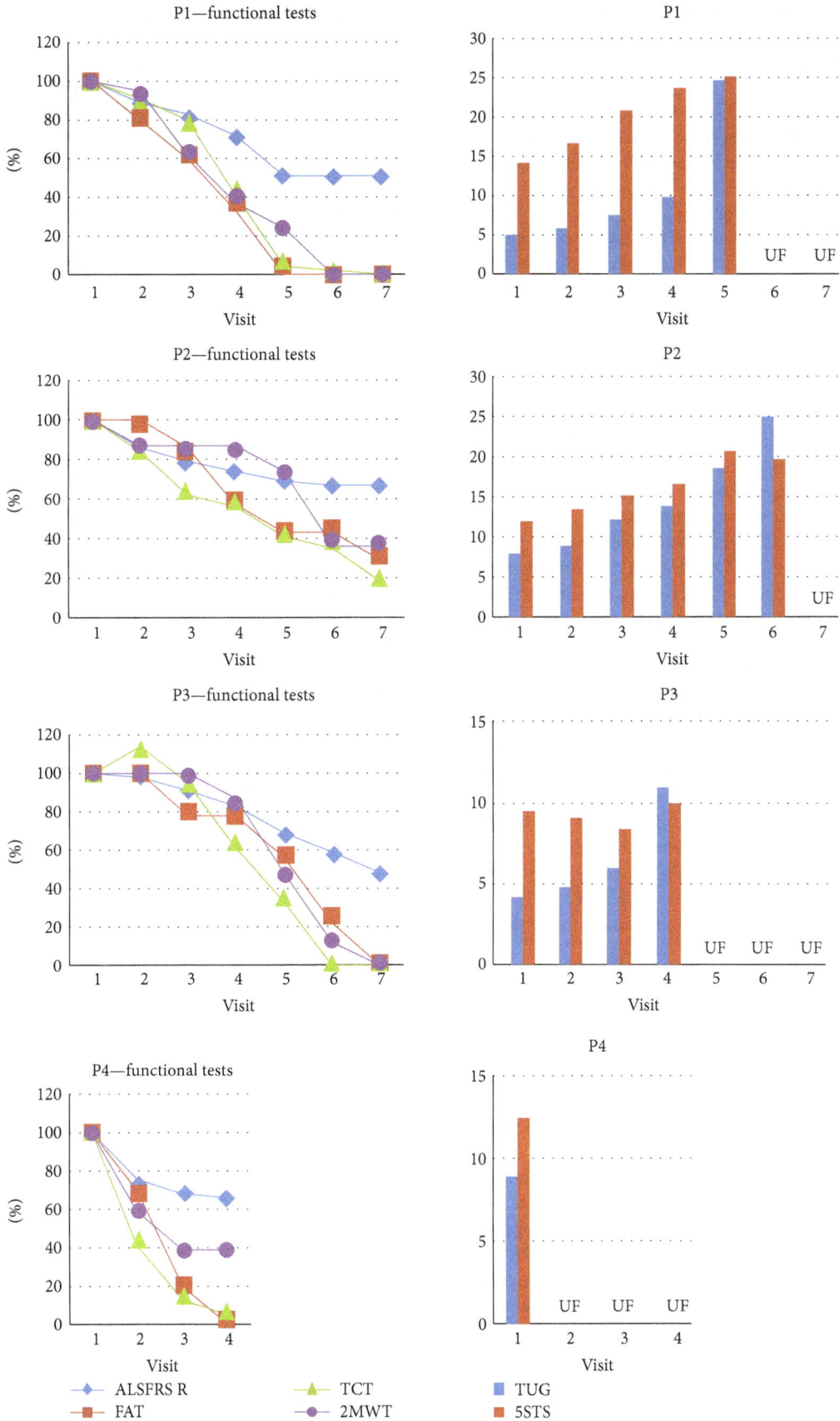

FIGURE 6: Comparison of the course of the disease before and after the cell therapy. The graphs show the course of disease preceding the use of ADRC (blue graph) and the course of disease during cell therapy.

a lesser extent, a similar correlation was found between the results of FAT, the only functional test assessing exclusively upper limbs, and MUNIX/HHD in the upper extremities (Figures 4–6).

Although 5STS and TUG showed good correlation with other functional parameters, their longitudinal use was limited in patients who were no longer able to stand up without the help of their arms/hands (on average 6–9 months after the first transplantation) (Figure 6).

The ALS patients differed in terms of spasticity, which—in all cases—increased with disease progression. The MAS results ranged from 1.06 (1.37 ± 0.25 in patient P1, 1.5 in P2, 0.0 in P3 and 1.37 ± 0.35 in P4) at the first visit to 1.84 (2.25 ± 0.7, 2.12 ± 1.06, 1 ± 1.4 and 2 ± 0.35, respectively) at the last follow-up visit (Vt). Due to spasticity, the MRC results could not be interpreted in P2 and P4. The spasticity did not correlate with fatigue (data not shown).

No differences in the progression rate of ALSFRS R was found between the pre- and posttransplantation observation period (Figure 5). There was a prominent increase in MUNIX results in P2 prior to intraspinal transplantation and 3 months after and in the posttransplantation period in the case of P4 (Figure 5). After intraspinal transplantation, MUNIX showed a higher progression rate in P1 and no changes in P3. The 2MWT decrease was stable in P1 and P3, whereas it was markedly increased in P2 and P4.

The FSS was found increased in all patients. It scored from the level of 39–50 at V1 to 50–68 at Vt.

The results of psychological assessment (ADI-2) showed mild depression (score 27) in two out of four patients prior to transplantation. It increased within the first 12 months of observation reaching the level of 30–33 (clinically relevant depression) in all patients (4/4) and required antidepressive treatment. None of the patients presented a wish for hastened death throughout the study. The QoL (ACSA) was very low in patients P2 and P4 (−5) and neutral in P1 (−1) and P3 (1). After 12 months, it markedly increased in the first two patients (1) and slightly decreased in P1 (−2) and P3 (−1).

3.2. Cell Culture: ADRC Parameters. Using a 1 ml suspension, we obtained approx. 14×10^6/ml ADRC with 95% viability, expressing CD73 (99.3% of cells), CD90 (99.6%), and CD105 (89.1%) as well as CD34, CD19, CD11b, and HLA-DR (all in 1.7% of cells) as surface markers which was in line with our previous experiments (10). According to ISCT recommendation, the ability of the MSC population to create CFU (colony-forming unit fibroblasts) was considered one of the most specific tests to define the content of stem/progenitor cells in the whole heterogeneous MSC population, thus predicting expansion and longevity of the ADRC cells. Our results indicate that ADRCs isolated with the described method do contain a relatively high fraction of the genuine stem cells to approx. 20% of total (Figure 2(c)).

In the next task, the factors involved in self-renewal, regeneration, and immunomodulatory capacity of ADRC were analyzed in all CSF samples gathered according to the scheme given in Material and Methods. We have performed analysis of 102 cytokines/chemokines in the CSF of ALS patients in the samples taken before cell transplantation

and then at 24 hours after each subsequent cell application, in order to correlate the change in their expression with course of the disease. Unfortunately, the pattern of their expression changed individually without any common trend neither for the whole group of patients nor for the particular stages of the disease (Figure 2(a)). Among these cytokines, only six factors have been identified, the levels of which would be correlated with the therapeutic effect of ADRC treatment. They exhibited a decrease in CSF levels of proinflammatory TNFα, IFN-γ, and IL-1β after MSC transplantation, but more interestingly with the exception of those taken 24 hours after the first ADRC injection when they remain unchanged or even elevated in comparison with the CSF samples from untreated patients. In contrast to this, growth factors and anti-inflammatory/regressive agents like IL-6, bFGF, and MMP-9 have been increased in most samples as well as those gathered at 24 hours after cell administration (Figure 2(b)).

4. Discussion

Qualification of ALS patients to controlled pharmacological clinical trials encounters a number of obstacles resulting from the disease character. They include prolonged diagnosis delay, variable clinical certainty at diagnosis, clinical phenotype conditioning disease progression, and a short ventilation-free survival [35]. Clinical trials including neurosurgical procedures, like in the case of intraspinal stem cell transplantation, additionally face the problem of bulbar and respiratory involvement interfering with anesthesia. In order to enable functional analysis, they also require a partially preserved function of muscles innervated by the studied part of the spinal cord. For these reasons, despite a high number of patients followed in our ALS center, their final eligibility for the current trial was only 3.2%. Our finding goes in line with recently published results from the French ALS registry where nearly 40% of patients had diagnosis delay > 12 months, over 30% of patients had a bulbar disease onset, 15% had other phenotype than classic ALS, and in nearly 30% of cases the diagnosis was only clinically possible [36]. When adding age limit, functional stage according to ALSFRS R, and the reduced FVC, the number of patients potentially eligible for a stem cell clinical trial dropped dramatically.

Intraspinal ADRC transplantation at the Th10/11 level was proved safe and well tolerated. In two patients, neurosurgery induced reduction of the muscle tone, which resulted in improved walking capacity of a one-month duration, objectively measured in one case. There was also a reduction in the progression rate of walking impairment within 3 months after the transplantation in the same patient. Both patients had a prevalent upper motor neuron involvement (UMN) with marked spasticity, and the effect was not observed after an intrathecal ADRC infusion. It suggests an intraspinal mechanism—either due to neurosurgical manipulation similar to postcontusion neurogenic shock or due to an immunomodulatory effect of the ADRC. Although the sedation effect could not be excluded within the first two days, both patients reported persistence of this state for the 4 following weeks. The phenomenon has not been previously reported following neurosurgical operations (if not after a pathologic mass removal). We did not observe any deterioration due to a reduced muscle tone in two other operated patients (including one with prevalent lower motor neuron (LMN) impairment) that could potentially decrease their physical performance.

Otherwise, the study did not prove effective in terms of reversing or relenting the disease progression. The limitations of the current study included an open-label character and a low patient number limiting the use of statistical analyses. However, a number of observations have been made. From all applied measures, MUNIX proved to be the first and the most sensitive tool in identifying fine changes at the muscle level. It was markedly more sensitive than ALSFRS R and MRC which was earlier found in electrophysiological studies in ALS [37]. Previous studies have also shown that unlike the majority of other ALS outcome measures (FVC, ALS-FRS, and survival), MUNIX has not been subject to high variability [38]. It also showed a high interrater reproducibility in patients with ALS [39]. Moreover, in longitudinal studies, it was reduced not only in paretic but also in presymptomatic muscles [40]. This feature is of utmost importance as it enables monitoring of fine changes during the stem cell therapies. The transplantations should however be planned earlier in the disease course since, as shown by the same group, at the time of diagnosis the total MUNIX score in ALS patients is reduced by 70% compared to healthy volunteers [41]. In an advanced process, the protective stem cell properties might not be sufficient to influence the clinical outcome.

Interestingly, in our hands MUNIX was higher in patients with prevalent UMN involvement. It may be due to the muscle fiber overwork accompanying spasticity. A similar phenomenon was described in Parkinson's disease. The authors found changed muscle's mechanical properties including increased muscle bulk related to structural changes within muscles accompanying pathological central neural drive [42]. Longitudinal studies on MUNIX in patients with marked UMN involvement as compared to those with preferential LMN damage should shed more light on this process. By that time, it is important to measure spasticity level in all patients who undergo intraspinal stem cell therapy. It might also be worth considering the use of averaging multiple MUNIX measures recently described in longitudinal assessment of ALS patients in order to further objectify results [43].

In our hand, the Modified Ashworth Scale was a sensitive tool in a potential patient stratification according to the spasticity level. A recent meta-analysis of studies regarding reliability of the scale showed a satisfactory inter- and intrarater agreement. MAS scores exhibited better reliability when measuring upper extremities compared to lower extremities [44]. It might explain the lack of score change in patient P4 who reported decreased muscle spasticity following the intraspinal transplantation procedure resulting in objective walking improvement.

In our current study, the dynamometry was the closest measurement to MUNIX, both on the upper and lower limb level. It was a fine tool in terms of slope and range of change in the course of the disease. The utility of this measure was proved in several other studies, showing a high reliability especially in early disease stages [19, 22, 42]. To our knowledge, to date it was not compared to MUNIX in longitudinal monitoring of the disease course.

Beside muscle and motor unit assessment, we found the functional tests very useful in a complex analysis of the preserved physical power of the limbs and trunk. ALSFRS R is the reference functional scale for all the clinical trials; it is simple and easy to use at every check-up visit. However, it asymmetrically addresses the functions of the bulbar muscles (12 points), upper (12 points), lower limbs (8 points), and trunk (4 points), together with respiratory functions (12 points). For this reason, an analysis of FAT, 2MWT, and TCT at the same time points allows for a more precise description of disease progression. By addressing the functions of one part of musculature at a time, this non-time-consuming examination (lasting up to 20 min altogether) gives a wider range of scores able to reflect more subtle changes over the disease course and applied treatment.

Although very useful in several neurologic conditions [45] as well as in elderly patients [30], 5STS and TUG have been found of limited use in monitoring the disease progression in patients with ALS. Since both techniques require standing up from a sitting position, patients with increased proximal muscles paresis were not able to perform the tests as early as 3 months after transplantation. Despite assessing trunk muscles in a more limited way, 2MTW was proved more easily applicable and showed a very early decrease with a wide range of change. Its combination with assessment of fatigability by RPE has given additional reassuring information (as p.ex. in P2 whose walking distance improved after the intraspinal transplantation which was accompanied by a marked decrease in fatigability by REP). Fatigue was reported by 83% of ALS patients [46]. It was the most prevalent symptom in the late stage of ALS, significantly decreasing the quality of life [47, 48]. It was also an important reason to give up physical activity [49]. In our study, all patients presented increased fatigue from the first visit. Longitudinal analysis showed its further increase with time. Despite close monitoring, multidisciplinary care, and participation in a clinical trial, all patients developed clinically relevant depression requiring pharmacological treatment. Since in the general ALS population, depression does not significantly increase with disease progression [50], the higher depression levels observed at the end of the study might have been due to the lack of improvement following the intervention. Interestingly, QoL did not go along with depression in individual cases. Primarily very low in 2 patients and neutral in the remaining two, it became neutral in all cases. The increase of QoL despite an apparent increase in motor impairment is probably due to the previously described adaptation process [51].

Beside a broad experience in patients' monitoring, there is still a need to find a correlation between the clinical management and quality of the used transplantation material. Analysis of MSC secretive properties in vitro and in vivo suggests the need for repeated/cyclic ADRC transplantation. It seems that the optimal time between consecutive transplantations in order to support their therapeutic effect is about

3 months [52]. This is in line with the first paper published in 2010 by our group, describing intracerebroventricular transplantation of cord blood-derived neural progenitors in a child with severe global brain ischemic injury. After a subsequent transplantation of the cells tagged with SPIO nanoparticles, we found them to have persisted at a wall of the lateral ventricle for about 4 months [53]. The levels of cytokines found in CSF at 3 months after ADRC transplantation are also in agreement with the data reported by others [54], stating that the route of intraspinal cell delivery is effective, feasible, and most probably optimal because of their strait vicinity or even incorporation into the host's neural network [55].

The cytokine and chemokine changes observed here after ADRC transplantation correspond well with the data published by Tyndall et al. [12]. Although abnormal levels of interleukin IL-6 are described mainly in relation to inflammatory processes [56], it should also be remembered that in reverse, IL-6 as belonging to the so-called dual-function cytokines may also inhibit TNF-alpha and IL-1β expression. Lu et al. [57] demonstrated in a cohort of ALS patients that IL-6 had a significantly increased expression at the end-stage of the disease. This may explain the increase found in our first patient (P1), the only one who has died during the course of observation. Conversely, in the other patients the level of IL-6 remained rather stable together with concomitant decrease of TNF-alpha and IL-1β. In light of the previously reported negative correlation between the levels of these cytokines and the duration and severity of ALS [58], this effect of ADRC which inhibits TNF-alpha and IL-1β expression seems to be therapeutically promising.

The above conclusion is also in line with other experiences gathered during preclinical experiments. They suggest that highly proliferating, undifferentiated, SRTF-expressing cells present in ADRC population are one of the most effective material in therapeutic transplantation.

To sum up, there is a strong need for an international collaborative effort facilitating an early and effective enrollment of ALS patients into stem cell clinical trials. It will help also to improve enrollment and monitoring criteria, which may result in more coherent and reliable data [59, 60].

Keeping in mind the limitations of the study, suggestions from the presented research indicate the following:

(1) Enlargement of the group of patients at the early stage of disease selected from several centers

(2) MUNIX analysis in patients with marked UMN involvement/together with MAS

(3) Combination of MUNIX, HHD, MAS, 2MWT (with BS), FSS, FAT, and TCT (approx. 1 h) which may help obtain results along the disease progression

Acknowledgments

This work was partially supported by National Centre for Research and Development Grant no. Strategmed 1/234261/2/NCBR/2014 as well as OnWebDuals and Needs in ALS projects (JPND-PS/0001/2013 and JPND 01ED1405). This is an EU Joint Programme-Neurodegenerative Disease Research (JPND) project. The project is supported through the following funding organisations under JPND (http://www.jpnd.eu): Germany, Bundesministerium für Bildung und Forschung (BMBF); Poland, Narodowe Centrum Badan i Rozwoju (NCBiR, DZP/2/JPND-II/2014 and JPND/02/2015); Portugal, Fundação a Ciência e a Tecnologia (FCT); and Sweden, Vetenskapsrådet (VR).

References

[1] L. J. Haverkamp, V. Appel, and S. H. Appel, "Natural history of amyotrophic lateral sclerosis in a database population. Validation of a scoring system and a model for survival prediction," *Brain*, vol. 118, no. 3, pp. 707–719, 1995.

[2] R. G. Miller, J. D. Mitchell, M. Lyon, and D. H. Moore, "Riluzole for amyotrophic lateral sclerosis (ALS)/motor neuron disease (MND)," *Cochrane Database of Systematic Reviews*, vol. 3, 2002.

[3] The Edaravone (Mci-186) Als 16 Study Group, "A post-hoc subgroup analysis of outcomes in the first phase III clinical study of edaravone (MCI-186) in amyotrophic lateral sclerosis," *Amyotrophic Lateral Sclerosis and Frontotemporal Degeneration*, vol. 18, no. sup1, pp. 11–19, 2017.

[4] T. M. Miller, A. Pestronk, W. David et al., "An antisense oligonucleotide against SOD1 delivered intrathecally for patients with SOD1 familial amyotrophic lateral sclerosis: a phase 1, randomised, first-in-man study," *Lancet Neurology*, vol. 12, no. 5, pp. 435–442, 2013.

[5] M. J. Crisp, K. G. Mawuenyega, B. W. Patterson et al., "In vivo kinetic approach reveals slow SOD1 turnover in the CNS," *The Journal of Clinical Investigation*, vol. 125, no. 7, pp. 2772–2780, 2015.

[6] H. Deda, M. C. Inci, A. E. Kürekçi et al., "Treatment of amyotrophic lateral sclerosis patients by autologous bone marrow-derived hematopoietic stem cell transplantation: a 1-year follow-up," *Cytotherapy*, vol. 11, no. 1, pp. 18–25, 2009.

[7] L. Mazzini, K. Mareschi, I. Ferrero et al., "Mesenchymal stromal cell transplantation in amyotrophic lateral sclerosis: a long-term safety study," *Cytotherapy*, vol. 14, no. 1, pp. 56–60, 2012.

[8] J. Riley, T. Federici, M. Polak et al., "Intraspinal stem cell transplantation in amyotrophic lateral sclerosis: a phase I safety trial, technical note, and lumbar safety outcomes," *Neurosurgery*, vol. 71, no. 2, pp. 405–416, 2012.

[9] N. Atassi, E. Beghi, M. Blanquer et al., "Intraspinal stem cell transplantation for amyotrophic lateral sclerosis: ready for efficacy clinical trials?," *Cytotherapy*, vol. 18, no. 12, pp. 1471–1475, 2016.

[10] W. Lech, A. Figiel-Dabrowska, A. Sarnowska et al., "Phenotypic, functional, and safety control at preimplantation phase of MSC-based therapy," *Stem Cells International*, vol. 2016, 13 pages, 2016.

[11] S. Dabrowska, J. Sypecka, A. Jablonska et al., "Neuroprotective potential and paracrine activity of stromal vs. culture-expanded hMSC derived from Wharton jelly under co-cultured with hippocampal organotypic slices," *Molecular Neurobiology*, vol. 55, no. 7, pp. 6021–6036, 2018.

[12] A. Tyndall, U. A. Walker, A. Cope et al., "Immunomodulatory properties of mesenchymal stem cells: a review based on an

interdisciplinary meeting held at the Kennedy Institute of Rheumatology Division, London, UK, 31 October 2005," *Arthritis Research & Therapy*, vol. 9, no. 1, p. 301, 2007.

[13] H. Kanno, "Regenerative therapy for neuronal diseases with transplantation of somatic stem cells," *World Journal of Stem Cells*, vol. 5, no. 4, pp. 163–171, 2013.

[14] B. Gornicka-Pawlak el, M. Janowski, A. Habich et al., "Systemic treatment of focal brain injury in the rat by human umbilical cord blood cells being at different level of neural commitment," *Acta Neurobiologiae Experimentalis*, vol. 71, no. 1, pp. 46–64, 2011.

[15] J. K. Fraser, K. C. Hicok, R. Shanahan, M. Zhu, S. Miller, and D. M. Arm, "The Celution® system: automated processing of adipose-derived regenerative cells in a functionally closed system," *Advances in Wound Care*, vol. 3, no. 1, pp. 38–45, 2014.

[16] G. Marino, M. Moraci, E. Armenia et al., "Therapy with autologous adipose-derived regenerative cells for the care of chronic ulcer of lower limbs in patients with peripheral arterial disease," *The Journal of Surgical Research*, vol. 185, no. 1, pp. 36–44, 2013.

[17] N. E. Krześniak and B. H. Noszczyk, "Autologous fat transfer in secondary carpal tunnel release," *Plastic and Reconstructive Surgery - Global Open*, vol. 3, no. 5, article e401, 2015.

[18] R. P. Kleyweg, F. G. A. Van Der Meché, and P. I. M. Schmitz, "Interobserver agreement in the assessment of muscle strength and functional abilities in Guillain-Barré syndrome," *Muscle & Nerve*, vol. 14, no. 11, pp. 1103–1109, 1991.

[19] J. M. Shefner, "Strength testing in motor neuron diseases," *Neurotherapeutics*, vol. 14, no. 1, pp. 154–160, 2017.

[20] J. M. Cedarbaum and N. Stambler, "Performance of the amyotrophic lateral sclerosis functional rating scale (ALSFRS) in multicenter clinical trials," *Journal of the Neurological Sciences*, vol. 152, Suppl 1, pp. S1–S9, 1997.

[21] A. Heller, D. T. Wade, V. A. Wood, A. Sunderland, R. L. Hewer, and E. Ward, "Arm function after stroke: measurement and recovery over the first three months," *Journal of Neurology, Neurosurgery, and Psychiatry*, vol. 50, no. 6, pp. 714–719, 1987.

[22] C. Collin and D. Wade, "Assessing motor impairment after stroke: a pilot reliability study," *Journal of Neurology, Neurosurgery, and Psychiatry*, vol. 53, no. 7, pp. 576–579, 1990.

[23] R. J. Butland, J. Pang, E. R. Gross, A. A. Woodcock, and D. M. Geddes, "Two-, six-, and 12-minute walking tests in respiratory disease," *BMJ*, vol. 284, no. 6329, pp. 1607-1608, 1982.

[24] G. A. V. Borg, "Psychophysical bases of perceived exertion," *Medicine & Science in Sports & Exercise*, vol. 14, no. 5, pp. 377–381, 1982.

[25] L. B. Krupp, N. G. LaRocca, J. Muir-Nash, and A. D. Steinberg, "The fatigue severity scale. Application to patients with multiple sclerosis and systemic lupus erythematosus," *Archives of Neurology*, vol. 46, no. 10, pp. 1121–1123, 1989.

[26] S. Mathias, U. S. Nayak, and B. Isaacs, "Balance in elderly patients: the "get-up and go" test," *Archives of Physical Medicine and Rehabilitation*, vol. 67, no. 6, pp. 387–389, 1986.

[27] D. Podsiadlo and S. Richardson, "The timed "up & go": a test of basic functional mobility for frail elderly persons," *Journal of the American Geriatrics Society*, vol. 39, no. 2, pp. 142–148, 1991.

[28] K. L. Newcomer, H. E. Krug, and M. L. Mahowald, "Validity and reliability of the timed-stands test for patients with rheu-matoid arthritis and other chronic diseases," *The Journal of Rheumatology*, vol. 20, no. 1, pp. 21–27, 1993.

[29] N. L. Ashworth, L. E. Satkunam, and D. Deforge, "Treatment for spasticity in amyotrophic lateral sclerosis/motor neuron disease," *The Cochrane Database of Systematic Reviews*, vol. 2, 2012.

[30] R. W. Bohannon, "Reference values for the five-repetition sit-to-stand test: a descriptive meta-analysis of data from elders," *Perceptual and Motor Skills*, vol. 103, no. 1, pp. 215–222, 2016.

[31] E. M. Hammer, S. Häcker, M. Hautzinger, T. D. Meyer, and A. Kübler, "Validity of the ALS-Depression-Inventory (ADI-12)— a new screening instrument for depressive disorders in patients with amyotrophic lateral sclerosis," *Journal of Affective Disorders*, vol. 109, no. 1-2, pp. 213–219, 2008.

[32] J. L. Bernham, "How to get serious answers to the serious question: "how have you been?": subjective quality of life (QOL) as an individual experiential emergent construct," *Bioethics*, vol. 13, no. 3-4, pp. 272–287, 1999.

[33] C. Neuwirth, M. Weber, E. Stålberg et al., "Motor Unit Number Index (MUNIX): a novel neurophysiological marker for neuromuscular disorders; test-retest reliability in healthy volunteers," *Clinical Neurophysiology*, vol. 122, no. 9, pp. 1867–1872, 2011.

[34] H. Mitsumoto, B. R. Brooks, and V. Silani, "Clinical trials in amyotrophic lateral sclerosis: why so many negative trials and how can trials be improved?," *The Lancet Neurology*, vol. 13, no. 11, pp. 1127–1138, 2014.

[35] B. Hamidou, B. Marin, G. Lautrette et al., "Exploring the diagnosis delay and ALS functional impairment at diagnosis as relevant criteria for clinical trial enrolment," *Amyotrophic Lateral Sclerosis and Frontotemporal Degeneration*, vol. 18, no. 7-8, pp. 519–527, 2017.

[36] W. A. Boekestein, H. J. Schelhaas, M. J. A. M. van Putten, D. F. Stegeman, M. J. Zwarts, and J. P. van Dijk, "Motor unit number index (MUNIX) versus motor unit number estimation (MUNE): a direct comparison in a longitudinal study of ALS patients," *Clinical Neurophysiology*, vol. 123, no. 8, pp. 1644–1649, 2012.

[37] C. Neuwirth, S. Nandedkar, E. StålBerg, and M. Weber, "Motor unit number index (MUNIX): a novel neurophysiological technique to follow disease progression in amyotrophic lateral sclerosis," *Muscle & Nerve*, vol. 42, no. 3, pp. 379–384, 2010.

[38] S. D. Nandedkar, P. E. Barkhaus, and E. V. Stålberg, "Reproducibility of MUNIX in patients with amyotrophic lateral sclerosis," *Muscle & Nerve*, vol. 44, no. 6, pp. 919–922, 2011.

[39] C. Neuwirth, P. E. Barkhaus, C. Burkhardt et al., "Motor unit number index (MUNIX) detects motor neuron loss in pre-symptomatic muscles in amyotrophic lateral sclerosis," *Clinical Neurophysiology*, vol. 128, no. 3, pp. 495–500, 2017.

[40] J. Marusiak, A. Jaskólska, M. Koszewicz, S. Budrewicz, and A. Jaskólski, "Myometry revealed medication-induced decrease in resting skeletal muscle stiffness in Parkinson's disease patients," *Clinical Biomechanics*, vol. 27, no. 6, pp. 632–635, 2012.

[41] A. B. Meseguer-Henarejos, J. Sánchez-Meca, J. A. López-Pina, and R. Carles-Hernández, "Inter- and intra-rater reliability of the Modified Ashworth Scale: a systematic review and meta-analysis," *European Journal of Physical and Rehabilitation Medicine*, vol. 13, 2017.

[42] M. Beck, R. Giess, W. Würffel, T. Magnus, G. Ochs, and K. V. Toyka, "Comparison of maximal voluntary isometric contraction and Drachman's hand-held dynamometry in evaluating patients with amyotrophic lateral sclerosis," *Muscle & Nerve*, vol. 22, no. 9, pp. 1265–1270, 1999.

[43] M. L. Escorcio-Bezerra, A. Abrahao, D. Santos-Neto, N. I. de Oliveira Braga, A. S. B. Oliveira, and G. M. Manzano, "Why averaging multiple MUNIX measures in the longitudinal assessment of patients with ALS?," *Clinical Neurophysiology*, vol. 128, no. 12, pp. 2392–2396, 2017.

[44] J. Visser, E. Mans, M. de Visser et al., "Comparison of maximal voluntary isometric contraction and hand-held dynamometry in measuring muscle strength of patients with progressive lower motor neuron syndrome," *Neuromuscular Disorders*, vol. 13, no. 9, pp. 744–750, 2003.

[45] Y. Mong, T. W. Teo, and S. S. Ng, "5-Repetition sit-to-stand test in subjects with chronic stroke: reliability and validity," *Archives of Physical Medicine and Rehabilitation*, vol. 91, no. 3, pp. 407–413, 2010.

[46] C. Ramirez, M. E. P. Piemonte, D. Callegaro, and H. C. A. Da Silva, "Fatigue in amyotrophic lateral sclerosis: frequency and associated factors," *Amyotrophic Lateral Sclerosis*, vol. 9, no. 2, pp. 75–80, 2009.

[47] The EFNS Task Force on Diagnosis and Management of Amyotrophic Lateral Sclerosis, P. M. Andersen, S. Abrahams et al., "EFNS guidelines on the clinical management of amyotrophic lateral sclerosis (MALS)- revised report of an EFNS task force," *European Journal of Neurology*, vol. 19, no. 3, pp. 360–375, 2012.

[48] A. Abraham and V. E. Drory, "Fatigue in motor neuron diseases," *Neuromuscular Disorders*, vol. 22, Supplement 3, pp. S198–S202, 2012.

[49] V. E. Drory, E. Goltsman, J. Goldman Reznik, A. Mosek, and A. D. Korczyn, "The value of muscle exercise in patients with amyotrophic lateral sclerosis," *Journal of the Neurological Sciences*, vol. 191, no. 1-2, pp. 133–137, 2001.

[50] N. J. Thakore and E. P. Pioro, "Depression in ALS in a large self-reporting cohort," *Neurology*, vol. 86, no. 11, pp. 1031–1038, 2016.

[51] D. Lulé, S. Pauli, E. Altintas et al., "Emotional adjustment in amyotrophic lateral sclerosis (ALS)," *Journal of Neurology*, vol. 259, no. 2, pp. 334–341, 2012.

[52] E. Syková, P. Rychmach, I. Drahorádová et al., "Transplantation of mesenchymal stromal cells in patients with amyotrophic lateral sclerosis: results of phase I/IIa clinical trial," *Cell Transplantation*, vol. 26, no. 4, pp. 647–658, 2017.

[53] S. Jozwiak, A. Habich, K. Kotulska et al., "Intracerebroventricular transplantation of cord blood-derived neural progenitors in a child with severe global brain ischemic injury," *Cell Medicine*, vol. 1, no. 2, pp. 71–80, 2010.

[54] L. Mazzini, K. Mareschi, I. Ferrero et al., "Autologous mesenchymal stem cells: clinical applications in amyotrophic lateral sclerosis," *Neurological Research*, vol. 28, no. 5, pp. 523–526, 2013.

[55] T. Tadesse, M. Gearing, D. Senitzer et al., "Analysis of graft survival in a trial of stem cell transplant in ALS," *Annals of Clinical Translational Neurology*, vol. 1, no. 11, pp. 900–908, 2014.

[56] C. Moreau, D. Devos, V. Brunaud-Danel et al., "Elevated IL-6 and TNF-α levels in patients with ALS: Inflammation or hypoxia?," *Neurology*, vol. 65, no. 12, pp. 1958–1960, 2005.

[57] C.-H. Lu, K. Allen, F. Oei et al., "Systemic inflammatory response and neuromuscular involvement in amyotrophic lateral sclerosis," *Neurology - Neuroimmunology Neuroinflammation*, vol. 3, no. 4, p. e244, 2016.

[58] Y. Hu, C. Cao, X. Y. Qin et al., "Increased peripheral blood inflammatory cytokine levels in amyotrophic lateral sclerosis: a meta-analysis study," *Scientific Reports*, vol. 7, no. 1, p. 9094, 2017.

[59] N. Katyal and R. Govindarajan, "Shortcomings in the current amyotrophic lateral sclerosis trials and potential solutions for improvement," *Frontiers in Neurology*, vol. 8, 2017.

[60] M. Kraemer, M. Buerger, and P. Berlit, "Diagnostic problems and delay of diagnosis in amyotrophic lateral sclerosis," *Clinical Neurology and Neurosurgery*, vol. 112, no. 2, pp. 103–105, 2010.

Permissions

All chapters in this book were first published in SCI, by Hindawi Publishing Corporation; hereby published with permission under the Creative Commons Attribution License or equivalent. Every chapter published in this book has been scrutinized by our experts. Their significance has been extensively debated. The topics covered herein carry significant findings which will fuel the growth of the discipline. They may even be implemented as practical applications or may be referred to as a beginning point for another development.

The contributors of this book come from diverse backgrounds, making this book a truly international effort. This book will bring forth new frontiers with its revolutionizing research information and detailed analysis of the nascent developments around the world.

We would like to thank all the contributing authors for lending their expertise to make the book truly unique. They have played a crucial role in the development of this book. Without their invaluable contributions this book wouldn't have been possible. They have made vital efforts to compile up to date information on the varied aspects of this subject to make this book a valuable addition to the collection of many professionals and students.

This book was conceptualized with the vision of imparting up-to-date information and advanced data in this field. To ensure the same, a matchless editorial board was set up. Every individual on the board went through rigorous rounds of assessment to prove their worth. After which they invested a large part of their time researching and compiling the most relevant data for our readers.

The editorial board has been involved in producing this book since its inception. They have spent rigorous hours researching and exploring the diverse topics which have resulted in the successful publishing of this book. They have passed on their knowledge of decades through this book. To expedite this challenging task, the publisher supported the team at every step. A small team of assistant editors was also appointed to further simplify the editing procedure and attain best results for the readers.

Apart from the editorial board, the designing team has also invested a significant amount of their time in understanding the subject and creating the most relevant covers. They scrutinized every image to scout for the most suitable representation of the subject and create an appropriate cover for the book.

The publishing team has been an ardent support to the editorial, designing and production team. Their endless efforts to recruit the best for this project, has resulted in the accomplishment of this book. They are a veteran in the field of academics and their pool of knowledge is as vast as their experience in printing. Their expertise and guidance has proved useful at every step. Their uncompromising quality standards have made this book an exceptional effort. Their encouragement from time to time has been an inspiration for everyone.

The publisher and the editorial board hope that this book will prove to be a valuable piece of knowledge for researchers, students, practitioners and scholars across the globe.

List of Contributors

Jonathan Lozano-Salgado, Maria Alexandra Rodriguez-Sastre and Emilio Rojas
Instituto de Investigaciones Biomédicas, Universidad Nacional Autónoma de México, C.U. 04510, Mexico

Mahara Valverde
Instituto de Investigaciones Biomédicas, Universidad Nacional Autónoma de México, C.U. 04510, Mexico
Department of Environment and Health, Istituto Superiore di Sanità, Viale Regina Elena 299, 00161 Roma, Italy

Paola Fortini and Eugenia Dogliotti
Department of Environment and Health, Istituto Superiore di Sanità, Viale Regina Elena 299, 00161 Roma, Italy

Shuaishuai Zhang, Junqin Li, Huijie Jiang, Yi Gao, Pengzhen Cheng, Tianqing Cao, Yue Song, Bin Liu, Hao Wu, Chunmei Wang, Liu Yang and Guoxian Pei
Department of Orthopaedics, Xijing Hospital, Fourth Military Medical University, Xi'an 710032, China

Donglin Li
Department of Orthopaedics, The 463rd Hospital of PLA, Shenyang 110042, China

Jimeng Wang
Department of Orthopaedics, The 251st Hospital of PLA, Zhangjiakou 075000, China

Jihye Kwak, Soo Jin Choi, Wonil Oh, Yoon Sun Yang, Hong Bae Jeon and Eun Su Jeon
Biomedical Research Institute, R&D Center, and MEDIPOST Co, Ltd, 21 Daewangpangyo-ro 644 Beon-gil, Bundang-gu, Seongnam-si, 13494 Gyeonggi-do, Republic of Korea

Jennifer Steens and Diana Klein
Institute for Cell Biology (Cancer Research), University Hospital Essen, University of Duisburg-Essen, Essen, Germany

Tingting Meng, Ying Zhou, Jingkun Li, Meilin Hu, Pingting Wang, Zhi Jia and Dayong Liu
Department of Endodontics & Laboratory of Stem Cells and Endocrine Immunology, Tianjin Medical University School of Stomatology, Tianjin 300070, China

Xiaomeng Li
Department of Prosthodontics, Tianjin Medical University School of Stomatology, Tianjin 300070, China

Liyu Li
Department of Intensive Care Unit, The Second Hospital of Tianjin Medical University, Tianjin 300211, China

Shuhui Zheng, Yongyong Li and Caixia Xu
Research Center for Translational Medicine, The First Affiliated Hospital of Sun Yat-sen University, Guangzhou, China

Hang Zhou, Taifeng Zhou and Peiqiang Su
Department of Orthopedic Surgery, The First Affiliated Hospital of Sun Yat-sen University, Guangzhou, China

Zhuohui Chen
Oral and Maxillofacial Surgery, Guanghua School of Stomatology, Hospital of Stomatology, Sun Yat-sen University,Guangzhou, China

Chengjie Lian and Bo Gao
Department of Spine Surgery, Sun Yat-Sen Memorial Hospital, Sun Yat-sen University, Guangzhou, China

Yunqian Guan, Chunsong Zhao and Zhiguo Chen
Cell Therapy Center, Xuanwu Hospital, Capital Medical University, and Key Laboratory of Neurodegeneration,Ministry of Education, Beijing, China

Xiaobo Li, Wenxiu Yu, Zhaohui Liang, Min Huang, Renchao Zhao and Yao Liu
Department of Neurology, Northern Jiangsu People's Hospital, Clinical Medical School of Yangzhou University, Yangzhou, China

Haiqiang Zou
Department of Neurology, The General Hospital of Guangzhou Military Command, Guangzhou, China

Yanli Hao
Department of Anatomy, Guangzhou Medical University, Guangzhou, China

Stefania Niada
IRCCS Istituto Ortopedico Galeazzi, Milan, Italy

Chiara Giannasi and Anna Teresa Brini
IRCCS Istituto Ortopedico Galeazzi, Milan, Italy
Department of Biomedical, Surgical and Dental Sciences, Università degli Studi di Milano, Milan, Italy

Giuseppe Banfi
IRCCS Istituto Ortopedico Galeazzi, Milan, Italy
Vita-Salute San Raffaele University, via Olgettina 58, 20132 Milan, Italy

Alice Gualerzi
Laboratory of Nanomedicine and Clinical Biophotonics, IRCCS Fondazione Don Carlo Gnocchi, via Capecelatro 66,20148 Milan, Italy

Emil Østergaard Nielsen, Jonas Overgaard Hansen, Søren Overgaard and Ming Ding
Orthopaedic Research Laboratory, Department of Orthopaedic Surgery and Traumatology, Odense University Hospital, Department of Clinical Research, University of Southern Denmark, Sdr. Boulevard 29, 5000 Odense, Denmark

Li Chen
Department of Endocrinology and Metabolism, Molecular Endocrinology Laboratory (KMEB), Odense University Hospital,University of Southern Denmark, J. B. Winsløws Vej 25.1, 5000 Odense, Denmark

Matilda Degn
Department of Pediatrics and Adolescent Medicine, University of Copenhagen, Rigshospitalet, Blegdamsvej 9,2100 Copenhagen, Denmark

Ling Zhou
Department of Endocrinology, The Affiliated Hospital, Southwest Medical University, Taiping Street, Luzhou 646000, China

Jiangyi Tu and Guangbi Fang
Department of Anatomy, Southwest Medical University, Zhongshan Road, Luzhou 646000, China

Li Deng, Xiaoqing Gao and Chaoxian Yang
Department of Anatomy, Southwest Medical University, Zhongshan Road, Luzhou 646000, China
Department of Neurobiology, Preclinical Medicine Research Center, Southwest Medical University, Zhongshan Road,Luzhou 646000, China

Kan Guo, Jing Lv and Weikang Guan
Department of Neurobiology, Preclinical Medicine Research Center, Southwest Medical University, Zhongshan Road,Luzhou 646000, China

Jiming Kong
Department of Human Anatomy and Cell Science, College of Medicine, University of Manitoba, Winnipeg, MB, Canada

Maria Andersson and Anne Hultquist
Hematopoietic Stem Cell Laboratory, Lund Stem Cell Center, Lund University, Klinikgatan 26, 221 84 Lund, Sweden

Farhan Basit
Hematopoietic Stem Cell Laboratory, Lund Stem Cell Center, Lund University, Klinikgatan 26, 221 84 Lund, Sweden
Department of Tumor Immunology, Radboud Institute for Molecular Life Sciences, Radboudumc, Nijmegen, Netherlands

H. Chopra
B.D.S., M.D.S. (Conservative Dentistry and Endodontics), Research Postgraduate Student, Discipline of Prosthodontics,Faculty of Dentistry, The University of Hong Kong, Pok Fu Lam, Hong Kong

M. K. Hung
BChinMed, Research Assistant, Department of Surgery, Queen Mary Hospital, The University of Hong Kong,Pok Fu Lam, Hong Kong

D. L. Kwong
MBBS, MD, FRCR, FHKCR, FHKAM, Clinical Professor, Department of Clinical Oncology, Li Ka Shing Faculty of Medicine,The University of Hong Kong, Pok Fu Lam, Hong Kong

C. F. Zhang
D.D.S, Ph.D.(Med), Clinical Professor, Discipline of Endodontics, Faculty of Dentistry, The University of Hong Kong,Pok Fu Lam, Hong Kong

E. H. N. Pow
B.D.S.,M.D.S.(Prosthetic Dentistry), MRACDS (Pros), FRACDS, FCDHK (Pros), FHKAM (Dental Surgery),Clinical Associate Professor, Discipline of Prosthodontics, Faculty of Dentistry, The University of Hong Kong,Pok Fu Lam, Hong Kong

Jie Yang, Zhuxiao Ren, Chunyi Zhang, Yunbei Rao, Junjuan Zhong and Zhu Wang
Department of Neonatology, Guangdong Women and Children Hospital, Guangzhou, China

Qi Wang
Department of Neonatology, Guangdong Women and Children Hospital, Guangzhou, China
Guangdong Cord Blood and Stem Cell Bank, Guangzhou, China

Zhipeng Liu and Wei Wei
Guangdong Cord Blood and Stem Cell Bank, Guangzhou, China

Lijuang Lu, Jiying Wen and Guocheng Liu
Department of Obstetrics, Guangdong Women and Children Hospital, Guangzhou, China

Kaiyan Liu
Institute of Hematology, People's Hospital, Peking University, Beijing, China

Michalina Alicka
Department of Experimental Biology, The Faculty of Biology and Animal Science, University of Environmental and Life Sciences Wroclaw, Wroclaw, Poland

Krzysztof Marycz
Department of Experimental Biology, The Faculty of Biology and Animal Science, University of Environmental and Life Sciences Wroclaw, Wroclaw, Poland
Faculty of Veterinary Medicine, Equine Clinic-Equine Surgery, Justus-Liebig-University, 35392 Gießen, Germany

Ross E. B. Fitzsimmons and Agnes Soos
Institute of Biomaterials and Biomedical Engineering, University of Toronto, 164 College Street, Toronto, ON, Canada M5S 3G9
Translational Biology and Engineering Program, Ted Rogers Centre for Heart Research, 661 University Ave, Toronto, ON, Canada M5G 1M1

Craig A. Simmons
Institute of Biomaterials and Biomedical Engineering, University of Toronto, 164 College Street, Toronto, ON, Canada M5S 3G9
Translational Biology and Engineering Program, Ted Rogers Centre for Heart Research, 661 University Ave, Toronto, ON, Canada M5G 1M1
Department of Mechanical and Industrial Engineering, University of Toronto, 5 King's College Road, Toronto, ON, Canada M5S 3G8

Matthew S. Mazurek
Division of Gastroenterology and Hepatology, Department of Medicine, University of Calgary, Calgary, AB, Canada T2N 4Z6

Magdalena Kuzma-Kozakiewicz, Anna Kaminska and Malgorzata Gawe
Department of Neurology, Medical University of Warsaw, Zwirki i Wigury 61 Str, 02-091 Warsaw, Poland
Neurodegenerative Diseases Research Group, Medical University of Warsaw, Zwirki i Wigury 61 Str, 02-091 Warsaw, Poland

Andrzej Marchel and Arkadiusz Nowak
Department of Neurosurgery, Medical University of Warsaw, Zwirki i Wigury 61 Str, 02-091 Warsaw, Poland

Jan Sznajder
Department of Rehabilitation, Józef Piłsudski University of Physical Education in Warsaw, Marymoncka Str. 34,00-968 Warsaw, Poland

Anna Figiel-Dabrowska, Krystyna Domanska-Janik, and Anna Sarnowska
Mossakowski Medical Research Centre, Polish Academy of Sciences, 5 Pawinskiego Str, 02-106 Warsaw, Poland

Edyta Maj
62nd Department of Clinical Radiology, Medical University of Warsaw, Zwirki i Wigury 61 Str, 02-091 Warsaw, Poland

Natalia Ewa Krzesniak and Bartlomiej H. Noszczyk
Department of Plastic and Reconstructive Surgery, Centre of Postgraduate Medical Education, Prof. W. Orlowski Memorial Hospital, Czerniakowska 231,00-416 Warsaw, Poland

Index

www.ingramcontent.com/pod-product-compliance
Lightning Source LLC
Chambersburg PA
CBHW050447200326

41458CB00014B/5099